Diagnostic
Endocrinology

Diagnostic Endocrinology

W. Tabb Moore, M.D.
Clinical Professor of Medicine

Richard C. Eastman, M.D.
Associate Professor of Medicine
Director, Division of Endocrinology

Georgetown University School of Medicine
Washington, D.C.

1990
B.C. Decker Inc • Toronto • Philadelphia

Publisher	**B.C. Decker Inc**	**B.C. Decker Inc**
	3228 South Service Road	320 Walnut Street
	Burlington, Ontario L7N 3H8	Suite 400
		Philadelphia, Pennsylvania 19106

Sales and Distribution

United States and Puerto Rico
The C.V. Mosby Company
11830 Westline Industrial Drive
Saint Louis, Missouri 63146

Canada
McAinsh & Co. Ltd.
2760 Old Leslie Street
Willowdale, Ontario M2K 2X5

Australia
McGraw-Hill Book Company Australia Pty. Ltd.
4 Barcoo Street
Roseville East 2069
New South Wales, Australia

Brazil
Editora McGraw-Hill do Brasil, Ltda.
rua Tabapua, 1.105, Itaim-Bibi
Sao Paulo, S.P. Brasil

Colombia
Interamericana/McGraw-Hill de Colombia, S.A.
Apartado Aereo 81078
Bogota, D.E. Colombia

Europe
McGraw-Hill Book Company GmbH
Lademannbogen 136
D-2000 Hamburg 63
West Germany

France
MEDSI/McGraw-Hill
6, avenue Daniel Lesueur
75007 Paris, France

Hong Kong and China
McGraw-Hill Book Company
Suite 618, Ocean Centre
5 Canton Road
Tsimshatsui, Kowloon
Hong Kong

India
Tata McGraw-Hill Publishing Company, Ltd.
12/4 Asaf Ali Road, 3rd Floor
New Delhi 110002, India

Indonesia
P.O. Box 122/JAT
Jakarta, 1300 Indonesia

Italy
McGraw-Hill Libri Italia, s.r.l.
Piazza Emilia, 5
I-20129 Milano MI
Italy

Japan
Igaku-Shoin Ltd.
Tokyo International P.O. Box 5063
1-28-36 Hongo, Bunkyo-ku,
Tokyo 113, Japan

Korea
C.P.O. Box 10583
Seoul, Korea

Malaysia
No. 8 Jalan SS 7/6B
Kelana Jaya
47301 Petaling Jaya
Selangor, Malaysia

Mexico
Interamericana/McGraw-Hill de Mexico, S.A. de C.V.
Cedro 512, Colonia Atlampa
(Apartado Postal 26370)
06450 Mexico, D.F., Mexico

New Zealand
McGraw-Hill Book Co. New Zealand Ltd.
5 Joval Place, Wiri
Manukau City, New Zealand

Panama
Editorial McGraw-Hill Latinoamericana, S.A.
Apartado Postal 2036
Zona Libre de Colon
Colon, Republica de Panama

Portugal
Editora McGraw-Hill de Portugal, Ltda.
Rua Rosa Damasceno 11A–B
1900 Lisboa, Portugal

South Africa
Libriger Book Distributors
Warehouse Number 8
''Die Ou Looiery''
Tannery Road
Hamilton, Bloemfontein 9300

Southeast Asia
McGraw-Hill Book Co.
348 Jalan Boon Lay
Jurong, Singapore 2261

Spain
McGraw-Hill/Interamericana de Espana, S.A.
Manuel Ferrero, 13
28020 Madrid, Spain

Taiwan
P.O. Box 87–601
Taipei, Taiwan

Thailand
632/5 Phaholyothin Road
Sapan Kwai
Bangkok 10400
Thailand

United Kingdom, Middle East and Africa
McGraw-Hill Book Company (U.K.) Ltd.
Shoppenhangers Road
Maidenhead, Berkshire
SL6 2QL England

Venezuela
McGraw-Hill/Interamericana, C.A.
2da. calle Bello Monte
(entre avenida Casanova y Sabana Grande)
Apartado Aereo 50785
Caracas 1050, Venezuela

NOTICE

The authors and publisher have made every effort to ensure that the patient care recommended herein, including choice of drugs and drug dosages, is in accord with the accepted standards and practice at the time of publication. However, since research and regulation constantly change clinical standards, the reader is urged to check the product information sheet included in the package of each drug, which includes recommended doses, warnings, and contraindications. This is particularly important with new or infrequently used drugs.

Diagnostic Endocrinology

ISBN 1-55664-079-X

Library of Congress catalog card number: 88–51914

10 9 8 7 6 5 4 3 2 1

For Rosie, Jonathan, and Ann.
For Susan, Nathan, and Crystal.

Contributors

DAVID K. ALSTER, M.D.

Assistant Professor of Medicine, Tulane University Medical School, New Orleans, Louisiana
Diabetes Mellitus

GUNNAR H. ANDERSON, Jr., M.D.

Associate Professor of Medicine, SUNY Health Science Center; Associate Attending in Medicine, University Hospital and Veterans Administration Medical Center, Syracuse, New York
Aldosterone Disorders

STEPHEN B. BAYLIN, M.D.

Professor of Oncology, The Johns Hopkins University School of Medicine; Active Staff, The Johns Hopkins Hospital, Baltimore, Maryland
Ectopic Hormone Production by Tumors

DANIEL G. BICHET, M.D., F.R.C.P.C., F.A.C.P.

Associate Professor of Medicine, University of Montreal Faculty of Medicine; Staff Nephrologist, Hôpital du Sacré-Coeur de Montréal, Montreal, Quebec, Canada
Diabetes Insipidus and Vasopressin

EMMANUEL L. BRAVO, M.D.

Head, Endocrine/Hypertension Research Laboratory, Research Institute, The Cleveland Clinic Foundation, Cleveland, Ohio
Adrenal Medullary Function

ANDRÉE de BUSTROS, M.D.

Assistant Professor of Oncology and Medicine, The Johns Hopkins University School of Medicine; Active Staff, The Johns Hopkins Hospital, Baltimore, Maryland
Ectopic Hormone Production by Tumors

GEORGE P. CHROUSOS, M.D.

Clinical Professor, Georgetown University School of Medicine and Health Sciences, Washington, D.C.; Senior Investigator and Head, Clinical Neuroendocrinology Unit, National Institute of Child Health and Human Development, National Institutes of Health, Bethesda, Maryland
Adrenal Diseases

RICHARD V. CLARK, M.D., Ph.D.

Assistant Professor of Medicine, Division of Endocrinology and Metabolism, Department of Internal Medicine, and Director of Andrology Laboratory, Emory University, Atlanta, Georgia
Disorders of Male Reproductive Function

RICHARD C. EASTMAN, M.D., F.A.C.P.

Associate Professor of Medicine and Director, Division of Endocrinology, Georgetown University School of Medicine, Washington, D.C.
Acromegaly, Hyperprolactinemia, Gonadotropin-Secreting Tumors, and Hypopituitarism
Hypoglycemia
Thyroid Diseases

MILTON D. GROSS, M.D., F.A.C.P.

Associate Professor of Internal Medicine, Division of Nuclear Medicine, Department of Internal Medicine, University of Michigan Medical Center; Director, Department of Nuclear Medicine, The Veterans Administration Medical Center, Ann Arbor, Michigan
Nuclear Medicine

EN-HUI HAO, M.D.

Visiting Fellow, Developmental Endocrinology Branch, National Institute of Child Health and Human Development, National Institutes of Health, Bethesda, Maryland; Associate Professor, Department of Endocrinology, Peking Union Medical College Hospital, Beijing, China
Acromegaly, Hyperprolactinemia, Gonadotropin-Secreting Tumors, and Hypopituitarism

JEROME E. HERBERS, Jr., M.D., MAJ MC

Assistant Professor of Medicine, Uniformed Services University of the Health Sciences, Bethesda, Maryland; Staff Internist, Walter Reed Army Medical Center, Washington, D.C.
Diagnostic Tests and Clinical Decisions

WELLINGTON HUNG, M.D., Ph.D., F.A.C.P., F.A.A.P.

Professor of Pediatrics, The George Washington University School of Medicine and Health Sciences; Chairman, Department of Endocrinology and Metabolism, Children's National Medical Center, Washington, D.C.
Growth

C. RONALD KAHN, M.D.

Mary K. Iacocca Professor of Medicine, Harvard Medical School; Director, Elliot P. Joslin Research Laboratory, Joslin Diabetes Center; Chief, Division of Diabetes and Metabolism, Brigham and Women's Medical Center, Boston, Massachusetts
Hypoglycemia

THEMISTOCLES C. KAMILARIS, M.D., Ph.D.

Adjunct Scientist, Clinical Neuroendocrinology Unit, National Institute of Child Health and Human Development, National Institutes of Health, Bethesda, Maryland
Adrenal Diseases

FREDERICK A. KHAFAGI, M.B., B.S., F.R.A.C.P.

Research Fellow, Division of Nuclear Medicine,
Department of Internal Medicine, University of Michigan
Medical Center, Ann Arbor, Michigan; Director,
Department of Nuclear Medicine, Royal Brisbane
Hospital, Brisbane, Queensland, Australia
Nuclear Medicine

MICHAEL A. LEVINE, M.D.

Associate Professor of Medicine and Laboratory Medicine
(Pathology), The Johns Hopkins University School of
Medicine; Physician, The Johns Hopkins Hospital,
Baltimore, Maryland
Diseases of Calcium Metabolism

TU LIN, M.D.

Professor of Medicine, University of South Carolina
School of Medicine; Chief, Endocrine Section, Medical
Service, William Jennings Bryan Dorn Veterans' Hospital,
Columbia, South Carolina
Disorders of Male Reproductive Function

JACQUELYN LOUGHLIN, M.D.

Assistant Professor of Obstetrics and Gynecology, Brown
University; Associate Director of Gynecologic
Endocrinology, Women and Infants Hospital of Rhode
Island, Providence, Rhode Island
The Hypothalamic-Pituitary-Ovarian Axis

SAMUEL P. MARYNICK, M.D., F.A.C.P.

Associate Clinical Professor, University of Texas
Southwestern Medical Center; Attending Physician, Baylor
University Medical Center, Dallas, Texas
Competitive-Binding Assays

GEORGE R. MERRIAM, M.D.

Head, Clinical Neuroendocrinology Unit, National
Institute of Child Health and Human Development,
National Institutes of Health, Bethesda, Maryland
*Acromegaly, Hyperprolactinemia, Gonadotropin-Secreting
Tumors, and Hypopituitarism*

W. TABB MOORE, M.D.

Clinical Professor of Medicine, Department of Internal
Medicine, Georgetown University School of Medicine,
Washington, D.C.
Thyroid Disease
*Acromegaly, Hyperprolactinemia, Gonadotropin-Secreting
Tumors, and Hypopituitarism*

HOWARD R. NANKIN, M.D.

Professor of Medicine and Director, Division of
Endocrinology and Metabolism, Department of Medicine,
University of South Carolina School of Medicine; Staff
Physician, Endocrine Section, Medical Service, William
Jennings Bryan Dorn Veterans' Hospital, Columbia,
South Carolina
Disorders of Male Reproductive Function

GORDON L. NOEL, M.D.

Professor of Medicine, Uniformed Services University of
the Health Sciences, Bethesda, Maryland
Diagnostic Tests and Clinical Decisions

YOLANDA C. OERTEL, M.D.

Professor of Pathology, The George Washington University
School of Medicine; Pathologist, The George Washington
University Medical Center, Washington, D.C.
Fine-Needle Aspiration of the Thyroid

MANUEL SAINZ DE LA PEÑA, M.D.

Senior Endocrine Fellow, Georgetown University Hospital,
Washington, D.C.
*Acromegaly, Hyperprolactinemia, Gonadotropin-Secreting
Tumors, and Hypopituitarism*

BRAHM SHAPIRO, M.B., Ch.B., Ph.D.

Professor of Internal Medicine, Division of Nuclear
Medicine, Department of Internal Medicine, University of
Michigan Medical Center, Ann Arbor, Michigan
Nuclear Medicine

DANIEL SPRATT, M.D.

Assistant Professor of Medicine, University of Vermont,
Burlington, Vermont; Attending in Endocrinology,
Maine Medical Center, Portland, Maine
The Hypothalamic-Pituitary-Ovarian Axis

DAVID H. P. STREETEN, M.B., D.Phil., F.R.C.P.

Professor of Medicine and Chief of Endocrine Section,
State University of New York Health Science Center;
Attending in Medicine, University Hospital and Veterans
Administration Medical Center, and Consultant in
Medicine, Crouse Irving Memorial Hospital, Syracuse,
New York
Aldosterone Disorders

ROBERT J. TANENBERG, M.D., F.A.C.P.

Clinical Associate Professor of Medicine, Georgetown
University; Medical Director, Diabetes Treatment
Center, Georgetown University Hospital, Washington,
D.C.
Diabetes Mellitus

MARILYN TUTTLEMAN, B.S., M.T.(ASCP)

Research Assistant, The George Washington University
Biostatistics Center, Washington, D.C.
Diabetes Mellitus

SAMUEL M. WOLPERT, M.B., B.Ch.

Professor of Radiology, Tufts University School of
Medicine; Chief, Section of Neuroradiology,
Department of Radiology, New England Medical
Center Hospitals, Boston, Massachusetts
Pituitary Imaging

Preface

During the past ten years the field of endocrinology has undergone remarkable change. With new techniques for measuring levels of hormones in serum using radioligands (Chapter 2, by Marynick), new imaging methods such as CT scans and MRI, and fine-needle aspiration of tissue (Chapter 8, by Oertel) have come more precise diagnosis and understanding of the pathophysiology of the disease process. At the same time, the number of available tests has expanded exponentially, challenging the skill of the practitioner in making sound decisions in ordering tests as well as in interpreting them.

The goal of our book, *Diagnostic Endocrinology*, is to bring to the practicing clinician as well as the student an understanding of the method of the various tests, their proper use and selection, and problems involved in their interpretation. To this end we have endeavored to look at endocrine testing in the context of sound pathophysiology. Important tests with their method, normal results, and pitfalls have been put in tabular form to provide a ready reference source for the busy clinician.

Where possible, we have included both specificity and sensitivity figures to help in the analysis of the tests involved. The first chapter, by Herbers and Noel, sets the tone for the thoughtful analysis of the clinical data in endocrinology.

We have tried to cover diseases that are most commonly encountered in the practice of endocrinology, emphasizing information that is new and developing, such as the use of MRI in pituitary imaging, sensitive TSH assays in the diagnosis of thyroid disorders, and C-peptide tests in diabetes.

The editors are grateful to a number of our colleagues who have taught us and to our students and Fellows who continue to stimulate our thinking. Doctors Daniel Federman, Bruce Weintraub, Paul Ladenson, Simeon Margolis, Terry Taylor, Jim Ramey, and Joanna Zawadzki have been helpful in their comments and criticisms. Our secretaries, Aleta Dubose, Lely Constantinople, and Kathlen Kelly, have done yeoman work. Finally, we express our gratitude to Brian Decker for his initial enthusiasm and encouragement as well as to our editor, Mary Mansor, who guided us so well.

It is our hope that the book will prove useful to the practitioner and lead to better diagnosis and care.

W. Tabb Moore, M.D.
Richard C. Eastman, M.D.

Contents

1 Diagnostic Tests and Clinical Decisions

Jerome E. Herbers Jr., M.D., MAJ MC
Gordon L. Noel, M.D.

At their best, diagnostic tests improve the clinician's assessment of the probability of disease in a patient so that therapeutic decisions can be made in the patient's best interest. At their worst, tests cause diagnostic error and increase the risk that treatment decisions will be incorrect. An understanding of how tests are effectively used is particularly important in endocrinologic diagnosis, where test results often greatly affect therapeutic decisions. This chapter discusses principles of test selection and interpretation and presents several approaches to clinical decision making, with examples drawn from clinical endocrinology. In general, tests are analyzed with respect to how they alter the clinician's view of the probability of disease. The focus is on the benefits and risks for the individual patient rather than for groups of patients or for society, although often no such distinction can be made.

PRETEST PROBABILITIES

When an individual presents for medical care, the clinician is frequently faced with uncertainty about which, if any, of myriad pathologic processes are responsible for signs, symptoms, or abnormal laboratory studies. Nevertheless, skilled clinicians rapidly narrow the range of probable diagnoses by analysis of data from the patient's history and physical examination (Elstein et al, 1978). The degree of certainty required before a clinician is willing to initiate therapy depends on the disease processes and therapeutic options being considered. Generally, extremely high degrees of certainty are attainable only with the use of invasive and expensive diagnostic tests. Since such high levels of certainty are often unnecessary in clinical decision making, diagnostic tests that are less accurate, but also relatively safer and less expensive, have proliferated in all fields of medicine. To know whether such tests can be beneficial when applied in a specific case, the diagnostician must consider the likelihood that a disease is present *before* applying any test. The potential for tests to affect management decisions can then be assessed. This approach assumes that the clinician is thinking in terms of probabilities.

Because diagnoses can only rarely be absolutely excluded or confirmed, clinical judgments are usually best expressed in terms of the clinician's degree of certainty. Such judgments have traditionally been stated in qualitative terms: *improbable, compatible with,* and *almost certain,* for example. Unfortunately, such expressions are inherently ambiguous. When asked to assign to these terms an approximate numerical value on a probability scale ranging from 0 to 1, physicians differ substantially among themselves (Bryant and Norman, 1979; Kong et al, 1986). This ambiguity is a potential source of miscommunication and unnecessary disagreement among physicians about strategies for patient management. Probabilistic thinking encourages explicit recognition of the degree of uncertainty inherent in the process of making a diagnosis. The use of numbers in the place of phrases in no way implies increased precision or confidence, but it does focus attention on the importance of carefully estimating the likelihood of disease prior to application of any test. By stating in numerical terms one's belief in the presence or absence of a condition, one avoids ambiguity and is prepared to quantitatively assess the potential usefulness of a test.

The probability of an event prior to the application of a test is known as the *pretest probability* and is generally expressed on a scale of 0 to 1. Figure 1–1 depicts the pretest probability as a point on a continuum from absent to present, expressed in probabilistic terms. A physician's estimate that the pretest probability is .95, for example, indicates a high degree of confidence in the presence of a disease, whereas a probability of .5 indicates that the chances of the disease being present are about the same as that it is absent, and .01 indicates confidence that the disease is absent. Positive test results increase the probability of a diagnosis, and negative test results decrease that probability. The probability of an event or condition following the application of a test is called the *post-test probability.* Knowledge of the pretest probability and of a test's ability to distinguish diseased from nondiseased persons allows calculation of the post-test probability by the use of a simple formula. We will first discuss the ways that clinicians obtain pretest probabilities and then address the accuracy of tests and how they are used to revise those probabilities.

In day-to-day practice, clinicians make numerous judgments about the presence or absence of disease in patients. Those judgments generally are reached by using several mental shortcuts or rules of thumb known as *heuristics* (from a Greek root meaning "to discover"). Several types of heuristics have been described, applying in general to how people solve problems (Tversky and Kahneman, 1974); in recent years attention has been given to their use in medical diagnosis (Sox et al, 1988). Heuristics serve the experienced and knowledgeable clinician extremely well by improving diagnostic efficiency. Unfortunately, when misapplied, heuristics can lead to inappropriate diagnostic testing and errors in management.

Perhaps the most commonly used heuristic is employed almost unconsciously by clinicians when they make a presumptive diagnosis of a disease in patients who have many signs and symptoms compatible with that disease. The physician who makes an initial diagnosis of Graves' disease in a young adult woman with tachycardia, exophthalmos, and a goiter will generally be well served by this heuristic. On the other hand, if the clinician is led to test for corticosteroid excess in every patient with obesity, hypertension, and glucose intolerance, many unnecessary tests will be performed. The difference in the two situations lies largely in the prevalence of the diseases: hyperthyroidism is relatively common, whereas noniatrogenic Cushing's syndrome is relatively rare. Medical diagnosis is optimized when clinicians take into account known prevalences of the diseases in their patient populations when thinking about pretest probabilities.

Another frequently used heuristic leads the physician to consider a diagnosis because of memorable past cases. If tests are ordered as a result, this heuristic may serve poorly. An example of such a use of this heuristic might be a clinician who discovered a large pituitary tumor when he ordered a serum prolactin level in an elderly man with impotence and subsequently requests serum prolactin determinations in all patients with impotence.

An additional type of heuristic is used by the clinician who makes an initial assessment of the likelihood of a disease and then adjusts that likelihood upward or downward on the basis of subsequent information from history, physical examination, or laboratory tests. When used appropriately, this heuristic is very helpful. The clinician who initially believes that the probability of pheochromocytoma in a young man with hypertension is very low and later substantially adjusts that probability upward when the patient calls to relate a pertinent family history has used this heuristic to the patient's benefit. Unfortunately, cognitive psychologists have shown that when decisions are being made in the face of uncertainty, there is a strong tendency to change probability assessments very little in light of new information (Tversky and Kahneman, 1974). If a physician fails to greatly change his initial impression that a young woman's hirsutism is due to an adrenal tumor when he later elicits the history that she is a serious athlete who may be using androgens, the use of this heuristic may result in unnecessary testing and delay in diagnosis.

An awareness of some common pitfalls involved in making decisions is an important first step in setting pretest probabilities so that diagnostic tests can be ordered and interpreted most effectively. These subjective, often intuitive techniques are used successfully by skillful clinicians, incorporating clinical experience and knowledge about disease processes. For a number of diseases, however, clinical research has provided more formal guidelines for establishing the probability of disease in individuals. Known as *clinical prediction rules*, these guidelines bring to bear information about signs and symptoms of disease from far more patients than could ever be seen by most individual physicians. For patients with suspected hypothyroidism, a prediction rule has been derived by Billewicz and colleagues, and is illustrated in Table 1–1. The probability of hypothyroidism is estimated on the basis of presenting signs and symptoms by tallying the applicable number of points for clinical findings in an individual patient (Billewicz et al, 1969).

Clinical prediction rules have been developed for a number of clinical disorders. Griner and co-workers (1986) have collected a number of prediction rules relevant to endocrinology. Caution must be exercised in applying such rules, however. The population in which the prediction rule was derived should have similar demographics and spectrum of disease to that from which the patient is drawn. Further, rules can serve as only a rough estimate to be used in conjunction with clinical judgment. With these caveats in mind, clinical prediction rules offer

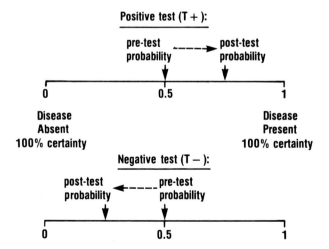

Figure 1–1 Continuum of probabilities expressing the degree of certainty in a diagnosis. The clinician's first step in applying a diagnostic test is to determine the pretest probability, here given to be .5 (there is a 50:50 chance that disease is present). Note that the diagnostic test (T) increases the probability that disease is present (positive test) or absent (negative test), but diagnostic uncertainty remains.

TABLE 1-1   The Billewicz Index for Estimating the Pretest Probability of
Hypothyroidism in Ambulatory Patients*

Symptom or Sign	Present	Absent
Diminished sweating	+ 6	− 2
Dry skin	+ 3	− 6
Cold intolerance	+ 4	− 5
Weight increase	+ 1	− 1
Constipation	+ 2	− 1
Hoarseness	+ 5	− 6
Paresthesias	+ 5	− 4
Deafness	+ 2	0
Slow movements	+ 11	− 3
Coarse skin	+ 7	− 7
Cold skin	+ 3	− 2
Periorbital puffiness	+ 4	− 6
Pulse rate < 75	+ 4	− 4
Delayed relaxation, ankle jerk	+ 15	− 6

* To use this clinical prediction rule, add all pertinent numbers to obtain the index. Index values less than 30 indicate a probability of hypothyroidism of less than .2%. Values greater than or equal to 30 strongly suggest the diagnosis (probability near 100%) (From Billewicz WZ, Chapman RS, Crooks J, et al. Statistical methods applied to the diagnosis of hypothyroidism. Q J Med 1969; 38:255; with permission.)

the potential for refined estimates of pretest probabilities. Facility in thinking about and deriving pretest probabilities prepares the diagnostician to use the characteristics of tests to determine post-test probabilities and thereby assess the potential usefulness of a test before ordering it.

TEST CHARACTERISTICS

The ideal diagnostic test discriminates perfectly between diseased and nondiseased individuals. The extent to which tests diverge from the ideal largely determines whether they will be useful. *Sensitivity*, or true-positive rate (TPR), describes the ability of a test to correctly identify diseased persons. *Specificity*, or true-negative rate (TNR), describes the ability of a test to correctly identify nondiseased persons. The false-negative rate (FNR) and false-positive rate (FPR) describe the tendency of a test to incorrectly classify patients who are, respectively, diseased and nondiseased. Table 1-2 indicates how all patients are classified by the results of a test and shows the relationships between sensitivity, specificity, and their related terms, FNR and FPR. Since all patients are in fact either diseased or nondiseased, knowledge of either measure of test discrimination in persons known to have or not have disease implies knowledge of the other measure. These relationships are summarized in the following expressions.

Persons with disease:

$$TPR + FNR = 1; \quad FNR = 1 - TPR$$

Persons without disease:

$$TNR + FPR = 1; \quad FPR = 1 - TNR$$

It is important to note that the degree to which tests deviate from ideal discrimination is generally different for diseased and nondiseased persons. Thus many tests have high sensitivities and low specificities, and others have high specificities and low sensitivities. The result of this observation is that in certain clinical situations, some tests are useful only if positive and others are useful only if negative. Further, there is frequently no need for a test to be extremely accurate in both diseased and nondiseased patients, since physicians are often most interested in being sure either that persons with disease are identified as such or that persons who are healthy are not incorrectly labeled as diseased.

Data on test characteristics are the result of studies in which all patients who undergo testing are also measured by an acceptable "gold standard" test which is assumed to be able to determine their true state. In this way all tested patients are categorized according to their actual state and according to whether they test positive or negative (see Table 1-2). The test being studied is usually cheaper, faster, or safer than the gold standard test and therefore a better option for the patient if it is sufficiently accurate. Hamberger and associates (1982) evaluated fine-needle aspiration of thyroid nodules as a diagnostic test for carcinoma of the thyroid. The sensitivity and specificity that they determined (87 percent and 73 percent, respectively) allow the clinician to determine in advance how aspiration might help in the management of a patient with a thyroid nodule. Just as they must do with clinical prediction rules, clinicians must take care that published test characteristics were obtained by studying patients similar to their own. This generally requires that studies include patients with a broad spectrum of diseases and disease severity (Sackett et al, 1985).

When published reports on diagnostic tests do not appear to be directly applicable in a given instance, it

TABLE 1–2 Classification of Patients Based on Test Results

| | True State of The Patient | | |
Test Result	Diseased	Nondiseased	Total
Positive	True-positives (TP)	False-positives (FP)	Patients with positive tests (TP + FP)
Negative	False-negatives (FN)	True-negatives (TN)	Patients with negative tests (FN + TN)
Total	All diseased patients (TP + FN)	All nondiseased patients (FP + TN)	All patients studied (TP + FP + FN + TN)

Sensitivity (true-positive rate, TPR) $= TP/(TP + FN) = 1 - FNR$
False-negative rate (FNR) $= FN/(TP + FN) = 1 - TPR$
Specificity (true-negative rate, TNR) $= TN/(FP + TN) = 1 - FPR$
False-positive rate (FPR) $= FP/(TN + FP) = 1 - TNR$

is often appropriate to adjust sensitivities and specificities upward or downward. The necessity of such adjustments can be illustrated by examining the history of the overnight dexamethasone suppression test for detecting Cushing's syndrome. This diagnostic test was originally studied in healthy volunteers and in persons with known Cushing's syndrome; applied to those subjects, the test was found to have a specificity of 99 percent (Nugent et al, 1965). However, when the test was later applied to hospital inpatients with a variety of medical problems, its specificity was found to be much lower (63 percent; Connolly et al, 1968). To apply the specificity of a test in the evaluation of a given patient, the clinician should ensure that the patient is identifiably similar to the control group in whom the test was studied. If the patient is generally less well than those in the control group, the specificity should probably be adjusted downward somewhat.

Published test characteristics may also not apply because diagnostic tests are often initially studied in tertiary-care referral centers, where patients have been filtered through referring physicians and thus tend to have more severe manifestations of disease. Since many tests are more likely to be positive in severe or advanced forms of disease than in milder forms, the sensitivity of a test in such an environment will often be falsely elevated, and the clinician practicing in a general community setting may need to adjust the sensitivity downward when applying the test. On the other hand, if a test is studied by applying it to patients who have numerous unrelated illnesses, the test specificity is likely to be lower than when applied to generally healthy people. Therefore, the clinician might wish to adjust the specificity upward when using the test in a primary care practice. The problems involved in the use of published test characteristics in clinical practice are discussed in detail by Sackett and colleagues (1985) and Sox and associates (1988).

DERIVING POST-TEST PROBABILITIES

Once the pretest probability is estimated and test characteristics obtained, calculation of the post-test probability is straightforward. Several approaches are possible. Presented here is a method that uses the 2-by-2 table shown in Table 1–2, followed by a simpler but less intuitive method. Starting with the framework of the 2-by-2 table, the diagnostician estimates the number of persons from a hypothetical cohort of 1,000 persons similar to the patient in question who would in fact have the disease in question (the number 1,000 is chosen for ease of calculation). This is a restatement of the pretest probability. The next step is to use published test characteristics to determine the numbers of true-positive, false-positive, true-negative, and false-negative results. Finally, for a positive test result, the post-test probability of disease is the fraction of positive test results that are true-positive; for a negative result, the post-test probability is the fraction of negative results that are false-negative.

For example, Figure 1–2 illustrates these calculations for hypercortisolism, with the test to be analyzed being a single plasma cortisol determination at 4 to 9 PM. The pretest probability of hypercortisolism can be estimated, and test characteristics are known. The effect of the test on the clinician's belief about the probability of hypercortisolism can be measured by inserting the appropriate numbers. If the pretest probability based on the patient's history, physical examination, and initial laboratory data is thought to be .1 (10 percent), this is equivalent to 100 of 1,000 similar persons having the disease, and the number 100 is placed at the bottom of the first column (total number with disease); 900 persons must be disease free, so this number is placed at the bottom of the second column (total number without disease). Assuming a sensitivity (TPR) of .83 (pooled data; Cra-

I. Assumptions:

Pre-test probability = 0.10
Sensitivity   = 0.83
Specificity   = 0.67

II. 2 × 2 Table:

HYPERCORTISOLISM (GOLD STANDARD)

PLASMA CORTISOL	Present	Absent	TOTAL
> 16	83	297	380
≤ 16	17	603	620
TOTAL	100	900	1000

III. Calculation of Post-test Probabilities:

If test is positive, probability of disease $= \dfrac{TP}{TP + FP} = \dfrac{83}{83 + 297} = 0.22$

If test is negative, probability of disease $= \dfrac{FN}{FN + TN} = \dfrac{17}{17 + 603} = 0.03$

IV. Summary of Probability Revisions:

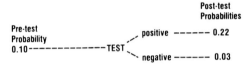

Post-test Probabilities

Pre-test Probability 0.10 ----------- TEST
positive ------ 0.22
negative ------ 0.03

Figure 1-2 Analysis of the single PM plasma cortisol measurement in the diagnosis of hypercortisolism (units are micrograms per deciliter). Since sensitivity = .83, 83 of 100 persons with hypercortisolism will have a positive test (plasma cortisol > 16) and 17 will have a negative test (cortisol ≤ 16); since specificity = .67, 603 of 900 persons without hypercortisolism will have a negative test and 297 will have a positive test.

po, 1979) and a specificity (TNR) of .67 (Griner et al, 1986), the 2-by-2 table can be completed by multiplying the sensitivity by the number with disease (.83 × 100 = 83) and the specificity by the number without disease (.67 × 900 = 603). These calculations yield the numbers of patients with true-positive and true-negative test results. The number of false-negative results is obtained by subtracting the number of true-positive results from the total number of persons with disease (100 − 83 = 17); the number of false-positive results is likewise obtained by subtraction (900 − 603 = 297).

With the 2-by-2 table completed, the physician is ready to answer the question, "Given that my patient has a positive or negative test result, what is the probability that he or she has hypercortisolism?" For a positive test, this is simply the number of true-positive results divided by the total number of patients testing positive [83 / (83 + 297) = .22]. If the test is negative, the probability that the patient has the disease is the number of false-negative results divided by the total testing negative [17 / (17 + 603) = .03]. Comparing these post-test probabilities with the pretest probability of .1 allows the

clinician to judge whether and how this test might be helpful in advising an individual patient. Note that most of the positive results occur in nondiseased persons. Thus, even though the PM cortisol is elevated, a patient with a pretest probability of Cushing's syndrome of 10 percent is still most likely not to have Cushing's. How much a probability must change from before to after a test for the clinician to take further action depends on several factors—cost, invasiveness of subsequent tests, consequences of missing or delaying a diagnosis, for example—and is discussed in the next section.

Once comfortable with the concepts of the 2-by-2 approach, the clinician can gain efficiency by using one of the several forms of Bayes' formula directly. These approaches are entirely equivalent algebraically to that described previously and are presented here for those interested in a faster method for finding post-test probabilities. Several alternative notations are in use for describing Bayes' formula. One set of notation employs the language of probability, with terms equivalent to those previously defined. Conditional probabilities are indicated by a vertical bar that is read "given." For example, the sensitivity (TPR) of a test can be expressed as $p(T+ \mid D+)$, read "probability of a positive test result given disease is present." The post-test probability of disease if the test is negative can be expressed $p(D+ \mid T-)$. Note that the vertical bar does not indicate division. Table 1–3 lists equivalent terms and their synonyms. Bayes' formula can thus be expressed:

$$P(D+ \mid T+) = \frac{p(D+) \times p(T+ \mid D+)}{p(D+) \times p(T+ \mid D+) + p(D-) \times p(T+ \mid D-)}$$

$$= \frac{(\text{Pretest prob.})(\text{TPR})}{(\text{Pretest prob.})(\text{TPR}) + (1 - \text{Pretest prob.})(\text{FPR})}$$

$$P(D+ \mid T-) = \frac{p(D+) \times p(T- \mid D+)}{p(D+) \times p(T- \mid D+) + p(D-) \times p(T- \mid D-)}$$

$$= \frac{(\text{Pretest prob.})(\text{FNR})}{(\text{Pretest prob.})(\text{FNR}) + (1 - \text{Pretest prob.})(\text{TNR})}$$

As described, post-test probabilities vary with sensitivity and specificity and with pretest probability. A positive test result has the greatest potential effect on post-test probabilities when the pretest probability is very low. Since the post-test probability given a positive test is the proportion of all positive tests that are true-positive, changes in test specificity (1 − FPR) most readily affect this probability (Fig. 1–3A). Similarly, negative test results are usually most important when the pretest probability is very high, and in this case sensitivity is the most important test characteristic (Fig. 1–3B).

THE THRESHOLD MODEL: DECIDING WHEN TESTS CAN HELP

When clinicians decide whether or not to initiate therapy, it is with the understanding that diagnostic error may lead to treatment for some patients who do

TABLE 1–3 Synonymous Terms and Expressions Used in Bayes' Theorem

Common Term	Alternative Term	Probability Expression
Test Characteristics		
Sensitivity: Probability of a positive test result when disease is present	True-positive rate (TPR) TP/(TP + FN)	$p(T+ \mid D+)$
Specificity: Probability of a negative test result when disease is absent	True-negative rate (TNR) TN/(TN + FP)	$p(T- \mid D-)$
False reassurance rate: Probability of a negative test result when disease is present	False-negative rate (FNR) FN/(FN + TP)	$P(T- \mid D+)$
False alarm rate: Probability of a positive test result when disease is absent	False-positive rate (FPR) FP/(FP + TN)	$p(T+ \mid D-)$
Pretest and Post-Test Probabilities		
Pretest probability of disease	Prior probability, prevalence* TP + FN	$p(D+)$
Post-test probability of disease if test result is positive	Posterior probability (positive test), positive predictive value TP/(TP + FP)	$p(D+ \mid T+)$
Post-test probability of disease if test result is negative	Posterior probability (negative test) FN/(FN + TN)	$p(D+ \mid T-)$
Post-test probability of no disease if test result is negative	Negative predictive value TN/(TN + FN)	$p(D- \mid T-)$

* Prevalence is often used to refer only to populations of patients; see Weinstein et al, 1980.

not have disease and to no treatment for other patients who in fact have disease. How sure of the diagnosis clinicians must be before initiating therapy, i.e., how willing they are to accept therapeutic error, defines a *threshold probability*. At this probability of disease, clinicians are indifferent between treating and not treating (Pauker and Kassirer, 1975). If the clinician believes that the probability of disease is greater than the threshold probability, treatment will, on average, yield the best outcome for the patient. If the probability of disease is believed to be less than the threshold probability, treatment should be withheld. A severely ill patient in an intensive care unit who has hyperkalemia and hypoglycemia may or may not have adrenal insufficiency. For most clinicians, however, the threshold probability for administering a glucocorticosteroid is probably low because the benefit of treating affected patients is large and the cost of treating unaffected individuals is small. If the probability of adrenal insufficiency exceeds the threshold for treatment, treatment may begin without awaiting the results of diagnostic tests.

Tests that do not alter the probability of disease enough to cross a threshold cannot change the physician's management plans and should not be ordered. As illustrated in Figure 1–4, this conceptualization applies equally well to situations in which physicians seek to rule in or rule out a diagnostic possibility. Attention is usually focused on the potential effect of either a positive or a negative test result, but not of both. By explicitly stating the probability of disease at which he or she will take action in a given case, the clinician can use the pretest probability and test characteristics to determine *in advance* whether a test could be worthwhile. This approach has been developed by Sox and co-workers (1988) for use by clinicians; its essential components can be summarized as follows:

1. Set a threshold at which you are indifferent between taking action and not taking action.
2. Assess the pretest probability of disease.
3. Obtain test characteristics (sensitivity and specificity).
4. Calculate the post-test probability, and compare it with the threshold probability:
   A. If the pretest probability of disease is less than

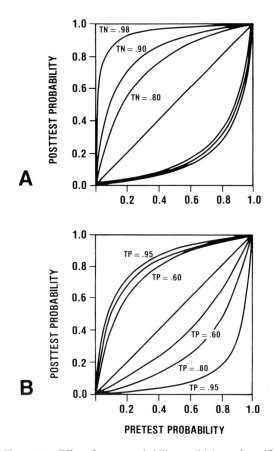

Figure 1–3 Effect of pretest probability, sensitivity, and specificity on post-test probability. *A*, The sensitivity of the test was assumed to be .90, and the calculations were repeated for several values of test specificity. *B*, The specificity of the test was assumed to be .90, and the calculations were repeated for several values of the sensitivity of the test. In both *A* and *B*, TP = true-positive rate; TN = true-negative rate. The top family of curves corresponds to positive test results, and the bottom family of curves corresponds to negative test results. (From Sox HC. Common diagnostic tests: Use and interpretation. Philadelphia: American College of Physicians, 1987; with permission.)

the threshold probability, calculate the post-test probability for a positive test result (positive predictive value). If the post-test probability is greater than the threshold probability, testing could affect patient care.

B. If the pretest probability of disease is greater than the threshold probability, calculate the post-test probability for a negative test result. If the post-test probability is less than the threshold probability, testing could affect patient care.

An example illustrates the use of this approach. A generally healthy 60-year-old woman being treated for a peptic ulcer was found to have a serum calcium level of 11.4 mg per deciliter. After this result was confirmed, her physician considered ordering a serum parathyroid hormone (PTH) level. Does this test have the potential to alter the management of this patient? An elevated PTH

level would presumably indicate primary hyperparathyroidism, whereas a low PTH level would indicate another cause, such as an underlying malignancy (levels in the normal range are considered subsequently).

As outlined previously, the first step is to determine the probability of disease at which further action will be taken: the threshold probability. If the action to be taken is the initiation of a formal work-up in anticipation of parathyroid surgery, a conservative clinician might require a probability of hyperparathyroidism of at least 80 percent. The next step is to estimate the pretest probability of disease, in this case taken to be primary hyperparathyroidism. A reasonable estimate in the absence of other information might be 45 percent (Fallon and Arvan, 1986). Test characteristics for the PTH assay are next required to calculate a post-test probability. These numbers depend on the assay used and on definitions of normal and abnormal. For the C-terminal assay, sensitivity is approximately 86 percent and specificity 91 percent (false-positive rate 9 percent) (Fallon and Arvan, 1986). Since the threshold probability (80 percent) exceeds the pretest probability, we are interested in whether a positive test result can raise the probability of disease above the threshold for action; if a positive test cannot increase the probability of hyperparathyroidism to at least 80 percent, there is no reason to order the test. The post-test probability given a positive test result is

$$\frac{(.45)(.86)}{(.45)(.86) + (.55)(.09)} = .89$$

A positive test result raises the probability of disease past the threshold probability (p*).

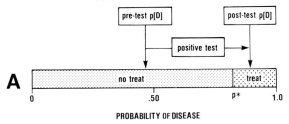

A negative test result lowers the probability of disease past the threshold probability (p*).

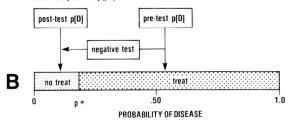

Figure 1–4 The use of thresholds when deciding whether to order a diagnostic test. (Reproduced with permission from Sox HC, Blatt M, Marton KI, et al. Medical decision making. Stoneham, MA: Butterworth Publishers, 1988.)

Because the threshold for action was crossed (.89 > .80), the test is potentially useful.

Since PTH levels in the normal range might be considered abnormal in the presence of hypercalcemia, a positive test could be taken to be any result in the normal range or greater. Although precise test characteristics are not available for this definition of positivity, the sensitivity must be greater than 86 percent and the specificity less than 91 percent (Sox et al, 1988; Weinstein et al, 1980). Assuming a sensitivity of 99 percent and a specificity of 60 percent, the post-test probability given a positive test is

$$\frac{(.45) \ (.99)}{(.45) \ (.99) \ + \ (.55) \ (.4)} = .67$$

If this latter cutoff point for defining a positive result is used, the PTH level would not be helpful and should not be ordered (0.67 < 0.80).

Of course, reasonable physicians will vary in their assessments of the pretest probability, threshold for action, and definition of tests positivity. With this approach, however, the important components of the decision to order or not to order the test can be scrutinized and altered as appropriate. In many cases, this type of analysis points to critical gaps in our knowledge of disease processes, test capabilities, and preferences of individual patients, with the result that the thoughtful clinician will be more circumspect in ordering and interpreting tests.

The concept of a threshold probability can be generalized to include any diagnostic or therapeutic action. Thus, in addition to thresholds for treatment, thresholds can be defined for further diagnostic testing. Figure 1–5 indicates these thresholds as points on a probability continuum. Within the "test" range of probabilities, testing has the potential to alter one's assessment of the probability of disease sufficiently to cross the threshold for taking further action.

The threshold probability in a given case is related to the benefits of treating diseased persons and to the

costs of treating well persons. Threshold probabilities are generally implicitly determined by clinicians using subjective assessments of costs and benefits. However, they can be calculated precisely in terms of the values patients place on each possible outcome, through application of the methods of decision analysis (Pauker and Kassirer, 1975; Greenes et al, 1984; Sox et al, 1988). An introduction to decision analysis is presented in the next section.

DECISION ANALYSIS IN TEST SELECTION

In many cases the decision to order a diagnostic test is not difficult because discomfort to the patient is minimal (as in most blood tests) and because monetary costs are not prohibitive. Indeed, some clinicians evince the belief that all reasonably inexpensive tests should be obtained if they have the potential to improve diagnostic accuracy. Aside from a tacit disregard for optimal use of resources, this attitude fails to account for tests' potential for harm. False-positive test results increase the risk that more invasive testing or inappropriate treatment will be recommended, and false-negative results increase the risk that appropriate treatment will be withheld. Thus, although diagnostic tests may be obtained to improve patient outcomes, patients may in fact fare less well as a result of the information provided.

If any diagnostic test can ultimately lead to improvement or deterioration of a patient's condition, the clinician must assess whether benefit or harm is more likely if testing is done. This assessment requires consideration of numerous probabilities that almost never can be stated with great confidence. Just as in setting pretest probabilities, however, the probabilities for the possible outcomes of a testing strategy can be estimated from clinical experience, from expert opinion, or from the medical literature. The primary difficulty in bringing all of this information to bear on a decision is that most people, including physicians, have difficulty assimilating large amounts of data, tending to rely on one or several pieces of information to the exclusion of others (Tversky and Kahneman, 1974). Further, easily lost amid the data are the values placed on clinical outcomes by the person most affected by the decision, the patient.

Decision analysis offers a systematic approach to decision making under conditions of uncertainty (Raiffa, 1970; Weinstein et al, 1980; Kassirer et al, 1987). Initially developed for use in business and industry and later introduced into clinical medicine, decision analysis examines all options available to the decision maker and explicitly incorporates judgments about the likelihoods of and preferences for all possible outcomes. When choices are difficult and/or stakes are high, decision analysis may be helpful by pointing to the alternative that, on average, offers the greatest chance for the best outcome.

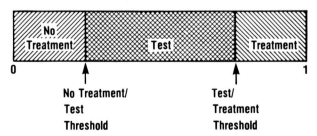

Figure 1–5   Testing (t) and test-treatment (t-Rx) thresholds expressed as points on a probability scale ranging from 0 to 1. (Adapted from Pauker SG, Kassirer JP. The threshold approach to clinical decision making. N Engl J Med 1980; 302:1109; reprinted with permission from *The New England Journal of Medicine.*)

To begin systematic analysis of a decision, one must clearly identify for whom the optimal course of action is being sought—patient, family, physician, health care system, society. In clinical settings, explicit measurement of patients' values and preferences may be required. This point is emphasized in decision analysis: "individual" or "decision maker" often replaces "clinician" or "physician" when patient preferences are the basis of decisions. Although infrequently discussed in medicine, the perspective from which decisions are made bears emphasis because patients and physicians often in fact have markedly different views with respect to risk taking and the values of clinical outcomes (McNeil et al, 1981).

Decisions are not difficult when future events can be predicted with certainty. However, because most events in nature (and medicine) occur unpredictably, the prospects for any patient can be described only in probability terms. Thus, although a future event may not be predicted with certainty, a statement can be made about the number of times the event would occur if the situation were faced repeatedly. The rational decision maker chooses from among alternatives the one alternative that is expected, on repeated repetition, to most often yield the best outcome. This way of thinking, known as *expected value decision making*, is fundamental to decision analysis. Its use can be illustrated by a simple monetary example.

Suppose a person is offered a choice between either receiving $5 or being given a chance at a gamble. The gamble involves a coin flip; if "heads" results, $12 is paid, and if "tails" results, nothing is paid. Although many persons would choose to receive a certain $5 rather than risk gaining nothing, it is clear that on average the gamble yields a greater return. The expected value of the gamble can be calculated exactly by multiplying the probability of each outcome (.5) by its value ($12, $0). and then adding the result for each outcome [(.5 × $12) + (.5 × $0) = $6]. These relationships and calculations can be expressed by analogy with a scale, as shown in Figure 1–6A. The option with the greatest expected value "tips the scale," indicating the optimal choice.

In clinical medicine, a patient may face a difficult choice between a shortened life expectancy due to disease and a gamble involving an operation that is risky but curative. If surgery is chosen, all possible care will be taken to ensure an optimal outcome, but the word *gamble* is nonetheless appropriate since surgical results for a given individual can never be precisely predicted: chances for cure can be expressed only in probabilistic terms. In this case the probability of surviving surgery replaces the probability of winning a coin toss. The values assigned to the possible outcomes (cure, death, disease) depend on the concerns of the decision maker and might be expressed as overall life expectancy, short-term life expectancy, quality of life, and/or monetary costs. Figure 1–6B depicts the situation in a way analogous to the coin

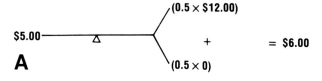

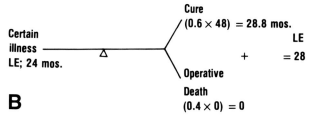

Figure 1-6 Expected value decision making. *A*, In the simple example of a choice between a coin toss, with the greatest and least possible gains ($12, $0), and a guaranteed intermediate gain ($5), the highest monetary yield on average results from choosing the gamble. *B*, In a hypothetical clinical example, an elderly patient must decide between two undesirable outcomes: decreased life expectancy (LE) due to illness (LE, 24 months) and a chance at cure (LE, 48 months), which also carries the risk of imminent death at surgery. Even with a 40 percent operative mortality, surgery is favored if the patient is only interested in maximizing overall life expectancy.

toss. In this example, a year of life is valued equally whether it is gained (or lost) in the very near or in the more distant future. Since most people place greater importance on gains and losses that accrue in the near future and vary significantly in their willingness to take risks, this representation of the problem is incomplete and inherently biased in favor of surgery.

Realistic clinical decisions ideally take into account all pertinent probabilities and outcomes and also include patients' propensities for risk taking in the present and in the future. Using the concept of expected value decision making, decision analysis offers a systematic way to analyze such decisions. The following sections outline the steps that a clinician might use to evaluate a test-ordering strategy. The reader interested in a more detailed description of the approach is referred to excellent texts by Sox and colleagues (1988), Sackett and associates (1985), and Weinstein and co-workers (1980). The current method is modified from that presented by Sox and co-workers.

In order to include all important aspects of a problem in an analysis, a *decision tree* is used as a schematic organizer. The first step in creating a tree is to define the problem requiring a decision and to identify all of the decision alternatives. A clinical example, familiar to all clinicians, modified and simplified from Molitch and associates (1984), illustrates the building of a typical decision tree. A patient with a solitary hypofunctioning thyroid nodule may be asked to consider the following options: (1) immediate surgical excision, which carries the risk of operative mortality and morbidity but offers the greatest potential for cure of cancer that may be present; (2) a trial of suppressive therapy, which carries the least immediate risk and also the least potential for cancer cure; and (3) aspiration biopsy, with intermediate apparent risks and benefits. In a decision tree, a decision point is called a *decision node* and is represented by a square (Figure 1–7). The initial outlining of the exact nature of the problem and of all reasonable options sometimes elucidates neglected possibilities. In many situations, no more detailed analysis will be necessary.

For particularly difficult decisions or when formulating a policy that will be applied many times, the next step in tree building is to list the clinical outcomes of each decision and to indicate the sequence of events leading to those outcomes. A final outcome is found in a decision tree at a *terminal node* and is indicated by a rectangle (see Figure 1–7). The outcomes possible in this example are: no malignancy or surgical cure of a small malignancy (BENIGN), malignancy remaining after surgery (MALIG), operative complications with a benign nodule (COMPLIC), operative complications with a malignant lesion that remains after surgery (MALCOMP), and death (DEAD). An intermediate future event that cannot be predicted precisely in advance, but that can be described in probabilistic terms, is represented as a branch emanating from a *chance node*, illustrated by a circle (see Fig. 1–7). Since the branches following a chance node must include all discrete possible subsequent events (i.e., they must be mutually exclusive and collectively exhaustive), when only two branches are present at a chance node, knowledge of the probability for one branch implies knowledge of the other.

For the thyroid nodule problem, the following events or conditions are possible if the surgery branch is chosen (the associated probabilities are indicated in parentheses): operative death (pOpDie) or survival, and surgical complications (pComp) or no complications (complications here are limited to the serious long-term complications of hypoparathyroidism and recurrent laryngeal nerve palsy); an excised nodule may be malignant (pMalig) or not, and malignant lesions will either be cured (pCure) or not cured. If a trial of suppressive therapy is chosen, the nodule may decrease in size, fail to decrease in size (pFail), or decrease in size initially only to later increase in size (pLateFl); nodules that fail to decrease in size are assumed to lead to surgical excision. For the choice of aspiration biopsy, pathologic examination may be positive (pBxPos) or negative for malignancy; positive results lead to surgery, and negative results lead to suppressive therapy. (Molitch and associates showed that "suspicious" results are best treated as negative.) If suppression or aspiration is chosen, it is possible that surgery may be performed subsequently. This possibility is displayed in the decision tree by the appearance of the OPERATE node, with all

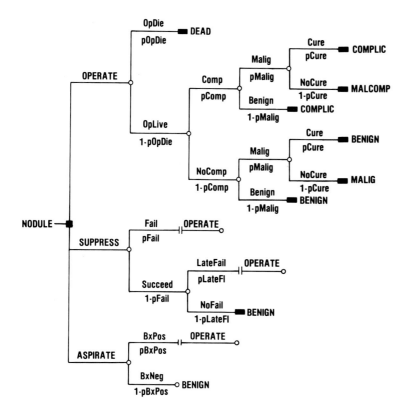

Figure 1–7   A decision tree for the problem of the hypofunctioning thyroid nodule. All reasonable decision alternatives are shown as branches from a decision node, indicated by the square. Circles indicate chance nodes; rectangles, terminal nodes (see text).

of the possible outcomes as if surgery were chosen initially. However, when these branches are found in different parts of the tree, different probabilities and utilities may pertain.

Again, by making assumptions about possible future events explicit, basic tree building may improve clinical decision making, without the need for quantitative analysis. If further study is warranted, however, the next step is to assign numerical probabilities to each possible event in the decision tree. These numbers are usually derived from the medical literature, but often expert opinion is required when published data are not available. It is at this point in tree building that the basis for clinical controversy often becomes clear: reasonable clinicians frequently make widely different assumptions about important probabilities. Assumed probabilities for this tree were modified from Molitch and associates and are listed in Table 1–4. As will be shown subsequently, any of these probabilities can be altered to test how they affect decisions.

The last numbers to be added to the tree represent the value of each outcome in the eyes of the decision maker. As mentioned, values can be described in terms of years of life remaining, quality of life, monetary costs, and other meaningful terms. For example, the value of having thyroid cancer discovered late can be expressed as years of life remaining if that state is reached. However, this expression does not account for the marked variability among patients in their willingness to take risks and trade off quantity for quality of life (McNeil et al, 1981).

A method of quantifying preferences, known as *utility assessment*, has been developed for determining preferences for outcomes in terms of gambles involving outcomes of known value. In a *standard reference gamble*, a decision maker is faced with a choice between a certain outcome of intermediate value and a gamble involving a better and a worse outcome. To set up standard reference gambles, one must identify the best and worst outcomes from among all the possible outcomes in a decision tree. These outcomes are assigned arbitrary numerical values of 100 and 0, respectively. As will be shown, all other outcomes can be assigned values relative to the best and worst outcomes. Along with assumptions about probabilities, values assigned to outcome states can be altered to test how decisions might be influenced.

In the thyroid nodule decision, most individuals would consider having a benign nodule to be clearly the best outcome and death the worst (because of very similar clinical significance, a small malignancy cured by surgery is considered here to have the same value as a benign nodule). The remaining possible outcomes—complications

TABLE 1–4   Baseline Probabilities Used in the Thyroid Nodule Decision Tree*

Event/State	Probability
Perioperative death (pOpDie)	.001
Surgical complication (pComp)	.003
Failure of suppressive therapy (pFail)	.78
Subsequent failure of suppressive therapy after initial success (pLateFl)	.02
Nodule is malignant— neither biopsy nor suppression done (pMalig)	.1
Aspiration biopsy shows malignancy (pBxPos)	.08
Malignancy is present if biopsy positive (pMIBxP)	.89
Malignancy is present if suppression fails (pMIFail)	.11
Surgical cure of malignant lesion (pCure)	.95
Surgical cure after late failure of suppression	.90

* See text for definitions of the events or conditions listed. Abbreviations are used in Figure 1–7. With sensitivity analysis, the effect of changes in any of these numbers on the decision to operate, give suppressive therapy, or perform aspiration biopsy can be determined. Modified from Molitch ME, Beck JR, Dreisman M, et al. The cold thyroid nodule: An analysis of diagnostic and therapeutic options. Endocr Rev 1984; 5:185.

of surgery and malignancy not cured by surgery—must be ranked relative to the best and worst.

The use of standard reference gambles in medicine requires careful preparation of scenarios that accurately describe what is at stake and careful preparation of the patient for the task of thinking abstractly about possible future events. A scenario for a young woman with a cold nodule might be as follows:

> Ms. X, we've discussed the options available for management of your thyroid nodule, and it would be helpful in advising you if we knew more about your feelings about the possibilities that lie ahead. To do this we'll need to play a sort of game. I'll be asking you questions about problems that might develop in the future, but that are distinctly unlikely to happen. I'm asking you about them just to find out more about your preferences.
>
> I want you to pretend you are in an unfamiliar situation, faced with a difficult choice: you have had thyroid surgery and cancer was found, but the surgeons were unable to remove all of the cancer. You will have to undergo further treatment and have frequent follow-up visits to the clinic. Given that you are now 30 years old, your life expectancy of approximately 49 years will be reduced by about 4 years. As an alternative to remaining in this circumstance, you may choose a gamble in which you blindly select a ball from an urn. This urn contains 1,000 balls, 999 of which are white and one of which is black. If you select a white ball, you will be cured of cancer, have no more thyroid problems, and have a normal life expectancy; if you select a black ball, you die immediately (painlessly). Which do you prefer, the gamble or the status quo? (Assuming she chooses the gamble, questioning proceeds.) Now suppose that there were 700 white balls and 300 black balls, which do you prefer? (Assuming the status quo is chosen, questioning proceeds.) What about 800 white balls and 200 black balls?

By repeatedly reframing the standard reference gamble scenario, a point is reached at which the patient is indifferent between the gamble (cure, death) and the status quo (thyroid cancer). This point indicates the *indifference probability*, at which the utilities of the gamble and of the status quo are identical. If an individual were indifferent when there were 850 white balls and 150 black balls in the urn, the indifference probability would be

.85. This is obtained by calculating the expected value of the gamble; since the gamble and the sure thing are equal in value as measured in the reference gamble, the expected value of the gamble equals the value of the intermediate state. On a scale ranging from 0 (death) to 100 (benign or cured lesion, no complications), the utility of a thyroid malignancy is thus 85 (see example in Figure 1–8). The utility of long-term postoperative morbidity due to surgical complications could be obtained in a similar way. In the current example this utility is also assumed to be 85. In essence, this number indicates the patient's belief that her quality of life after a complication is on average worth approximately 85 percent of what it would be worth without complications.

For persons unable to participate in the abstract thinking required by standard reference gambles, other forms of utility assessment are available. The *time trade-off* method elicits patient views on the lesser number of years in good health that they believe is equivalent to a greater number of years in poor health. The *direct scaling* method simply uses a linear scale on which a patient indicates preferences for outcomes. These alternate methods may provide critical insights useful in decision making, but their use is not so firmly founded in decision theory and may not be directly applicable to expected value decision making. Finally, it should be noted that individuals' preferences vary over time and with subtle changes in how questions are framed. For instance, Llewellyn-Thomas and co-workers (1982) showed that measured preferences for different states of health varied depending on whether death was used as a possible outcome in standard reference gambles. These and other problems make utility assessment difficult to apply universally in clinical settings. Nonetheless, with proper care and preparation this approach can, in selected cases, contribute to decision making in a way that improves physician-patient communication and optimizes clinical outcomes.

Utility determinations complete the building of the decision tree. Table 1–5 lists the utilities assumed for the current problem. Using the concept of expected value de-

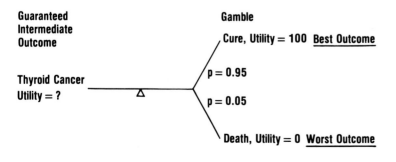

Utility (Thyroid Cancer) = (0.95 × 100) + (0.05 × 0) = 0.95.

Figure 1–8 Measurement of patient preferences for the possible outcomes in the thyroid nodule decision tree. The utility of thyroid cancer is measured by finding the indifference probability between the intermediate outcome and the gamble. In this case, the patient is indifferent when the urn contains 950 white balls and 50 black balls, as described in the text. Thus, the utility of thyroid cancer for this patient is .95.

TABLE 1-5   Baseline Utilities for the Thyroid Nodule Decision Tree*

Outcome State	Utility
Benign lesion or small cancer cured, no complications (BENIGN)	100
Malignancy (MALIG)	85
Benign lesion, complications (COMPLIC)	85
Malignancy, complications (MALCOMP)	70
Death (DEAD)	0

* Abbreviations are used in Figure 1–7.

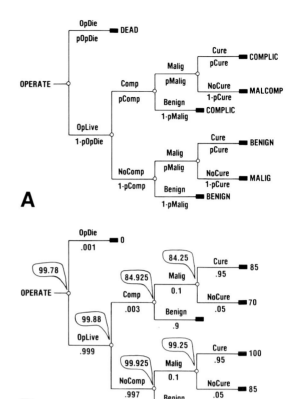

A

B

Figure 1-9   Averaging out and folding back. The expected value of the decision to operate immediately is calculated starting from the right-hand side of this subtree and working back to the decision node.

cision making, the clinician is now ready to calculate which of the decision alternatives maximizes chances of achieving the most desirable outcome, i.e., the greatest utility.

Just as was the case for the coin toss example described previously, the expected value at any chance node is calculated by multiplying the probability of each outcome by its utility, then adding the products for all outcomes. In decision trees the process is repeated at each chance node in a process known as "averaging out and folding back," beginning at the terminal nodes and working backward. For the OPERATE branch in Figure 1–7, one of the final chance nodes pertains to the probability of cure in a patient who has complications after undergoing surgery for a malignant nodule.

To calculate the expected value of that chance node, one multiplies the number corresponding to pCure by the value of COMPLIC, and this product is added to the product of (1-pCure) and MALCOMP (Fig. 1–9A). Applying the appropriate numbers from Tables 1–4 and 1–5,

$$
\begin{aligned}
.95 \times 85 &= 80.75 \\
&\qquad + \qquad = \qquad 84.25 \\
.05 \times 70 &= 3.5
\end{aligned}
$$

Once the value of a chance node has been determined (by "averaging out"), the branches to the right of that node are no longer needed and can be "folded back." Attention is then directed to the next chance node, and the process is repeated until the beginning of the OPER-ATE branch is reached (Fig. 1–9B), thus establishing the expected value of the decision to operate. The expected value is here expressed in relative units based on the previously mentioned scale bounded by the best (BE-NIGN) and worst (DEATH) outcomes. When all calculations are completed, each decision branch has an associated expected value that can be compared with other branches (Fig. 1–10). The decision with the highest expected value is the best option for the patient.

The most obvious result of this analysis is that no option offers a significant advantage over any other; the decision is essentially a "toss-up," and individuals may best decide on the basis of monetary, emotional, or other factors (Kassirer and Pauker, 1981). However, any clinician might reasonably doubt the validity of any of the numbers used in the decision tree and wish to substitute values believed to be more appropriate. Further, when different experts or studies estimate different probabilities for key events (e.g., operative mortality or incidence of recurrent laryngeal nerve damage), a wide range of possible values may need to be evaluated. *Sensitivity*

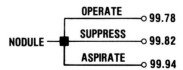

Figure 1-10   Expected values for the possible options in the thyroid nodule problem. The decision to perform aspiration biopsy has the highest expected value and is thus the favored choice. Because the differences are small, however, this decision might be considered a "toss-up" (see text).

analysis allows the decision maker to test whether conclusions remain stable when the numbers in a decision tree are varied. For example, if the probability of cure of a malignancy immediately removed surgically were thought to be .8 instead of .95, the expected value at the chance node evaluated above would be

$$
\begin{array}{r}
.80 \times 85 = 68.0 \\
+ \\
.20 \times 70 = 14.0
\end{array} \quad = \quad 82.0
$$

The resulting branch for the OPERATE option is shown in Figure 1–11. As expected with a decreased chance of surgical success, the OPERATE option now has a lower utility and would compare even less favorably with the other options.

Computer programs are available that allow the probabilities in a decision tree to be varied repeatedly to test the effect of changes on decisions (Hollenberg, 1989). Graphic displays of sensitivity analyses provide rapid insight into the importance of various factors. Figures 1–12A and 1–12B show sensitivity analyses for single variables. In Figure 1–12A the probability of surgical cure of a cancer is varied from 0 to 1 and expected utilities for each decision alternative are plotted against that probability. Where the suppression and aspiration biopsy lines cross indicates a threshold: when the probability of cure exceeds 0.84, aspiration biopsy is favored. Because the aspiration biopsy line is at all points higher than the operation line, aspiration biopsy is favored even if surgery is always curative. Figure 1–12B depicts a sensitivity analysis in which the probability of failure of suppressive therapy is varied from 0 to 1. Aspiration biopsy is favored as long there is more than a 27 percent chance of failure of suppression.

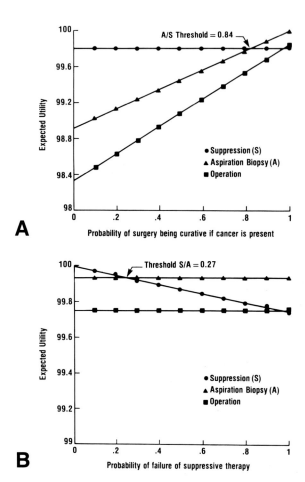

Figure 1–12 One-way sensitivity analysis: the effect on expected utility when one value in the decision tree is varied while all others are held constant. *A*, The probability of surgery being curative (pCure) is varied across the entire range of possibilities (0 to 1). Suppressive therapy yields the highest expected value when the probability of cure is less than .83. *B*, The effect of changes in the probability that suppressive therapy will fail to cause a reduction in size of a "cold" thyroid nodule (pFail). Aspiration biopsy is favored when this probability is greater than .27.

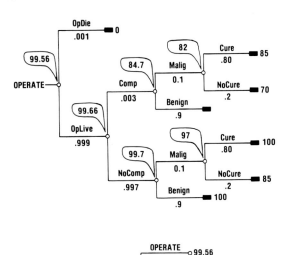

Figure 1–11 Sensitivity analysis. The expected value of the OPERATE branch is recalculated with the assumption that the probability of surgical cure of a thyroid malignancy (pCure) is .8 instead of .95. After recalculation for the other tree branches, it is clear that the decision to defer surgery is not sensitive to this change.

Graphic representations of up to three variables changing simultaneously are possible. Other, nongraphic, techniques allow all of the variables in a tree to be varied over pertinent ranges, giving the decision maker an idea of how confident he should be in choosing one of several alternatives.

Formal quantitative decision analysis is most often unnecessary in clinical practice. Furthermore, few clinicians have the time or expertise required to perform a thorough analysis. The decision tree framework, however, can provide useful insights into the elements of a decision. In a very few minutes the clinician can easily sketch a tree to be sure that all possible options and outcomes are being considered. This can be very useful for counseling patients and discussing management with consultants. In addition, explicit consideration of probabilities and utilities can point out where clinicians disagree, where further research is needed, and where explicit input from the patient is critical to decision making—all without performing any calculations. Aside from work with individual patients, an understanding of the principles of decision analysis permits one to read the profusion of articles in the current medical literature which use this approach, especially inasmuch as this literature addresses recurrent and/or difficult clinical problems for which formal quantitative analyses can be particularly helpful.

SUMMARY

This chapter has presented a way of thinking about how diagnostic tests can benefit patients. The most important principle is that of thinking in probabilistic terms. The clinician who carefully considers the likelihood of disease in a patient *before* ordering a test can decide whether the test has the potential to alter his management strategy. In addition to thinking about pretest probability, the approach requires the clinician to set a threshold probability—the probability of disease at which management plans will change—and to ascertain how well the test discriminates between persons with and without disease. If a test can alter the probability of disease such that a threshold is crossed, it can potentially alter management so that the patient's condition is improved. A test which cannot sufficiently alter the probability of disease should, in general, not be ordered.

For difficult, controversial, and/or recurring diagnostic problems, decision analysis is useful because it explicitly takes into account all important management options and possible clinical occurrences. Its use may be particularly appropriate since it can explicitly include patients' preferences for different health states. In everyday clinical practice, decision analysis offers a qualitative approach to considering all important variables. An understanding of how detailed quantitative analyses are conducted also allows the clinician to garner useful information from the growing body of medical literature which uses these techniques.

Acknowledgments. The authors wish to thank Dr. Robert Golub of Northwestern University for careful review of the manuscript, and Drs. Kelley Skeff and Harold Sox of Stanford University for encouragement and for introducing us to effective approaches to teaching medical decision making.

BIBLIOGRAPHY

Billewicz WZ, Chapman RS, Crooks J, et al. Statistical methods applied to the diagnosis of hypothyroidism. Q J Med 1969; 38:255.

Bryant GD, Norman GR. The communication of uncertainty. Annu Conf Res Med Educ 1979; 18:205.

Connolly CK, Gore MBR, Stanley N, et al. Single-dose dexamethasone suppression in normal subjects and hospitalized patients. Br Med J 1968; 2:665.

Crapo L. Cushing's syndrome: A review of diagnostic tests. Metabolism 1979; 28:955.

Elstein AS, Shulman LS, Sprafka SA. Medical problem solving: An analysis of clinical reasoning. Cambridge, MA: Harvard University Press, 1978.

Fallon MA, Arvan DA. Hypercalcemia. In: Griner PF, Panzer RJ, Greenland P, eds. Clinical diagnosis and the laboratory. Chicago: Year Book, 1986.

Greenes RA, Cain KC, Begg CB, et al. Patient-oriented performance measures of diagnostic tests. Med Decis Making 1984; 4:7.

Griner PF, Panzer RJ, Greenland P. Clinical diagnosis and the laboratory: Logical strategies for common medical problems. Chicago: Year Book, 1986.

Hamberger B, Gharib H, Melton LJ, et al. Fine-needle aspiration biopsy of thyroid nodules. Am J Med 1982; 73:381.

Hollenberg JP. SMLTREE. Boston: Pratt Medical Group, 1989.

Kassirer JP, Moskowitz AJ, Lau J, Pauker SG. Decision analysis: A progress report. Ann Intern Med 1987; 106:275.

Kassirer JP, Pauker SC. The toss-up (editorial). N Engl J Med 1981; 305:1467.

Kong A, Barnett GO, Mosteller F, Youtz C. How medical professionals evaluate expressions of probability. N Engl J Med 1986; 315:740.

Llewellyn-Thomas H, Sutherland HJ, Tibshirani R, et al. The measurement of patient values in medicine. Med Decis Making 1982; 2:449.

McNeil BJ, Weichselbaum R, Pauker SG. Speech and survival: tradeoffs between quality and quantity of life in laryngeal cancer. N Engl J Med 1981; 305:982.

Molitch ME, Beck JR, Dreisman M, et al. The cold thyroid nodule: An analysis of diagnostic and therapeutic options. Endocr Rev 1984; 5:185.

Nugent CA, Nichols T, Tyler FH. Diagnosis of cushing's syndrome—single dose dexamethasone suppression test. Arch Intern Med 1965; 116:172.

Pauker SG, Kassirer JP. Therapeutic decision making: A cost-benefit analysis. N Engl J Med 1975; 293:229.

Pauker SG, Kassirer JP. The threshold approach to clinical decision making. N Engl J Med 1980; 302:1109.

Raiffa H. Decision analysis: Introductory lectures on choices under uncertainty. Reading, MA: Addison-Wesley, 1970.

Sackett DL, Haynes RB, Tugwell P. Clinical epidemiology: A basic science for clinical medicine. Boston: Little, Brown, 1985.

Sox HC. Common diagnostic tests: Use and interpretation. Philadelphia: American College of Physicians, 1987.

Sox HC, Blatt M, Marton KI, Higgins M. Medical decision making. Boston: Butterworth, 1988.

Tversky A, Kahneman D. Judgement under uncertainty: Heuristics and biases. Science 1974; 185:1124.

Weinstein MC, Fineberg HV, Elstein AS, et al. Clinical decision analysis. Philadelphia: WB Saunders, 1980.

2 Competitive-Binding Assays

Samuel P. Marynick, M.D., F.A.C.P.

HISTORY OF LIGAND COMPETITIVE-BINDING ASSAY

The observations in the 1950s of Yalow and Berson on the behavior of insulin-binding antibodies gave rise to the technique known as competitive assay (1959). Yalow has stated that the development of technology that allowed for hormones to be obtained of sufficient purity and quantity to permit labeling with radioisotopes and for immunization was essential in the development of competitive assay techniques (Yalow, 1985).

Ligand assay has been appreciated for about three decades and over that time has penetrated most areas of medicine. The technique of ligand assay has proliferated because it permits sensitive and specific (accurate) quantitation of a variety of compounds (e.g., peptides, steroid hormones, vitamins, thyroid hormones, medications) of biologic importance over a wide range of concentrations (Howanitz and Howanitz, 1984).

Before development of ligand assay technology, many hormonal substances were measured by crude chemical or in vivo assays using various laboratory animals, or they were not measurable at all. Indeed, the development of clinical endocrinology as we know it today is dependent on and parallels that of ligand assay technology.

PRINCIPLES OF LIGAND COMPETITIVE-BINDING ASSAY

Ligand competitive-binding assays have several principles in common. They depend on similar behavior of the standard to be measured and the unknown. They depend on laws of mass action to partition the compound to be measured between the free state and the state of being bound to a binding reagent with a specific but limited capacity to bind the compound. They depend on a means of distinguishing bound compound from free compound.

Many specific binding agents have been used in ligand-binding assays, including antibodies, naturally occurring proteins, hormone receptors, and enzymes (Howanitz and Howanitz, 1984). All of these binding reagents have advantages and disadvantages. The most important differences in the binding agents relate to their affinity (how avidly they bind the compound to be measured) and specificity (how specifically they bind only the compound being measured).

The association constant (K_a) of a binding reagent is obtained by measuring how strongly a compound is bound to a binding reagent. K_a is expressed in liters per mole. Generally, the greater the K_a of a binding reagent, the more stable is the association of the binding reagent and the specifically bound compound (Thompson, 1984).

DESCRIPTION OF LIGAND COMPETITIVE-BINDING ASSAY CHARACTERISTICS

Principles of Radioimmunoassay

Radioimmunoassay (RIA) is based on an interaction between a radioisotope-labeled compound and an antibody directed against it that can be inhibited by a similar but unlabeled compound (Fig. 2–1) (Yalow, 1973). It is the most commonly used form of ligand competitive-binding assay because antibodies can be prepared for a wide variety of compounds, including peptides, steroids, and medications (Yalow, 1973).

Potential drawbacks to RIA include (1) cross-reactivity of antibody with compounds other than the one to be measured, (2) difficulty of inducing antibody formation to some compounds, (3) multiple antibody for-

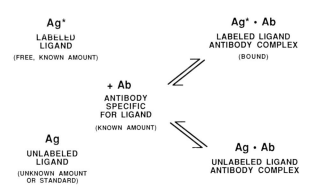

Figure 2–1 Schematic representation of the principle of RIA.

mation to the antigenic compound in each individual immunized animal and the resultant differences in characteristics or immunologic properties of different antibodies in one animal for a specific compound, (4) varying properties of antibodies induced to the same specific antigen in different animals of the same species, making it necessary to characterize the individual properties of antibodies from different animals to the same compound (antigen). Finally, in RIA, one is looking at immunologic reactivity rather than biologic activity, and these two functions for a compound may differ (Howanitz and Howanitz, 1984).

It is important in RIA to show that both the standard and the unknown compound decrease in concentration as measured by the assay in a fashion that parallels the dilution of the compound and that both the standard and compound being measured in an unknown sample react similarly in the RIA as their concentrations decrease because of sample dilution (Yalow, 1978; Felber, 1978).

Historically and to the present, antigen-specific antibodies have been obtained by injecting an animal with the compound for which a specific antibody is desired. If a compound is too small to induce antibody formation, it can be attached to a larger molecule (such as a protein) prior to injection; because of the increase in antigen size, antibody formation to the small compound results (Howanitz and Howanitz, 1984; Midgley and Niswender, 1970).

When an animal is injected with an antigen, that animal may begin to produce more than one antibody to the antigen. This often results in complex antibody characteristics to an antigen in a previously immunized animal (Thompson, 1984). Recently, cell lines have been developed that make antibodies to one antigenic deter-

minant. These monoclonal antibody-forming cell lines, called hybridomas, are produced by fusing an antibody-forming mouse spleen cell with myeloma cells. Such cell lines are capable of producing large quantities of monoclonal or homogeneous antibody. This can be contrasted to heterogeneous or polyclonal antibodies that recognize different antigenic determinants of the same compound, which are formed when an animal is immunized (Sevier et al, 1981).

RIA is performed by preparing mixtures of a fixed amount of a radioisotope-labeled antigen (compound) and its antibody with standard concentrations of the antigen that is not labeled or with a sample whose content of unlabeled antigen is not known. These mixtures are incubated for a defined amount of time, and then the antibody-bound, labeled antigen (bound, B) is separated from the unbound, labeled antigen (free, F) by one of a variety of techniques (Felber, 1978).

Once bound antigen is separated from free antigen, one must decide how to present the results of the assay. A variety of methods have been used to present immunoassay data. Frequently, the standard curve (data obtained using known amounts of unlabeled antigen) is constructed placing either the percentage of labeled antigen bound (% B) or the ratio labeled antigen bound to that bound in the absence of unlabeled antigen (B/B_0) on the ordinate and relating this to the amount of unlabeled antigen added to the mixture on the abscissa.

The plot generated using the preceding method is usually nonlinear, but if one uses logarithmic or semilogarithmic plotting for the concentrations of unlabeled antigen added to the reaction, linearity is sometimes produced. Schematic representations of these methods of plotting RIA data are shown in Figure 2–2. If one plots

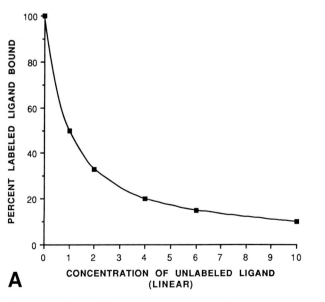
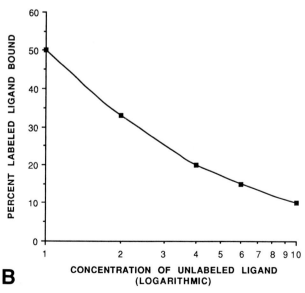

Figure 2–2   Plotting RIA data for the same assay with the concentration of unlabeled ligand in the assay plotted linearly (*A*) or logarithmically (*B*).

RIA data placing the logit of B/B_0 on the ordinate and the log of the concentration of unlabeled ligand on the abscissa, linearization of RIA standard curves is possible (Felber, 1978; Rodbard et al, 1968, 1969).

Principles of Radioassay

Binding proteins that occur in nature may be used as specific binding reagents. Compared with RIA, radioassays using binding proteins are less sensitive (lower binding affinity) and less specific (more interaction with compounds not being measured) (Murphy, 1970). Serum normally contains proteins that bind cortisol, thyroid hormone, testosterone, and vitamin B_{12}. When these binding proteins are used in assays, it is key to destroy any similar binding protein in the sample to be measured. Generally, this is accomplished by heating the unknown sample or by precipitating interfering binders from the sample to be analyzed by exposing the sample to organic solvents, such as ethanol, prior to radioassay analysis (Murphy, 1970).

The advantages of radioassays using naturally occurring binding proteins relate to their availability, relative inexpensiveness, ease of preparation, storage stability, and consistency in properties from one preparation to another.

The disadvantage of these naturally occurring proteins relates to their lower affinity (sensitivity) and specificity compared with RIA. Also, binding proteins are available for a limited number of compounds (Howanitz and Howanitz, 1984; Murphy, 1970).

Principles of Receptor Assays

Receptors for various compounds have been localized on cellular membranes, in the cytoplasm of cells, and in their nuclei. These receptors can specifically interact with compounds such as medications, peptide hormones, steroid hormones, and smaller substances, such as thyroid hormones, catecholamines, and other neurotransmitters. These receptors are generally directed more toward the biologically active portion of a molecule, which may not necessarily be the most immunologically active portion (Howanitz and Howanitz, 1984; Gorden and Weintraub, 1985).

Disadvantages of receptor assays include:

1. Receptors tend not to be stable.
2. Receptors must be prepared from a source in which they are often present in small amounts, then concentrated.
3. The techniques used to separate receptors often diminish the number of intact receptors isolated and may adversely affect the binding characteristics of these receptors.
4. Receptors may be able to recognize small changes in compounds produced by radioisotope labeling, making the labeled compound a less than optimal tracer for a particular assay.
5. Receptor assays are generally less sensitive than RIAs.
6. Receptors may be occupied by nonspecific binding agents (Howanitz and Howanitz, 1984).

Advantages of receptor assays include uniformity of characteristics from preparation to preparation and assessment of biologic activity as opposed to immunologic activity (Howanitz and Howanitz, 1984; Gorden and Weintraub, 1985).

LABELS FOR LIGAND COMPETITIVE-BINDING ASSAY

General Principles

Indicators employed in ligand competitive-binding assay systems have included radioactive isotope-labeled molecules, enzymatic activity, and fluorescence. The labeled molecule need not biochemically behave precisely as the unlabeled compound, but the two compounds must show similar behavior in the assay system being used (Howanitz and Howanitz, 1984; Thompson, 1984; Hunter, 1974).

Immunoassays can be divided into two types: (1) homogeneous, in which free label can be distinguished from bound label without prior physical separation, and (2) heterogeneous, in which free and bound labels must be separated physically before the assay is performed (Howanitz and Howanitz, 1984; Thompson, 1984).

It is desirable for the labeled compound to have an affinity for its binder equivalent to the nonlabeled compound being measured. If the affinity of the labeled compound for the binding site is less than that of unlabeled compounds, the sensitivity of the assay will be impaired. Also, if the labeled compound interacts with the binder in a manner different from that of the unlabeled compound or has biochemical properties different from those of the unlabeled compound, assay results may not be predictable (Howanitz and Howanitz, 1984; Thompson, 1984; Hunter, 1974).

Radioactive Labels

Radio labels have been used in immunochemical assays because they offer great flexibility in how they can be used and allow for very sensitive assays. The two main types of radio labels used are beta emitters such as tritium (^3H) and gamma emitters such as iodine 125 (^{125}I).

Radioisotopes have different properties that influence why they are chosen for particular assays. The beta emitter tritium has a long half-life, 12.3 years, when compared with the gamma emitter iodine 125, which has a half-life of 60.2 days, and tritium is easily incorporated into organic compounds (Howanitz and Howanitz, 1984; U.S. Department of Health, Education and Welfare, 1970).

However, beta emitters have several disadvantages. For example, the specific activity (amount of radioactivity per unit mass of labeled compound) of tritium is much less than that for ^{125}I-labeled compounds, and beta-emitter radioactivity can be assessed only by using a liquid scintillation counting system (Howanitz and Howanitz, 1984; Landon, 1976). Scintillation counting systems are cumbersome. They require that the beta-emitter compound be added to scintillation fluid. When beta irradiation is emitted by the decaying radioactive isotope, the scintillation fluid is excited or fluor occurs. When the fluor returns to the unexcited state, light is emitted, and the excitation of a photoelectric tube by this light signifies that a beta emission has occurred. The time and expense necessitated by the scintillation counting method and quenching (internal interference with light transmission from the scintillation fluid to a photoelectric tube) make beta emitters less than optimal for use in immunoassays (Howanitz and Howanitz, 1984; Finlayson, 1969).

Gamma-emitting radioisotopes have several advantages over beta-emitting radioisotopes when used in immunoassays. First, gamma detection can be obtained directly from the test tube in which the assay occurs and does not require the placing of the material to be assessed into special scintillation vials to which scintillation fluid must be added. Second, because of its high specific activity, less gamma-emitting radioisotope is required for reliable determination of the quantity of isotope present in a sample, and counting time for gamma-labeled samples is reduced (Howanitz and Howanitz, 1984; Gorden and Weintraub, 1985; Landon, 1976). At this time, ^{125}I is the most commonly used gamma-emitter isotope in immunoassays (Howanitz and Howanitz, 1984).

Though high specific activity is a desirable characteristic of a radioisotope-labeled compound, too high a specific activity can actually be harmful and may result in loss of immunoreactivity of the compound because of radiation-induced intramolecular damage. When the number of radioactive ^{125}I atoms per molecule of labeled antigen is increased from one to two, disintegration and gamma emission from one of the ^{125}I atoms may disrupt the labeled molecule, resulting in molecular fragments that may possess radioactivity and have reduced immunoreactivity. This phenomenon, called decay catastrophe, results in an unreliable assay (Yalow, 1973).

Labeled Binders—Immunoradiometric Assay

Immunoradiometric assays (IRMAs) differ from RIAs and radioassays in that the compound to be measured binds with a labeled antibody that is present in the reaction mixture in an excessive quantity (Woodhead et al, 1974; Baker et al, 1985). Free antibody is separated from bound antibody, often by exposing the reaction mixture to antigen that is coupled to a solid phase. The radioactive-labeled antibody that is not bound to the solid-phase attached antigen reflects the concentration

of antigen in the sample being measured (Figs. 2–3 and 2–4). In some IRMAs, two antibodies are reacted with the same antigen. One of these antibodies is absorbed onto a solid phase, and the other, which is radioisotope labeled, is added to the assay after incubation of the antigen with the solid-phase-bound, antigen-specific unlabeled antibody. This type of assay is referred to as a two-site IRMA or sandwich IRMA (Woodhead et al, 1974; Baker et al, 1985). In two-site IRMA, the amount of a radiolabeled antibody attached to the solid phase reflects the concentration of antigen present. Variations on the IRMA sandwich have been developed. These include fluorescence labeling of the compound being measured that has been previously bound to a solid-phase attached antibody, immunofluorometric assay, and enzymatic measurement of solid-phase attached antibody-bound substances, immunoenzymometric assay (Howanitz and Howanitz, 1984). IRMA assays using three antibodies have been developed. The third antibody, which is labeled, is directed to the second antibody that was added after the compound being measured was bound to a solid-phase attached antibody (Howanitz and Howanitz, 1984).

An important point in IRMA is that if the concentration of the compound to be measured exceeds the binding capacity of the compound-specific antibody, the assay becomes meaningless (Howanitz and Howanitz, 1984).

Enzyme Labels, Enzyme-Linked Immunosorbent Assays

In enzyme-linked immunosorbent assays (ELISAs), enzymes are used in place of radioactive isotopes to label antigens or antibodies to specific antigens. In a method

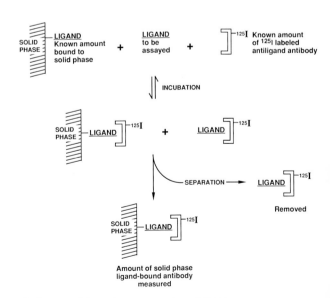

Figure 2–3   Schematic representation of IRMA.

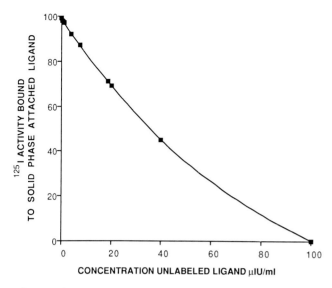

Figure 2-4   Graphic representation of IRMA for TSH.

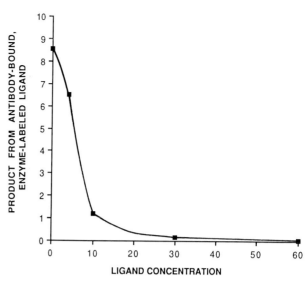

Figure 2-6   Graphic depiction of ELISA.

analogous to RIA, the enzyme is linked to the antigen to be studied. The enzymatic activity is then determined in either bound or free antigen fraction after a procedure to separate antibody bound from free antigen (Figs. 2–5 and 2–6) (Engvall et al, 1971). Enzymes that are convenient to use because they are commercially available and have a reliable and rapid method of assay include glucose-6-phosphate dehydrogenase, alkaline phosphatase, and lysozyme (Howanitz and Howanitz, 1984). Enzymes may be bound to antigen-specific antibodies and used in a method analogous to the IRMA sandwich technique (Fig. 2-7) (Engvall and Perlmann, 1972).

In enzyme-labeled systems in which the antigen is covalently linked to the enzyme, binding of the antigen to antibody may result in diminished or lost enzymatic

activity (Rubenstein et al, 1972). Thus, by determining enzymatic activity, one can assess the amount of antibody-bound and free enzyme-labeled antigen in the sample being analyzed. This particular type of ELISA, called enzyme-multiplied immunoassay technique (EMIT) (Figs. 2–8 and 2–9), is a homogeneous assay because it is not necessary to separate bound from free antigen before assessing enzymatic activity. The inhibition of enzyme activity in antibody-bound enzyme-labeled antigen is believed to be the result of conformational changes occurring in the enzyme either because of antibody binding to the antigen-enzyme complex or because of antibody prevention of conformational changes required before enzymatic activity can be manifest (Howanitz and Howanitz, 1984; Rowley et al, 1975).

Figure 2-5   Schematic representation of ELISA with ligand labeled.

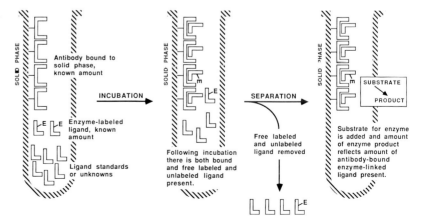

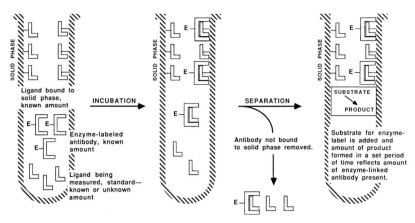

Figure 2-7 Schematic representation of ELISA with antibody labeled.

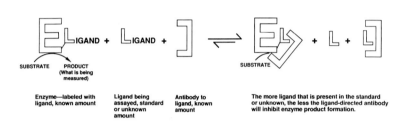

Figure 2-8 Schematic representation of EMIT.

There are some disadvantages to ELISAs. Enzyme labels can hinder the necessary antigen-antibody binding and decrease the sensitivity of the assay. Also, enzymatic labeling of antigens and antibodies is technically difficult, and naturally occurring substances may inhibit or interfere with quantitation of enzymatic activity (Howanitz and Howanitz, 1984; Yalow, 1978; Wisdom, 1976).

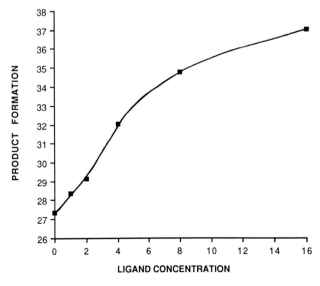

Figure 2-9 Graphic representation of EMIT.

Fluorescent Labels

The advantages of fluorescent labels include their stability, their low cost, the relative inexpensiveness of the instruments used to measure fluorescence, and the speed of assay performance (Howanitz and Howanitz, 1984; Soini and Hemmilä, 1979).

Fluorescent label immunoassays are inherently less sensitive than RIAs. Additionally, the sensitivity of these assays is adversely influenced by background fluorescence and scattering of fluorescence. Instrumentation has been developed to attempt to minimize the adverse effects of background fluorescence and fluorescence scatter on the sensitivity of these immunoassays. Time-resolved fluorometry minimizes background fluorescence by using a pulse of light to excite the fluorescent label. Fluorescence is then measured during a specific time after this excitation (Soini and Hemmilä, 1979).

Some fluorescent immunoassays do not require separation of free from bound label to quantitate the unknown compound being measured. This technology includes the fluorescence polarization method of immunoassay and homogeneous assays using nonfluorescent precursors as enzyme substrates that are changed to fluorescent compounds. These homogeneous assays utilize not only ELISA technology, but fluorescent immunoassay technology as well (Schall and Tenoso, 1981).

In fluorescent polarization method of assay, polarized light excites a fluorescent label. As this label is

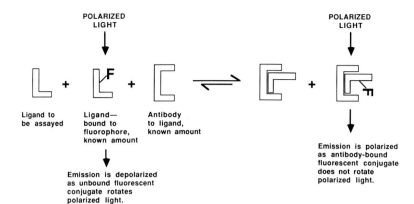

Figure 2-10 Schematic representation of FPIA.

bound, the degree of polarization of the fluorescent emission from the label increases. Disadvantages of this method are a nonlinear assay when the concentration of the test compound is related to polarization of the fluorescent emission. Also, this type of assay has a limited range of concentrations over which the compound being assayed can be accurately measured (Soini and Hemmilä, 1979). A schematic representation of a fluorescence polarization immunoassay (FPIA) is shown in Figure 2-10, and a graphic representation of how data are presented for FPIA is shown in Figure 2-11.

SEPARATION SYSTEM

The purpose of all ligand-binding assays is to determine the relative portion of an antigen that is free and to determine which portion is bound to a specific and saturable binding agent. Often a physical separation of the bound from the free fraction of the substance being measured is required to distinguish the two (Yalow, 1985;

Howanitz and Howanitz, 1984; Yalow, 1973; Ratcliffe, 1974); however, a separation step is not necessary in some homogeneous enzyme and fluorescent immunoassay systems (Howanitz and Howanitz, 1984; Thompson, 1984; Sevier et al, 1981; Rubenstein et al, 1972; Rowley et al, 1975; Soini and Hemmilä, 1979).

Several criteria must be met for a separation step not to adversely influence the quality of an immunoassay (Table 2-1) (Yalow, 1985; Howanitz and Howanitz, 1984; Yalow, 1973; Ratcliffe, 1974). Some separatory systems that have been utilized are listed in Table 2-2 (Howanitz and Howanitz, 1984; Yalow, 1978; Ratcliffe, 1974). Generally, more cumbersome separatory systems, such as electrophoresis, have been replaced by less complicated systems.

Separation methods using adsorption of free moiety have been achieved for compounds with a molecular weight of less than 30,000 daltons (Yalow, 1978). Adsorption separation is influenced by many factors, including (1) surface area of the adsorbent, (2) size of the ligand, (3) charge of the adsorbent and ligand, (4) protein con-

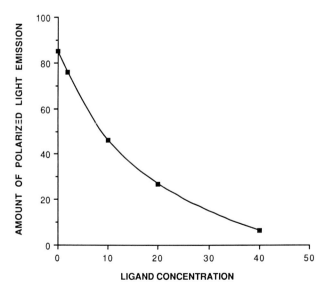

Figure 2-11 Graphic representation of FPIA.

TABLE 2-1 Characteristics of Ideal Separation Systems in Ligand Competitive-Binding Assays

1. Separation should be fast, uncomplicated, and inexpensive (performed with easily obtainable reagents using equipment that is present in a clinical chemistry laboratory).
2. The separating agent must not alter the equilibrium present in the reaction medium and yet must completely separate the substrate being measured into bound and free fractions.
3. The separation process must be reproducible from assay to assay and uniform in the same assay run.
4. The system must be able to achieve separation despite wide variation in the concentrations of moieties to be separated.
5. Nonspecific substances in the sample being assayed should not alter the quality of separation.
6. The system of separation should be usable in different assays.
7. The system of separation should be able to delineate damaged from undamaged label.

TABLE 2-2   Systems Utilized to Separate a Compound Being Analyzed into Bound (B) and Unbound or Free (F) Fractions

	Principle Utilized	*System*	*Example*
1.	Nonspecific adsorption of free ligand	Adsorption	a. Charcoal b. Silicates c. Resins (Amberlite)
2.	Adsorption of bound	Adsorption	Resins (diethylaminoethyl cellulose)
3.	Nonspecific precipitation	Precipitation of bound ligand	a. Ammonium sulfate b. Polyethylene glycol (PEG) c. Ethanol
4.	Immunologic precipitation	Precipitation of bound ligand	Double antibody or second antibody
5.	Antibody attached to a solid moiety	Solid phase	a. Antibody-coated test tube or disk b. Antibody-coated dextran or cellulose particles
6.	Difference in charge of bound and free ligand	Differential electrical migration of bound and free ligand	Electrophoresis
7.	Difference in bound and free ligand molecular weight	Differential migration of bound and free ligand	Gel filtration
8.	Two or more of the above	Combinations	a. Ammonium sulfate and second antibody b. Second antibody bound to solid phase c. Etc.

centrations in the assay system, (5) temperature at separation, and (6) pH of and ionic constituents in the assay system (Ratcliffe, 1974). Charcoal is commonly used in adsorption systems and is a reliable substance. However, it must be used in specific concentrations, at a relatively low temperature, and for defined extraction-reaction times; otherwise, it has a tendency to remove bound as well as free ligand, a phenomenon known as stripping (Howanitz and Howanitz, 1984; Ekins, 1974; Binoux and Odell, 1973).

Various agents have been utilized for precipitation of bound substrate, leaving the free fraction in solution. Ammonium sulfate, ethanol, polyethylene glycol, and other agents have been used in these nonspecific precipitation systems (Howanitz and Howanitz, 1984; Yalow, 1978; Ratcliffe, 1974).

Second antibody or double antibody reactions can precipitate substrate that is bound to a first antibody. The first antibody may be exposed to the second after the first antibody reacts with its ligand (postprecipitation method) (Morgan and Lazarow, 1963) or before it reacts with its ligand (preprecipitation method) (Hales and Randle, 1963). These methods depend on the second antibody recognizing antigenic sites on only the first antibody in the system. If the second antibody reacts with compounds or proteins other than the first antibody, the assay does not generate accurate data (Howanitz and Howanitz, 1984). Double antibody systems are frequently used to measure peptide hormones. Because interfering factors often prolong the time for adequate separation of bound from free substrate in this type of assay, incubation times

are often as long as 1 or 2 days (Ratcliffe, 1974). In some double antibody systems, the concentrations of the antibodies used do not favor precipitation. In such cases, ammonium sulfate may produce successful precipitation of the antibody complex and reduce the amount of second antibody necessary for an adequate ligand separation (Ratcliffe, 1974).

In solid-phase systems of separation, antibody is irreversibly bound to some nonsoluble structure of large size. These systems provide an efficient, rapid, and adaptable way to separate free from bound antigen. The problems encountered in these systems relate to the large amount of antibody required to coat the solid phase and to the variation in antibody coating that may occur (Howanitz and Howanitz, 1984). The kinetics of solid-phase systems generally allow more rapid completion than conventional liquid-phase radioimmunoassays (Ratcliffe, 1974).

In radial partition radioimmunoassay, a process in which all of an immunoassay occurs in a solid phase, a known amount of antibody is bound to the solid phase. When this antibody has the unknown sample applied, it binds and immobilizes the antigen. Enzyme-labeled antigen is then applied and occupies the remaining antibody sites where no antigen has been bound previously. Finally, when the solid phase is washed with a solution to activate the label enzyme, unbound enzyme-labeled antigen is washed away, leaving bound non-enzyme-labeled and bound enzyme-labeled antigen to be quantitated (Giegel et al, 1982).

It must be stressed that separation systems are

fraught with many potential problems, and opportunities for the generation of inaccurate data are numerous. Every step of a separation technique must be studied carefully and possible causes for error controlled. One general principle is that the protein concentrations in a system must be constant. Also, systems must produce minimal alteration or damage to the reactants. For example, if a damaged label is adsorbed to precipitated complexes in a double antibody system, the amount of bound label may erroneously appear increased. Conversely, if the antibody binding the label is damaged so that it no longer binds its antigen, the amount of labeled antigen precipitated will decrease, making the amount of unlabeled antigen appear more than it really is (Howanitz and Howanitz, 1984; Ratcliffe, 1974).

STANDARDS, ASSAY DEVELOPMENT, AND VALIDATION

Validation of assays depends on a reliable standard that behaves similarly to the substance being studied in an assay and on control of factors that influence assay reactions. To minimize nonspecific factors, items such as pH, ionic concentration, protein concentration, buffer used, and other influences must remain constant within an assay system (Howanitz and Howanitz, 1984; Yalow, 1978). Some problems may occur over time as a result of spontaneous changes in stored standard, antibody, and testing solutions (Yalow, 1978). Vigilance must be maintained to appreciate when an assay develops inaccuracies in the data it generates (Felber, 1978).

The sensitivity of an assay relates to the minimal amount of antigen that can be measured with acceptable precision (Ekins, 1971, 1974). Sensitivity is a characteristic of the affinity of a binding agent for the substance it is binding. In RIA, maximum sensitivity occurs in an antibody concentration that binds between 20 and 70 percent of a given amount of labeled antigen, in the absence of unlabeled antigen (Howanitz and Howanitz, 1984). Other measures that enhance the sensitivity of an assay include small quantities of label, increased incubation time, and addition of label after unlabeled-antigen antibody reaction in the absence of labeled antigen (nonequilibrium assay) (Chard, 1971). Generally, nonequilibrium assays are more sensitive, but less precise, than equilibrium assays where antibody is incubated simultaneously with labeled and unlabeled antigen (Rodbard et al, 1971).

Efforts have been made to extract and concentrate antigen to increase assay sensitivity; however, attempts to obtain meaningful data from ligand-binding assays at their limits of sensitivity are generally unrewarding (Howanitz and Howanitz, 1984).

Several parameters must be observed for an immunoassay to have validity. First, one must show that added antigen is recovered in and appreciated by the assay. Also, when a sample is diluted, the concentration of ligand in the sample must diminish in a linear fashion, and the dilution curve of the unknown amount of ligand must be the same as that of the ligand standard. Additionally, to be valid, an assay must demonstrate that compounds similar to the ligand being measured are minimally or not at all appreciated by the assay (Yalow, 1985; Howanitz and Howanitz, 1984; Yalow, 1978). As all polyclonal antibodies differ, each antibody to a given substance must be characterized individually. Finally, analysis of samples obtained under varying physiologic circumstances is important to demonstrate an assay's ability to appreciate in vivo increases and decreases in the level of the substance being assayed (Howanitz and Howanitz, 1984). In RIAs, other factors must be included in the overall performance of the assay to ensure accuracy and validity. Two blanks must be used in every assay, one containing only labeled ligand and antibody, the other containing labeled ligand and ligand-free plasma or serum, but no antibody (Howanitz and Howanitz, 1984; Challand et al, 1974). The first blank allows for assessment of ligand reaction with antibody and ability to separate ligand from antibody. The second blank generates information on nonspecific protein binding of labeled ligand. Both factors must be considered in immunoassay characterization (Howanitz and Howanitz, 1984; Challand et al, 1974).

When data obtained from immunoassays are used in the clinical practice of medicine, one must be cognizant that these data relate to immunologic properties of an agent and not necessarily in vivo biologic activity. For example, proinsulin may react significantly with an insulin antibody, and patients with immunologically reactive but biologically inactive thyroid-stimulating hormone (TSH) have been described (Gavin et al, 1975; Faglia et al, 1983). Other examples of disparity in immunologic and biologic activity are presented in the section of this chapter on clinical applications of hormonal assays. Also, naturally occurring antibodies in the sera of patients may produce erroneous imunoassay results by binding with the ligand being assayed or the ligand-specific antibody being used in the assay (Howanitz et al, 1982).

The precision that is achievable in other laboratory chemical assays should not be expected in ligand assays. Variation of intra-assay duplicate samples often exceeds 10 percent, and precision varies at different locations on standard curves, a phenomenon called nonuniformity of variance (Challand et al, 1974; Rodbard and Hutt, 1974).

The graphic descriptions of ligand assay standard curves use many methods of plotting. Some formats tend to display the standard curve in linear form. A common technique available in computerized assay programs is logit-log plotting. The logit of bound labeled ligand (B), divided by the amount of labeled ligand bound in the absence of unlabeled ligand (B_0), is placed on the ordinate, and the log of the concentration of unlabeled ligand is placed on the abscissa (Rodbard and Hutt, 1974). Though this logit-log plotting gives a linear configuration to the standard curve, it does not influence the pre-

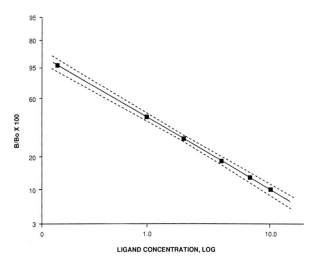

Figure 2–12   Logit-log plotting of an RIA, with same data as in Figure 2–2. Broken lines represent 95 percent confidence limits of the assay.

cision of the assay (Howanitz and Howanitz, 1984; Felber, 1978). In Figure 2–12, the hatched lines on either side of the logit-log plot represent the 95 percent confidence limits of the assay at varying concentrations of ligand (Felber, 1978).

CLINICAL APPLICATIONS OF COMPETITIVE-BINDING LIGAND ASSAYS

Discrepancies in Hormonal Competitive-Binding Ligand Assay

Hormonal ligand assays have greatly increased the understanding of endocrine systems. However, data obtained from ligand-binding assays must be evaluated carefully to avoid incorrect conclusions (Odell and Ross, 1971).

Examples of discrepancy when clinical observations and bioassay data are compared to results obtained in ligand-binding assays are numerous. Confusing factors may include (1) immunologic or binder-active hormones with diminished biologic activity (Faglia et al, 1983), (2) biologically active hormones that, in a given assay, are immunologically or binder nonreactive (Zapf et al, 1978), (3) immunologically related hormones with different biologic functions (Greenwood et al, 1964), (4) hormonal fragments that are immunologically active but biologically inactive (Faglia et al, 1983; Kahn et al, 1977), (5) the influence of medication or other substances that interfere with an assay, such as native antibody against the ligand being assayed or against the binding agent (Morrow, 1983; Kahn et al, 1988), and (6) the influence of disease or an unusual circumstance on hormonal production or clearance (Morrow, 1983; Cohen, 1977; Friedman, 1980; Emmanouel et al, 1980; Schussler et al, 1978). These and other potential problems in the use of ligand

assays will be discussed to convey concepts rather than to give a complete listing of all the assay problems that have been appreciated.

Peptide Hormone Heterogeneity

When a sample of plasma or serum is treated by various separation techniques and then assayed for ligand-binding activity, many polypeptide hormones are found to exist in multiple or heterogeneous forms (Yalow, 1970, 1971, 1973, 1978, 1985; Berson and Yalow, 1968; Silverman and Yalow, 1973).

Insulin has been studied carefully to determine why immunologic potency may not correlate well with insulin receptor binding and biologic potency (Gavin et al, 1975). It has been found that if a significant amount of the insulin prehormone (proinsulin) is found in the plasma, proinsulin is appreciated to a greater degree by RIA than by radioreceptor assay; thus, its immunologic activity exceeds its receptor-binding activity and expressed biologic potency. Consequently, if an appreciable level of proinsulin is present in plasma, it may produce a false elevation in insulin assessed by RIA, and the amount of immunologically detectable insulin will exceed that assessed in biologic assays or using clinical data.

A common assay in evaluating calcium metabolism is that for parathyroid hormone. Immunologic heterogeneity has been observed when parathyroid hormone was quantitated in different assays (Berson and Yalow, 1968). These discrepancies were increased following parathyroidectomy or in uremia (Emmanouel et al, 1980; Berson and Yalow, 1968). When these phenomena were investigated, the reasons for the discrepancies were appreciated. Parathyroid hormone immunologic activity was found to be present in humans, not only for the intact molecule but also for the metabolic products of parathyroid hormone degradation (carboxy or C-terminal fragment and amino or N-terminal fragment). The N-terminal fragment was shown to be metabolized more quickly than the C-terminal fragment, and levels of C-terminal fragment usually exceeded levels of intact parathyroid hormone (Berson and Yalow, 1968; Silverman and Yalow, 1973). Generally, in clinical situations, an assessment of C-terminal activity was useful in monitoring parathyroid gland activity. However, in conditions such as uremia, in which C-terminal fragments of parathyroid hormone accumulate in the blood because of diminished renal clearance, C-terminal parathyroid hormone assays are misleading (Yalow, 1977, 1985). In such a condition, hyperparathyroidism would seem to be present when it was not. By understanding the metabolism of parathyroid and other hormones, the clinician can predict certain instances in which routine hormonal assays will not be helpful. For example, in the case of parathyroid hormone, the clinician could use an assay that measures the level of intact hormone or one that will separate hormonal fragments from intact hormone prior to the determination of the hormone level in patients with renal insufficiency (Hackeng et al, 1986).

Other common assays in which clinical observation may not correlate with biochemical analysis include adrenocorticotropic hormone (ACTH) and gastrin (Yalow, 1985). Neoplasms often produce a very large peptide molecule called big ACTH (Gewirtz and Yalow, 1974). Though this molecule has only about 4 percent of the biologic activity of native ACTH (a 39-amino-acid peptide), it often produces Cushing's syndrome (Gewirtz et al, 1974). If native ACTH is assessed following sample fractionation in such cases, the amount of biologically active ACTH present might be underestimated. Conversely, if ACTH is assayed without separation of different-sized molecules, high levels of ACTH might be found in the absence of any clinical illness. This would be caused by the presence of an increased amount of the immunologically reactive but relatively biologically inactive big ACTH.

In the case of gastrin, though the normally produced hormone is a 34-amino-acid peptide, following feeding there is an increase not only in the 34-amino-acid hormone but also in a 17-amino-acid hormone. It is biologically as active as the 34-amino-acid hormone but has a considerably greater metabolic clearance rate (Yalow, 1985). Consequently, a clinical condition such as a gastrinoma theoretically could exist that would produce the 17-amino-acid hormone, and immunologic reactivity for gastrin might be normal in the presence of hypersecretion of gastrin and gastric acid (Zollinger-Ellison syndrome) (Yalow, 1985).

Immunologically Related Hormones with Different Functions

Many hormones in nature are immunologically related but different in their physiologic function (Yalow, 1985; Greenwood et al, 1964; Pierce, 1971). Understanding that such situations exist is essential for drawing correct conclusions from assay data. Examples of these situations include hormones composed of two subunits, such as the glycoprotein hormones luteinizing hormone (LH), follicle-stimulating hormone (FSH), TSH, and human chorionic gonadotropin (hCG), in which all of the hormone contains the same alpha subunit but different beta subunits. Although these hormones have different beta subunits, there is some degree of homology in these subunits (Vaitukaitis et al, 1972). Consequently, for an assay to be capable of immunologically distinguishing these hormones, it must appreciate areas on the beta subunit that are unique to the hormone in question.

Clinically available assays for LH generally cross-react with hCG in a manner indistinguishable from LH. Consequently, an elevated LH level in a patient with primary or secondary amenorrhea might indicate ovarian failure or pregnancy if hCG is detected in an LH assay. In such

a situation, an elevated level of hCG must be suspected, and an assay specific for the unique portion of the beta subunit of hCG must be used to confirm or eliminate the presence of hCG (Pierce, 1971).

Systems revealing immunologic cross-reactivity but biologically distinct functions include growth hormone–human placental lactogen, gastrin-cholecystokinin, and ACTH–melanocyte-stimulating hormone (Yalow, 1985; Greenwood et al, 1964).

Receptor Ligand Competitive-Binding Assays

Receptor ligand competitive-binding assays help to distinguish immunoreactivity from bioactivity. If an immunologically reactive agent will not bind to its receptor, that agent is unlikely to have bioactivity. However, the fact that an agent binds to a hormonal receptor does not dictate that the agent will have biologic activity per se. When bound to a receptor, an agent has the potential to produce several actions. It may block the receptor and make it more difficult for the native receptor binder to react with the receptor (antagonists). It may stimulate the receptor to produce the same response induced by the native receptor binder (agonist). It may change in the way that other similar receptors on a cell bind similar agents (negative or positive cooperativity). It may produce an agonist effect and then remain receptor bound and produce an antagonist effect (Gorden and Weintraub, 1985).

Using receptor-binding data, the study of compounds in vitro has made possible predictions of their in vivo characteristics. For example, when luteinizing hormone–releasing hormone analogs were studied in vitro, superagonist status was predicted that was confirmed in vivo (Loumaye et al, 1982; Bergquist et al, 1982).

Ligand Competitive-Binding Assay of Steroid Hormones

Ligand competitive-binding and other assays for steroid hormones and their metabolites are fraught with difficulties. Minor alterations in steroid structure may produce vastly different biologic functions in these compounds. Binding agents may detect different steroid compounds with similar sensitivity, unless directed at a site that is unique to that particular steroid. Techniques to maximize the specificity of steroid hormone assays include separation of steroid compounds using their intrinsic chemical properties (e.g., charge, hydrophilic or hydrophobic tendency) prior to analysis (Mikhall et al, 1970).

Another problem is the marked differences in steroid production that may occur on a daily basis (cortisol secretion) (Brandenberger and Follenius, 1973) or on a monthly basis (estrogen, progesterone, and other fluctuations in the normal menstrual cycle) (Ross et al, 1970) or may be related to a given period of life (high levels of adrenal androgen at birth, puberty, and adulthood but low levels in childhood and in the elderly) (Odell and Parker, 1980; Vermeulen, 1980).

Steroid hormones have specific binding proteins that may increase or decrease to reflect other conditions. For example, the glucocorticoid-binding protein, cortisol-binding globulin (CBG), is increased in pregnancy (Rosner, 1986). Thus, cortisol levels may appear to be increased in pregnancy as a result of increased CBG when, in fact, the amount of biologically active or free cortisol is unchanged (Brien, 1980). Additionally, a pregnant individual may have levels of cortisol normal for a nonpregnant individual and actually be cortisol deficient (Jaffe, 1986).

Another steroid hormone–binding protein—sex hormone–binding globulin (SHBG or TeBG) (Anderson, 1974)—can significantly influence the level of steroid hormones that it binds. For example, the majority of testosterone is SHBG bound; thus, in the presence of increased SHBG, testosterone levels may appear to be elevated when the free and biologically active fraction of testosterone is normal or diminished. Conversely, if SHBG is diminished, a normal level of total testosterone might be found in a patient in whom an increased amount of free and biologically active testosterone was producing clinical findings such as hirsutism, acne, and menstrual irregularities (Mathus et al, 1981).

Urinary metabolites of steroid hormones provide insight into many clinical situations. For example, urinary total estrogen measurement was used to monitor ovarian stimulation during ovulation induction with human menopausal gonadotropin until a specific and sensitive assay for serum estradiol was devised (Gemzell, 1969). Urinary free cortisol determination still gives information on cortisol production (Rosner et al, 1963). Urinary assays are no longer used as frequently as previously because they require complete collection over a period of time to generate meaningful data. Creatinine should be analyzed in timed urine collections to assess the adequacy of collection.

Steroid hormone receptor assays have allowed insight into many clinical situations that otherwise would be difficult to elucidate such as cortisol resistance (Chrousos et al, 1983). Digitalis glycosides were known to produce gynecomastia for many years before they were shown to be an agonist at the estrogen receptor level. This relatively unopposed estrogen effect occurs in susceptible individuals taking this medication (Rifka et al, 1976). Also, if there is an absence or a diminished number of androgen receptors or biologically ineffective androgen receptors, such individuals will express varying degrees of relative estrogen excess and/or androgen deficiency such as feminizing of the external genitalia, gynecomastia, and female body habitus, even in the presence of normal or frankly elevated levels of androgen (Griffin and Wilson, 1980). Indeed, clinical syndromes relating to deficien-

cies of steroid receptors for all major groups of steroid hormones have been reported (Armanini et al, 1985).

Ligand Competitive-Binding Assay of Thyroid Hormones

Ligand competitive-binding assay is one of the main tools used in assessing thyroid function. As with steroid hormones, a plasma-binding protein for thyroid hormones was the basis for some of the early thyroid hormone ligand competitive-binding assays (Murphy and Pattee, 1964). As is true for CBG and SHBG, estrogen exposure and liver disease increase hepatic production of thyroxine-binding globulin (Schussler et al, 1978; Malkasian and Mayberry, 1970). Thus, one would expect thyroid hormone levels to increase in pregnancy, during estrogen therapy, and in chronic liver disease (Schussler et al, 1978; Malkasian and Mayberry, 1970). However, the free fraction of thyroxine would remain normal or might even decrease in such instances (Schussler et al, 1978; Malkasian and Mayberry, 1970). As is the case in other hormones in which plasma-binding proteins are present, absolute certainty whether an individual has a normal, high, or low value of a hormone is difficult unless the free fraction of the hormone is assessed.

Abnormalities in thyroid hormone receptors have been reported. Generally, the defect is expressed by development of an enlarged thyroid gland and elevated levels of thyroid hormone in the presence of a normal metabolic state (Menezes-Ferreira et al, 1984).

Numerous hormones not discussed in this chapter (including catecholamines) have been characterized using ligand competitive-binding assays. The principles listed here apply to this large body of data, only a small fraction of which has been mentioned.

During use of the preceding techniques, numerous discrepancies may occur if an attempt is made to correlate data revealed by immunologic, receptor, and biologic assays. These discrepancies generally relate to differences in (1) receptor and immunoglobulin affinity for precursor and product hormone, (2) mixtures of hormones with some similarities but from different DNA sites of origin, and (3) changes that have occurred to the structure of a hormonal peptide following its synthesis (posttranslation modification) (Gorden and Weintraub, 1985).

Autoantibodies and Ligand Competitive-Binding Assays

Assay problems and pathophysiologic states can arise as a result of antibody production to either an antigen (hormone or ligand), the immunoglobulin used to assay an antigen, or the antigen's receptor site.

The first RIA for insulin was possible because recipients of insulin therapy produced polyclonal antibodies to insulin (Yalow and Berson, 1959). Indeed, most individuals who receive nonhuman insulin, and some who receive human insulin, develop insulin antibodies (Fineberg et al, 1983). If an attempt is made to measure insulin levels in a subject having insulin antibodies, misleading data may be obtained because excessive antibody in the reaction mixture binds not only the labeled ligand, but unlabeled ligand as well (Scarlett et al, 1977). Thus, quantitation of bound labeled ligand would give a high value; measurement of free labeled ligand would yield a low value. However, if the separation technique used in an insulin assay is a second antibody directed to nonhuman gamma globulin, a falsely low assessment of antibody-bound labeled ligand would result, since the majority of this labeled ligand would be bound to human gamma globulin. Consequently, the amount of insulin in the sample would be overestimated.

Antibodies induced when peptides are administered in clinical practice generally are not of clinical significance. However, when such antibodies are made to exogenously administered growth hormone, antihormonal antibodies may become clinically significant (Tanner et al, 1971).

Antibodies to hormonal receptor sites can be instigators of clinical illness. These antibodies may bind to the hormonal receptor portion of the receptor and act as an agonist or block the site so that it is no longer available to its hormone ligand, a hormone antagonist (Gorden and Weintraub, 1985). Also, antibodies may react at locations on a receptor other than the hormone-binding site to produce receptor malfunction (Blecher and Bar, 1981).

Antibodies directed at the hormonal binding site of a receptor can be appreciated by competitive ligand assay. However, appreciation of antibodies directed against nonhormonal binding portions of hormonal receptors requires other methods of assessment, such as immunoprecipitation of receptor antibody complexes (Harrison et al, 1979; Kahn et al, 1981). The most common syndromes produced by antireceptor antibodies are those related to the TSH receptor and associated with Graves' disease. In Graves' disease, antibodies that stimulate production of thyroid hormone have been found (Adams and Purves, 1956; Bitensky et al, 1974; McKenzie and Williamson, 1966), and antibodies have been reported that block the ability of TSH to bind to its receptor site, but do not stimulate thyroid hormone formation (a TSH receptor-blocking antibody) (Sugenoya et al, 1979). In general, an assay of these receptor antibodies is not required in the clinical management of immune-mediated thyroid diseases but may be helpful in confirming a diagnosis (Peterson et al, 1975; Endo et al, 1978; Zakarija et al, 1980). Additionally, some data suggest that these assays may be helpful in predicting the activity of Graves' disease (Teng et al, 1980).

As with TSH receptor antibodies, measurement of insulin receptor antibodies is infrequently required in clinical practice. In unusual cases of insulin-resistant hyperglycemia, insulin receptor antibody assay may be helpful in understanding the pathophysiology (Dons et al, 1983). Additionally, insulin receptor antibodies have been implicated in the induction of hypoglycemia (Taylor et al, 1982), in which the anti-insulin receptor antibody is acting as a receptor agonist and mimicking insulin in its activity. In such cases, plasma insulin levels have been found to be normal (Taylor et al, 1982).

BIBLIOGRAPHY

Adams DD, Purves HD. Abnormal response in assay of thyrotropin. Proc Univ Otago Med Sch 1956; 34:11.

Anderson DC. Sex-hormone-binding globulin. Clin Endocrinol (Oxf) 1974; 3:69.

Armanini D, Kuhnle V, Strasser T, et al. Aldosterone-receptor deficiency in pseudohypoaldosteronism. N Engl J Med 1985; 313:1178.

Baker TS, Abbott SR, Daniel SG, Wright JF. Immunoradiometric assays. In: Collins WP, ed. Alternative immunoassays. Chichester, England: John Wiley, 1985:59.

Bergquist C, Nillius SJ, Wide L. Intranasal luteinizing hormone-releasing hormone agonist treatment for inhibition of ovulation in women: clinical aspects. Clin Endocrinol (Oxf) 1982; 17:91.

Berson SA, Yalow RS. Immunochemical heterogeneity of parathyroid hormone in plasma. J Clin Endocrinol Metab 1968; 28:1037.

Binoux MA, Odell WD. Use of dextran-coated charcoal to separate antibody-bound from free hormone: a critique. J Clin Endocrinol Metab 1973; 36:303.

Bitensky L, Alaghband-Zadeh J, Chayen J. Studies on thyroid stimulating hormone and long-acting thyroid stimulating hormone. Clin Endocrinol (Oxf) 1974; 3:363.

Blecher M, Bar RS. Acetylcholine receptors: myasthenia gravis. In: Blecher M, Bar RS, eds. Receptors and human disease. Baltimore: Williams & Wilkins, 1981:237.

Brandenberger G, Follenius M. Day-time variations of plasma cortisol and glucose and of urinary cortisol excretion in normal subjects at rest. J Physiol (Paris) 1973; 66:271.

Brien TG. Free cortisol in human plasma. Horm Metab Res 1980; 12:643.

Challand G, Goldie D, Landon J. Immunoassay in the diagnostic laboratory. Br Med Bull 1974; 30:38.

Chard T. Observations on the uses of a mathematical model in radioimmunoassays. In: Kirkham RE, Hunter WM, eds. Radioimmunoassay methods. Edinburgh: Churchill Livingstone, 1971:595.

Chrousos GP, Vingerhoeds ACM, Loriaux DL, Lipsett MB. Primary cortisol resistance: a family study. J Clin Endocrinol Metab 1983; 56:1243.

Cohen KL. Metabolic, endocrine and drug interference with pituitary function tests: a review. Metabolism 1977; 28:1165.

Dons RF, Harlik R, Taylor SI. Clinical disorders associated with autoantibodies to the insulin receptor. J Clin Invest 1983; 72:1072.

Ekins RP. Basic principles and theory. Br Med Bull 1974; 30:3.

Ekins RP. Mathematical treatment of data. In: Kirkham KE, Hunter WM, eds. Radioimmunoassay methods. Edinburgh: Churchill Livingstone, 1971:607.

Emmanouel DS, Lindbreimer MD, Keitz AI. Pathogenesis of endocrine abnormalities in uremia. Endocr Rev 1980; 1:28.

Endo K, Kasagi K, Konishi J. Detection and properties of TSH-binding inhibitor immunoglobulins in patients with Graves' disease and Hashimoto's thyroiditis. J Clin Endocrinol Metab 1978; 46:734.

Engvall E, Jonsson K, Perlmann P. Enzyme-linked immunosorbent assay. II. Quantitative assay of protein antigen, immunoglobulin G, by means of enzyme-labeled antigen and antibody-coated tubes. Biochim Biophys Acta 1971; 251:427.

Engvall E, Perlmann P. Enzyme-linked immunosorbent assay, ELISA. III. Quantitation of specific antibodies by enzyme-labeled anti-immunoglobulin in antigen-coated tubes. J Immunol 1972; 109:129.

Faglia G, Beck-Peccoz P, Ballabio M, Nava C. Excess of β-subunit of thyrotropin (TSH) in patients with idiopathic central hypothyroidism due to the secretion of TSH with reduced biological activity. J Clin Endocrinol Metab 1983; 56:908.

Felber JP. Radioimmunoassay in the clinical chemistry laboratory. Adv Clin Chem 1978; 20:129.

Fineberg SE, Galloway JA, Fineberg NS, et al. Immunogenicity of recombinant DNA human insulin. Diabetologia 1983; 25:465.

Finlayson JS. Basic biochemical calculations: related procedures and principles. Reading, MA: Addison-Wesley Publishing, 1969:250.

Friedman RB. Effects of disease on clinical laboratory tests. Clin Chem 1980; 26:1D.

Gavin JR III, Kahn CR, Gorden P. Radioreceptor assay of insulin: comparison of plasma and pancreatic insulins and proinsulins. J Clin Endocrinol Metab 1975; 41:438.

Gemzell C. Treatment of female and male sterility with human gonadotropins. Acta Obstet Gynecol Scand 1969; 48 (Suppl 1):17.

Gewirtz G, Schneider B, Krieger DT. Big ACTH: conversion to biologically active ACTH by trypsin. J Clin Endocrinol Metab 1974; 38:227.

Gewirtz G, Yalow RS. Ectopic ACTH production in carcinoma of the lung. J Clin Invest 1974; 53:1022.

Giegel JL, Brotherton MM, Cronin P, et al. Radial partition immunoassay. Clin Chem 1982; 28:1894.

Gorden P, Weintraub BD. Radioreceptor and other functional hormone assays. In: Wilson JD, Foster DW, eds. Williams textbook of endocrinology. 7th ed. Philadelphia: WB Saunders, 1985:133.

Greenwood FC, Hunter WM, Klopper A. Assay of human growth hormone in pregnancy, at parturition and in lactation: detection of a growth-hormone-like substance from the placenta. Br Med J 1964; 1:22.

Griffin JE, Wilson JD. The syndromes of androgen resistance. N Engl J Med 1980; 302:198.

Hackeng WHL, Lips P, Netelenbos JC, Lips CJM. Clinical implications of estimation of intact parathyroid hormone (PTH) versus total PTH in normal subjects and hyperparathyroid patients. J Clin Endocrinol Metab 1986; 63:447.

Hales CN, Randle PJ. Immunoassay of insulin with insulin-antibody precipitate. Biochem J 1963; 88:137.

Harrison LC, Flier JS, Itin A. Radioimmunoassay of insulin receptor: a new probe of receptor structure and function. Science 1979; 203:544.

Howanitz JH, Howanitz PJ. Immunoassay and related techniques; tumor markers. In: Henry JB, ed. Clinical diagnosis and management by laboratory methods. 17th ed. Philadelphia: WB Saunders, 1984:283.

Howanitz PJ, Howanitz JH, Lamberson HV, Ennis KM. Incidence and mechanism of spurious increases in serum thyrotropin. Clin Chem 1982; 28:427.

Hunter WM. Preparation and assessment of radioactive tracers. Br Med Bull 1974; 30:18.

Jaffe RB. Integrative maternal-fetal endocrine control systems. In: Yen SSC, Jaffe RB, eds. Reproductive endocrinology. 2nd ed. Philadelphia: WB Saunders, 1986:770.

Kahn CR, Baird KL, Flier JS. Insulin receptors, receptor antibodies, and the mechanism of insulin action. Recent Prog Horm Res 1981; 37:477.

Kahn CR, Rosen SW, Weintraub BD, et al. Ectopic production of chorionic gonadotropin and its subunits by islet-cell tumors. N Engl J Med 1977; 297:565.

Kahn BB, Weintraub BD, Csako G, Zweig MH. Factitious elevation of thyrotropin in a new ultrasensitive assay: implications for the use of monoclonal antibodies in "sandwich" immunoassay. J Clin Endocrinol Metab 1988; 66:526.

Landon J. The radioimmunoassay of drugs. Analyst 1976; 101:225.

Loumaye E, Naor Z, Catt KU. Binding affinity and biological activity of gonadotropin-releasing hormone agonsits in isolated pituitary cells. Endocrinology 1982; 111:730.

Malkasian GD, Mayberry WE. Serum total and free thyroxine and thyrotropin in normal and pregnant women, neonates, and women receiving progestogens. Am J Obstet Gynecol 1970; 108:1234.

Mathus RS, Moody LO, Landgrebe S, Williamson, HO. Plasma androgens and sex hormone–binding globulin in the evaluation of hirsute females. Fertil Steril 1981; 35:29.

McKenzie JM, Williamson A. Experience with the bioassay of the long-acting thyroid stimulator. J Clin Endocrinol Metab 1966; 26:518.

Menezes-Ferreira MM, Wortsman J, Weintraub BD. Decreased nuclear uptake of [^{125}I] triiodo-L-thyronine in fibroblasts from patients with peripheral thyroid hormone resistance. J Clin Endocrinol Metab 1984; 59:1081.

Midgley AR, Niswender GD. Radioimmunoassay of steroids. In: Diczfalusy E, ed. Steroid assay by protein binding. Stockholm: Karolinska sjukhuset, 1970:320.

Mikhall G, Chung H-W, Ferin M, Vande Wielc RL. Radioimmunoassay of plasma estrogens: use of polymerized antibodies. In: Péron FG, Caldwell BV, eds. Immunologic methods in steroid determination. New York: Appleton-Century-Crofts, 1970:113.

Morgan CR, Lazarow A. Immunoassay of insulin: two antibody system-plasma insulin levels of normal, subdiabetic and diabetic rats. Diabetes 1963: 12:115.

Morrow LB. Interference in endocrine testing. In: Streck WF, Lockwood DH, eds. Endocrine diagnosis: clinical and laboratory approach. Boston: Little, Brown, 1983:297.

Murphy BEP. Methodological problems in competitive protein-binding techniques; the use of sephadex column chromatography to separate steroids. Stockholm: Karolinska sjukhuset, 1970:37.

Murphy BEP, Pattee CJ. Determination of thyroxine utilizing the property of protein-binding. J Clin Endocrinol Metab 1964; 24:187.

Odell W, Parker L. Control of adrenal androgen secretion. In:Genazzani AR, Thijssen JHH, Siiteri PK, eds. Adrenal androgens. New York: Raven Press, 1980:27.

Odell WD, Ross GT. Correlation of bioassay and immunoassay potencies for FSH, LH, TSH and HCG. In: Odell WD, Daughaday WH, eds. Principles of competitive protein binding assays. Philadelphia: JB Lippincott, 1971:401.

Peterson VB, Smith BR, Hall RA. A study of thyroid stimulating activity in human serum with the highly sensitive cytochemical bioassay. J Clin Endocrinol Metab 1975; 96:199.

Pierce JG. The Lilly lecture: the subunits of pituitary thyrotropin—their relationship to other glycoprotein hormones. Endocrinology 1971; 89:1331.

Ratcliffe JG. Separation techniques in saturation analysis. Br Med Bull 1974; 30:32.

Rifka SM, Pita JC Jr, Loriaux DL. Mechanism of interaction of digitalis with estradiol binding sites in rat uteri. Endocrinology 1976; 99:1091.

Rodbard D, Bridson W, Rayford PL. Rapid calculation of radioimmunoassay results. J Lab Clin Med 1969; 74:770.

Rodbard D, Hutt DM. Statistical analysis of radioimmunoassays and immunoradiometric (labelled antibody) assays. A generalized weighted, iterative, least-squares method for logistic curve fitting. In: Radioimmunoassay and related procedures in medicine. Vienna: International Atomic Energy Agency (Proc Symp Istanbul 1973) 1974:165.

Rodbard D, Rayford PL, Cooper JA, Ross GT. Statistical quality control of radioimmunoassays. J Clin Endocrinol 1968; 28:1412.

Rodbard D, Ruder JH, Vaitukaitis J, Jacobs HS. Mathematical analysis of kinetics of radioligand assays: improved sensitivity obtained by delayed addition of labeled ligand. J Clin Endocrinol Metab 1971; 33:343.

Rosner W. The endocrinology of human plasma steroid-binding proteins. Am Assoc Clin Chem Endo 1986; 4:1.

Rosner JM, Cos JJ, Biglieri EG, et al. Determination of urinary unconjugated cortisol by glass fiber chromatography in the diagnosis of Cushing's syndrome. J Clin Endocrinol Metab 1963; 23:820.

Ross GT, Cargille CM, Lipsett MB, et al. Pituitary and gonadal hormones in women during spontaneous and induced ovulatory cycles. Recent Prog Horm Res 1970; 26:1.

Rowley GL, Rubenstein KE, Huisjen J, Ullman EF. Mechanism by which antibodies inhibit hapten-malate dehydrogenase conjugates. J Biol Chem 1975; 250:3759.

Rubenstein KE, Schneider RS, Ullman EF. "Homogenous" enzyme immunoassay. A new immunochemical technique. Biochem Biophys Res Commun 1972; 47:846.

Scarlett JA, Mako ME, Rubenstein AH, et al. Factitious hypoglycemia-diagnosis by measurement of serum C-peptide immunoreactivity and insulin-binding antibodies. N Engl J Med 1977; 297:1029.

Schall RF, Tenoso JH. Alternatives to radioimmunoassay: labels and methods. Clin Chem 1981; 27:1157.

Schussler GC, Schaffner F, Newmark SR. Increased serum thyroid hormone binding and decreased free hormone in chronic active liver disease. N Engl J Med 1978; 299:510.

Sevier ED, David GS, Martinis J, et al. Monoclonal antibodies in clinical immunology. Clin Chem 1981; 27:1797.

Silverman R, Yalow RS. Heterogeneity of parathyroid hormone: clinical and physiological implications. J Clin Invest 1973; 52:1958.

Soini E, Hemmilä I. Fluoroimmunoassay: present status and key problems. Clin Chem 1979; 25:356–361.

Sugenoya A, Kidd A, Row VV. Correlation between thyrotropin displacing activity and human thyroid-stimulating activity by immunoglobulins from patients with Graves' disease and other thyroid disorders. J Clin Endocrinol Metab 1979; 48:398.

Tanner JM, Whitehouse RH, Hughes PCR, Vince FP. Effect of human growth hormone treatment for 1 to 7 years on growth of 100 children with growth hormone deficiency, low birth weight, inherited smallness, Turner's syndrome, and other complaints. Arch Dis Child 1971; 46:745.

Taylor SI, Grunberger G, Marcus-Samuels B. Hypoglycemia associated with antibodies to the insulin receptor. N Engl J Med 1982; 307:1422.

Teng CS, Tong TC, Hutchison JH. Thyroid stimulating immunoglobulins in neonatal Graves' disease. Arch Dis Child 1980; 55:894.

Thompson SG. Competitive-binding assays. In: Kaplan LA, Pesce AJ, eds. Clinical chemistry. St. Louis: CV Mosby, 1984:211.

U.S. Department of Health, Education and Welfare. Radiological health handbook. Rockville, MD: U.S. Department of Health Education and Welfare, 1970:231, 297.

Vaitukaitis JL, Braunstein GD, Ross GT. A radioimmunoassay which specifically measures human chorionic gonadotropin in the presence of human luteinizing hormone. Am J Obstet Gynecol 1972; 113:751.

Vermeulen A. Adrenal androgens and aging. In: Genazzani AR, Thijssen JHH, Siiteri PK, eds. Adrenal androgens. New York: Raven Press, 1980:207.

Wisdom GB. Enzyme immunoassay. Clin Chem 1976; 22:1243.

Woodhead JS, Addison GM, Hales CN. The immunoradiometric assay and related techniques. Br Med Bull 1974; 30:44.

Yalow RS. Heterogeneity of peptide hormones. Its relevance in clinical radioimmunoassay. Adv Clin Chem 1978; 20:1.

Yalow RS. Radioimmunoassay methodology: application to problems of heterogeneity of peptide hormones. In: Cotten M deV, ed. New York Heart Association Symposium on Immunopharmacology. Baltimore: Williams & Wilkins, 1973:161.

Yalow RS. Radioimmunoassays of hormones. In: Wilson JD, Foster DW, eds. Williams textbook of endocrinology. 7th ed. Philadelphia: WB Saunders, 1985:123.

Yalow RS. Significance of heterogeneity of parathyroid hormone. In: Copp DH, Talmage RV, eds. Endocrinology of calcium metabolism. Excerpta Medica International Congress Series No. 421; 1977:308.

Yalow RS, Berson SA. Assay of plasma insulin in human subjects by immunological methods. Nature 1959; 184:1648.

Yalow RS, Berson SA. Further studies on the nature of immunoreactive gastrin in human plasma. Gastroenterology 1971; 60:203.

Yalow RS, Berson SA. Size and charge distinctions between endogenous human plasma gastrin in peripheral blood and heptadecapeptide gastrins. Gastroenterology 1970; 58:609.

Zakarija M, McKenzie JM, Banovac K. Clinical significance of assay of thyroid-stimulating antibody in Graves' disease. Ann Intern Med 1980; 93:28.

Zapf J, Rinderknecht E, Humbel RE. Nonsuppressible insulin-like activity (NSILA) from human serum: recent accomplishments and their physiologic implications. Metabolism 1978; 27:1803.

3

Acromegaly, Hyperprolactinemia, Gonadotropin-Secreting Tumors, and Hypopituitarism

Richard C. Eastman, M.D., F.A.C.P.
Manuel Sainz de la Peña, M.D.
W. Tabb Moore, M.D.
En-hui Hao, M.D.
George R. Merriam, M.D.

In the last two decades many scientific advances have led to a fuller understanding of hypothalamic and pituitary function. These advances have included the identification and sequencing of growth hormone releasing hormone (GH-RH), somatostatin, and the insulin-like growth factors IGF-I (somatomedin-C) and IGF-II. An outgrowth of these advances is that assays for IGF-I are available to the clinician, and GH-RH and somatostatin analogues have become available for diagnostic testing and for therapy. This section discusses the evaluation of acromegaly from the point of view of the traditional approach to diagnosis, and incorporates the new tests now and soon to be available to the clinician.

GROWTH HORMONE PHYSIOLOGY

The radioimmunoassay for growth hormone (GH) was described in 1962, shortly after the development of the insulin assay in the laboratory of Berson and Yalow. GH assays have changed little since that time, and reliable assays are available through many commercial laboratories (Table 3–1). The radioimmunoassay for GH and newer assays for IGF-I (somatomedin-C) are the measures used by the clinician for diagnosis and follow-up of acromegaly. Bioassays and radioreceptor assays of GH are used for research studies.

In normal man, GH is secreted episodically, with three to eight major secretory bursts occurring daily during the growth years, and a subsequent progressive decline in frequency through adult life. Most GH is secreted at night, in association with stage-4 (slow-wave) sleep. Other GH pulses follow meals or exercise or occur spontane-

ously. Females secrete greater amounts than males, probably because of the effects of estrogen, which sensitizes the hypothalamus to diverse stimuli of GH secretion. GH is normally suppressed during the first 2 hours postprandially, and then increases during the subsequent 3 to 5 hours. It is also increased by exercise, acute hypoglycemia, and chronic (3 to 5 days) fasting. Glucose suppresses GH secretion under these circumstances. After major surgery or other severe stress, and after administration of pyrogens or amino acids, GH is also increased but is not suppressible by glucose. Secretion of GH is also stimulated by the administration of dopaminergic agents (L-dopa, bromocriptine), glucagon, alpha-adrenergic agonists, and GH-RH. GH is reduced in obesity and by the administration of somatostatin.

The final common pathway through which diverse inputs to the central nervous system affect GH secretion is through regulation of GH-RH and somatostatin secre-

TABLE 3–1 Growth Hormone Assay

Methods	Radioimmunoassay Radioreceptor assay Bioassay
Normal range	Fasting basal < 5 ng/ml
Uses	Diagnosing acromegaly Evaluating treatment of acromegaly Evaluating anterior pituitary function
Problems	Acromegaly with values in the normal range Basal concentrations are impractical to obtain on outpatients and may be increased by stress or minimal exertion, especially in females

tion by neurosecretory cells in the hypothalamus. Of the two factors, stimulation by GH-RH is dominant, and stalk section leads to markedly reduced GH secretion. This distinguishes GH secretion from that of prolactin, which is under tonic inhibition. GH-RH is a 44-amino-acid peptide present in extracts of the pituitary and hypothalamus, as well as in the pancreas and other tissues. It stimulates GH release and synthesis through adenylate cyclase in a dose-dependent fashion. Maximal responses in humans occur at an administered dose of 1 μg per kilogram of body weight. At this dosage the response is unaffected by age, sex, or hormonal status. GH-RH–stimulated growth hormone release is acutely suppressible by glucose, suggesting that glucose stimulates somatostatin. Other factors that affect the GH response to GH-RH are shown in Table 3–2.

Stimulation of growth hormone secretion by GH-RH is balanced by suppression of secretion by somatostatin. Somatostatin is a 14-amino-acid peptide that is present in the hypothalamus as well as in many peripheral tissues. The physiologic pattern of GH secretion probably reflects variations in the secretion of both hypothalamic GH-RH and somatostatin; stimulation of GH secretion is mediated by a brisk increase in GH-RH and a lesser decrease in somatostatin, and suppression is mediated by reciprocal changes in these peptides.

GH circulates in plasma primarily in the unbound state. Although binding to plasma proteins has been demonstrated recently, the biological significance of this is uncertain. A major portion of the binding appears to be to soluble fragments of the GH receptor. There is considerable heterogeneity in the circulating forms of GH. The principal species in circulation is a 22,000 molecular weight (MW) peptide with 191 amino acids. A 20,000 MW variant that lacks residues 32 to 46 is also present. It is cleared more slowly than the 22,000 MW variant, and has decreased lipolytic and insulin-like activity. Higher molecular weight forms consisting of dimers and oligomers are also present and are largely biologically inactive.

Until recently GH was thought to have no direct effects on growth. It was widely held that GH stimulated production of IGFs by the liver and by other tissues, and that circulating IGFs mediated the growth effects. This is now known to be only partly true. In vitro GH stimulates local production of IGF-I in target tissues; these affect growth processes by autocrine or paracrine mechanisms.

IGF-I (somatomedin-C) is the principal somatomedin through which GH action is expressed. IGF-I is a basic peptide with 70 amino acid residues and a molecular weight of 7,649 daltons. Secretion of IGF-I is GH dependent: The concentration is decreased in hypopituitarism, rises with GH treatment, and is increased in acromegaly. The hormone shows a high degree of homology with proinsulin and with IGF-II.

IGF-II is a weakly acidic peptide with 67 amino acid residues and a molecular weight of 7,471 daltons. Its

TABLE 3–2   Factors Affecting the Growth Hormone Response to Growth Hormone Releasing Hormone

Decreased response
  Obesity
  Hypothyroidism
  Acute hyperglycemia
  IGF-I and IGF-II
  Estrogens
  Somatostatin
  Fatty acids
  Acute glucose load

Increased response
  Suppression of somatostatin
    Beta-adrenergic antagonists (propranolol,
      atenolol, metoprolol)
    Dopaminergic agonists (L-dopa, bromocriptine)
    Cholinergic agents (pyridostigmine)
    Hypoglycemia

secretion is only partially GH dependent, being decreased in GH deficiency and normal in patients with acromegaly. The principal clinical importance of IGF-II is in patients with hypoglycemia associated with non-islet-cell neoplasms. The role of IGF-II in normal growth and development has not been determined.

The insulin-like growth factors circulate in blood bound to carrier proteins. A major species that binds about 70 percent of the circulating IGF has a molecular weight of 150,000 daltons. The secretion of this protein is GH dependent, being decreased in GH deficiency and increased in acromegaly. A minor species of binding protein with a molecular weight of 50,000 binds about 25 percent of the circulating IGFs. The unbound or free IGF is believed to be the biologically active moiety, but this has not been fully established.

ACROMEGALY

Clinical Features

Acromegaly is the clinical syndrome caused by excess GH secretion. Although less common than prolactinoma, acromegaly occurs with a frequency similar to that of Cushing's syndrome. GH hypersecretion occurring in childhood causes an increase in linear growth and tall stature in the syndrome of gigantism. Most patients with GH-secreting pituitary adenomas, however, develop the syndrome as adults, when fusion of the epiphyses precludes further linear growth, and the bone changes then are most prominent in bones without epiphyses (such as the facial bones) and in the form of lateral growth at the ends of long bones. In addition, changes occur in cartilage and soft tissues.

Patients with acromegaly manifest characteristic enlargement of the distal extremities and coarsening of the facial features, fatigue, increased sweating, headache, nerve compression syndromes, cardiac disease, and osteoarthropathy. Hypertrophy of many internal organs can be detected by sensitive methods and may be associated with hyperfunction (Table 3–3). Impaired glucose tolerance or frank diabetes mellitus, insulin resistance, and phosphate retention are biochemical features of the disease. Most patients have evidence of a pituitary macroadenoma, and the mass effects of large tumors may dominate the clinical presentation. Hyperprolactinemia is the most common abnormality of the other pituitary hormones in acromegaly, occurring in 30 to 40 percent of patients. Only a small number of patients show evidence of panhypopituitarism at the time of presentation.

Classification of Growth Hormone Excess

GH levels are elevated in diverse conditions, only some of which are associated with acromegaly (Table 3–4). Patients with uncontrolled diabetes, illness, malnutrition, and severe stress all have increased concentrations of GH. Excessive growth is not present in these conditions, and the concentrations of IGF-I are typically low. It has been suggested that reduced production of IGF-I may stimulate an increase in GH in these individuals by release of negative feedback. The overwhelming majority (probably more than 99 percent) of acromegalic persons have a GH-producing pituitary adenoma. Hypersecretion of GH-RH by gangliocytomas of the hypothalamus or pituitary, or by carcinoids, pancreatic adenomas, or other neoplasms, are rare causes of acromegaly. Ectopic secretion of GH itself by pulmonary neoplasms has been reported but is exceedingly rare. With the increasing availability of biosynthetic GH, the use of exogenous GH

TABLE 3–4   Etiologic Classification of Growth Hormone Excess

Growth Increased (acromegaly and gigantism)
  Pituitary adenoma secreting GH
  Ectopic GH secretion (rare)
  GH-RH mediated
    Gangliocytoma
    Ectopic GH-RH
  Exogenous GH
  Exogenous releasing substances
    Amino acids
    GH-RH
  Polyostotic fibrous dysplasia
Growth Not Increased
  Uncontrolled diabetes
  Malnutrition
    Anorexia nervosa
  Severe stress
  GH resistance

and large amounts of amino acid supplements may potentially lead to some cases of acromegaly, although this has not yet been documented. There appears to be an increased prevalence of acromegaly in patients with polyostotic fibrous dysplasia.

Growth Hormone Secretion in Acromegaly

Secretion of GH in acromegaly is characterized by abnormal responses to a wide variety of stimuli. Typically, basal GH concentrations are continuously elevated, whereas in normal persons GH falls to low values and

TABLE 3–3   Ancillary Tests Used in Evaluating Acromegaly

Test	Reported Findings
Metabolic tests	
Glucose tolerance	Normal, impaired, diabetes mellitus
Insulin tolerance	Insulin resistance
Serum phosphate	Increased (except in parathyroid hyperplasia)
Creatinine clearance	Increased
Urine calcium	Increased
BSP clearance	Increased
Cardiac function	
Electrocardiography	Arrhythmias, conduction disturbances, left ventricular hypertrophy, arteriosclerotic heart disease
Echocardiography	Concentric left ventricular hypertrophy Asymmetric septal hypertrophy
Pulmonary function	Increased lung volume Upper airway obstruction
Salivary gland function	Increased size Normal sialography Normal scintigraphy
Pituitary function	Anterior pituitary hormone deficiency Hypogonadism frequent; ACTH, TSH deficiency rare Hyperprolactinemia
Visual fields	Any defect possible
Pituitary imaging	Normal, microadenoma, macroadenoma

is undetectable at many times during the day. This profile of continuously measurable GH secretion can lead to acromegaly even if peak GH levels are not elevated. Some patients demonstrate highly variable GH secretion, making it impossible to establish an accurate baseline value from single or even several samples drawn during the day. In individual patients the diurnal profiles may be surprisingly reproducible.

Although most GH-secreting adenomas are relatively well differentiated and remain responsive to many normal stimuli and inhibitors, they are less completely suppressed than normal somatotrophs and continue to secrete GH even in the absence of external stimuli. Failure of GH to suppress normally after ingestion of glucose is typical of acromegaly. In some cases the GH may paradoxically increase after meals. Abnormal responses to a variety of other stimuli are observed. GH may be stimulated by thyrotropin-releasing hormone (TRH) or luteinizing hormone releasing hormone (LH-RH), responses which are not usually observed in normal persons. Dopaminergic agents that stimulate GH secretion in normal subjects often lead to suppression in acromegalic patients. Finally, the responses to GH-RH and somatostatin are variable. Most acromegalics with pituitary adenomas respond to GH-RH, although the response may be blunted in patients who have previously received pituitary irradiation. Somatostatin acutely suppresses GH secretion in most but not all cases. The abnormal secretory responses to various stimuli form the basis for several tests that are used for diagnosis and follow-up after treatment (Table 3–5).

Diagnosis

The diagnosis of acromegaly is based on abnormal laboratory studies in conjunction with a positive history or abnormal physical examination. A history of soft tissue growth (even if the physical findings are equivocal) or clear-cut evidence of soft tissue changes (even if the history of progression cannot be established) is required (Table 3–6). The following tests are most commonly used for biochemical confirmation of the diagnosis.

Basal Growth Hormone

The majority of patients with acromegaly have GH concentrations greater than 5 ng per milliliter on fasting basal samples drawn with the patient at bedrest, before morning ambulation (see Table 3–1). However, minimal exercise, especially in females, may elevate the GH level significantly in normal subjects. As a result, no single elevated GH value can confirm the diagnosis of acromegaly unless it is above the maximum of a normal peak of secretion (greater than 150 ng per milliliter); nor does a value of less than 5 ng per milliliter exclude mild acromegaly. After repeated measurement or extended series of samples, however, normal persons frequently also show low values below the detection limit (0.5 to 1.0 ng

TABLE 3–5   Tests for Evaluating Growth Hormone Excess

Basal GH
Oral glucose tolerance test
IGF-I/somatomedin-C plasma levels
Stimulation tests
  TRH
  GH-RH
GH-RH assay

per milliliter) of most clinical assays between secretory peaks, whereas values in acromegalics remain continuously detectable and may or may not fluctuate. Since extended frequent sampling can be difficult in an outpatient setting, in most clinical settings an abnormal glucose suppression test and elevated IGF-I (somatomedin-C) concentration are simpler chemical indicators of disease to obtain.

Glucose Suppression Test

The glucose suppression test (Table 3–7) is practical to perform and reliable on an outpatient basis in all but the severely ill or stressed. In normal persons GH falls to less than 2 ng per milliliter 1 or 2 hours after administration of glucose. Values greater than 5 ng per milliliter are consistent with acromegaly, provided that clinical features of the disease are present (see Table 3–6). However, some patients with acromegaly do have values that suppress to below 5 ng per milliliter after glucose administration, and other tests are required to confirm the diagnosis if one's clinical index of suspicion remains high.

IGF-I (Somatomedin-C)

Assays for IGF-I are available through several commercial laboratories, and are internally reliable if care is taken in drawing and handling the samples (Table 3–8). There are, however, significant differences between standards and normal ranges in different laboratories. Outside the normal range the concentration correlates roughly with the integrated concentration of GH during 24-hour sampling, and also with other clinical and biochemical parameters of disease activity. Values are elevated in virtually all patients with active disease, including the majority of patients with mild acromegaly and GH values less than 10 ng per milliliter basally or below 5 ng per milliliter after glucose administration. A normal IGF-I concentration in a patient with clinical features of acromegaly should suggest deficiency in the binding proteins for IGF, spontaneous infarction of the GH-secreting tumor, effective treatment of the disease, or acromegaloidism (see later).

The test is not without pitfalls, however. Assays of unextracted sera are subject to false readings if the samples are not collected properly. Plasma should be sepa-

TABLE 3-6 Diagnostic Criteria for Acromegaly

	False Positives	False Negatives
I. Clinical criteria		
A. History of progressive acral enlargement	Acral enlargement due to obesity, pulmonary osteoarthropathy	
or		Mild acromegaly
B. Physical findings of acromegaly	Familial or racial acromegalic features, heavy manual labor, normal aging	
II. Laboratory criteria		
A. Fasting, basal GH > 10 ng/ml	Exercise; ambulation, especially in estrogenized females, stress, surgery, hypoglycemia	
and		Mild acromegaly Pituitary infarction Prior therapy
B. GH > 5 ng/ml, 2 hr after a 100 g oral glucose load	Stress, surgery	

1. If 1A or 1B is present and 2A plus 2B are present (and if false-positive elevations of GH have been excluded), the diagnosis is acromegaly.

2. If 1A or 1B is present, but fasting GH is < 5 ng/ml, the diagnosis is in doubt. Other supportive evidence of acromegaly such as elevated IGF-I/somatomedin-C levels or response to TRH stimulation should be sought.

3. If 1A or 1B is present, but fasting GH is 5 to 10 ng/ml on multiple occasions, and if the IGF-I/somatomedin-C concentration is elevated, the diagnosis is acromegaly.

4. If 1A or 1B is absent, the diagnosis is doubtful irrespective of the plasma GH values.

rated from cells within 20 minutes of sample collection. Degradation of IGF activity may occur in patients with low levels of binding proteins. Addition of trypsin inhibitor to sample collection tubes, immediate separation from cells in the cold, and storage at −70°C may prevent degradation in such instances. Other factors that may affect IGF-I determinations are shown in Table 3–9.

TRH-Stimulated Growth Hormone Secretion

Approximately 80 percent of patients with acromegaly show GH responses to TRH (Table 3–10). Responses occur in patients with pituitary adenomas as well as in patients with ectopic GH-RH, but are uncommon (less than 10 percent) in normal persons. This test may be useful in documenting abnormal GH secretory dynamics in patients with equivocal values for GH or

TABLE 3-7 Glucose Suppression Test

Method	GH radioimmunoassay after oral glucose
Normal	GH < 2 ng/ml 2 hr after oral glucose load
Acromegaly	GH > 5 ng/ml 2 hr after oral glucose load
Procedure	A 100-g oral glucose load is given, and GH determined at baseline, 1, and 2 hr
Uses	Diagnosis of acromegaly Evaluating patients after treatment of acromegaly
Limitations	Lack of suppression in the chronically ill and after surgery Acromegaly with GH values < 5 ng/ml after glucose

TABLE 3-8 IGF-I/Somatomedin-C

Methods	Radioimmunoassays of extracted or unextracted plasma Competitive protein binding assays Radioreceptor assays Bioassays
Normal	0.5–2.5 U/ml in healthy adults 50–250 ng/ml Normal range highly age dependent Increases with puberty, decreases with age, menopause
Uses	Diagnosis of acromegaly and GH deficiency
Limitations	False-positive elevations may occur if the plasma is not collected in EDTA and separated soon after drawing False-negative values due to degradation of activity if samples are not properly handled during storage and transport Results affected by changes in binding proteins, which are increased during anabolic processes and decreased during catabolic processes Assays using monoclonal antibodies against synthetic fragments of IGF-I lack sensitivity at the low end

TABLE 3-9   Factors Affecting IGF-I/Somatomedin-C Measurements

Factor	Reported Change
Age/Sex	Values at different ages: Birth — 0.4 U/ml Puberty — Boys 2.2 U/ml Girls 2.6 U/ml Ages 18–20 — 1.3 U/ml Seventh decade — 0.7 U/ml
Nutritional status	Decreased by fasting
Thyroid status	Decreased in hypothyroidism
Pregnancy	Increased progressively
Prolactin	Increased by hyperprolactinemia in hypopituitary patients
Renal failure	Increased affinity of binding proteins
Estrogen	Increased by physiologic amounts of estrogen

Since the half-life is long, concentrations change slowly. Time of day, relationship to meals, testosterone, and pharmacologic doses of glucocorticoids have little or no effect.

IGF-I. The TRH test is useful for determining whether residual neoplasm is present after surgery in some cases. Stimulation of GH by TRH is consistent with the presence of residual neoplasm. Since response to TRH may occur in patients with ectopic GH-RH secretion, this test does not reliably distinguish patients with ectopic GH-RH secretion from patients with pituitary adenomas. Also, the response to TRH may persist for several weeks after removal of the nonpituitary neoplasm in patients with ectopic GH-RH.

Patients who respond to TRH are more likely to show acute suppression of GH by bromocriptine. Neither acute response, however, appears to predict accurately which patients will respond to long-term bromocriptine treatment.

GH-RH Assay and GH-RH Stimulation Test

Although rare, "ectopic" secretion of GH-RH may present as classic acromegaly and be impossible to distinguish from GH secretion by a pituitary adenoma on

TABLE 3-10   TRH Stimulation Test for Growth Hormone

Method	GH radioimmunoassay after administration of TRH
Normal	No response
Procedure	Serial GH samples are obtained at intervals of 15 minutes for 1 hour after administration of an intravenous bolus of TRH (500 μg)
Uses	Diagnosis and follow-up of treatment of acromegaly
Limitations	Hypotensive/hypertensive reactions to TRH Failure of some acromegalic patients to respond

the basis of clinical criteria, tests for GH secretion mentioned previously, or pituitary imaging, since GH-RH excess may cause pituitary hyperplasia (Table 3–11). Short of a costly and potentially invasive search for an extrapituitary neoplasm, the most direct way to confirm ectopic GH-RH secretion is to measure the peripheral level of GH-RH (Table 3–12). This assay is available through a small number of commercial and academic endocrine laboratories. Whether it is necesary to measure GH-RH in every patient with acromegaly in order to rule out ectopic GH-RH has not been firmly established. Several surveys have shown that perhaps only 1 in 200 patients with acromegaly has ectopic GH-RH. However, the diagnosis of ectopic GH-RH should be considered in patients with normal pituitary imaging and in patients with evidence of extrapituitary neoplasm such as Zollinger-Ellison or carcinoid syndrome. Since therapy directed at the pituitary is expensive, inappropriate, and usually unsuccessful in patients with ectopic GH-RH syndrome, we believe that the modest extra cost of a GH-RH measurement is probably justified in the work-up of a patient with newly diagnosed acromegaly. The level of GH-RH in normal persons is less than 1 ng per milliliter in peripheral blood using conventional assay techniques. Patients with ectopic GH-RH secretion have had values greater than 1 ng per milliliter in all cases reported to date.

The role of the GH response to GH-RH in evaluating patients with acromegaly is unclear at this time. On the basis of studies in a very small number of patients, it appears that patients with ectopic GH-RH syndrome usually do not respond to exogenous GH-RH, whereas most pituitary adenomas seem to respond. This seems intuitively reasonable, since there are already high levels of GH-RH in circulation in these patients. However, exceptions have been reported, and the value of the GH-RH stimulation test for distinguishing ectopic GH-RH from pituitary adenoma requires further validation.

TABLE 3–11   Differentiation of Acromegaly Due to Pituitary Adenoma from Ectopic Growth Hormone Releasing Hormone

	Pituitary Adenoma	Ectopic GH-RH
Clinical features	Typical acromegaly	Typical acromegaly
GH	Increased	Increased
IGF-I/somatomedin-C	Increased	Increased
Glucose load	No suppression or increase	No suppression or increase
TRH stimulation	Increase or no response	Increase or no response
Bromocriptine	Suppression or no response	Suppression or no response
Pituitary size	Normal or increased	Normal or increased
GH-RH assay	< <1 ng/ml	≥1 ng/ml
Pituitary histology	Adenoma	Hyperplasia

Acromegaly With Normal Growth Hormone

Occasionally patients have symptoms or physical findings suggesting acromegaly, but have normal or equivocal biochemical tests (Table 3–13). This may occur in patients with acromegaly with intermittent pulses of GH and low basal levels, normal basal concentrations of GH and abnormal secretory dynamics, or spontaneous infarction of the adenoma leaving the patient with only the residue of past GH excess. The term "acromegaloidism" should be reserved for patients with clinical features of acromegaly and normal GH secretion: These patients may have overproduction of other growth factors (such as IGF-II in patients with extrapancreatic neoplasms), or may have features of acromegaly due to severe insulin resistance resulting in hyperinsulinemia. It seems possible that in these patients the high concentrations of insulin are acting through cross-reactivity at IGF-I receptors to stimulate growth processes. Insulin concentrations on fasting and post-glucose samples are markedly elevated in these patients. Bioassays for growth factors, available in some research laboratories, have identified growth factor activity in samples from patients with acromegaloidism, although the exact nature of this material remains to be determined.

Evaluation of Efficacy of Treatment

Patients should be followed indefinitely after treatment of acromegaly to assess the efficacy of control of GH excess and of tumor mass, and to detect hypo-pituitarism following radiotherapy (Table 3–14). GH secretion should be reassessed after surgery in all cases. After successful removal of tumor, GH secretion may initially be reduced, but then recovers rapidly. Typically the patients are evaluated 3 months postoperatively. The glucose suppression test is performed and IGF-I levels are obtained. Patients with macroadenomas and with initial GH levels greater than 50 ng per milliliter are those most likely to have residual neoplasm, and to have recurrence. In most of these patients the GH and IGF-I levels gradually increase with time, and additional treatment is necessary. In some cases the basal and post-glucose GH levels may be normal after surgery, and the IGF-I level may be increased. Residual neoplasm is present in most of these cases, and future recurrence is likely. Laboratory error due to improper sample handling should be excluded. Persistence of a GH response to TRH several months after surgery is consistent with the presence of residual neoplasm, even if the post-glucose GH and IGF-I are normal. If all three tests are normal, the likelihood of recurrence is small.

Pituitary anatomy should also be evaluated periodically after treatment. Patients who have undergone surgery should have pituitary imaging repeated 3 to 6 months postoperatively. Magnetic resonance imaging (MRI) or computed tomography (CT) is used to establish a baseline for future comparison. Patients with evi-

TABLE 3–12   Growth Hormone Releasing Hormone Assay

Method	Radioimmunoassay
Normals	GH-RH < 1 ng/ml
Uses	Differentiation of pituitary adenoma from ectopic GH-RH secretion
Limitations	Variable sensitivity of available assays; assay not widely available

TABLE 3–13   Acromegaly With Normal Growth Hormone

GH mediated
    Episodic secretion
    Normal basal GH, abnormal secretory dynamics
    Infarction of a GH-secreting adenoma
    Increased end-organ sensitivity
Not mediated by GH (acromegaloidism)
    Severe insulin resistance
    Mediated by growth factors
        Extrapancreatic neoplasms
        Non-neoplastic

TABLE 3-14 Follow-up Testing for Treated Acromegaly

Frequency	3 mo, 6 mo, 1 yr, 3 yr, 5 yr, then every 5 yr
GH secretion	Glucose suppression test
	IGF-I/somatomedin-C
	TRH (if positive before treatment)
Pituitary function	Prolactin (may increase if initially normal)
	Adrenal function (Cortrosyn stimulation test)
	Thyroid function (total T_4, free T_4)
	Gonadal function
	LH, FSH
	Testosterone (males)
	Estradiol (females)
Pituitary anatomy	Visual field testing
	Pituitary imaging
	CT
	MRI

dence of residual neoplasm should have repeat imaging studies during follow-up. The optimal frequency for performing imaging studies has not been demonstrated. Pituitary imaging before surgery, 3 to 6 months after surgery, and at 1, 3, 5, and 10 years after surgery is reasonable. Patients with clinical or biochemical evidence of progressive disease should be studied more frequently, if necessary. Visual fields should be followed, particularly in patients who have demonstrated abnormalities on baseline study.

Pituitary function should be assessed periodically in all patients with acromegaly, regardless of the treatment modality. The evaluation should include measurement of thyroid and adrenal function, prolactin, and gonadal function (see Table 3-14). Hypopituitarism due to surgery is usually apparent in the immediate postoperative period. Nevertheless, pituitary function should be evaluated 3 months after surgery. Late development of hypopituitarism occurs after pituitary irradiation. The development of hypopituitarism is insidious in these patients, and may be overlooked if pituitary function tests are not obtained periodically during follow-up. Patients may variably manifest hypogonadism, adrenal insufficiency, and hypothyroidism due to loss of trophic hormones. Diabetes insipidus is unusual except as a complication of surgery. In patients with hyperprolactinemia prior to irradiation, the prolactin level tends to fall more slowly than GH. Prolactin may increase with time in patients who have normal concentrations initially.

HYPERPROLACTINEMIA

The development of a sensitive and specific radioimmunoassay by Frantz and co-workers in 1970 was the basis for the identification of human prolactin as a distinct pituitary hormone. Since then hyperprolactinemia has been recognized as one of the most common pituitary hormonal abnormalities and a frequent cause of reproductive dysfunction. Improving the detection and management of prolactin-secreting tumors has been the focus of intensive study. Furthermore, many pituitary tumors formerly classified as nonfunctioning chromophobe adenomas are now known to synthesize and secrete prolactin. This section focuses on the application of clinical laboratory testing to the diagnosis and management of hyperprolactinemia.

Physiology

Prolactin is a 198-amino-acid peptide synthesized and secreted by lactotrophs located in the anterior lobe of the pituitary gland. Within the pituitary, the lactotrophs are located in the posterolateral wings in close proximity to the somatotrophs and the gonadotrophs. Lactotrophs and somatotrophs emerge from a common embryonal precursor cell and show similar staining properties. In adult life a small population of cells, the "somatolactotrophs," remain capable of secreting both GH and prolactin.

Three predominant species of prolactin with molecular weights of 23,000, 48,000, and 170,000 are detected in the peripheral circulation. Glycosylated forms of prolactin also account for some of the heterogeneity.

Prolactin secretion is episodic with a sleep-entrained diurnal rhythm. Maximal concentrations in blood usually occur between 12 midnight and 8AM. Daytime pulses of prolactin may follow meals, stress, or exercise or may occur spontaneously. Prolactin levels in normal persons are influenced by many factors, including age, sex, and reproductive status (Table 3-15). Before puberty, prolactin levels are the same in males and females. After puberty, females have higher levels than males, presumably because of the stimulatory effects of estrogen. During the menstrual cycle, a small increase is seen during the luteal phase. Prolactin levels rise during pregnancy and may reach levels of 500 ng per milliliter in the third

TABLE 3-15 Physiologic Factors That Can Produce
Hyperprolactinemia

Sleep	Dehydration
Sex	Food
Females > males	Menstrual cycle?
Nipple stimulation	Pregnancy
Coitus	Neonatal period
Stress	Coitus
Exercise	Hypoglycemia
General anesthesia	

trimester. The basal concentrations remain elevated in the early postpartum period and may increase markedly during nursing. After several months the basal concentration returns to normal, even if lactation and nursing continue. Breast stimulation during fondling or intercourse can stimulate a lesser rise in prolactin in nonpregnant females. After menopause, differences between males and females disappear. Prolactin concentrations are also increased by a variety of stresses, including anxiety, pain (even the minor pain of venipuncture), general anesthesia, dehydration, hypoglycemia, exercise, coitus, and illness.

Control of Prolactin Secretion

Unique among the pituitary hormones, prolactin secretion is under tonic inhibition by dopamine secretion from the hypothalamus and possibly other prolactin inhibitory factors whose existence remains uncertain. There are numerous other neuronal and hormonal factors involved in the regulation of secretion of this hormone. Stimulation of neural afferents from the breast plays an important role in the maintenance of normal lactation. Irritation of the chest wall by skin lesions or other pathology may produce galactorrhea or hyperprolactinemia through a similar mechanism.

Dopamine is synthesized and secreted by neurosecretory cells in the tuberoinfundibular regions of the basal hypothalamus. From there it is transported via the hypothalamic-pituitary portal system to the anterior pituitary. Dopamine interacts with specific receptors on the surface of the lactotrophs and through a cyclic AMP–dependent mechanism leads to decreased secretion and synthesis of prolactin.

Estrogen has a stimulatory effect on lactotroph growth and probably also acts at the hypothalamic level to modulate dopamine secretion. Vasoactive intestinal polypeptide (VIP) has also been shown to release prolactin and may be another physiologic regulator of prolactin secretion. Histamine, acetylcholine, serotonin, and gonadotropin releasing hormone (Gn-RH) also have some prolactin releasing activity; in normal subjects and patients being treated with pulsatile Gn-RH, many of the prolactin pulses are entrained to Gn-RH–induced pulses of luteinizing hormone (LH). Interaction of histamine with H_1 and H_2 receptors has different effects; activated H_1 receptors stimulate and H_2 receptors inhibit prolactin secretion. TRH in pharmacologic doses has long been known to stimulate prolactin secretion, but probably plays a minor role, if any, in the physiologic regulation of prolactin secretion.

In addition to the above factors, short-loop feedback of prolactin on the hypothalamus has been demonstrated. Centrally, prolactin stimulates dopamine production by hypothalamic neurons, leading to suppression of prolactin secretion.

Clinical Manifestations of Hyperprolactinemia

Hyperprolactinemia may cause reproductive dysfunction in both sexes. Females may manifest subtle abnormalities of the menstrual cycle or may present with oligomenorrhea or amenorrhea with or without galactorrhea. Conversely, prolactin levels are normal in the majority of women with normal menses and isolated galactorrhea. Isolated galactorrhea with normal menses and normal prolactin level is reported in 2 to 20 percent of the normal female population. It is more common in parous women than in women who have not completed a pregnancy. About 30 percent of females with oligomenorrhea or amenorrhea due to hyperprolactinemia manifest galactorrhea. The majority of women with hyperprolactinemia have microadenomas. The gonadotropin disturbance may be subtle, and mean gonadotropin levels are not necessarily low.

Males with hyperprolactinemia may present with erectile dysfunction, signs of hypogonadism, or infertility. Pituitary tumors are often larger and invasive at the time of diagnosis in men with tumoral hyperprolactinemia, although this is not a universal finding. In contrast to women, gonadotropin levels are usually clearly reduced. It is not clear whether the difference in tumor size at presentation reflects a true sex-related difference in the natural history of the disease, or whether it simply indicates the lack of a discrete marker such as menstrual irregularity to indicate the presence of the lesion at an earlier stage. Symptoms and signs of hypogonadism develop more gradually in men and may not become obvious unless the tumors become large or the hyperprolactinemia and gonadotropin deficiency severe. Males rarely demonstrate galactorrhea because of the need for estrogen priming of the breast.

There are several mechanisms by which hyperprolactinemia can produce alterations in the hypothalamic-pituitary-gonadal axis. Centrally, prolactin appears to inhibit pulsatile release of Gn-RH; this may be an exaggeration of a normal regulatory mechanism, since Gn-RH can stimulate prolactin release (see earlier). This is inferred from the observation that the pituitary response to Gn-RH in patients with hyperprolactinemia is normal.

In addition to the central effect, prolactin is also known to have peripheral effects on the adrenal glands and ovary. Prolactin stimulates adrenal androgen production and blocks steroid synthesis by the gonads, particularly the conversion of testosterone to dihydrotestosterone by 5 α-reductase. Since gonadotropin levels are low to normal in hyperprolactinemia, however, this is clearly less important than the Gn-RH disorder. Hyperprolactinemic women treated with Gn-RH can ovulate normally.

In addition to these effects, patients with macroadenomas may also have pituitary dysfunction due to the mass lesion.

Evaluation of Hyperprolactinemia

Prolactin concentrations can be measured by bioassay, radioreceptor assay, and radioimmunoassay (Table 3–16). Most commercial laboratories offer prolactin radioimmunoassays. Samples for prolactin are ideally drawn in the resting basal state without prior breast examination. If samples are drawn under less than optimal conditions, the levels may be elevated in normal individuals. Since most patients with pathologic hyperprolactinemia have persistent hyperprolactinemia through the day, samples may be drawn at the time of a routine office visit. Even the stress of a general medical examination and venipuncture can raise the prolactin level to greater than 50 ng per milliliter, especially in women. If a random prolactin sample is modestly elevated, it may be wise to obtain an "unstressed" level to confirm this value before more extensive studies are done. One inserts a needle or catheter with a saline drip or a heparin lock and has the patient rest in a chair for 90 to 120 minutes before the sample is drawn through the line. The patient should be advised to rest and fast, but not sleep, and should be told in advance that the sample will be drawn through the existing line without another needle stick to avoid anticipatory stress. Breast examination should not be performed before samples are obtained for prolactin assay.

Measurement of prolactin is indicated in patients with oligomenorrhea or amenorrhea. In addition, hyperprolactinemia should be sought in patients with a wide variety of lesions affecting the hypothalamus and pituitary, even in the absence of symptoms, since hyperprolactinemia can be a sensitive marker of hypothalamic dysfunction.

Not all hyperprolactinemic patients have a prolactinoma. An evaluation of the possible causes is directed toward the goal of detecting mass lesions in the pituitary and hypothalamus and finding readily treatable causes such as hypothyroidism.

Differential Diagnosis

Once hyperprolactinemia is documented, additional studies are indicated to establish a diagnosis. Hyperprolactinemia may be due to physiologic or pathologic processes (Table 3–17). An important consideration is

TABLE 3–16   Prolactin Assay

Methods	Radioimmunoassay Radioreceptor assay Bioassay
Uses	Evaluation of pituitary and hypothalamic disease, amenorrhea, galactorrhea, male infertility, impotence, and hypogonadism
Normals	Males < 15 ng/ml Females < 20 ng/ml Pregnancy < 500 ng/ml
Limitations	Variability between laboratories False-positive elevations due to stress, time of day, recent breast examination

whether hyperprolactinemia is the manifestation of a pituitary or hypothalamic mass lesion or pressure effect. Some of the specific conditions associated with hyperprolactinemia are discussed in the following sections.

Pharmacologic Agents

Many drugs can produce hyperprolactinemia (see Table 3–17) by varied mechanisms. Reserpine and alphamethyldopa lead to dopamine depletion in the hypothalamus. The phenothiazines, butyrophenones, tricyclics, and metoclopramide block dopamine receptors at the level of the pituitary. Cimetidine blocks H_2 receptors, decreasing the prolactin-inhibitory effect of H_2 receptor activation. Estrogens and TRH appear to stimulate the lactotroph directly; estrogens also inhibit dopamine production at the hypothalamic level. Calcium channel blockade with verapamil also produces hyperprolactinemia. Many opiates elevate prolactin at the hypothalamic level.

Patients with elevations in prolactin level caused by pharmacologic agents usually have prolactin concentrations of less than 150 ng per milliliter. If prolactin levels are much higher, another cause should be carefully sought. Since prolactinomas and hypothyroidism are both common, the presence of hyperprolactinemia in a patient taking one of the drugs should not be presumed to result from the drug unless it can be withdrawn and prolactin retested, or these other causes reasonably excluded.

Hyperprolactinemia due to macroprolactinemia has been reported in otherwise normal males and females. Diagnosis can be confirmed by gel filtration.

Other Disease States

Hyperprolactinemia may occur as a concomitant of other disease states. Patients with renal failure or, to a lesser degree, hepatic failure may develop hyperprolactinemia due to altered neurotransmitter function and in part to decreased clearance of prolactin. Patients with

TABLE 3-17   Etiologic Classification of Hyperprolactinemia

Pituitary Isolation Syndrome	Pharmacologic Agents	Disease States	Tumoral
Stalk section or	Phenothiazines	Liver disease	Prolactinoma
hypothalamic dysfunction	H₂ blockers	Renal failure	GH and prolactin secretion
Trauma	Butyrophenones	Hypothyroidism	TSHoma
Surgery	Reserpine	Adrenal insufficiency	Multiple endocrine neoplasia type I
Radiotherapy	alpha-Methyldopa	Thyrotoxicosis	Nelson's syndrome
Central nervous system	Estrogens	Anorexia nervosa	Metastatic tumor
neoplasms	Opiates		Ectopic prolactin
Infiltrative diseases	Metoclopramide		
Tuberculosis	Verapamil		
Sarcoidosis	Tricyclic		
Eosinophilic granuloma	antidepressants		
(Hand-Schüller-Christian)			
Hypophysitis			
Empty sella			
syndrome			
Hydrocephalus			
Arteriovenous malformations			

hypothyroidism may also develop hyperprolactinemia. In general, hypothyroidism does not cause significant hyperprolactinemia until the concentration of thyroxine (T_4) is less than 2 μg per deciliter and that of thyroid-stimulating hormone (TSH), greater than 50 μU per milliliter. Treatment of the hypothyroidism rapidly normalizes the prolactin level. Hyperprolactinemia can cause increases in adrenal androgens and may be present in some patients with polycystic ovary syndrome or idiopathic hirsuitism.

Pituitary Isolation Syndrome

Structural pathology that impairs the production or transport of dopamine from the hypothalamus to the pituitary may lead to hyperprolactinemia. Hyperprolactinemia due to anatomic pathology affecting the hypothalamus or pituitary stalk has been termed the pituitary isolation syndrome. At the level of the hypothalamus, infiltrative diseases, neoplasms, inflammatory and infectious diseases, trauma, or damage due to radiation or surgery may lead to destruction of the cells that produce dopamine. The same wide range of pathologic processes can affect the transport of dopamine through the hypothalamic pituitary portal system. Stalk section due to nonfunctioning pituitary neoplasm or pressure effects due to hydrocephalus or the empty sella syndrome are additional considerations. Stalk dysfunction usually does not produce prolactin levels greater than 200 ng per milliliter, and patients with much higher levels probably have prolactin-producing tumors (Table 3–18). Distinguishing between stalk compression and prolactinoma in patients with lesser degrees of hyperprolactinemia may be difficult, but has important implications for

TABLE 3-18   Classification and Natural History of Prolactinoma

Classification	Size (mm)	Natural History
Microprolactinoma	< 10	< 30% grow to macro size 30% disappear spontaneously Non-invasive Most are stable during pregnancy
Macroprolactinoma	> 10	Larger potential for growth if left untreated Need to check visual fields Pituitary insufficiency
Invasive prolactinoma	> 10	Destruction of parasellar structures Local extension, frequent involvement of optic chiasm Pituitary insufficiency
Pseudoprolactinoma	> 10	No prolactin release by tumoral tissue Altered anatomy produces loss of prolactin-inhibiting factor/dopamine activity on residual lactotrophs

the long-term follow-up and treatment of the patient. Pseudoprolactinoma is a term used to describe any pituitary tumor whose cells do not directly secrete prolactin, but where hyperprolactinemia is present on the basis of loss of dopamine effects on the stalk or on the hypothalamus.

Laboratory Evaluation of Patients with Hyperprolactinemia

The laboratory evaluation of patients with hyperprolactinemia is outlined in Table 3–19. Thyroid function tests, including TSH, are always indicated to exclude hypothyroidism. Additional endocrine studies are indicated if there is evidence of a hypothalamic or pituitary mass lesion. These studies are rarely abnormal in patients with microadenomas. Formal visual-field testing is indicated in the presence of macroadenomas and other suprasellar lesions, and during pregnancy in patients with known prolactinomas.

Anteroposterior and lateral skull radiographs and sellar tomograms were previously used to define abnormalities in the bony margins of the sella. It is now recognized that many of the changes attributed to microadenomas, such as depression of the floor on one side of the sella, may be normal variations. A postmortem study of sellar tomograms in accident victims showed a high incidence of abnormalities in subjects who had no symptoms during life, and this technique has been largely superseded. At present, CT and MRI are the methods of choice for delineating the sella contents. Of the two, MRI gives better contrast and anatomic detail and better definition of structures such as the optic chiasm and the cavernous sinus. Gadolinium (Gd) diethylene triamine penta-acetic acid (DTPA) is a paramagnetic material recently released for use as a contrast material during MRI studies. MRI with Gd-DTPA provides better imaging of small, intrasellar lesions. It should be emphasized that many hormonally active microadenomas may be invisible in current CT and MRI studies.

The optimal frequency of follow-up imaging in patients with documented pituitary tumors is uncertain. Most prolactinomas do not increase in size. Some lesions may spontaneously remit, and a small percentage of the lesions are aggressive and may show appreciable increases in size during follow-up. Although the optimal frequency for imaging patients is not known, a reasonable approach is to do a scan at the time of diagnosis, after 6 months, and then yearly for several years until the rate of growth of the lesion is established. Less frequent imaging may be satisfactory if it is clear that the lesion is not progressing rapidly. Patients should undergo repeat imaging if they have signs of pituitary apoplexy, including sudden headache or change in headache pattern, signs of other pituitary hormone defects, or visual abnormalities.

TABLE 3–19   Tests for Evaluating Hyperprolactinemic Patients

Endocrine studies
  Thyroid function tests
  LH/FSH
  Testosterone (male)
  Estradiol (female)
  Progestin withdrawal
  Bone densitometry
    (selected cases)
Imaging studies
  Skull film
  CT or MRI with Gd-DTPA
    (selected cases)
Mass effect
  Visual fields

Prolactinoma and Pregnancy

The pituitary enlarges and prolactin levels rise significantly during normal pregnancy. Lactotroph hypertrophy due to estrogen stimulation is the accepted mechanism for this physiologic change. The intrasellar volume more than doubles by the end of the third trimester. This complicates the evaluation of patients with pituitary adenomas who become pregnant, since it may be difficult to distinguish between physiologic enlargement of the pituitary and tumor progression. However, the experience of treated prolactinoma patients who have carried pregnancies is reassuring. Enlargement to the point at which symptoms appear occurs in less than 5 percent of patients with previous microadenomas. Most authors believe that patients with small tumors can be followed expectantly during pregnancy.

In patients with antecedent macroadenomas, symptomatic growth is more common, with headaches or visual-field abnormalities occurring in 15 to 35 percent. Although bromocriptine is not currently registered for use during pregnancy, it is as effective in reversing these changes during pregnancy and has not been linked with an excess of fetal abnormalities. Surveillance of patients who became pregnant while taking bromocriptine but did not immediately discontinue the drug has shown no increase in the incidence of birth defects.

GONADOTROPIN-SECRETING ADENOMAS

During the era when pituitary adenomas were classified by their staining characteristics under light microscopy, the majority of tumors were classified as nonfunctioning chromophobe adenomas. When the prolactin radioimmunoassay was developed in the early 1970s, it became clear that the majority of the neoplasms previously classified as "nonfunctioning" were prolactinomas. Because of the rarity of elevated concentrations of LH and follicle-stimulating hormone (FSH) in patients with pituitary adenomas, gonadotropin secretion by pituitary adenomas has been considered rare. With the application of assays for alpha subunit, and through immunohistochemistry, it has become clear that many of these apparently "nonfunctioning" tumors synthesize gonadotropin subunits or intact gonadotropins. Snyder has reported an incidence of 17 percent in a series of men presenting with pituitary macroadenomas.

The typical patient with this type of tumor is a male with a history of normal puberty and fertility who presents with a large pituitary tumor. There is usually evidence of visual impairment, and imaging usually shows extrasellar extension. Hypogonadism may be present. The diagnosis of these tumors in women is more difficult because elevated FSH/LH levels at the menopause may be a normal finding. Those cases which have been reported have shown high FSH levels with normal or low LH levels.

The characteristic hormonal pattern of these tumors is secretion of the intact FSH molecule. Concentrations of alpha and beta subunits of FSH may also be elevated. The levels of FSH-beta are significantly higher than those seen in men with primary hypogonadism. High levels of intact LH occur much less frequently in patients with gonadotroph adenomas.

Administration of TRH to patients with gonadotroph adenomas often elicits a characteristic pattern. Typically there is an increase in intact FSH and an increase in the LH subunits. When FSH is the primary product, the testosterone level is low or normal. In the few patients with high LH secretion the testosterone level is often elevated; estradiol may also be elevated, which may lead to gynecomastia. The former patients demonstrate a testosterone response when stimulated with human chorionic gonadotropin (hCG), whereas the patients with LH hypersecretion, who are already maximally stimulated, do not.

Patients with gonadotropin secreting adenomas can be distinguished from patients with primary hypogonadism and secondary hypersecretion of FSH/LH (Table 3–20). The latter patient will have a history of prolonged hypogonadism usually beginning before puberty, with evidence on examination of inadequate virilization and with small testes. An exception is Klinefelter's syndrome,

in which the defect in androgenization may be partial and does not occur prior to puberty. Both FSH and LH levels are elevated, in contrast to the patient with a gonadotroph adenoma, in whom FSH and alpha and beta subunits are elevated. The patient with primary hypogonadism will not show FSH/LH responsiveness to stimulation with TRH, nor does the testosterone level increase with hCG administration. The levels of FSH and its subunits and the response of the tumor to TRH can be used to follow patients undergoing treatment.

HYPOPITUITARISM

Patients with hypopituitarism may be deficient in a single hormone (unitrophic defect), multiple hormones, or have complete pituitary failure (panhypopituitarism). The loss of hormonal function often occurs in a predictable sequence, with early loss of GH and gonadotropin function, only later progressing to adrenocorticotropic hormone (ACTH) and TSH deficiency. Most adults with hypopituitarism present with symptoms and signs of gonadal insufficiency or infertility, and children usually present with growth failure. Occasionally the presentation is acute, with signs of adrenal insufficiency. This may occur if there is an acute injury to the hypothalamic-pituitary axis from pituitary apoplexy, trauma, or surgery, or may occur in the patient with chronic hypopituitarism who is subjected to severe stress, illness, or surgery. The different types of clinical presentation often direct the selection of initial laboratory tests. For example, when a child presents with growth retardation or short stature, testing for GH deficiency is the critical issue. For men or women with signs of hypogonadism, the evaluation of prolactin, FSH, LH, and testosterone or estrogen would take precedence. Generally, if a deficiency in any single pituitary hormone is detected, a more complete evaluation of anterior pituitary function is undertaken. In addition, since the clinical manifestations of hypopituitarism may be mild, patients with known lesions of the hypothalamus, stalk, or pituitary should undergo an

TABLE 3–20 Hormonal Patterns in Hypergonadotropic States

	LH	FSH	Testosterone or Estrogen	TRH Response
Primary hypogonadism	High	High	Low	None
FSH-secreting tumor	Normal or low	High	Normal or low	Increased FSH
LH-secreting tumor	High	Normal	Normal-high (men) Low (women)	Increased subunits

evaluation of pituitary function at least once, and perhaps have selected tests at regular intervals.

Approach to Analyzing Pituitary Function

For evaluating pituitary function, the clinician has a wide range of basal and dynamic endocrine tests to consider (Table 3–21). The types of tests that provide the most diagnostic information with the least cost vary among the different pituitary hormone systems. Often a combination of measurements of basal hormone concentrations from the relevant peripheral target organs and basal or stimulated levels of the pituitary hormones is required. The approach to diagnosis for each of the pituitary hormones is discussed in the following sections.

Hypogonadotropic Hypogonadism

Oligomenorrhea or secondary amenorrhea in women carries a very different connotation from hypogonadism in men. The former is very common, often transient and unassociated with significant pituitary-hypothalamic disease, and so can initially be followed expectantly; the latter almost always reflects a significant underlying disorder and mandates a thorough evaluation. In part this reflects the "all or nothing" character of the menstrual cycle, which can be interrupted even by subtle changes in hormonal signals, providing an immediate clinical marker of the disturbance. Many such women have normal estrogen and gonadotropin levels and are not hypogonadal, although they are anovulatory. In contrast, gonadal function in men is continuously graded to the gonadotropin stimulation and may remain clinically silent until the hypogonadism becomes severe. Thus, although the basic physiologic principles underlying gonadal function are similar in men and women, their evaluation often proceeds differently.

The presence of regular menstrual cycles in a woman who is not taking cyclic estrogen therapy excludes gonadotropin deficiency. Since oligoamenorrhea may be a response to stress, exercise, weight reduction, drugs, or intercurrent illness, these factors should be explored prior to obtaining extensive laboratory tests in a woman with irregular or absent menses. Since the commonest cause of secondary amenorrhea is pregnancy, a pregnancy test is always indicated.

In men, or in women in whom it appears that further evaluation is indicated, as with prolonged or primary amenorrhea, the work-up should include gonadotropins (especially FSH) and gonadal steroids—a testosterone level in men and a measure of estrogen levels in women. Besides an estradiol assay, the latter can be assessed by progestin challenge: A positive response, with bleeding, indicates an intact endometrium, a patent outflow tract, and estrogen levels sufficient to induce endometrial proliferation, about 40 to 50 pg per milliliter. In addition to its diagnostic value, this test can provide psychological reassurance to patients that many functions are normal. Even with a negative pregnancy test, it is safest to use progesterone itself rather than a synthetic progestin, because of the reports of genitourinary anomalies in babies born to mothers who received these drugs during early pregnancy.

Gonadotropin levels are obtained to distinguish primary gonadal failure, in which they are high, from pituitary-hypothalamic disease, in which they are low in men and low or normal in women. High levels of gonadotropins in women are also consistent with the midcycle

TABLE 3-21   Tests for Evaluating Anterior Pituitary Function

	Screening Tests	Secondary Tests
Gonadotropin deficiency		
Male	LH, FSH, testosterone	Sperm count Gn-RH test
Female	LH, FSH Progestin withdrawal	Gn-RH test
GH deficiency	Exercise test Somatomedin-C	Insulin tolerance test Arginine infusion L-Dopa Propranolol-glucagon Sleep test Clonidine test ? GH-RH test
TSH deficiency	T₄, Free T₄ TSH	TRH test
ACTH deficiency	1-hr ACTH stimulation test	ACTH level Insulin tolerance test CRH test
Prolactin deficiency	Prolactin	TRH test Insulin tolerance test Chlorpromazine test

LH surge (with elevated estrogens) or with pregnancy. Menopause or ovarian failure is not a single event; ovarian function can progress and intermit over several years, and it is important to obtain several gonadotropin measurements at intervals before concluding that ovarian failure is present. FSH is a more sensitive indicator of this process than LH, rising with more subtle degrees of hypogonadism; thus, if cost is a concern, the LH measurements can often be eliminated. Whether the increased FSH reflects changes in gonadal factors other than sex steroids, such as inhibin, is controversial and does not alter the clinical evaluation.

Hyperprolactinemia is a common cause of hypothalamic amenorrhea and hypogonadism. Once pregnancy and primary gonadal failure are excluded, prolactin should be measured early in the evaluation.

Gn-RH directly stimulates pituitary gonadotropin release, and when it became available for clinical use it was hoped that the presence or absence of a response could be used to distinguish pituitary from hypothalamic hypogonadism. Unfortunately, this has not proven to be true. Unresponsivity can occur with lesions at either site; with hypothalamic lesions, this may be due to gonadotroph atrophy and reduced releasable stores of gonadotropins in pituitaries which have long been unstimulated. Repeated administration of Gn-RH can often induce a response in these patients.

On a finer level of distinction, attention is sometimes paid to the relative LH versus FSH responses to Gn-RH. Prepubertal children have a brisker FSH response, and at puberty this shifts to an LH-predominant response. However, these changes probably reflect increases in sex steroid levels rather than more fundamental neuroendocrine processes, and their clinical value is limited.

In a child with delayed puberty it would be extremely helpful to be able to distinguish simple pubertal delay from hypogonadotropic hypogonadism, allowing earlier treatment in the latter case. Besides the Gn-RH test, a variety of provocative tests—for example, chlorpromazine or metaclopramide stimulation of prolactin—have been proposed, and in some studies differences between the two diagnostic categories have been found. However, as with the gonadotropin responses to Gn-RH, the changes in prolactin responses probably reflect sex steroid levels, with responses failing as steroids fall to low values, rather than neuroendocrine abnormalities, and so indicate the severity rather than the etiology of the hypogonadism. This factor and substantial overlap between groups suggest that these tests usually do not add useful diagnostic information.

Growth Hormone Deficiency

The diagnosis of GH deficiency (GHD) has traditionally been made by the measurement of GH responses after provocative stimuli. The measurement of spontaneous secretion of GH or levels of IGF-I (somatomedin-C)

are newer approaches, but it has yet to be demonstrated that they offer significant diagnostic advantages.

Since GH secretion is episodic and levels are often undetectable between pulses, single GH measurements may be low even in normal subjects and so do not distinguish the normal state from GHD. For this reason a variety of stimulation tests have been devised (Table 3–22). A significant proportion of normal subjects will fail to show a response to any of these tests (except GH-RH), and therefore the traditional approach has been to make the diagnosis of GHD only if the response is abnormal in at least two independent tests. By the same traditional criteria, passing any test with a satisfactory GH response excludes the diagnosis. How a satisfactory GH response should be defined, however, is controversial, and the interpretation of these tests is subject to some debate (see below).

Physiologic stimulation of GH by exercise, sleep, or amino acids and pharmacologic stimuli with hypoglycemia or a variety of drugs have all been employed for testing. Of these, the measurement of GH after exercise is simple and safe and is commonly used as an initial screening test. The child should be vigorously exercised under supervision. If the response is normal, further testing is not indicated. A second test is performed if the response is borderline or low.

None of these tests is ideal, and most have significant side effects. Insulin-induced hypoglycemia is a potent stimulus to GH secretion but carries a risk from hypoglycemia. Since the frequency of severe hypoglycemia is increased in hypopituitarism, this test is most risky in the patients most likely to have GHD. Therefore, close monitoring by nurse and physician, intravenous access, and dextrose for intravenous administration must be available.

Various other tests for the diagnosis of GHD have been devised. The infusion of arginine and the administration of L-dopa, glucagon (alone or with propranolol), and clonidine are some of the tests used (see Table 3–22). Responses to all these tests can be blunted by factors such as hypothyroidism, obesity, and hyperglycemia. In evaluating a child who may have multiple pituitary deficiencies, one should exclude hypothyroidism before doing GH testing.

With the recent availability of GH-RH, this hormone has been evaluated as another diagnostic test for GHD. This test differs in principle from the others in that it provides a direct pituitary stimulus, while the other tests activate all or part of the hypothalamic GH-RH release mechanisms. This means that while the traditional indirect tests may fail to stimulate GH in some normal subjects, GH-RH testing has the opposite problem: Many patients with hypothalamic GHD (the majority of cases) respond to GH-RH testing, and in 30 to 50 percent of GHD children the response overlaps the normal range. This means that GH-RH testing is not very useful in the diagnosis of GHD. In principle it could be used to differentiate between hypothalamic and pituitary causes

TABLE 3-22   Stimulation Tests for Evaluating Growth Hormone Secretion*

Exercise Test

    Method: Measure GH at 0, 10, 20, 40, and 60 min after vigorous exercise (e.g., running subject up 5–6 flights of stairs). Best if the exercise challenge can be calibrated, as with a treadmill ergometer.

    Problems: Contraindicated in patients with cardiac disease or other conditions that would limit the ability to exercise.

Insulin Tolerance Test

    Method: Regular insulin is given IV (0.1–0.15 U/kg). Glucose, GH, and cortisol are measured at 0, 30, 60, 90, and 120 min. A 50% decrease in glucose concentration and symptoms of hypoglycemia are required for the test to be interpretable.

    Problems: Contraindicated in patients with seizures or known cardiovascular or cerebrovascular disease. Patients must be monitored continuously during the test. Obesity, thyroid dysfunction, hypogonadism, and Cushing's syndrome may result in blunted responses.

Arginine Infusion Test

    Method: Arginine is infused IV at a dose of 0.5 g/kg to a maximal dose of 30 g over 30 min. Measure GH at 0, 30, 60, 90, and 120 min.

    Problems: False-negative rate of 30–35% in patients with hypopituitarism. Contraindicated in patients with liver or renal failure.

L-Dopa Test

    Method: 500 mg L-dopa is given PO to adults and 10 mg/kg to children to a maximum of 500 mg. Measure GH at 0, 1, 2, and 3 hr. Keep patient recumbent during test.

    Problems: Nausea, vomiting, vertigo, and hypotension.

Propranolol-Glucagon Test

    Method: 40 mg of propranolol is given PO at 7 AM and glucagon 1 mg IM or SQ at 9 AM. Measure GH and plasma cortisol at 0, 1, 2, and 3 hr

    Problems: Nausea, vomiting, weakness, and apprehension. Contraindicated in patients with asthma, heart block, congestive heart failure, or diabetes.

Sleep Test

    Method: Measure GH with indwelling catheter 60 and 90 min after onset of deep sleep.

    Problems: Difficult to perform on an outpatient basis; 10% of normals have low values.

Clonidine Test

    Method: Administer 0.15 μg/kg (maximum dose 0.25 mg PO). GH is measured at 0 and 75 min.
    Problems: Postural hypotension and drowsiness.

Responses to Stimulation Tests for GH

    Normal: stimulated GH > 10 ng/ml
    Borderline: stimulated GH 7–10 ng/ml
    Abnormal: stimulated GH < 7 ng/ml

Growth Hormone Releasing Hormone Test

    Method: Administer 1 μg/kg of GH-RH IV. GH is measured at 0, 30, 60, 90, 120 min.

    Problems: 30–50% of patients with idiopathic GH deficiency exhibit a normal response. Range of normal very broad: any measurable rise compatible with normal.

* Because of the suppressive effect of glucose on GH secretion, all tests should be performed after an overnight fast.

of GHD, but in practice many of the same problems found with Gn-RH testing are encountered. A patient with hypothalamic GHD may fail to respond initially because of somatotroph atrophy, but then develop a response after repeated stimuli. Thus at present GH-RH testing in GHD seems useful only to identify candidates for therapy with GH-RH as an alternative to GH, a treatment which is currently only available experimentally in a few centers.

The growth retardation of GHD reflects a reduction in GH secretion, and therefore it has been suggested that measuring physiologic GH secretion might provide a better diagnostic tool than the rather artificial provocative tests. Because of pulsatile and circadian variations in GH, this requires overnight or even 24-hour-long sampling to estimate average GH levels and perhaps characterize the pulses. Some investigators have argued that a substantial proportion of children with retarded growth but normal responses to GH testing have a "neurosecretory defect" with reduced spontaneous secretion but retained ability to respond to pharmacologic stimuli. This issue is controversial, with some investigators claiming that many such cases can be diagnosed by extended sampling, and others finding little or no further diagnostic yield beyond the responses to provocative testing. Because this kind of testing is laborious and expensive, even if the samples are pooled before assay, and because its value is still unproven, we believe that it should be undertaken only in the context of a research study.

In addition to measurements of GH, GH biological activity can be assessed by measuring IGF-I/somatomedin-C. For several reasons these assays have not replaced measurements of GH, although IGF-I has a long half-life in plasma and so in principle could serve as a measure of integrated GH action. IGF-I assays differ considerably from one laboratory to another, and normal ranges differ with age and pubertal development. Thus results can only be interpreted against the background of extensive normative data in that assay. Normal values in children less than 6 years old are very low, and most assays do not reliably distinguish between normal and GHD in this age group. Also, malnutrition and a variety of systemic illnesses can inhibit IGF-I production even when GH levels are normal, making low values difficult to interpret. In GHD, IGF-I levels may not reflect the severity of the deficiency, and changes in IGF-I during GH therapy do not correlate well with the growth response. In part these problems may reflect the fact that IGF-I is produced locally in many tissues to act in a paracrine fashion, and levels in the circulation may just reflect unregulated "spillover" and not GH action in the relevant biological compartment.

The typical patient with GH deficiency demonstrates low GH responses to provocative testing and low IGF-I levels. Rarely, growth failure may reflect other abnormalities in the hypothalamic-pituitary-IGF axis (Table 3–23). Growth failure due to malnutrition is associated with normal or high levels of GH and low levels of IGF-I. The Laron dwarf has high GH levels and low IGF-I concentrations, thought to be due to abnormal GH receptors. By contrast, the African pygmy has normal IGF-I levels but appears to be resistant to its action.

GHD may reflect a variety of underlying causes (Table 3–24). For a fuller discussion of disorders of growth, see also Chapter 4.

The difficulties with GH testing for GHD are part of a more general problem: Although classical GHD can be clear-cut, the majority of children with growth failure and evidence of GHD have a partial deficiency and retain some GH responses, and the boundaries between normal and GH deficiency are not well established. There is growing dissatisfaction with using arbitrary cutoffs to distinguish "idiopathic short stature" from "growth hormone deficiency." Recent studies of responses to treatment with synthetic GH suggest that none of the measures in current use reliably predicts which children will respond to GH. If this is true, it may not be clinically helpful to try to insist on such a distinction. It may be that idiopathic short stature and GHD lie on a continuum, and that after the initial tests and the clinical setting have been assessed, a trial of GH therapy may be more useful than further testing. Because the possible side effects and the effect of GH on final stature in patients who are not GH deficient are unknown, this should be undertaken only as part of a study protocol.

TSH Deficiency

The diagnosis of TSH deficiency is based on the measurement of in vitro tests of thyroid function (T_4, free T_4) and of TSH. A low free T_4 and an elevated TSH level indicates primary hypothyroidism. A low free T_4 with a normal or low TSH level is consistent with a lesion of either the pituitary (secondary hypothyroidism) or hypothalamus (tertiary hypothyroidism). It may be difficult to distinguish secondary (or tertiary) hypothyroidism from the euthyroid sick syndrome. Occasionally patients with secondary hypothyroidism are found to have elevated concentrations of TSH, a surprising finding. This has been found to be due either to antibodies that cross-react in supersensitive TSH assays or to secretion of a form of the hormone with reduced biological activity.

When TRH became available for clinical use, it was hoped that TSH response to the releasing hormone would distinguish hypothalamic from pituitary hypothyroidism. A delayed response to TRH was initially reported as characteristic of tertiary hypothyroidism. In fact, it is now

TABLE 3–23   Classification of Growth Hormone Deficiency by GH, IGF-I, and Response to Treatment

Type	GH Level	IGF-I Level	Response to Treatment
Congenital	Low	Low	Respond to GH
Isolated type Ia	Low	Low	Initial response to GH, then failure due to development of antibodies
Biologically inactive GH	Low radioreceptor assay/radioimmunoassay ratio	Low	Respond to GH
Laron Dwarf	High	Low	No response
Pygmy	Normal	Normal	No response
"Neurosecretory dysfunction"	Low (integrated) 24-hr secretory pattern	Low	Respond to GH
Protein-calorie malnutrition	High	Low	Respond to refeeding
Psychosocial dwarfism	Low	Low	Respond to change in environment

TABLE 3-24   Growth Hormone Deficiency

Congenital
  Multiple pituitary hormone defects
  Idiopathic
  Embryologic—midline defects, aplasia
  Familial
	Cerebral irradiation
	
	Trauma
	
	Psychosocial deprivation

Hormone resistance
  Biologically inactive hormone
  Laron dwarf
  Pygmy
	Infections
	  Tuberculosis
	  Meningitis
	  Encephalitis
	  Syphilis
	  Fungal infection

Pituitary and central nervous system tumors
  Craniopharyngioma
  Germinoma
  Pituitary adenoma
	Vascular
	  Aneurysm
	  Pituitary infarction

Granulomatous and infiltrative diseases
  Sarcoidosis
  Histiocytosis
  Hemochromatosis
  Leukemia
  Lymphoma
	Surgical ablation

clear that a delayed response does not indicate the anatomic level of the lesion, and that failure to respond to TRH does not exclude hypothalamic disease.

Secondary Adrenal Insufficiency

Because of overlap in basal cortisol levels between normal subjects and patients with ACTH deficiency, it is necessary to assess adrenal reserve to establish the diagnosis of secondary adrenal insufficiency. Of the many tests that have been devised for this purpose, the adrenal response to the administration of 250 μg of ACTH is considered by most to be the test of choice, and is also entirely safe even in patients who may have adrenal insufficiency. The secretory reserve of the adrenal cortex is a sensitive integrator of the stimulation to which it has been subjected; conditions that suppress ACTH lead to a blunted response to ACTH testing within a few days. A plasma cortisol increase to more than 18 μg per milliliter 1 hour after administration of ACTH is normal. If the value is greater than 10 but less than 18 μg per milliliter, adrenal insufficiency may be present, but usually replacement is required for stress only. Peak values of less than 10 μg per milliliter signify the need for chronic replacement with hydrocortisone.

If there is an abnormality in the rapid ACTH test, the plasma ACTH should be measured. In primary adrenal insufficiency the level is quite high—usually more than 250 pg per milliliter. If the rapid ACTH test is abnormal with a normal or low ACTH level, secondary or tertiary adrenal insufficiency is present. The distinction between these two entities can be made by prolonged infusion of ACTH for several days, or with the CRH (corticotropin-releasing hormone) test. Failure of ACTH to respond to CRH is indicative of pituitary disease. An increase in the plasma cortisol of more than 10 μg per

milliliter at 30 to 60 minutes implicates the hypothalamus as the site of insufficiency.

Insulin-induced hypoglycemia and the metyrapone test have also been used to evaluate the pituitary-adrenal axis. The cortisol response to insulin-induced hypoglycemia correlates highly with the cortisol response to stress and has the advantage that GH can be measured at the same sitting. However, if the patient has adrenal insufficiency, severe and prolonged hypoglycemia may occur. In addition, the test is contraindicated in the presence of cardiac and cerebrovascular disease.

Metyrapone blocks the 11-hydroxylation of 11-deoxycortisol (compound S), resulting in a fall in cortisol. If the hypothalamic-pituitary axis is intact, ACTH is released and results in increased plasma 11-deoxycortisol. A normal response is an increase in plasma 11-deoxycortisol of at least 7 μg per milliliter in the presence of a documented decrease in cortisol to below 10 μg per milliliter. Failure of the cortisol to decrease indicates an inadequate test. This test may have a role in the evaluation of hypercortisolism but runs the risk of provoking acute adrenal insufficiency in a patient with diminished adrenal reserve. We therefore believe that it has little place in the evaluation of suspected adrenal insufficiency.

The recent administration of glucocorticoids suppresses the pituitary, making test responses difficult to interpret. Therefore, patients should have stopped taking replacement glucocorticoids at least 1 month before testing.

Prolactin Deficiency

Diseases of the hypothalamus and pituitary more often produce hyperprolactinemia than prolactin deficiency. Although prolactin is secreted in a pulsatile fashion, levels remain detectable even between pulses, and an undetectable prolactin level is always abnormal unless the patient is taking a drug such as L-dopa or bromocriptine. Prolactin deficiency has been reported rarely, and is usually a result of complete or partial pituitary failure occurring at the time of parturition (Sheehan's syndrome). Although this has most often been ascribed to hemorrhage, ischemia, and pituitary infarctions, an autoimmune hypophysitis is also possible. Prolactin deficiency is manifested as failure to lactate post partum. The finding of a normal prolactin level excludes the diagnosis. In the case of low-normal values, provocative testing may be helpful. The most useful test is the TRH stimulation test. A normal response is a twofold increase in the prolactin level at 15 to 30 minutes. Estrogen is trophic for lactotrophs; patients with hypogonadism may have low (but detectable) prolactin levels that return to normal when gonadal replacement therapy is begun.

Sequential Testing of Anterior Pituitary Function

As described by Sheldon and his colleagues and modified by others, pituitary function can be assessed in one sitting by the sequential administration of the four available hypothalamic releasing hormones, TRH, Gn-RH, CRH, and GH-RH (Table 3–25). This is convenient if the circumstances would mandate testing all these systems; however, because Gn-RH and GH-RH testing are of limited proven utility, such testing is rarely required. As noted, atrophy may lead to blunted or even absent responses to Gn-RH or GH-RH, even when the primary disorder is of hypothalamic origin and a normal pituitary is present. In these circumstances, repeated "priming" with the releasing hormone may induce a response and so demonstrate the presence of functional pituitary cells. For example, approximately half of children with idiopathic GH deficiency and no response to GH-RH acquire a response after 5 to 7 days of daily GH-RH priming (1 µg per kilogram intravenously), and some patients with hypogonadotropic hypogonadism and no response to Gn-RH acquire a response after 1 week of wearing a Gn-RH pulsatile infusion pump (200 µg per kilogram subcutaneously every 90 to 120 minutes). The diagnostic utility of this maneuver is limited to very selected cases; it may be of value to demonstrate responsivity in this way if a patient is being considered for GH-RH or Gn-RH therapy.

Differential Diagnosis of Hypopituitarism

There are numerous causes to consider in the patient with hypopituitarism (Table 3–26). When diabetes insipidus is associated with anterior pituitary hormonal

---

TABLE 3–25   Sequential Pituitary Testing

Uses:	Rapid one-sitting evaluation of hormone pituitary function.
Method:	The following releasing hormones are infused sequentially at 20-sec intervals: CRH 1 µg/kg.; Gn-RH 100 µg; GH-RH 1 µg/kg; TRH 200 µg. Samples are obtained for hormone assays according to the following table.

	Time after infusion (min)						
	0	10	15	30	45	60	90
ACTH	X	X				X	X
Cortisol	X				X	X	
FSH	X					X	X
LH	X			X		X	
TSH	X			X		X	
Prolactin	X	X		X			
GH	X			X		X	X

Mean incremental responses in normals.

	Men	Women
ACTH (pg/ml)	40 ± 7.6	40 ± 6.6
Cortisol (µg/dl)	9.5 ± 1.0	9.8 ± 1.2
FSH (mIU/ml)	2.7 ± 0.6	3.0 ± 0.2
LH (mIU/ml)	21 ± 2.6	13.9 ± 1.9
TSH (µU/ml)	12 ± 1.2	15 ± 2.1
Prolactin (ng/ml)	46 ± 5.0	92 ± 15
GH (ng/ml)	23 ± 7.1	55 ± 20

Problems:	Facial flushing, nausea, and urinary urgency. A large number of assays are necessary and the expense is considerable. May provide more information than clinically necessary to collect in a given patient.

Adapted from Sheldon et al. J Clin Endocrinol Metab 1985; 60:623–628.

deficiency(ies), a lesion of the hypothalamus is suggested. Infiltrative diseases such as eosinophilic granuloma (e.g., Hand-Schüller-Christian disease) or sarcoidosis, and primary or metastatic tumors of the hypothalamus, often present in this manner. An exception to this rule is when there is surgical injury to the pituitary stalk, which may lead to diabetes insipidus without a lesion of the hypothalamus. In many cases a careful history and physical examination and screening laboratory studies will yield important clues to the diagnosis. Detailed imaging of the hypothalamic area using CT, MRI, and occasionally arteriography may be necessary to define the pathologic lesion.

In the cases of GH and gonadotropin regulation, some apparent deficiency states may represent a reversible response to systemic illness, stress, weight loss, or physical exertion. Children deprived of normal parental interactions (maternal deprivation syndrome) may show retarded growth, reduced GH secretion, and low plasma levels of IGF-I, closely mimicking true GH deficiency, but rapidly return to normal when hospitalized or placed in a supportive foster home. Malnutrition and anorexia nervosa can also be associated with growth failure and low IGF-I levels, but in this case IGF-I synthesis is primarily blocked and GH levels are normal to high.

TABLE 3-26 Causes of Hypopituitarism

Pituitary tumors
    Primary
    Metastatic (breast, other)
Tumors involving the stalk and hypothalamus
    Craniopharyngioma
    Meningioma
    Glioma
    Hamartoma
Infections
    Tuberculosis
    Syphilis
    Fungal
    Meningitis
    Malaria
Vascular
    Postpartum infarction
    Infarction of a pituitary tumor
    Vasculitis—temporal arteritis
    Aneurysm of the internal carotid artery
    Cavernous sinus thrombosis
    Sickle cell disease
    Arteriosclerosis
Infiltrative disease
    Hemochromatosis
    Histiocytosis
        (e.g., Hand-Schüller-Christian disease)
    Sarcoidosis
Miscellaneous
    Basal skull fracture
    Empty sella syndrome
    Idiopathic hypothalamic defect, usually monotrophic
    Functional (usually amenorrhea only)
Iatrogenic
    Exogenous glucocorticoids
    Irradiation
    Surgical hypophysectomy or stalk section

Stress, exercise, and weight change can also inhibit gonadotropin secretion, perhaps because of an effect of opiate peptides on Gn-RH. This rarely causes clinical hypogonadism in men but often produces amenorrhea in women, probably because a more tightly regulated sequence of events must occur to trigger follicular development and ovulation. Hypothalamic amenorrhea commonly occurs in the absence of apparent hypothalamic-pituitary disease; gonadotropins and estradiol levels may be normal. In the absence of hypogonadotropism, severe estrogen deficiency, or thyroid or adrenal hypofunction, a full work-up with radiographic studies of the hypothalamus and pituitary may not be necessary.

BIBLIOGRAPHY

Growth Hormone Physiology

Baumann G, Stolar MW, Amburn H, et al. A specific growth hormone-binding protein in human plasma: Initial characterization. J Clin Endocrinol Metab 1986; 62:134.

Daughaday WH, Kapadia M, Mariz I. Serum somatomedin binding proteins: Physiologic significance and interference in radioligand assay. J Lab Clin Med 1987; 109:355.

Efendic S, Hokfelt T, Luft R. Somatostatin. Adv Metab Disord 1978; 9:367.

Gelato MC, Merriam GR. Growth hormone releasing hormone. Annu Rev Physiol 1986; 48:569.

Goodman HM. Basic medical endocrinology. New York: Raven Press, 1988:236.

Guyda HJ, Corvol MT, Rappaport R, Posner BI. Radioreceptor assay of insulin-like peptides in human plasma: Growth hormone dependence and correlation with sulfation activity by two bioassays. J Clin Endocrinol Metab 1979; 48:739.

Hendricks CM, Eastman RC, Takeda S, et al. Plasma clearance of intravenously administered pituitary growth hormone: Gel filtration studies of heterogeneous components. J Clin Endocrinol Metab 1985; 60:864.

Lundbaek K. Somatostatin: Clinical importance and outlook. Metabolism 1978; 27(Suppl 1):1463.

Pawel MA, Sassin JF, Weitzman ED. The temporal relation between HGH release and sleep stage changes at nocturnal sleep onset in man. Life Sci 1972; 11:587.

Quabbe HJ. Chronobiology of growth hormone secretion. Chronobiologia 1977; 4:217.

Stolar MW, Amburn K, Baumann G. Plasma "big" and "big-big" growth hormone(GH) in man: An oligomeric series composed of structualy diverse GH monomers. J Clin Endocrinol Metab 1984; 59:212.

Thorner MO, Vance ML, Evans WS, et al. Physiological and clinical studies of GRF and GH. Recent Prog Horm Res 1986; 42:589.

Thorner MO, Vance ML, Evans WS, et al. Clinical studies with GHRH in man. Horm Res 1986; 24:91.

Utiger RD, Parker ML, Daughaday WH. Studies on human growth hormone. I. A radio-immunoassay for human growth hormone. J Clin Invest 1962; 41:254.

Zapf J, Froesch ER. Pathophysiological and clinical aspects of the insulin-like growth factors. Horm Res 1986; 24:160.

Acromegaly

Clinical Features

Baumann G. Acromegaly. Endocrinol Metab Clin North Am 1987; 16:685.

Eastman RC, Roth J. Growth hormone. In: Melmon KL, Morrelli HF, eds. Clinical pharmacology. New York: Macmillan, 1978:560.

Eskildsen PC, Parving HH, Mogensen CE, Christiansen JS. Kidney function in acromegaly. Acta Med Scand [Suppl] 1979; 624:79.

Evans CC, Hipkin LJ, Murray GM. Pulmonary function in acromegaly. Thorax 1977; 32:322.

Harrison BD, Millhouse KA, Harrington M, Naborro JD. Lung function in acromegaly. Q J Med 1978; 47:517.

Hart TB, Radow SK, Blackard WG, et al. Sleep apnea in active acromegaly. Arch Intern Med 1985; 145:865.

McGuffin WS, Sherman BM, Roth J, et al. Acromegaly and cardiovascular disorders. A prospective study. Ann Intern Med 1974; 81:11.

Muggeo M, Bar RS, Roth J, et al. The insulin resistance of acromegaly: Evidence for two alterations in the insulin receptor on circulating monocytes. J Clin Endocrinol Metab 1979; 48:17.

O'Duffy JD, Randall RV, MacCarty CS. Median neuropathy (carpal-tunnel syndrome) in acromegaly. Ann Intern Med 1973; 78:379.

Roth J, Glick SM, Cuatrecasas P. Acromegaly and other disorders of growth hormone secretion. Ann Intern Med 1967; 66:760.

Savage DD, Henry WL, Eastman RC, et al. Echocardiographic assessment of cardiac anatomy and function in acromegalic patients. Am J Med 1979; 67:823.

Slatopolsky E, Rutherford WE, Rosenbaum R, et al. Hyperphosphatemia. Clin Nephrol 1977; 7:138.

Sober AJ, Gorden P, Roth J, AvRuskin TW. Visceromegaly in acromegaly. Arch Intern Med 1974; 134:415.

Thomson JA, McCrossan J, Mason D. Salivary gland enlargement in acromegaly. Clin Endocrinol 1974; 3:1.

Etiology

Asa SL, Bilbao JM, Kovacs K, Linfoot JA. Hypothalamic neuronal hamartoma associated with pituitary growth hormone cell adenoma and acromegaly. Acta Neuropathol (Berl) 1980; 52:231.

Barkan AL, Shenker Y, Grekin RJ, et al. Acromegaly due to ectopic growth hormone (GH)–releasing hormone (GHRH) production: Dynamic studies of GH and ectopic GHRH secretion. J Clin Endocrinol Metab 1986; 63:1057.

Boizel R, Halimi S, Labat F, et al. Acromegaly due to a growth hormone–releasing hormone–secreting bronchial carcinoid tumor: Further information on the abnormal responsiveness of the somatotroph cells and their recovery after successful treatment. J Clin Endocrinol Metab 1987; 64:304.

Leedman PJ, Cohen AK, Matz LR. The complex of myxomas, spotty pigmentation and endocrine overactivity. Clin Endocrinol 1986; 25:527.

Scheithauer BW, Kovacs K, Randall RV, et al. Pathology of excessive production of growth hormone. Clin Endocrinol Metab 1988; 15:655.

Toshiaki S, Asa SL, Kovacs K. Growth hormone-releasing hormone-producing tumors: Clinical, biochemical, and morphological manifestations. Endocr Rev 1988; 9:357.

Growth Hormone Secretion in Acromegaly

Bala RM, Bhaumick B. Radioimmunoassay of a basis somatomedin: Comparison of various assay techniques and somatomedin levels in various sera. J Clin Endocrinol Metab 1979; 49:770.

Baxter RC, Brown AS, Turtle JR. Radioimmunoassay for somatomedin C: Comparison with radioreceptor assay in patients with growth-hormone disorders, hypothyroidism, and renal failure. Clin Chem 1982; 28:488.

Belchetz PE. Growth hormone responses to hp GRF 1-44 amide, bromocriptine and stress in acromegaly are correlated. Postgrad Med J 1987; 63:241.

Best JD, Alford FP, Chisholm DJ, et al. An evaluation of dynamic pituitary function tests in patients with pituitary tumours. Aust NZ J Med 1982; 12:231.

Burrin JM, Paterson JL, Sharp PS, Yeo TH. Monoclonal and polyclonal antibodies compared for radioimmunoassay of somatomedin-C in patients with acromegaly or hypopituitarism. Clin Chem 1987; 33:1593.

Camanni F, Massara F, Belforte L, et al. Effect of dopamine on plasma growth hormone and prolactin levels in normal and acromegalic subjects. J Clin Endocrinol Metab 1977; 44:465.

Chiodini PG, Liuzzi A, Dallabonzana D, et al. Changes in growth hormone (GH) secretion induced by human pancreatic GH releasing hormone-44 in acromegaly: A comparison with thyrotropin-releasing hormone and bromocriptine. J Clin Endocrinol Metab 1985; 60:48.

Christensen SE, Weeke J, Orskov H, et al. Plasma growth hormone in acromegalic patients. Demonstration of highly reproducible diurnal profiles in individual patients. Acta Endocrinol 1987; 116:49.

Clemmons DR, Underwood LE. Somatomedin-C/insulin-like growth factor I in acromegaly. Clin Endocrinol Metab 1986; 15:629.

Clemmons DR, Underwood LE, Ridgway EC, et al. Hyperprolactinemia is assoicated with increased somatomedin-C in hypopituitarism. J Clin Endocrinol Metab 1981; 52:731.

Clemmons DR, Van Wyk JJ, Ridgway EC, et al. Evaluation of acromegaly by radioimmunoassay of somatomedin-C. N Engl J Med 1979; 301:1138.

Coutant G, Vandeweghe M, Vermeulen A. Comparison of TRF, propranolol-glucagon, insulin and glucose stimulation tests in acromegaly. Horm Metab Res 1977; 9:17.

Cozzi R, Dallabonzana D, Oppizzi G, et al. Bromocriptine does not alter growth hormone (GH) responsiveness to GH-releasing hormone in acromegaly. J Clin Endocrinol Meab 1986; 62:601.

Earll JM, Sparks LL, Forsham PH. Glucose suppression of serum growth hormone in the diagnosis of acromegaly. JAMA 1967; 291:134.

Furlanetto RW, Underwood LE, Van Wyk JJ, D'Ercole AJ. Estimation of somatomedin-C levels in normals and patients with pituitary disease by radioimmunoassay. J Clin Invest 1977; 60:648.

Gelato MC, Rock J, Oldfield EH, et al. Effects of growth hormone-releasing factor on growth hormone secretion in acromegaly. J Clin Endocrinol Metab 1985; 60:251.

Glass AR, Schaaf M, Dimond RC. Amitriptyline-induced suppression of growth hormone in acromegaly. Psychoneuroendocrinology 1980; 5:81.

Hanew K, Sasaki A, Sato S, et al. Growth hormone inhibitory and stimulatory actions of L-dopa in patients with acromegaly. J Clin Endocrinol Metab 1987; 64:255.

Hintz RL, Liu F, Seegan G. Characterization of an insulin-like growth factor-I/somatomedin-C radioimmunoassay specific for the C-peptide region. J Clin Endocrinol Metab 1982; 55:927.

Ikuyama S, Nawata H, Katok, et al. Plasma growth hormone responses to somatostatin (SRIH) and SRIH receptors in pituitary adenomas in acromegalic patients. J Clin Endocrinol Metab 1986; 62:729.

Ishibashi M, Yamaji T, Kosaka K. Effect of bromoergocriptine on TRH-induced growth hormone and prolactin release in acromegalic patients. J Clin Endocrinol Metab 1977; 45:275.

Ishibashi M, Yamaji T, Kosaka K. Induction of growth hormone and prolactin secretion by luteinizing hormone-releasing hormone and its blockade by bromoergocriptine in acromegalic patients. J Clin Endocrinol Metab 1978; 47:418.

Lamberts SW, Klijn JG, Kwa GH, Birkenhager JC. The dynamics of growth hormone and prolactin secretion in acromegalic patients with "mixed" pituitary tumours. Acta Endocrinol 1979; 90:198.

Lindholm J, Dige-Petersen H, Hummer L, et al. Effect of thyrotrophin releasing hormone (TRH) in patients with pituitary disorders. Acta Endocrinol 1977; 85:479.

Muller EE, Salerno F, Cocchi D, et al. Interaction between the thyrotrophin-releasing hormone-induced growth hormone rise and dopaminergic drugs: Studies in pathologic conditions of the animal and man. Clin Endocrinol 1979; 11:645.

Nakagawa K, Ohara T. Failure of growth hormone-suppressing agents to affect TSH-releasing hormone– and LH-releasing hormone-induced growth hormone release in acromegaly. J Clin endocrinol Metab 1977; 44:189.

Oppizzi G, Petroncini MM, Dallabonzana D, et al. Relationship between somatomedin-C and growth hormone levels in acromegaly: Basal and dynamic evaluation. J Clin Endocrinol Metab 1986; 63:1348.

Penny ES, Penman E, Price J, et al. Circulating growth hormone releasing factor concentrations in normal subjects and patients with acromegaly. Br Med J 1984; 289:453.

Rieu M, Girard F, Bricaire H, Binoux M. The importance of insulin-like growth factor (somatomedin) measurements in the diagnosis and surveillance of acromegaly. J Clin Endocrinol Metab 1982; 55:147.

Roelfsema F, Frolich M, Van Dulken H. Somatomedin-C levels in treated and untreated patients with acromegaly. Clin Endocrinol 1987; 26:137.

Shibasaki T, Hotta M, Masuda A, et al. Studies on the response of growth hormone (GH) secretion to GH-releasing hormone, thyrotropin-releasing hormone, gonadotropin-releasing hormone, and somatostatin in acromegaly. J Clin Endocrinol Metab 1986; 63:167.

Smals AE, Pieters GF, Smals AG, et al. Growth hormone responses to the releasing hormones GHRH and GnRH and the inhibitors somatostatin and bromocriptine in TRH-responsive and non-responsive acromegalics. Acta Endocrinol 1987; 116:53.

Smals AE, Pieters GF, Smals AG, et al. The higher the growth hormone response to growth hormone releasing hormone the lower the response to bromocriptine and thyrotrophin releasing hormone in acromegaly. Clin Endocrinol 1987; 27:43.

Teale JD, Marks V. The measurement of insulin-like growth factor I: Clinical applications and significance. Ann Clin Biochem 1986; 23:413.

Thorner MO, Frohman LA, Leong DA, et al. Extrahypothalamic growth-hormone-releasing factor (GRF) secretion is a rare cause of acromegaly: Plasma GRF levels in 177 acromegalic patients. J Clin Endocrinol Meab 1984; 59:846.

Werner S. Regulation of growth hormone secretion during normal conditions and in patients with acromegaly. Acta Endocrinol 1978; 216:179.

Pseudoacromegaly

Ashcroft MW, Van Herle AJ, Bersch N, Golde DW. A new growth stimulatory factor in patients with acromegaly. J Clin Endocrinol Metab 1983; 57:272.

Daughaday WH, Starkey RH, Saltman S, et al. Characterization of serum growth hormone (GH) and insulin-like growth factor I in active acromegaly with minimal elevation of serum GH. J Clin Endocrinol Metab 1987; 65:617.

Feingold KR, Goldfine ID, Weinstein PR. Acromegaly with normal growth-hormone levels and pituitary histology. Case report. J Neurosurg 1979; 50:503.

Hoffenberg R, Howell A, Epstein S, et al. Increasing growth with raised circulating somatomedin but normal immunoassayable growth hormone. Clin Endocrinol 1977; 6:443.

Evaluation of Treatment

Aloia JF, Archambeau JO. Hypopituitarism following pituitary irradiation for acromegaly. Horm Res 1978; 9:201.

Arafah BM, Rosenzweig JL, Fenstermaker R, et al. Value of growth hormone dynamics and somatomedin C (insulin-like growth factor I) levels in predicting the long-term benefit after transsphenoidal surgery for acromegaly. J Lab Clin Med 1987; 109:346.

Daggett PR, Nabarro JD. Measurement of the 24 hour intergrated plasma concentration of growth hormone, in assessing the response of acromegalic patients to treatment. Clin Endocrinol 1977; 7:437.

De Pablo F, Eastman RC, Roth J, Gorden P. Plasma prolactin in acromegaly before and after treatment. J Clin Endocrinol Metab 1981; 53:344.

Eastman RC, Gorden P, Roth J. Conventional supervoltage irradiation is an effective treatment for acromegaly. J Clin Endocrinol Metab 1979; 48:931.

Faglia G, Paracchi A, Ferrari C, Beck-Peccoz P. Evaluation of the results of trans-sphenoidal surgery in acromegaly by assessment of the growth hormone response to thyrotrophin-releasing hormone. Clin Endocrinol 1978; 8:373.

Giusti M, Lomeo A, Monachesi M, et al. The GH-releasing hormone (GHRH) test in acromegaly before and after adenomectomy. J Endocrinol Invest 1987; 10:143.

Hulting AL, Werner S, Wersall J, et al. Normal growth hormone secretion is rare after microsurgical normalization of growth hormone levels in acromegaly. Acta Med Scand 1982; 212:401.

Karashima T, Kato K, Nawata H, et al. Postoperative plasma GH levels and restoration of GH dynamics in acromegalic patients surgically treated by the transsphenoidal approach. Clin Endocrinol 1986; 25:157.

Karashima T, Kato K, Nawata H, et al. Long-term bromocriptine therapy and predictive tests in acromegaly. Endocrinol Jpn 1986; 33:163.

Shalet SM, MacFarlane IA, Beardwell CG. Radiation-induced hyperprolactinaemia in a treated acromegalic. Clin Endocrinol 1979; 11:169.

Snyder PJ, Fowble BF, Norman JS, et al. Hypopituitarism following radiation therapy of pituitary adenomas. Am J Med 1986; 81:457.

Hyperprolactinemia

Prolactin Physiology

Armeanu MC, Frolich M, Lequin RM. Circadian rhythm of prolactin during the menstrual cycle. Fertil Steril 1986; 46:315.

Blank MS, Dufau ML. Definition of bioactive prolactin pulsations during the menstrual cycle. Clin Endocrinol 1986; 24:1.

Brisson GR, Peronnet F, Ledoux M, et al. Temperature-induced hyperprolactinemia during exercise. Horm Metab Res 1986; 18:283.

Conti A, Togni E, Travaglini P, et al. Vasoactive intestinal polypeptide and dopamine: Effect on prolactin secretion in normal women and patients with microprolactinomas. Neuroendocrinology 1987; 46:241.

Jordan RM, Tresp NM, Kohler PO. Human prolactin heterogeneity in pituitary effluent blood. Horm Metab Res 1985; 17:598.

Kato Y, Shimatsu A, Matsushita N, et al. Role of vasoactive intestinal polypeptide (VIP) in regulating the pituitary function in man. Peptides 1984; 5:389.

Liu JH, Park KH. Gonadotropin and prolactin secretion increases during sleep during the puerperium in nonlactating women. J Clin Endocrinol Metab 1988; 66:839.

Malarkey WB, Jackson R, Wortsman J. Long-term assessment of patients with macroprolactinemia. Fertil Steril 1988; 50:413.

Markoff E, Lee DW. Glycosylated prolactin is a major circulating variant in human serum. J Clin Endocrinol Metab 1987; 65:1102.

Markoff E, Lee DW, Hollingsworth DR. Glycosylated and nonglycosylated prolactin in serum during pregnancy. J Clin Endocrinol Metab 1988; 67:519.

Rolandi E, Ragni N, Fanceschini R, et al. Possible role of vasoactive intestinal polypeptide on prolactin release during suckling in lactating women. Horm Res 1987; 27:211.

Salvador J, Dieguez C, Scanlon MF. The circadian rhythms of thyrotrophin and prolactin secretion. Chronobiol Int 1988; 5:85.

Sassin JF, Frantz AG, Weitzman ED, Kapen S. Human prolactin: 24-hour pattern with increased release during sleep. Science 1972; 177:1205.

Mechanism of Action

Clapp DH, Wiebe RH. The effect of hyperprolactinemia on the diurnal variation of adrenal androgens. Fertil Steril 1983; 39:749.

Cutie E, Andino NA. Prolactin inhibits the steroidogenesis in midfollicular phase human granulosa cells cultured in a chemically defined medium. Fertil Steril 1988; 49:632.

Whitworth NS. Lactation in humans. Psychoneuroendocrinology 1988; 13:171.

Clinical Manifestations

Chang RJ. Hyperprolactinemia and menstrual dysfunction. Clin Obstet Gynecol 1983; 26:736.

Gomez F, Reyes FI, Faiman C. Nonpuerperal galactorrhea and hyperprolactinemis. Am J Med 1977; 62:648.

Kleinberg D, Noel GL, Frantz AG. Galactorrhea; a study of 285 cases, including 48 patients with pituitary tumors. N Engl J Med 1977; 296:589.

Sakiyama R, Quan M. Galactorrhea and hyperprolactinemia. Obstet Gynecol Surv 1983; 38:689.

Vanrell JA, Balasch J. Prolactin in the evaluation of luteal phase in infertility. Fertil Steril 1983; 39:30.

Assay

Frantz AG, Kleinberg DL. Prolactin: Evidence that it is separate from growth hormone in human blood. Science 1970; 170:745.

Rose DP, Berke B, Cohen LA. Serum prolactin and growth hormone determined by radioimmunoassay and a two-site immunoradiometric assay: Comparison with the Nb2 cell bioassay. Horm Metab Res 1988; 20:49.

Tanaka T, Shiu RPC, Gout PW, et al. A sensitive and specific bioassay for lactogenic hormones; measurement of prolactin and growth hormone in human serum. J Clin Endocrinol Metab 1980; 51:1058.

Specific Causes

Anderson RE, Ben-Rafael Z, Flickinger GL, et al. Secretory dynamics of bioactive and immunoreactive prolactin in polycystic ovary syndrome. Fertil Steril 1988; 49:239.

Barbarino A, De-Marinis L, Mancini A, et al. Prolactin dynamics in normoprolactinemic primary empty sella: Correlation with intracranial pressure. Horm Res 1987; 27:141.

Bauer AG, Wilson JH, Lamberts SW, Blom W. Hyperprolactinemia in hepatic encephalopathy: The effect of infusion of an amino acid mixture with excess branched chain amino acids. Hepatogastroenterology 1983; 30:174.

Biasioli S, D'Andrea G, Micieli G, et al. Hyperprolactinemia as a marker of neurotransmitter imbalance in uremic population. Int J Artif Organs 1987; 10:245.

Celani MF, Giambuzzi G, Simoni M, Montanini V. Subnormal prolactin responsiveness to thyrotropin-releasing hormone (TRH) in women with primary empty sella syndrome. J Endocrinol Invest 1987; 10:421.

Fish LH, Mariash CN. Hyperprolactinemia, infertility, and hypothyroidism. A case report and literature review. Arch Intern Med 1988; 148:709.

Green AI, Brown WA. Prolactin and neuroleptic drugs. Neurol Clin 1988; 6:213.

Hershon KS, Kelly WA, Shaw CM, et al. Prolactinomas as part of the multiple endocrine neoplastic syndrome type 1. Am J Med 1983; 74:713.

Kapcala LP, Molitch ME, Jackson IMD, et al. Galactorrhea, amenorrhea with craniopharyngioma. J Clin Endocrinol Metab 1980; 51:798.

Malarkey WB, Goodenow TJ, Lanese RR. Diurnal variation of prolactin secretion differentiates pituitary tumors from the primary empty sella syndrome. Am J Med 1980; 69:886.

Mastrogiacomo I, De-Besi L, Serafini E, et al. Hyperprolactinemia and sexual disturbances among uremic women on hemodialysis. Nephron 1984; 37:195.

Mastrogiacomo I, De-Besi L, Zucchetta P, et al. Male hypogonadism of uremic patients on hemodialysis. Arch Androl 1988; 20:171.

Mayer G, Koverik J, Pohanka E, et al. Serum prolactin levels after kidney transplantation. Transplant Proc 1987; 19:3724.

Molitch ME, Schwartz S, Mukherji B. Is prolactin secreted ectopically? Am J Med 1981; 70:803.

Muller EE, Locatelli V, Cella S, et al. Prolactin-lowering and -releasing drugs. Mechanisms of action and therapeutic applications. Drugs 1983; 25:399.

Serri O, Robert F, Comtois R, et al. Distinctive features of prolactin secretion in acromegalic patients with hyperprolactinaemia. Clin Endocrinol 1987; 27:429.

Spitz IM, Sheinfeld M, Glasser B, Hirsch HJ. Hyperthyroidism due to inappropriate TSH secretion with associated hyperprolactinaemia—a case report and review of the literature. Postgrad Med J 1984; 60:328.

Wortsman J, Carlson HE, MaLarkey WB. Macroprolactinemia as the cause of elevated serum prolactin in men. Am J Med 1989; 86:704.

Dynamic Testing

Boyd AE, Reichlin S, Turksoy RN. Galactorrhea-amenorrhea syndrome: Diagnosis and therapy. Ann Intern Med 1977; 87:165.

Friesen H, Guyda H, Hwang P, et al. Functional evaluation of prolactin secretion: A guide to therapy. J Clin Invest 1972; 51:706.

Iannotta F, Fachinetti P, Fachinetti A, et al. Nomifensine, TRH and insulin-induced hypoglycemia tests in the diagnosis of prolactinomas. J Endocrinol Invest 1983; 6:353.

Evaluation of Treatment

Murphy FY, Vesely DL, Jordan RM, et al. Giant invasive prolactinomas. Am J Med 1987; 83:995.

Rodman EF, Molitch ME, Post KD, et al. Long-term follow-up of transsphenoidal selective adenomectomy for prolactinoma. JAMA 1984; 252:921.

Serri O, Rasio E, Beauregard H, et al. Recurrence of hyperprolactinemia after selective transsphenoidal adenomectomy in women with prolactinoma. N Engl J Med 1983; 309:280.

Pregnancy and Hyperprolactinemia

Gangemi M, Meneghetti G, Benato M, et al. Hyperprolactinemia and pregnancy. Clinical series. Clin Exp Obstet Gynecol 1983; 10:108.

Husami N, Jewelewicx R, Vande Wiele RL. Pregnancy in patients with pituitary tumors. Fertil Steril 1977; 28:920.

Magyar DM, Marshall JR. Pituitary tumors and pregnancy. Am J Obstet Gynecol 1978; 132:739.

Rigg LA, Lein A, Yen SSC. Pattern of increase in circulating prolactin levels during human gestation. Am J Obstet Gynecol 1977; 129:454.

Samaan NA, Leavens ME, Sacca R, et al. The effects of pregnancy on patients with hyperprolactinemia. Am J Obstet Gynecol 1984; 148:466.

Gonadotropin-Secreting Neoplasms

Beckers A, Stevenaert A, Mashiter K, Hennen G. Follicle-stimulating hormone-secreting pituitary adenomas. J Clin Endocrinol Metab 1985; 61:525.

Demura R, Jibiki K, Kubo O, et al. The significance of alpha-subunit as a tumor marker for gonadotropin-producing pituitary adenomas. J Clin Endocrinol Metab 1986; 63:564.

Klibanski A. Nonsecreting pituitary tumors. Endocrinol Metab Clin North Am 1987; 16:793.

Lawton NF, Evans AJ, Pickard JD, et al. Secretion of neuron-specific enolase, prolactin, growth hormone, luteinising hormone and follicle stimulating hormone by "functionless" and endocrine-active pituitary tumours in vitro. J Neurol Neurosurg Psychiatry 1986; 49:574.

Lamberts SW, Verleun T, Oosterom R, et al. The effects of bromocriptine, thyrotropin-releasing hormone, and gonadotropin-releasing hormone on hormone secretion of gonadotropin-secreting pituitary adenomas in vivo and in vitro. J Clin Endocrinol Metab 1987; 64:524.

Snyder PJ. Gonadotroph cell pituitary adenomas. Endocrinol Metab Clin North Am 1987; 16:755.

Snyder PJ, Muzyka R, Johnson J, Utiger RD. Thyrotropin releasing hormone provokes abnormal follicle-stimulating hormone (FSH) and luteinizing hormone responses in men who have pituitary adenomas and FSH hypersecretion. J Clin Endocrinol Metab 1980; 51:744.

Hypopituitarism
Hypogonadotropic Hypogonadism

Arafah BM. Reversible hypopituitarism in patients with large nonfunctioning pituitary adenomas. J Clin Endocrinol Metab 1986; 62:1173–9.

Snyder PJ, Bigdeli H, Gardner DF, et al. Gonadal function in fifty men with untreated pituitary adenomas. J Clin Endocrinol Metab 1979; 48:309.

Snyder PJ, Rudenstein RS, Gardner DF, Rothman JG. Repetitive infusion of gonadotropin-releasing hormone distinguishes hypothalamic from pituitary hypogonadism. J Clin Endocrinol Metab 1979; 48:864.

Vigersky RA, Loriaux DL, Andersen AE, et al. Delayed pituitary hormone response to LRF and TRF in patients with anorexia nervosa and with secondary amenorrhea associated with simple weight loss. J Clin Endocrinol Metab 1976; 43:893.

Woolf PD, Hamill RW, McDonald JV, et al. Transient hypogonadotropic hypogonadism caused by critical illness. J Clin Endocrinol Metab 1985; 60:444.

Growth Hormone Deficiency

Baxter RC, Brown AS, Turtle JR. Radioimmunoassay for somatomedin C: Comparison with radioreceptor assay in patients with growth-hormone disorders, hypothyroidism, and renal failure. Clin Chem 1982; 28:488.

Clemmons DR, Van Wyk JJ. Factors controlling blood concentration of somatomedin C. Clin Endocrinol Metab 1984; 13:113.

Eddy RL, Gilliland PF, Ibarra JD Jr, et al. Human growth hormone release. Comparison of provocative test procedures. Am J Med 1974; 56:179.

Jackson IM. Thyrotropin releasing hormone. N Engl J Med 1982; 306:145.

Laron Z, Gilad I, Topper E, et al. Low oral dose of clonidine: An effective screening test for growth hormone deficiency. Acta Paediatr Scand 1982; 71:847.

Laron Z, Keret R, Bauman B, et al. Differential diagnosis between hypothalamic and pituitary hGH deficiency with the aid of synthetic GH-RH 1-44. Clin Endocrinol 1984;21:9.

Schriock EA, Lustig RH, Rosenthal SM, et al. Effect of growth hormone (GH)-releasing hormone (GRH) on plasma GH in relation to magnitude and duration of GH deficiency in 26 children and adults with isolated GH deficiency or multiple pituitary hormone deficiencies: Evidence for hypothalamic GRH deficiency. J Clin Endocrinol Metab 1984; 58:1043.

Topper E, Gilad I, Bauman B, et al. Plasma growth hormone response to oral clonidine as compared to insulin hypoglycemia in obese children and adolescents. Horm Metab Res 1984; 16:127.

Williams T, Maxon H, Thorner MO, Frohman LA. Blunted growth hormone (GH) response to GH-releasing hormone in hypothyroidism resolves in the euthyroid state. J Clin Endocrinol Metab 1985; 61:454.

Williams T, Berelowitz M, Joffe SN, et al. Impaired growth hormone responses to growth hormone-releasing factor in obesity. A pituitary defect reversed with weight reduction. N Engl J Med 1984; 29:1403.

ACTH Deficiency

Borst GC, Michenfelder HJ, O'Brian JT. Discordant cortisol response to exogenous ACTH and insulin-induced hypoglycemia in patients with pituitary disease. N Engl J Med 1982; 306:1462.

DeBold C, Orth DN, DeCherney GS, et al. Corticotropin-releasing hormone: Stimulation of ACTH secretion in normal man. Horm Metab Res [Suppl] 1987; 16:8.

Hermus AR, Pieters GF, Pesman GJ, et al. CRH as a diagnostic and heuristic tool in hypothalamic-pituitary diseases. Horm Metab Res 1987; 16:68.

Lindholm J, Kehlet H, Blichert-Toft M, et al. Reliability of the 30-minute ACTH test in assessing hypothalamic-pituitary-adrenal function. J Clin Endocrinol Metab 1978; 47:272.

Nelson JC, Tindall DJ Jr. A comparison of the adrenal responses to hypoglycemia, metyrapone and ACTH. Am J Med Sci 1978; 275:165.

Schurmeyer TH, Tsokos GC, Avgerinos PC, et al. Pituitary-adrenal responsiveness to corticotropin-releasing hormone in patients receiving chronic alternate-day glucocorticoid therapy. J Clin Endocrinol Metab 1985; 61:22.

Spiger M, Jubiz W, Meikle AW, et al. Single-dose metyrapone test: Review of a four-year experience. Arch Intern Med 1975; 135:698.

Multiple Releasing Hormone Tests

Cohen KL. Metabolic, endocrine, and drug induced interference with pituitary function tests: A review. Metabolism 1977; 26:1165.

Goldzieher JW, Dozier TS, Smith KD, Steinberger E. Improving the diagnostic reliability of rapidly fluctuating plasma hormone levels by optimized multiple-sampling techniques. J Clin Endocrinol Metab 1976; 43:824.

Holl RW, Loos U, Hetzel WD, et al. Combined pituitary stimulation test: Interactions of hypothalamic releasing hormones in man. J Endocrinol Invest 1988; 11:219.

Mortimer CH, Besser GM, McNeilly AS, et al. Interaction between secretion of the gonadotrophins, prolactin, growth hormone, thyrotrophin and corticosteroids in man: The effects of LH, FSH-RH, TRH and hypoglycaemia alone and in combination. Clin Endocrinol 1973; 2:317.

Sheldon WR Jr, DeBold CR, Evans WS, et al. Rapid sequential intravenous administration of four hypothalamic releasing hormones as a combined anterior pituitary function test in normal subjects. J Clin Endocrinol Metabl 19854; 60:623.

Etiology

Asa SL, Bilbao JM, Kovacs K, et al. Lymphocytic hypophysitis of pregnancy resulting in hypopituitarism: A distinct clinicopathologic entity. Ann Intern Med 1981; 95:166.

Cardoso ER, Peterson EW. Pituitary apoplexy: A review. Neurosurgery 1984; 14:363.

Mohr G, Hardy J. Hemorrhage, necrosis, and apoplexy in pituitary adenomas. Surg Neurol 1982; 18:181.

Pelkonen R, Kuusisto A, Salmi J, et al. Pituitary function after pituitary apoplexy. Am J Med 1978; 65:773.

Stocks AE, Powell LW. Pituitary function in idiopathic haemochromatosis and cirrhosis of the liver. Lancet 1972; 2:298.

Williams TC, Frohman LA. Hypothalamic dysfunction associated with hemochromatosis. Ann Intern Med 1985; 103:550.

4

Growth

Wellington Hung, M.D., Ph.D., F.A.C.P., F.A.A.P.

GROWTH HORMONE PHYSIOLOGY

Growth is a complex physiologic process regulated by the interaction of genetic, hormonal, nutritional, and psychological influences. Aberrations in human growth can result from many endocrine diseases as well as from chronic organic diseases. Central in the endocrine control of growth is growth hormone (GH), a protein with 191 amino acids, the gene for which is located on chromosome 17. GH is secreted by the somatotrope cell of the anterior pituitary gland. Neural control of GH is mediated by GH-releasing hormone (GRH or GH-RH) and somatostatin (GH-releasing inhibiting hormone, SRIF), both of which are secreted into the hypophyseal-portal circulation from neurons in the hypothalamus. The GH-regulating neurons are influenced by monoaminergic and peptidergic neurons and by feedback hormonal effects.

Secretion of GH is pulsatile. In normal children the levels are low for most of the day and cannot be distinguished from those in GH-deficient children. In growing children there are five to nine discrete pulses every 24 hours. After 3 to 6 months of age, the most consistent pulses occur 45 to 90 minutes after the onset of sleep. GH circulates unbound in plasma.

The actions of GH include stimulation of skeletal and muscle growth, promotion of cellular uptake of amino acids, and regulation of lipolysis. GH has insulin-like effects and is also diabetogenic, with anti-insulin effects. Most of the effects of GH on growth are mediated indirectly through a basic peptide, somatomedin-C, which is synthesized in the liver and kidney and circulates in plasma bound to carrier proteins. It is now known that somatomedin-C and insulin-like growth factor I (IGF-I) are identical single-chain proteins with 70 amino acids coded for by a gene on chromosome 12. Somatomedin C stimulates proliferation of cartilage and synthesis of cartilage matrix chondroitin sulfate. Another somatomedin has been identified as a neutral peptide, insulin-like growth factor II (IGF-II), which is a single-chain protein with 67 amino acids coded for by a gene on the short arm of chromosome 11.

INTRAUTERINE GROWTH RETARDATION

Intrauterine growth retardation is a term that can be applied to newborn infants whose birth length and weight are more than two standard deviations below the mean for gestational age, sex and race. The causes are multiple, and some of the more common causes are listed in Table 4-1. Intrauterine growth retardation may be transient or permanent. Hypoxemia, malnutrition, and inadequate intrauterine space due to twinning are associated with transient growth retardation. Most chromosomal abnormalities (except multiple X and Y syndromes); fetal infections such as rubella, toxoplasmosis, and herpes simplex; and maternal consumption of heroin, hydantoin, and excessive tobacco and alcohol are usually associated with permanent stunting. In cases of alcoholism, rubella, heroin addiction, and fetal trisomy syndromes, the physical appearance at birth often suggests the specific cause of the intrauterine growth retardation.

TABLE 4-1 Etiology of Intrauterine Growth Retardation

Maternal factors
  Infections such as rubella, toxoplasmosis,
    herpes simplex
  Toxemia or chronic hypertension
  Short stature (height less than 150 cm)
  Severe malnutrition
  Alcohol abuse
  Cigarette smoking
  Narcotic use
  Ingestion of drugs such as hydantoins

Environmental factors
  Exposure to teratogens
  Residence at high altitude

Placental factors
  Thrombosis of fetal vessels
  Infarcts

Fetal factors
  Multiple fetuses
  Chromosomal abnormalities
  Inborn errors of metabolism

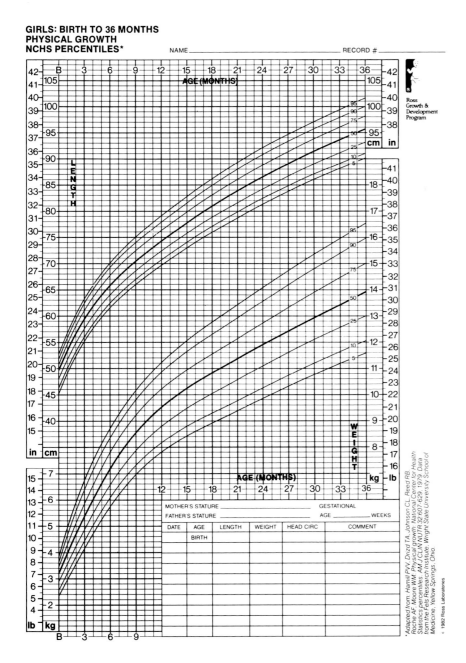

GIRLS: BIRTH TO 36 MONTHS PHYSICAL GROWTH NCHS PERCENTILES*

Figure 4–1 Growth curves for girls, from birth to 36 months of age, developed by the National Center for Health Statistics, 1977.

Neonates with permanent intrauterine growth retardation have head circumferences that may be normal or below normal. After birth these infants' growth rates are below but parallel to the third percentile. Plasma growth hormone levels are usually normal but may be elevated; in some, the plasma somatomedin C levels are subnormal. Most patients have bone ages that correspond to the chronologic age or are only mildly delayed.

NORMAL LINEAR GROWTH AND GROWTH CHARTS

Growth charts have been developed to demonstrate the progressive changes in height and weight with age. These charts consider the range of growth, as expressed either in percentiles or as standard deviation from the mean for average height or weight for age. Growth charts or curves, developed for accumulated height and for growth velocity, are based on either cross-sectional data (in which a number of individuals are measured at different ages) or longitudinal data (in which the same individual is measured at different ages). The cross-sectional curves should be used to determine the position of an individual at a given age, in relation to the general population. In the study of individual children over a period of time, longitudinal curves should be used.

At present, standards for growth for infants, children, and adolescents are based on data compiled by the National Center for Health Statistics of the United States Public Health Service and published in 1977 (Figs. 4–1 to 4–4). More recently, Tanner and Davies (1985) devel-

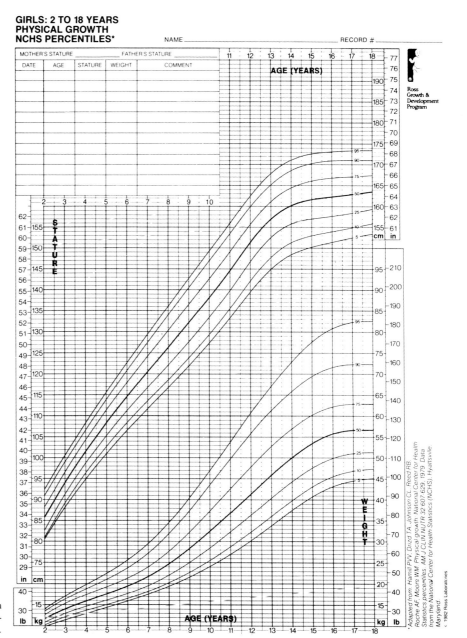

GIRLS: 2 TO 18 YEARS
PHYSICAL GROWTH
NCHS PERCENTILES*

Figure 4-2 Growth curves for girls, from 2 to 18 years of age, developed by the National Center for Health Statistics, 1977.

oped longitudinally derived height and height velocity charts for North American children based on the National Center for Health Statistics data (Figs. 4–5 and 4–6). The National Center for Health Statistics study was based on measurements of 7,000 normal children and adolescents of different ethnic backgrounds. In the last decade, data have been published demonstrating that the growth patterns of black American children differ from those of white children. Growth charts for black American boys and girls are available (Figs. 4–7 and 4–8).

Usually, the linear growth curve of a child from 2 to 3 years of age until puberty follows a specific percentile. Changes in percentile during infancy reflect, in part, intrauterine influences, whereas during puberty they represent variability in the timing and extent of the adolescent growth spurt.

Methods of Linear Measurements

Infants

The most commonly used growth charts for infants up to 3 years of age utilize the length of the infant and require accurate measurement in the supine position. The head should be held firmly against a stationary headboard; the legs should be straight; and a metal tape measure should be extended from the top of the head to the soles of the feet.

Children Over 2 Years of Age

The growth charts for patients over 2 years of age use stature or height. Measuring devices are available to ensure accurate measurement. They include a horizon-

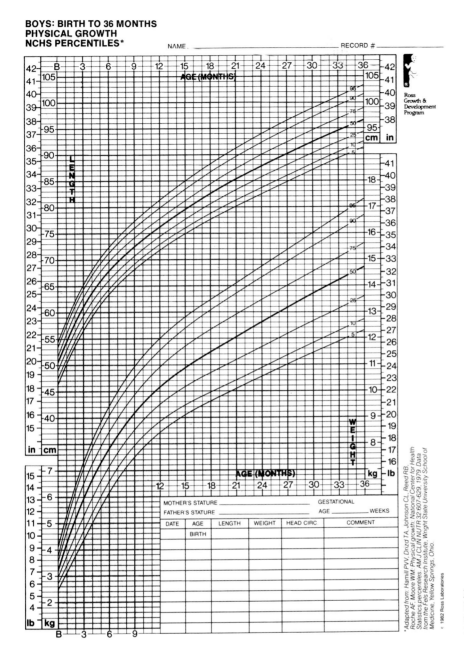

BOYS: BIRTH TO 36 MONTHS
PHYSICAL GROWTH
NCHS PERCENTILES*

Figure 4-3 Growth curves for boys, from birth to 36 months of age, developed by the National Center for Health Statistics, 1977.

tal board that is lowered onto the top of the head and a stationary vertical metal tape measure or a counter attached to the horizontal board to give a digital readout. The patient stands with his or her head firm against the tape measure, knees straightened, and head held erect.

Measurement using the height rod attached to the usual weight scale in the physician's office is not very accurate.

Height Velocity Charts

Linear growth can be evaluated in terms of an increase in height per unit of time, i.e., an increase in centimeters per 6-month period (Figs. 4-9 and 4-10). These charts clearly show significant deviations from average growth for age before the clinician can detect the devia-

tion from standard growth charts. Growth velocity varies with age and sex. Between birth and 6 months of age, boys should grow at least 17 cm and girls at least 16 cm. Between 1 and 2 years of age, boys should grow at least 10 cm and girls at least 11 cm. Boys and girls should grow 6 cm per year between 2 and 5 years of age. After 5 years of age and up to the beginning of the adolescent growth spurt, a growth velocity of less than 5 cm per year is subnormal in both sexes.

BODY PROPORTIONS

Determination of body proportions can provide information that is useful in classifying children and adolescents with short stature. The proportions that have been most widely used are the ratio of the upper body seg-

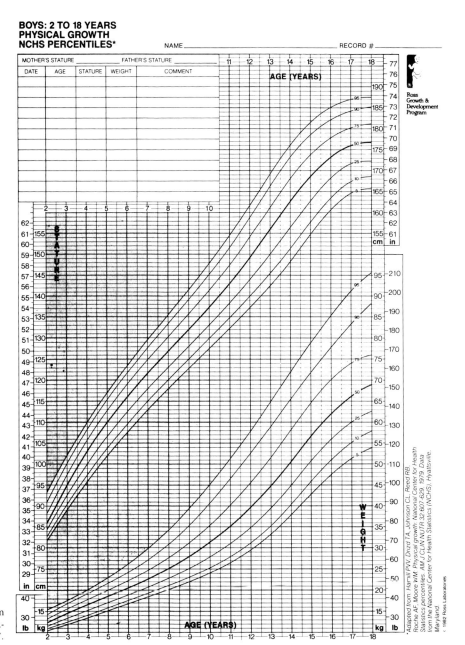

Figure 4-4 Growth curves for boys, from 2 to 18 years of age, developed by the National Center for Health Statistics, 1977.

ment to the lower body segment and the relationship between arm span and height. The lower segment is the distance from the top of the symphysis pubis to the heel. The upper segment measurement is obtained by subtracting the lower segment measurement from the height. Arm span is obtained by measuring across the chest with the upper extremities fully extended. The normal upper to lower segment ratio is different in both sexes at different ages. At birth, the upper to lower segment ratio is 1.7 and gradually decreases with age to 0.05 to 1.01 at the conclusion of growth. The upper to lower segment ratio at 10 years of age is 1.0. McKusick (1972) has published standard upper to lower segment ratios for both

white and black children and for adolescents. Blacks have relatively long limbs and upper to lower segment ratios of approximately 0.85 as adults. Short patients with primary disorders of bone and cartilage or long-standing hypothyroidism have short extremities, giving upper to lower segment ratios higher than expected for age and decreased arm spans. Short children with disorders of nonendocrine organ systems other than bone or cartilage and children with GH deficiency, constitutional delays in growth and maturation, familial short stature, intrauterine growth retardation, psychosocial short stature, and short stature due to a genetic or chromosomal abnormality usually are normally proportioned.

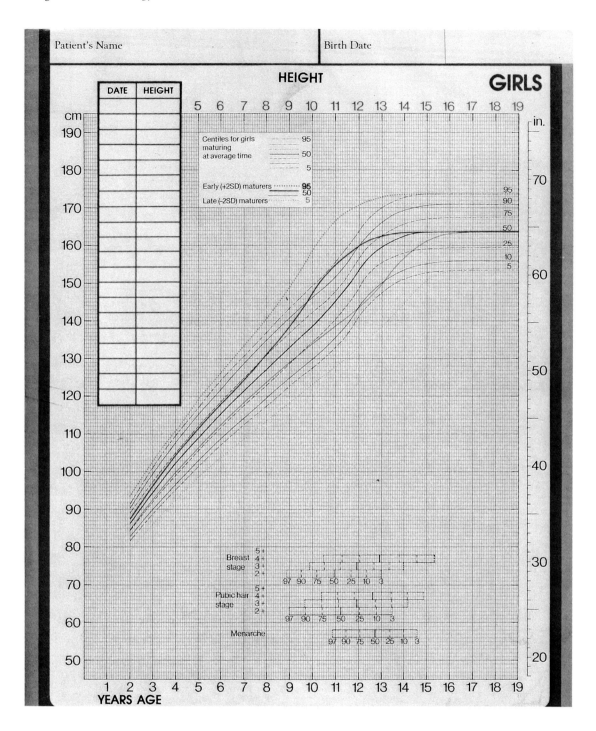

Figure 4-5   Height curve for girls. (From Tanner JM, Davies PW. Clinical longitudinal standards for height and height velocity for North American children. J Pediatr 1985; 107:317–329.) © Castlemead Publications. Distributed by Serono Laboratories, Inc., Randolph, Massachusetts.

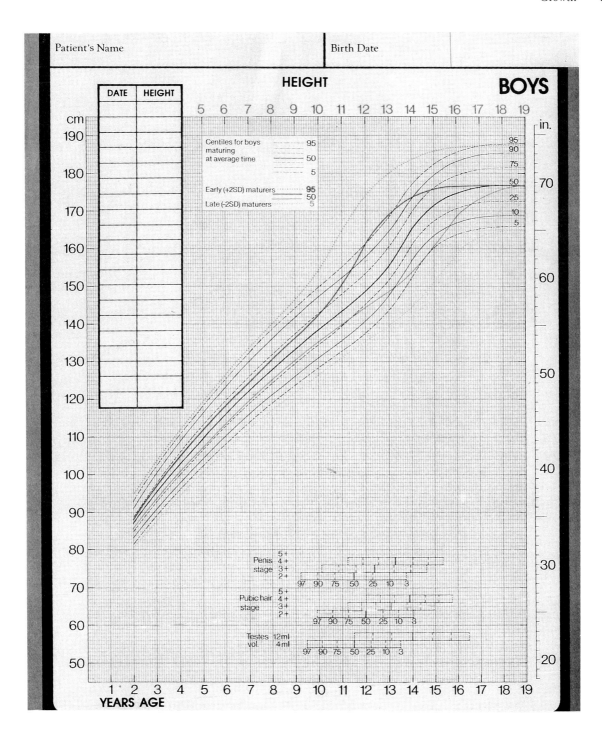

Figure 4-6 Height curve for boys. (From Tanner JM, Davies PW. Clinical longitudinal standards for height and height velocity for North American children. J Pediatr 1985; 107:317–329.) © Castlemead Publications. Distributed by Serono Laboratories, Inc., Randolph, Massachusetts.

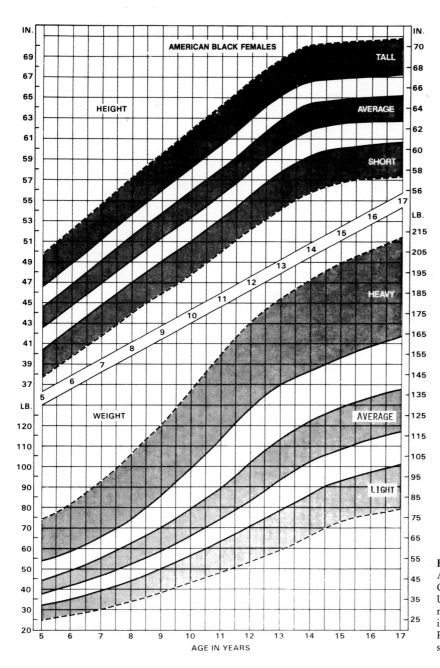

Figure 4-7 Height and weight chart for black American females. (From John H. Spurgeon, College of Health and Physical Education, University of South Carolina, 1977, with permission.) Charts may be obtained by contacting Professor John H. Spurgeon, Dept. of Physical Education, College of Health, University of South Carolina, Columbia, SC 29208.

STAGES OF SEXUAL DEVELOPMENT

Pubertal development, which typically begins between 9 and 14 years of age, consists of several interrelated processes that are initiated and regulated by hormones. Although the increase in circulating hormone levels and the physical changes of sexual maturation are age related, it is well known that the age at onset of puberty and the rate of progression through puberty vary widely. The sequence and age range of onset of physical changes occurring during female and male sexual maturation are illustrated in Figures 4–11 and 4–12.

During clinical examination of males and females, it is frequently necessary to designate how far they have

progressed pubertally, and various rating systems for judging this have been proposed. The most commonly used standards are those of Tanner (1962). He developed standards for stages of genital development in males; pubic hair growth in both sexes; and breast development in females. The standards are presented in Figures 4–13 to 4–16. All ratings are on a scale of 1 to 5, with 1 representing the prepubescent state. The size of the testes is best assessed by palpation in comparison with testicular-shaped models with specific volumes, known as the Prader orchidometer (Fig. 4–17). The models are marked according to their volumes in milliliters: sizes 1, 2, and 3 are prepubertal; 4 indicates the beginning of puberty; and 10 and 12 are usually midpubertal. Most adults reach the size of 15, 20, or 25.

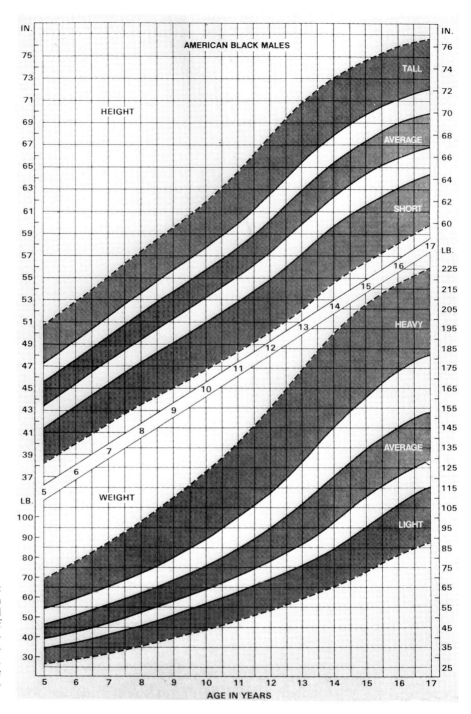

Figure 4-8 Height and weight chart for black American males. (From John H. Spurgeon, College of Health and Physical Education, University of South Carolina, 1977, with permission.) Charts may be obtained by contacting Professor John H. Spurgeon, Dept. of Physical Education, College of Health, University of South Carolina, Columbia, SC 29208.

DELAYED PUBERTY

Delayed puberty may be considered in girls if breast development has not occurred by 13 years of age or if more than 5 years have elapsed between the beginning of breast development and menarche. In boys, the first pubertal event to occur is testicular growth. A boy may be considered to have delayed puberty if testicular enlargement has not begun by 13.5 years of age or if more than 5 years have elapsed between the beginning and completion of genital growth. Delayed puberty is estimated to occur in 2 to 3 percent of adolescents.

Causes of delayed puberty based on serum gonadotropin levels are listed in Table 4–2. The most common cause is constitutional delay in growth and development, which represents retardation in activation of the hypothalamic-pituitary-gonadal axis at the time of puberty. These patients have a normal growth rate that is below but parallel to the fifth percentile until 10 to 12 years of age, when deceleration occurs. The bone age is delayed and usually is consistent with the height age.

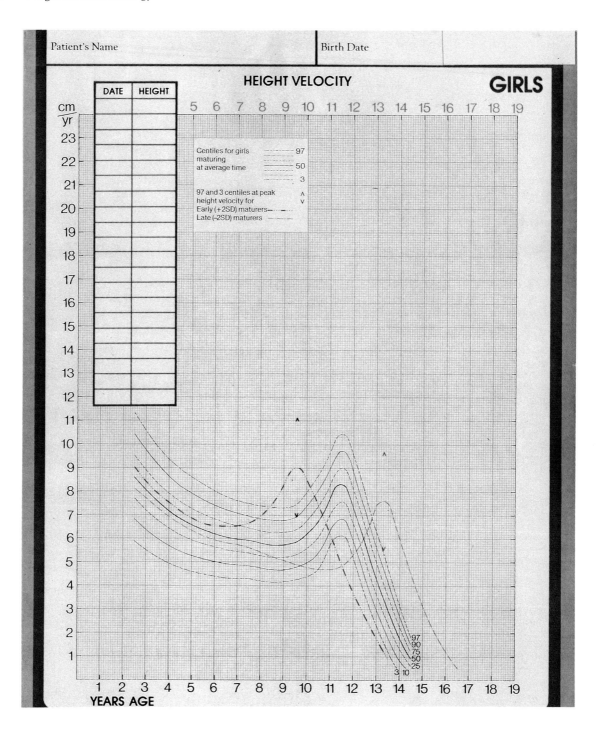

Figure 4-9   Height velocity chart for girls. (From Tanner JM, Davies PW. Clinical longitudinal standards for height, and height velocity for North American children. J Pediatr 1985; 107:317–329.) © Castlemead Publications. Distributed by Serono Laboratories, Inc., Randolph, Massachusetts.

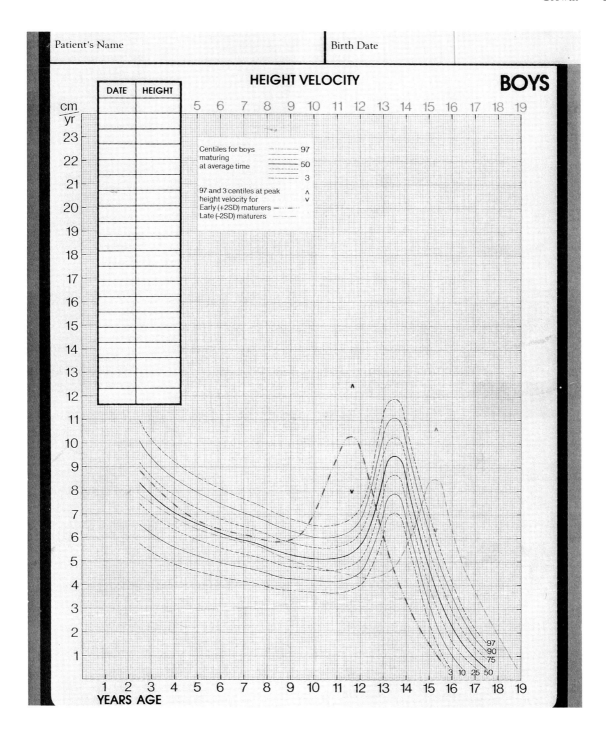

Figure 4-10 Height velocity chart for boys. (From Tanner JM, Davies PW. Clinical longitudinal standards for height and height velocity for North American children. J Pediatr 1985; 107:317–329.) © Castlemead Publications. Distributed by Serono Laboratories, Inc., Randolph, Massachusetts.

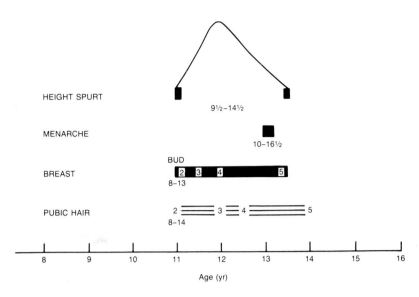

Figure 4–11 Sequence of development of physical changes associated with puberty in girls. Large numbers refer to Tanner stages of pubic hair and breast development. (From Tanner JM. Growth at adolescence. Oxford: Blackwell Scientific Publications, 1962, with permission.)

Frequently, there is a family history of delayed puberty. It may be difficult to differentiate constitutional delayed growth and development from permanent isolated hypogonadotropic hypogonadism initially.

Evaluation of the patient with delayed puberty, after a thorough history has been obtained, is presented in Figure 4–18. In the family history, the times of onset and patterns of growth and sexual development must be obtained. In addition, evidence of a perinatal or postnatal insult to the gonads or a systemic or familial disorder should be sought.

BONE AGE

The concept of bone age is based on the skeletal changes that occur with the physical growth and maturation of the child and adolescent. These skeletal changes include the calcification, growth, and shaping of the epiphyseal centers of the bones and the eventual fusion with the diaphyses. The most widely used standards for bone age calculation in this country are those of Greulich and Pyle (1959), in which an x-ray film of the patient's left hand and wrist is compared with a series of standard x-ray films. In Europe, the Tanner-Whitehouse method (TW2RUS) is used to calculate bone age through the use of maturity indicators for each bone, thus giving a composite score. The bone age is different in males and females at the same chronologic age. As is true with other laboratory studies, the bone age has a normal range and standard deviation (Table 4–3).

A delayed bone age does not provide specific diagnostic information. It occurs in all of the endocrine disorders that cause short stature, in constitutional delayed growth, and in sexual maturation and frequently accom-

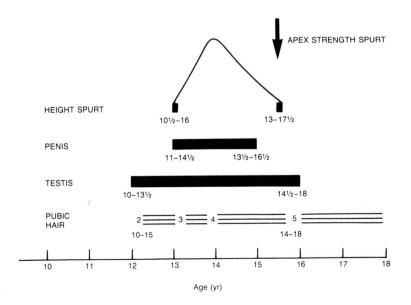

Figure 4–12 Sequence of development of physical changes associated with puberty in boys. Large numbers refer to Tanner stages of pubic hair and penis development. (From Tanner JM. Growth at adolescence. Oxford: Blackwell Scientific Publications, 1962, with permission.)

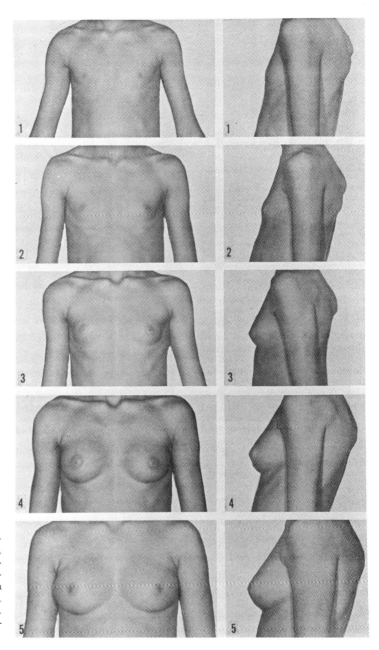

Figure 4-13 Stages of pubertal breast development in females. Numbers refer to Tanner stages. 1, Prepubertal. 2, Elevation of breast and papilla as small mound. Enlargement of areolar diameter. 3, Further enlargement and elevation of breast and areola. 4, Projection of areola and papilla to form a secondary mound above the level of the breast. 5, Mature stage. (From Tanner JM. Growth at adolescence. Oxford: Blackwell Scientific Publications, 1962, with permission.)

panies intrauterine growth retardation and psychosocial short stature. The bone age is usually normal in genetic or familial short stature. The major value of determining bone age is prognostic. Short children whose bone age is delayed have a much better prognosis for ultimate height than do children whose bone age is consistent with their chronologic age.

HEIGHT PREDICTION

Height prediction can be used to confirm suspicion of abnormal growth. Midparental height (average of both parents' height, at any age between 25 and 45 years) probably provides the best correlation for the appropriateness of the height of the patient. Tanner and associates (1983) devised a formula for determining the adjusted midparental height. It is obtained by averaging the parents' height after first adding 13 cm to the mother's height if the patient is a boy or by subtracting 13 cm from the father's height if the patient is a girl. Any patient whose height is less than 2.4 SD from midparental height represents a significant deviation from the norm.

Several methods of height prediction for *normal* children and adolescents have been developed, but none is perfect. Current height, weight, bone age, midparental height, growth velocity, and pubertal stage are variably included in the prediction equations.

In 1952, Bayley and Pinneau (BP) published a set of 11 tables for predicting adult height from the bone

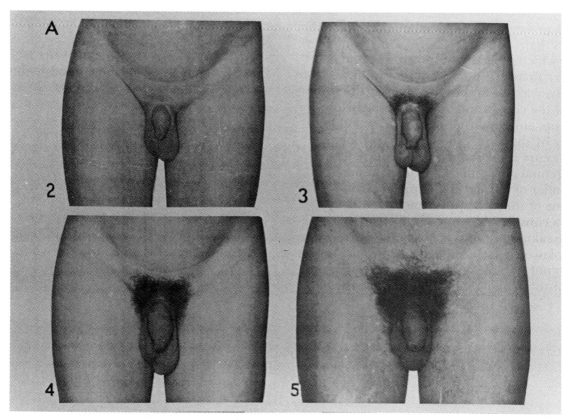

Figure 4-14 Stages of pubic hair growth in males. Numbers refer to Tanner stages. 1, No pubic hair (not shown). 2, Sparse growth of long, slightly pigmented downy hair, straight or slightly, curled, chiefly at the base of the penis. 3, Hair is considerably darker, coarser, and more curled. The hair spreads sparsely over the junction of the pubis. 4, Hair now adult in type, but area covered is less than in the adult. No spread to medial aspects of thighs. 5, Adult in quantity, type, and distribution. (From Tanner JM. Growth at adolescence. Oxford: Blackwell Scientific Publications, 1962, with permission.)

age, as determined by Greulich and Pyle standards, and current height for average, early, and late maturers. This method is the least complicated.

The Roche-Wainer-Thissen (RWT) method utilizes recumbent length, nude weight, midparental height, and bone age as determined by the Greulich and Pyle method (Roche, Wainer, and Thissen, 1975).

The Tanner and Whitehouse Mark II (TW Mark II; Table 4-4) method requires the use of regression equations that contain coefficients for chronologic age, height, and bone age as determined by TW2RUS. The TW Mark II method is a revision of the original TW Mark I method, and the regression equations were developed from a source sample that does not include very short and very tall children. The TW Mark II method uses regression equations developed from a source sample that included very short and very tall children.

The accuracy of these three methods for prediction of adult height varies and depends on the diagnosis. Zachmann and associates (1978) compared the three methods and concluded that the RWT and TW Mark I methods gave accurate results and were superior to the BP methods in *normal* children and in patients with normal growth potential in relation to their skeletal matu-

ration was inherently reduced and could not be corrected by treatment.

GUIDELINES FOR ASSESSMENT OF SHORT STATURE AND RETARDED LINEAR GROWTH

History and Physical Examination

In the evaluation of short stature, certain aspects of the history and physical examination must be emphasized, and these are outlined in Tables 4-4 and 4-5. The growth pattern of the patient may be extremely useful in establishing the diagnosis (Fig. 4-19). Three characteristic patterns of growth retardation are as follows:

1. Children with intrinsic short stature have an inherent limitation to linear growth. The growth curve for these children is below but approximately parallel to normal percentiles, the growth velocity is usually within normal limits, and the bone age is approximately equal to the chronologic age. Their adult height is subnormal.

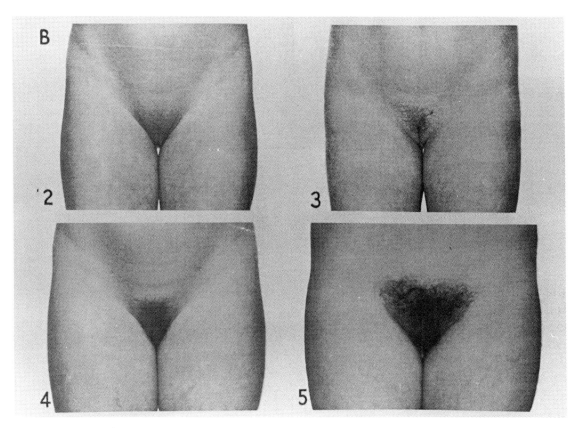

Figure 4-15 Stages of pubic hair growth in females. Numbers refer to Tanner stages. 1, No pubic hair (not shown). 2, Sparse growth of long, slightly pigmented downy hair, straight or slightly curled, chiefly along the labia. 3, Hair is considerably darker, coarser, and more curled. The hair spreads sparsely over the junction of the pubis. 4, Hair now adult in type, but area covered is less than in the adult. No spread to medial aspects of thighs. 5, Adult in quantity, type, and distribution. (From Tanner JM. Growth at adolescence. Oxford: Blackwell Scientific Publications, 1962, with permission.)

2. Children with a delayed growth pattern experience deceleration in growth during the first 2 years of life, and the growth curve from 2 years of age parallels the fifth percentile. These children have delayed puberty, continue to grow for a longer period of time than do their peers, and reach normal adult heights. The growth velocity is usually normal, and the bone age approximates the height age, which is the age at which the measured height is at the 50th percentile. This growth pattern most often occurs with constitutional delayed growth and puberty. However, this growth pattern can result from pathologic conditions.

3. Children with acquired growth failure have a definite subnormal growth rate, and their heights deviate progressively from the standard percentiles. The bone age is approximately equal to the height age; therefore, the adult height potential is normal. Children with acquired growth failure almost always have endocrine, metabolic, or systemic disease. The normal height potential is reached only if the underlying disorder is treated promptly and correctly.

Numerous classifications of short stature have been proposed based on a variety of clinical, radiographic, genetic, and biomedical criteria. The following discussion assumes that chronic illness of a nonendocrine organ system has been ruled out of diagnostic consideration. Comparison of the relationship between chronologic age, height age, growth velocity, and bone age can be used to give a differential diagnosis of growth disorders. On the basis of these variables, short stature can be categorized as intrinsic shortness, delayed growth, and acquired growth failure (Table 4-6).

If the short stature is unexplained by history and physical examination and is accompanied by significant delayed bone age, laboratory tests to rule out subclinical chronic organic diseases are indicated. Evaluation of children whose height is below the fifth percentile for age should include careful measurement of the growth rate for 6 to 12 months after the initial evaluation. If the growth pattern is consistent with intrinsic short stature, a radiographic skeletal survey for bone dysplasia should be obtained, and in girls, karyotyping of peripheral lymphocytes should be obtained to rule out Turner's syndrome or one of its variants (Fig. 4-20). If acquired growth failure is present and the growth rate is subnormal, all disorders that cause such a growth pattern should be investigated. The possibility of GH deficiency must be excluded; the tests used are discussed in another chapter.

Text continues on page 76

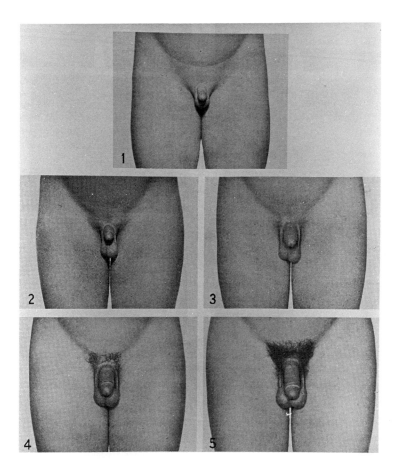

Figure 4-16 Stages of genital development during puberty for males. Numbers refer to Tanner stages. 1, Preadolescent. Testes, scrotum, and penis are approximately the same size and shape as in early childhood. 2, Scrotum slightly enlarged, with skin reddened and changed in texture. Little or no enlargement of penis. 3, Penis slightly enlarged in length. Scrotum further enlarged. 4, Penis further enlarged, with growth in width and development of glands. Scrotum further enlarged and scrotal skin darkened. 5, Genitalia adult in size and shape. (From Tanner JM. Growth at adolescence. Oxford: Blackwell Scientific Publications, 1962, with permission.)

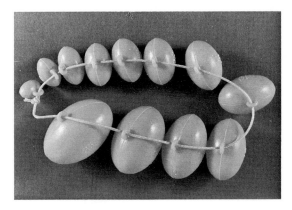

Figure 4-17   Prader orchidometer.

TABLE 4-2 Causes of Delayed Puberty

I. Normal or low serum gonadotropin levels
  A. Constitutional delay in growth and development
  B. Hypothalamic and/or pituitary disorders
    1. Isolated deficiency of growth hormone
    2. Isolated deficiency of Gn-RH*
    3. Isolated deficiency of LH and/or FSH†
    4. Multiple anterior pituitary hormone deficiencies
    5. Associated with congenital anomalies: Kallmann's syndrome; Prader-Willi syndrome; Laurence-Moon-Biedl syndrome; Friedreich's ataxia
    6. Trauma
    7. Postinfection
    8. Hyperprolactinemia
    9. Postirradiation
    10. Infiltrative disease (histiocytosis)
    11. Tumor
    12. Autoimmune hypophysitis
    13. Idiopathic
  C. Functional
    1. Chronic endocrinologic or systemic disorders
    2. Emotional disorders
    3. Drugs—cannabis
II. Increased serum gonadotropin levels
  A. Gonadal abnormalities
    1. Congenital
      a. Gonadal dysgenesis
      b. Klinefelter's syndrome
      c. Bilateral anorchism
      d. Resistant ovary syndrome
      e. Myotonia dystrophy in males
      f. 17-Hydroxylase deficiency in females
      g. Galactosemia
    2. Acquired
      a. Bilateral gonadal failure due to trauma or infection or following surgery, irradiation, or chemotherapy
      b. Oophoritis—isolated or with other autoimmune disorders
III. Uterine or vaginal disorders
  A. Absence of uterus and/or vagina
  B. Testicular feminization—complete or incomplete androgen insensitivity

* Gn-RH = gonadotropin-releasing hormone
† LH = luteinizing hormone; FSH = follicle-stimulating hormone

TABLE 4-3 Normal Ranges of Age of Appearance of Principal Centers

Range × 2 SD	Chronologic Age of Patient (in years)	
	Male	Female
± 3–6 months	0–1	0–1
± 1–1.5 years	3–4	2–3
± 2 years	7–11	6–10
± 2 years plus	13–14	12–13

From Graham CB. Assessment of bone maturation. Radiol Clin North Am 1972; 10:185–202.

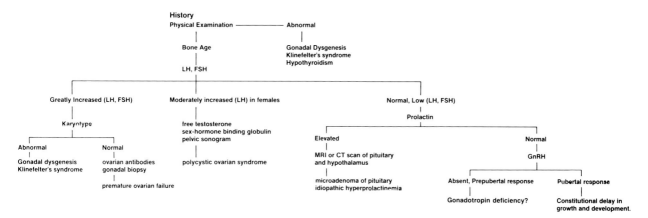

Figure 4-18 Evaluation of patient with delayed puberty.

TABLE 4-4   Important Historical Features in the Evaluation of Short Stature

Historical Features	Diagnostic Implications
Maternal history	
Length of gestation, previous abortions, complications of pregnancy, smoking, alcohol and drug use	Fetal alcohol syndrome, fetal hydantoin syndrome, TORCH infection (toxoplasmosis, rubella, cytomegalovirus, and herpes simplex)
Anthropometric values	
Birth length and weight, dysmorpholism	Intrauterine growth retardation, Turner's syndrome, Down syndrome, other short stature syndromes
Neonatal and developmental history	
Neonatal hypoglycemia, prolonged neonatal jaundice, developmental milestones	Hypopituitarism, hypothyroidism
Nutritional history	
Inadequate caloric intake	Failure to thrive
Psychosocial history	
Child abuse or neglect	Psychosocial short stature
Family history	
Genetic syndromes	Skeletal dysplasias, inborn errors of metabolism
Family heights, ages of onset of puberty, ages of menarche	Familial short stature, constitutional delayed growth, sexual maturation
Review of systems	
Specific chronic organic disorders	Cardiac, pulmonary, hepatic, renal disorders
Medical history	
Glucocorticoids, stimulants	Drug-induced growth retardation

Modified from Brunader REA, Moore DC. Evaluation of the child with growth redardation. Am Fam Physician 1987; 35:165–176.

TABLE 4-5   Important Physical Findings in the Evaluation
of Short Stature

Physical Findings	Diagnostic Implications
Upper to lower segment ratio	Skeletal dysplasias or disorders resulting in infantile proportions (hypothyroidism, hypopituitarism)
Head circumference	Poor cerebral growth due to malnutrition
Jaundice, goiter, large fontanelles	Hypothyroidism
Micropenis, abnormal neurology findings	Hypopituitarism
Chronic ill appearance, pallor, heart murmur, hypertension, cyanosis	Evidence of chronic organic disease
Stigmata of short stature syndromes	Turner's syndrome, Down syndrome

Modified from Brunader REA, Moore DC. Evaluation of the child with growth retardation. Am Fam Physician 1987; 35:165–176.

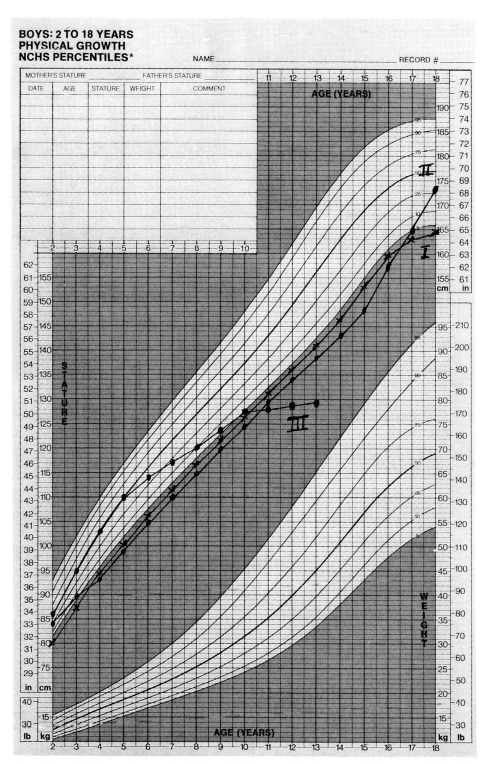

Figure 4-19 Height growth curves in children and adolescents with three types of short stature. I, Intrinsic short stature; II, constitutional delay in growth and sexual maturation; III, acquired growth failure, such as may be seen in growth hormone deficiency.

TABLE 4-6   Differential Diagnosis of Short Stature

Type of Growth Pattern	Chronologic Age, Height Age, and Bone Age	Growth Rate	Differentiate Diagnosis
Intrinsic short stature	CA = BA > HA*	Normal range[†]	Familial short stature Intrauterine growth retardation Chromosomal anomalies, especially Turner's syndrome or one of its variants Bone dysplasias Dysmorphic syndromes Secondary to spinal irradiation
	CA > BA > HA		Constitutional delay in growth and puberty with familial short stature Intrauterine growth retardation Chromosomal anomalies
Delayed growth	CA > BA = HA	Normal range[†]	Constitutional delayed growth and puberty Chronic disorders Malnutrition

Acquired growth failure	CA > HA ≥ BA	Subnormal	Endocrinopathies
			  Growth hormone deficiency
			  Non–growth hormone deficient, GH-responsive growth failure (biologic inactive GH, or GH and/or somatomedin-C resistance)
			Hypothyroidism
			Cushing's syndrome
			Sex hormone deficiency after 10 years of age
			Severe chronic organic diseases
			Severe malnutrition
			Psychosocial short stature

	CA > HA ≥ BA	Subnormal	Hypopituitarism Hypothyroidism

* CA = chronologic age; HA = height age; BA = bone age
[†] Slightly subnormal growth rate may occur occasionally.
Modified from Schaff-Blass E et al. Advances in diagnosis and treatment of short stature, with special reference to the role of growth hormone. J Pediatr 1984; 104:801–813, and Brunader RA, Moore DC. Evaluation of the child with growth retardation. Am Fam Physician 1987; 35:165–176.

TALL STATURE

Tall stature is a term that can be applied to those patients whose height is above the 95th percentile for chronologic age. There are many causes of tall stature during childhood and adolescence, and some of them are listed in Table 4–7. The most common cause is constitutional or familial tall stature. Tall children usually have tall parents, and their heights have been above the 95th percentile since early infancy or early childhood. They may have increased growth hormone responses to some stimuli or increased levels of somatomedin-C. In patients with gigantism, the sella turcica is usually enlarged and serum levels of growth hormone are elevated and often not suppressed by hyperglycemia. Some of the manifestations of acromegaly may be present in gigantism, with onset in late adolescence.

Increased levels of basal serum growth hormone may be present in conditions other than gigantism that have in common a disturbance in nutrition. These conditions include anorexia nervosa, starvation, kwashiorkor, renal failure, and hepatic cirrhosis.

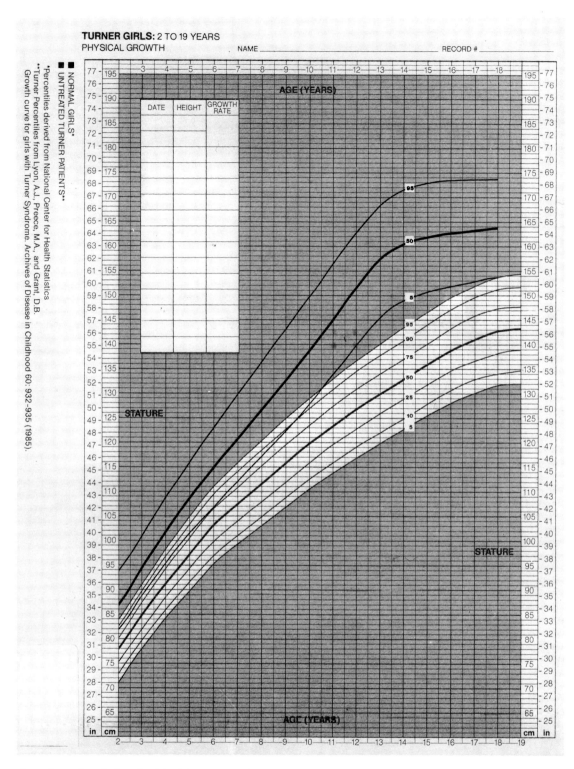

TURNER GIRLS: 2 TO 19 YEARS
PHYSICAL GROWTH   NAME _____   RECORD # _____

■ NORMAL GIRLS*
■ UNTREATED TURNER PATIENTS**

*Percentiles derived from National Center for Health Statistics
**Turner Percentiles from Lyon, A.J., Preece, M.A., and Grant, D.B.
Growth curve for girls with Turner Syndrome. Archives of Disease in Childhood 60: 932–935 (1985).

Figure 4-20   Growth chart for girls with Turner's syndrome. (From Lyon AJ, Preece MA, Grant DB. Growth curve for girls with Turner syndrome. Arch Dis Child 1985; 60:932–935, with permission.)

TABLE 4-7   Causes of Tall Stature

Constitutional (familial or genetic)—most common cause
Endocrine causes
    Growth hormone excess—gigantism
    Sexual precocity (tall as children, short as adults)
        True sexual precocity
        Pseudosexual precocity
    Androgen deficiency
        Klinefelter's syndrome
        Bilateral anorchism
Genetic causes
    Klinefelter's syndrome
    Syndromes of XYY, XXYY
Miscellaneous syndromes and disorders
    Cerebral gigantism or Sotos's syndrome: prominent forehead, hypertelorism, high arched palate, dolichocephaly, mental retardation, large hands and feet, and premature eruption of teeth. Large at birth, with most rapid growth in first 4 years of life.
    Marfan's syndrome: disorder of mesodermal tissues, subluxation of the lenses, arachnodactyly, and aortic aneurysm.
    Homocystinuria: same phenotype as Marfan's syndrome.
    Obesity: tall as infants, children, and adolescents.
    Total lipodystrophy: large hands and feet, generalized loss of subcutaneous fat, insulin-resistant diabetes mellitus, and hepatomegaly.
    Beckwith-Wiedemann syndrome: neonatal tallness, omphalocele, macroglossia, and neonatal hypoglycemia.
    Weaver-Smith syndrome: excessive intrauterine growth, mental retardation, megalocephaly, widened bifrontal diameter, hypertelorism, large ears, micrognathia, camptodactyly, broad thumbs, and limited extension of elbows and knees.
    Marshall-Smith syndrome: excessive intrauterine growth, mental retardation, blue sclerae, failure to thrive, and early death.

BIBLIOGRAPHY

Bailey JA. Disproportionate short stature, diagnosis and treatment. Philadelphia: WB Saunders, 1975.

Bayley N, Pinneau SR. Tables for predicting adult height from skeletal age: Revised for use with the Greulich-Pyle hand standards. J Pediatr 1952; 40:432.

Brunader REA, Moore DC. Evaluation of the child with growth retardation. Am Fam Physician 1987; 35:165.

Greulich WW, Pyle SI. Radiographic atlas of skeletal development of the hand and wrist. Stanford: Stanford University Press, 1959.

Hamill PVV, Drizd TA, Johnson CL, et al. NCHS growth curves for children from birth to 18 years. United States DHEW Pub. No. (PHS) 78–1650. Vital Health Stat 1977; 165:1.

Hung W, August GP, Glasgow AM. Pediatric endocrinology. New Hyde Park, NY: Medical Examination Publishing, 1983.

McKusick VA. Heritable disorders of connective tissue. St. Louis: CV Mosby, 1972.

Monthly Vital Statistics Report. National Center for Health Statistics, HRA 76–1120. Vol. 25, No. 3, Supplement, June 22, 1976. United States DHEW, PHS, Health Resources.

Roche AF, Wainer H, Thissen D. The RWT method for the prediction of adult stature. Pediatrics 1975; 56:1026.

Schaff-Blass, Burnstein S, Rosenfield RL. Advances in diagnosis and treatment of short stature, with special reference to the role of growth hormone. J Pediatr 1984; 104:801.

Schutter JE. Growth standards for blacks: Current status. J Natl Med Assoc 1980; 72:973.

Smith DW. Growth and its disorders: Basics and standards, approach and classifications, growth deficiency disorders, growth excess disorders, obesity. Philadelphia: WB Saunders, 1977.

Tanner JM. Growth at adolescence. Oxford: Blackwell Scientific Publications, 1962.

Tanner JM, Davies PW. Clinical longitudinal standards for height and height velocity for North American children. J Pediatr 1985; 107:317.

Tanner JM, Landt KW, Cameron N, et al. Prediction of adult height and bone age in childhood. Arch Dis Child 1983; 58:767.

Zachmann M, Prader A, Kind HP, et al. Testicular volume during adolescence: Cross-sectional and longitudinal studies. Helv Paediatr Acta 1974; 29:61.

Zachmann M, Sobradillo B, Frank M, et al. Bayley-Pinneau, Roche-Wainer-Thissen, and Tanner height predictions in normal children and in patients with various pathologic conditions. J Pediatr 1978; 93:749.

5

Adrenal Diseases

Themistocles C. Kamilaris, M.D., Ph.D.
George P. Chrousos, M.D.

In the past few years, considerable advances have been made in the diagnosis and management of the various disorders of the hypothalamic-pituitary-adrenal (HPA) axis. These include the ability to measure almost every steroid secreted by the adrenal cortex, the development of specific immunoassays for adrenocorticotropic hormone (ACTH) and corticotropin-releasing hormone (CRH), and the establishment of new dynamic endocrine tests and techniques in radiologic and magnetic resonance imaging (MRI).

Although many tests are currently available to aid the clinician in the diagnosis of adrenocortical diseases, occasionally neither the clinical nor the laboratory evaluation of patients is conclusive. This is particularly true in patients with Cushing's syndrome. The purpose of this chapter is to review the current diagnostic evaluation of adrenocortical disorders and to place special emphasis on situations with contradictory or equivocal results.

ADRENAL PHYSIOLOGY

The adrenal glands lie at the superior pole of each kidney and are composed of two distinct parts, the cortex and the medulla. The adrenal cortex consists of three anatomic zones: the outer zona glomerulosa, the intermediate zona fasciculata, and the inner zona reticularis. The zona glomerulosa is responsible for the production of aldosterone, the zona fasciculata for the production of cortisol, and the zona reticularis for the production of adrenal androgens. The adrenal medulla is functionally related to the sympathetic nervous system and secretes the hormones epinephrine and norepinephrine in response to stress.

Cholesterol is the biosynthetic precursor for all steroid hormones. The conversion of cholesterol to adrenocortical steroids occurs by a series of enzyme-mediated reactions (Fig. 5-1). ACTH is the primary regulator of fasciculata and reticularis cells and angiotension II of glomerulosa cells. ACTH is secreted by the anterior pituitary corticotropes. Hypothalamic control of ACTH secretion is exerted primarily by CRH, a 41-amino-acid peptide produced mainly in the paraventricular nucleus and secreted into the hypophyseal-portal system. Another hypothalamic hormone involved in the regulation of ACTH is vasopressin, which is secreted into both the hypophyseal-portal system and the systemic circulation.

The activity of the HPA axis is regulated by several major influences. Under unstressed conditions, it is under the influence of one or more circadian pacemakers. During stress, the HPA axis is activated in response to a variety of stressors. There are also several regulatory negative feedback loops that function to constrain the activity of the HPA axis. Prominent negative feedback loops are those exerted by glucocorticoids upon CRH and ACTH secretion.

Adrenal androgens (dehydroepiandrosterone [DHEA] and its sulfate, DHEAS; delta⁵-androstenediol; and delta⁴-androstenedione) are C19 steroids. They are synthesized by the adrenal cortex under the influence of ACTH and possibly other factors acting synergistically with ACTH. The latter have been called adrenal androgen-stimulating factors.

Four major factors influence aldosterone secretion in healthy men. These are the renin-angiotensin system (via angiotensin II), plasma potassium, sodium status (perhaps via atrial natriuretic factors), and ACTH. Angiotensin II is the predominant regulator of aldosterone secretion, whereas ACTH perhaps modulates the observed circadian rhythm. (Highest plasma aldosterone concentrations are observed in the early morning.)

The cortisol and aldosterone present in plasma either circulate in the free form or are bound to corticosteroid-binding globulin (CBG) and albumin. Steroid metabolism occurs mainly in the liver. The inactivated metabolites are excreted in the urine. Only a relatively small fraction (approximately 1 percent) of cortisol secreted daily is excreted unchanged in the urine as "free" cortisol. Urinary free cortisol excretion over 24 hours represents a time-integrated measure of plasma free cortisol during the period of urine collection.

ADRENAL FUNCTION TESTS

Basal Plasma Hormone Measurements

CRH

Measurement of human CRH immunoreactivity (IR-CRH) by radioimmunoassay (RIA), immunoradiometric assay (IRMA), and immunohistochemical tech-

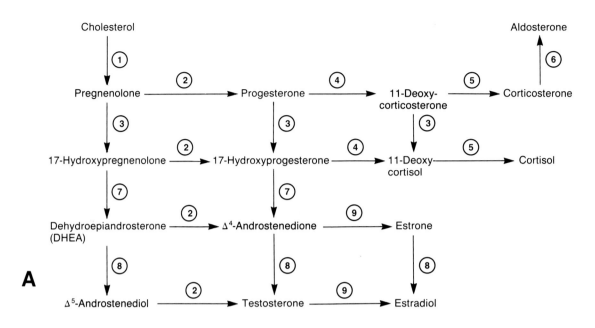

Figure 5-1 *A*, Steroid biosynthesis pathway. Each enzyme is represented by a number. *B*, Enzymes and associated deficiency syndromes are indicated. (CAH = congenital adrenal hyperplasia.)

niques has been restricted to research laboratories. Whereas normally IR-CRH in plasma is undetectable (< 8 pg per milliliter) for most available assays, measurement of plasma IR-CRH in patients with Cushing's syndrome is compatible with the diagnosis of ectopic CRH production. It should be noted that in the latter part of pregnancy IR-CRH of placental origin is detected in plasma. Levels reach 4,000 pg per milliliter. Interestingly, major stress and Addison's disease are not associated with significant elevations of circulating IR-CRH.

ACTH

Measurement of ACTH (Table 5-1) became widely available in the early 1960s when Berson and Yalow (1968) developed an ACTH radioimmunoassay. ACTH, a 39-amino-acid single-chain peptide, is normally synthe-

sized and secreted by the anterior pituitary corticotropes. It is part of a larger precursor molecule of 245 amino acids referred to as proopiomelanocortin (POMC). POMC is metabolized primarily into ACTH and beta-lipotropin and secondarily into beta-endorphin. Several forms of IR-ACTH circulate in blood. The majority of IR-ACTH in normal individuals and patients with Cushing's disease, Nelson's syndrome, and Addison's disease is of the 1-39 form (approximately 4,500 dalton). In a proportion of patients with the ectopic ACTH syndrome, IR-ACTH is found in larger molecules. The biologic activity of ACTH resides in the 24 amino acids in the N-terminal region; the first 13 amino acids are required for minimum corticotropic activity.

The methods that have been employed for the measurement of ACTH include bioassays, radioreceptor assays, RIAs, and recently a two-site IRMA and high-

TABLE 5–1   Plasma ACTH

Method:	RIA Two-site IRMA Bioassays (steroid response of dispersed adrenal cells)
Normal:	8 to 25 pg/ml at 8:00 AM
Uses:	Dynamic adrenal function tests Differential diagnosis of Cushing's syndrome Differential diagnosis of adrenal insufficiency As a tumor marker
Problems:	Requires antibody of high specificity and affinity Association of the episodic secretion and short plasma half-life with wide and rapid fluctuations Expense Errors in blood collection and storage

TABLE 5–2   Plasma Cortisol

	Plasma Total Cortisol
Method:	RIA Competitive protein-binding radioassay Fluorimetric assay High-pressure liquid chromatography
Normal:	8:00 AM: 10–20 μg/dl (range, 3–20μg/dl) 4:00 PM: Approximately 50% of morning values 11:00 PM: < 5 μg/dl
Uses:	Dynamic adrenal function tests Monitoring the rate of HPA axis recovery
Problems:	Changes in corticosteroid-binding globulin affect total plasma cortisol concentrations. Stress may influence values.
	Plasma Free Cortisol
Method:	Separation of bound and free steroid by equilibrium dialysis, gel filtration, or ultrafiltration followed by radioligand competition assay
Normal:	0.3–0.4 μg/dl
	Salivary Cortisol "Concentration"
Normal:	8:00 AM: 0.4 μg/dl

performance liquid chromatography (HPLC). RIA is the most sensitive and useful method used in clinical laboratories. In general, ACTH is measured following extraction or directly in unextracted plasma. The antiscra employed have been mostly raised against the active 1-24 sequence of human ACTH.

It must be noted that ACTH is secreted episodically, has a half-life of about 10 minutes, and is inactivated by proteases. Thus, blood samples for measurement of IR-ACTH must be collected in prechilled tubes containing EDTA and centrifuged in a refrigerated centrifuge. Plasma should remain frozen ($-20\,^{\circ}$C) until assayed.

Determination of plasma IR-ACTH is useful in the diagnosis and differential diagnosis of adrenal insufficiency and Cushing's syndrome and as a marker of tumors secreting ectopically bioactive or bioinactive ACTH.

Cortisol

Determination of plasma cortisol concentrations (Table 5–2) is a convenient method of evaluating adrenocortical function. Current methods for plasma cortisol determination include RIAs, competitive protein-binding assays, fluorescence assays, and rarely enzyme immunoassays and chromatography. Prior to assay, the steroid is extracted from the plasma with an organic solvent such as dichloromethane. For IR-cortisol determination several antisera are available that have limited cross-reactivity with other circulating natural steroids. Most antisera, however, cross-react with circulating prednisone-prednisolone and methylprednisolone, but not with dexamethasone.

In normal individuals, the highest plasma cortisol levels are found between 6:00 and 8:00 AM and the lowest at around midnight. Morning plasma cortisol levels measured by RIA have a significant variability, ranging from 5 to 25 μg per deciliter at 8:00 AM. The values fall during the day and by 11:00 PM are less than 5 μg per deciliter. Plasma cortisol concentrations are elevated during physical or emotional stress, including acute illness, trauma, surgery, infectious disease, and starvation. Plasma cortisol elevation is also noted in anorexia nervosa,

depression, alcoholism, withdrawal from alcohol and narcotics, and chronic liver and renal failure. In patients with Cushing's syndrome, plasma cortisol levels are elevated throughout the day, usually without the presence of circadian variation. Patients with adrenal insufficiency have low concentrations of plasma cortisol in the morning, which, however, can be within the low normal range.

Since the available assays for cortisol measure total plasma cortisol levels, conditions that alter cortisol-binding globulin concentrations can influence cortisol determinations. Thus, cortisol levels are elevated in conditions associated with increased CBG levels, such as pregnancy, obesity, hyperthyroidism, estrogen therapy, and therapy with mitotane (o,p'-DDD), and are decreased in conditions associated with low CBG levels, such as hypothyroidism, multiple myeloma, and congenitally decreased CBG. Salivary cortisol concentrations have been considered a good index of plasma free cortisol level, accurately reflecting its diurnal fluctuations. It is especially useful in patients with CBG abnormalities. The normal unstimulated salivary cortisol level at 8:00 AM is about 0.4 μg per deciliter.

Other Plasma Steroids

Determinations of steroid precursors (Table 5–3) of cortisol biosynthesis and/or measurements of adrenal androgens can be useful (see Fig. 5–1). Steroid precursor concentrations are necessary for the evaluation of patients with congenital adrenal biosynthetic defects. The most frequently employed measurements include pregnenolone, 17-alpha-hydroxypregnenolone, 17-alpha-hydroxyprogesterone, and 11-beta-deoxycortisol. Determinations are performed by RIA or by HPLC following separation by solvent extraction and/or chromatography.

TABLE 5-3   Determination of Other Plasma Steroids

	Steroidogenesis Precursors: Pregnenolone, 17-alpha-hydroxypregnenolone, progesterone, 17-alpha-hydroxyprogesterone, 11-deoxycortisol, 11-deoxycorticosterone, corticosterone
Method:	Extraction and/or chromatography followed by RIA-binding assay High-pressure liquid chromatography Adrenal Androgens: DHEA, DHEAS, Delta⁵-androstenediol, and delta⁴-androstenedione
Uses:	Diagnosis, differential diagnosis, and follow-up of adrenal biosynthetic defects Detection of adrenal carcinoma After administration of inhibitors of adrenal steroid biosynthesis (metyrapone test)

TABLE 5-4   Urinary 17-Hydroxycorticosteroids

Method:	Porter-Silber chromogen reaction (steroids with a 17-, 21-dihydroxyacetone configuration react with phenylhydrazine to form compounds that are measured colorimetrically)
Normal:	2–7 mg/g creatinine/day
Uses:	Screening and monitoring of patients with hypercortisolism Screening and monitoring of patients with 11-hydroxylase deficiency As end point in both adrenal stimulation and suppression tests
Problems:	Errors in urine collection can occur. Uncorrected values are dependent on body size. Drugs and diseases affect values. Values overlap in patients with and without hypercortisolism.

Urinary Steroid Measurements

The determinations of steroid levels in 24-hour urine collections include 17-hydroxycorticosteroids, urinary free cortisol, 17-ketosteroids, pregnanetriol, and tetrahydrocompound S (THS). Of course, to obtain meaningful results, the 24-hour urine collections must be complete. The creatinine content should be measured to confirm completeness of collection and/or to correct for patient size.

17-Hydroxycorticosteroids (Porter-Silber Chromogens)

One of the earliest procedures for estimating cortisol production rate is measurement of 17-hydroxycorticosteroid excretion in urine (Table 5-4). Normally, about one-third of the daily secreted cortisol is excreted in the urine as 17-hydroxycorticosteroid. The latter represents all cortisol metabolites with a 17-dihydroxyacetone side chain, which in the presence of phenylhydrazine produces a yellow color with an absorption maximum at 410 nm (Porter-Silber reaction).

Cortisol is metabolized by the liver to tetrahydrocortisol and glucuronic or sulfuric acid conjugates. Some cortisol is converted to cortisone, which is similarly metabolized to tetrahydrocortisone and glucuronic and sulfuric acid conjugates. Following hydrolysis and organic solvent extraction, the two cortisol metabolites tetrahydrocortisol and tetrahydrocortisone and the reduced metabolite of 11-beta-deoxycortisol (compound S) THS are measured in the urine by the Porter-Silber reaction.

Certain drugs that directly interfere with the color of the Porter-Silber reaction, such as spironolactone, chlordiazepoxide, hydroxyzine, and meprobamate, may result in artificially increased values. Other drugs, such as phenobarbital, phenytoin (Dilantin), pyrimidine, and mitotane (o,p'-DDD), may result in artificially decreased values. This is because these drugs increase conversion of cortisol to 6-hydroxylated metabolites, which are not extracted efficiently and therefore fail to be detected as 17-hydroxycorticosteroid.

When 17-hydroxycorticosteroid excretion is normalized for creatinine excretion, it is constant throughout life with a normal range of about 2 to 7 mg per gram of creatinine per day. Excretion of 17-hydroxycorticosteroids can be increased in hyperthyroidism and decreased in hypothyroidism, starvation, and renal and liver failure. The greatest diagnostic value of urinary 17-hydroxycorticosteroid measurements is in the context of dynamic adrenal tests used in the differential diagnosis of Cushing's syndrome and adrenal insufficiency. Basal secretion of 17-hydroxycorticosteroid is also frequently employed in the diagnosis of hypercortisolism and in the monitoring of patients with Cushing's syndrome.

Urinary Free Cortisol

The unbound or "free" fraction of plasma cortisol enters the renal glomerulus as plasma is filtered by the kidney. Once plasma cortisol levels exceed the values of 17 to 25 μg per deciliter, which is the upper 8:00 AM reference value, there is a disproportionate increase of unbound cortisol as a result of cortisol-binding globulin saturation. Plasma unbound cortisol is filtered and excreted by the kidney and appears in the urine as free cortisol. Urinary free cortisol represents approximately 1 percent of the cortisol secreted by the adrenals and about 2 to 4 percent of the time-integrated free plasma cortisol.

Urinary free cortisol can be measured by RIA or competitive protein-binding (CPB) radioassay, after extraction of the steroid from the urine with an organic solvent (Table 5-5). Frequently, a chromatographic step is necessary to separate cortisol from cross-reacting steroid metabolites. In adults, the normal upper range of urinary free cortisol by RIA or CPB radioassay is less than 100 μg per 24 hours.

This test is the best screening device to discriminate normal from hypercortisolemic states. In contrast to urinary 17-hydroxycorticosteroids, urinary free cortisol levels are normal in obesity and almost always elevated in patients with Cushing's syndrome. Urinary free cortisol values are not affected by drugs or changes in cortisol-

TABLE 5-5   Urinary Free Cortisol

Method:	Extraction and/or chromatography followed by RIA or competitive protein-binding assay
Normal:	< 100 μg/24h (age-dependent until age 21) Discrimination between normal and hypercortisolemic states
Uses:	Screening and monitoring of adrenal hyperfunction Dynamic tests in Cushing's syndrome
Problems:	Errors in urine collection can occur. Depression, alcoholism, stress, strenuous exercise, and pregnancy affect the values. Values below 15 μg/24h are unreliable.

binding globulin. However, emotional or physical stress, acute illness, severe depression, alcoholism, and withdrawal from alcohol or narcotics may increase the values.

17-Ketosteroids (Zimmerman Reaction)

Urinary 17-ketosteroids represent the excretory products of a number of androgens principally derived from the adrenal cortex and to a lesser extent from the gonads. The urinary 17-ketosteroids primarily comprise androgens with the 17-keto configuration. These include DHEA, DHEAS, delta⁴-androstenedione, delta⁵-androstenediol, androsterone, and etiocholanolone. Testosterone, however, is not included in the precursors of 17-ketosteroids.

The Zimmerman reaction (m-nitrobenzene reaction) is the standard method for colorimetrically quantifying 17-ketosteroids (Table 5–6). The steroids are first extracted from a 24-hour urine specimen with an organic solvent. They are then allowed to react with m-dinitrobenzene in the presence of alkali to produce a red color complex with an absorption maximum at 520 nm. The normal range for urinary 17-ketosteroids is generally 7 to 17 mg per 24 hours in adult males and 5 to 15 mg per 24 hours in adult females.

Medications such as cephalosporins, erythromycin, meprobamate, nalidixic acid, chlorpromazine, ethinamate, spironolactone, testolactone, testosterone, and troleandomycin can interfere with this assay and give ar-

TABLE 5-6   Urinary 17-Ketosteroids

Method:	Zimmerman chromogen reaction detecting androgens with the 17-keto configuration
Normal:	Males, 7–17 mg/24h Females, 5–15 mg/24h
Uses:	Diagnosis and differential diagnosis of virilization Congenital adrenal biosynthetic defects (primarily to monitor adequacy of treatment in the virilizing forms of congenital adrenal hyperplasia) As a screening test for adrenocortical carcinoma
Problems:	Errors in urine collection can occur. Normal range is age-dependent.

tificially elevated or decreased values. Similarly, reserpine, chlordiazepoxide, erytromine acetate, progestins, and propoxyphene interfere with the assay. For reliable results, these drugs should be discontinued several days before urinary 17-ketosteroids are determined.

Determinations of basal excretion of 17-ketosteroids are used primarily in the evaluation of hyperandrogenic states such as the 21-hydroxylase, 11-beta-hydroxylase, and 3-beta-hydroxysteroid dehydrogenase varieties of congenital adrenal hyperplasia, polycystic ovary syndrome, idiopathic hirsutism, and androgen-secreting tumors. As outlined earlier, urinary 17-ketosteroids include steroids from both the adrenal glands and the gonads. Therefore, in the polycystic ovary syndrome, the ovarian contribution of androgens (androstenedione) can be considerable. The test is also important as a screening device for adrenocortical carcinoma and in certain pathologic situations in which the production of an androgen cannot be recognized by the usual battery of available RIAs.

Pregnanetriol, THS

Pregnanetriol is the major metabolite of plasma 17-hydroxylated compounds (17-hydroxyprogesterone and 17-hydroxypregnenolone). Urinary pregnanetriol is measured chromatographically after incubation of an aliquot of urine with beta-glucuronidase, then by extraction of the liberated steroids with benzene, and finally by colorimetric quantification. Normal adults excrete 0.2 to 1.9 mg per day.

Determinations of pregnanetriol have been useful in the diagnosis and monitoring of the 21-hydroxylase form of congenital adrenal hyperplasia. Direct measurements of plasma 17-hydroxyprogesterone have started to supplant the urinary assay.

THS is the major urinary metabolite of compound S (11-deoxycortisol). Measurements of urinary excretion of THS have been useful in diagnosing and monitoring the therapy of 11-hydroxylase deficiency.

Dynamic Tests of Adrenal Function

Stimulation Tests

Insulin-Induced Hypoglycemia or Insulin Tolerance Test.   Plasma ACTH and cortisol response to hypoglycemia is a measure of HPA integrity. The insulin tolerance test (ITT) (Table 5–7) is performed after an overnight fast with measurement of plasma glucose, ACTH, and cortisol values before and at 30, 60, and 90 minutes after regular insulin is given intravenously. Plasma ACTH values are not necessary to measure since an adequate cortisol response would suggest a normal HPA axis. The recommended dose of insulin is 0.15 units per kilogram of body weight.

CRH Stimulation Test.   Ovine CRH (oCRH) and recently human CRH (hCRH) have proved to be valuable in the evaluation of patients with pituitary-adrenal

TABLE 5-7 Insulin Tolerance Test

Method:	After an overnight fast, 0.15 unit/kg body weight of regular insulin is given intravenously as a bolus. Blood samples for glucose and plasma values of ACTH and cortisol are drawn at 0, 30, 60, and 90 minutes. An experienced physician should be in attendance. Side effects include nervousness, sweating, drowsiness, tachycardia, hunger, and fatigue. Glucose must be available for immediate IV administration, if significant symptoms of neuroglycopenia such as confusion or disorientation occur. The test is generally contraindicated in patients older than 65 years of age, patients with cardiovascular or cerebrovascular disease or seizure disorders, and acutely ill patients.
Normal:	A rise in plasma ACTH or cortisol to levels above 4 coefficients of variation of the assay for the basal value is considered a positive response.
	NOTE: *The test is not safe in suspected adrenal insufficiency.*
Uses:	Differential diagnosis of pseudo–Cushing's syndrome from Cushing's syndrome
Problems:	An adequate degree of hypoglycemia must be obtained. This usually is defined as a drop in blood glucose concentration to $\leq$40 mg/dl or a decrease in blood glucose to < 50% of the fasting level.

TABLE 5-8 CRH Stimulation Test

Method:	CRH (ovine or human), 1 μg/kg body weight, is given intravenously over 1 minute. Plasma for measurements of ACTH and cortisol is drawn at -15, 0, 5, 15, 30, 60, 90, and 120 minutes. The late afternoon or evening is a better time than morning to perform the test, especially if one is using plasma cortisol as an index of response (plasma cortisol level is high in the morning and thus the increment is lower). With a CRH dose of 1 μg/kg body weight there are no signs or symptoms other than a mild flush occurring immediately after the injection in 15% of subjects tested.
Response:	Plasma ACTH rises within 2 minutes after CRH injection, reaching a peak within 10–15 minutes, whereas cortisol rises more slowly, beginning 10 minutes or more after injection and reaching peak values at 30–60 minutes. A rise in plasma ACTH or cortisol to levels above 4 coefficients of variation of the assay for the basal values is considered a positive response.
Uses:	Differential diagnosis of Cushing's disease from adrenal and ectopic Cushing's syndrome Differential diagnosis of pseudo–Cushing's syndrome from Cushing's syndrome Differential diagnosis of adrenal insufficiency Monitoring the rate of adrenal recovery after surgical cure of Cushing's syndrome
Interactions with other agents:	Arginine vasopressin and angiotensin II potentiate the effects of CRH.
Problems:	CRH is a new agent. hCRH stimulation is not as good a diagnostic test as oCRH.

disorders (Table 5–8). CRH directly stimulates pituitary corticotropes to secrete ACTH and other POMC-derived peptides such as beta-lipotropin and beta-endorphin.

The test is performed using an intravenous bolus administration of 1 μg per kilogram of body weight of CRH. Plasma ACTH and cortisol levels are measured before and after CRH administration. Although there is no significant difference in peak plasma ACTH and cortisol responses to CRH given early in the morning or late in the evening, the late afternoon or evening is a better time than morning to perform the test because of lower baseline values of ACTH and cortisol. With the CRH dose of 1 μg per kilogram of body weight there are no serious side effects. Facial warmth and flushing of the face, neck, and upper chest as well as transient shortness of breath, tightness in the chest, tachycardia, and mild decrease in blood pressure can be observed in approximately 15 percent of patients having the test.

Metyrapone Test. The standard metyrapone test was introduced by Liddle in 1959 and has since been widely used in the assessment of pituitary-adrenal reserve and in the differential diagnosis of Cushing's syndrome. By blocking 11β-hydroxylation of steroids in the adrenal cortex, metyrapone inhibits cortisol synthesis, thus stimulating ACTH production; as a result, plasma concentrations of 11-deoxycortisol and urinary excretion of 17-hydroxycorticosteroids increase. The latter is due to increased excretion of the tetrahydrometabolite of 11-deoxycortisol.

The standard metyrapone test involves administration of 750 mg of metyrapone orally every 4 hours for

24 hours and measurements of plasma cortisol (to confirm adrenal blockade), ACTH, 11-deoxycortisol (to assess response), and urinary 24-hour excretion of 17-hydroxysteroids (Table 5–9). 17-Hydroxysteroids represent metabolites of 11-deoxycortisol. It must be noted that a small group of normal subjects and patients on phenytoin and other drugs have an increased rate of degradation of metyrapone in the liver. Adequate inhibition of 11-beta-hydroxylase may not occur in these individuals.

Because the standard metyrapone test requires 3 days to perform and has been associated with severe side effects, it has fallen into disfavor. Different, single-dose metyrapone tests conducted at various times of the day have been suggested but not widely accepted. The most useful is the "rapid" single-dose overnight metyrapone test that provides similar information as the standard test without requiring urine collections (Table 5–10).

ACTH Stimulation Tests. The most convenient procedure for screening and studying patients suspected of having hypocortisolism is the injection of a commercially available ACTH analogue, cosyntropin (Table 5–11). This synthetic analogue has the 1-24 amino acid sequence of human ACTH 1-39 and contains the full biologic activity of ACTH 1-39.

TABLE 5-9   Standard Metyrapone Test

Method: A dose of 750 mg metyrapone every 4 hours for 24 hours is given orally, commencing at 8:00 AM. (Pediatric dose is 430 mg/m² every 4 hours for 24 hours.) Urine collections for 17-hydroxycorticosteroid are performed on the day before, day of, and day after metyrapone administration. Blood is taken for plasma ACTH, 11-deoxycortisol, and cortisol at 0, 1, 2, 3, 4, and 24 hours of metyrapone treatment. Side effects that the patient may experience include nausea, abdominal discomfort, gastric irritation, dizziness, sedation, headache, hypotension, and allergic rash.

Response: A positive response has been defined as a two- to fourfold increase of 17-hydroxycorticosteroid excretion or a rise in plasma 11-deoxycortisol from $< 1 \mu g/dl$ to $> 10 \mu g/dl$ (while the 8:00 AM plasma cortisol level drops to $< 6 \mu g/dl$).

Uses: Differential diagnosis of Cushing's disease from Cushing's syndrome due to functioning adrenal tumor.
Differential diagnosis of Cushing's disease from Cushing's syndrome due to ectopic ACTH secretion.

NOTE: *The test should be avoided in patients with adrenal insufficiency.*

Problems: Occasionally severe side effects occur.
Conditions of drugs that affect metyrapone metabolism affect the response.
Test takes 3 days to perform.
Errors with urine collections occur.

TABLE 5-11   ACTH Stimulation Tests

Rapid ACTH Stimulation Test

Method: 250 μg of cosyntropin (Cortrosyn) is given intravenously as a bolus.
Plasma samples for measurement of cortisol or steroidogenesis precursors are drawn at 0, 30, and 60 minutes

Normal: A plasma cortisol concentration of $\geq 18 \mu g/dl$ is a sufficient criterion for normal adrenal function. Stimulated plasma concentrations of 17-hydroxypregnenolone, 17-hydroxyprogesterone, and 11-deoxycortisol of $\geq 2,000$ ng/dl, 1,500 ng/dl and 1,500 ng/dl, respectively, indicate 3 beta-hydroxysteroid dehydrogenase, 21-hydroxylase, and 11-hydroxylase deficiency.

Uses: As a screening procedure for adrenal insufficiency
As a diagnostic procedure for adrenal biosynthetic defects

Prolonged ACTH Stimulation Test

Method: The test begins with a baseline 24-hour urine collection for creatinine and 17-hydroxycortico-steroids. After the baseline period, ACTH (cosyntropin), 800 $\mu g/24h$ is continuously infused intravenously for 2 to 3 consecutive days with concurrent 24-hour urine collections for 17-hydroxycortico-steroid determination.

Normal: An increase in the urinary 17-hydroxycorticosteroid excretion two to three times or greater of baseline levels in the first day.

Uses: Differential diagnosis of primary from secondary adrenal insufficiency

Rapid ACTH Stimulation Test.   The rapid ACTH stimulation test is the most useful screening procedure for suspected adrenal insufficiency and congenital adrenal hyperplasia. It can be performed on an outpatient basis at any time of the day and does not require fasting. Because of its simplicity, speed, and lack of side effects, the test has received wide acceptance. A subnormal cortisol response is consistent with either primary or secondary adrenal insufficiency and merely suggests that further investigation is needed.

TABLE 5-10   Single-Dose Overnight Metyrapone Test

Method: A single dose of metyrapone, 30 mg/kg body weight, is given orally at 11:00 PM with a snack to minimize gastrointestinal irritation. Blood for plasma ACTH, 11-deoxycortisol, and cortisol is drawn at 8:00 the morning before and the morning after administration of metyrapone.

Response: A postmetyrapone level of plasma ACTH greater than 100 pg/ml and an 11-deoxycortisol level greater than 7 $\mu g/dl$ (while plasma cortisol level is less than 10 $\mu g/dl$)

Uses: The same as with the classic test (see Table 5-9)

Problems: The same as with the classic test (see Table 5-9) but without severe side effects and the problems related to urine collection

Prolonged ACTH Stimulation Test.   The prolonged ACTH stimulation test has been traditionally used in the differential diagnosis of primary versus secondary adrenal insufficiency. A continuous intravenous infusion of ACTH 1-24 is administered for 2 to 3 days. In normal individuals, urinary excretion of 17-hydroxycorticosteroids increases two to three times above the baseline value even from the first day, whereas patients with primary adrenal insufficiency show no response. Patients with secondary adrenal insufficiency usually have an inadequate response of 17-hydroxycorticosteroid on the first day of testing but a progressively increased response in the next 2 days.

Suppression Tests

Dexamethasone Suppression Tests.   Dexamethasone suppression testing procedures can be divided into two groups—those in which only a single 8:00 AM plasma cortisol is obtained following a single dose of dexamethasone given 8 hours earlier, at midnight (1-mg or 8-mg overnight tests), and those in which plasma cortisol and 24-hour urine are collected prior to and during administration of two daily doses (low- and high-dose) of dexamethasone given consecutively for 2 days each. The rationale for all dexamethasone suppression tests is the same. In normal subjects in whom glucocorticoid negative feedback control of the HPA axis is normal, dexamethasone suppresses pituitary ACTH release and consequently adrenal cortisol secretion, whereas in patients with Cushing's syndrome in whom feedback control of ACTH by glucocorticoids is impaired, dexamethasone does not adequately suppress ACTH and cortisol secretion.

Dexamethasone, a synthetic steroid that has 40 times the glucocorticoid potency of cortisol, is administered orally. Dexamethasone in plasma and urine has little interference with cortisol or cortisol metabolite measure-

ments. Normally, after dexamethasone administration, there is a fall in plasma ACTH and cortisol that is reflected in low urinary free cortisol and 17-hydroxycorticosteroid excretion.

Overnight 1-mg Dexamethasone Suppression Test. A useful screening procedure for subjects suspected of having hypercortisolism is the overnight 1-mg dexamethasone suppression test (Table 5–12). The test can be performed on an outpatient basis and requires only one morning plasma specimen. It is a good screening test but has a significant proportion of false-positive results. Meas-

TABLE 5–12   Dexamethasone Suppression Tests

Overnight 1-mg Dexamethasone Suppression Test

Method: 1 mg dexamethasone is given orally at 11:00 PM. A plasma sample for measurement of cortisol is drawn at 8:00 the following morning.

Interpretation: Suppression of basal plasma cortisol level to < 5 μg/dl is defined as a normal suppression. A plasma cortisol level >5 μg/dl suggests hypercortisolism, and further evaluation to explore the possibility of Cushing's syndrome is required.

Uses: As a screening test for subjects suspected of having hypercortisolism

Problems: Technical errors such as failure to take the agent, poor sleeping, administration at the wrong time, and rapid or slow metabolism of dexamethasone. Pediatric standards have not been established.

Overnight 8-mg Dexamethasone Suppression Test

Method: Baseline plasma cortisol level is measured at 8:00 AM, and a single 8-mg oral dose of dexamethasone is given at 11:00 PM. A plasma sample for measurement of cortisol is drawn at 8:00 the following morning.

Interpretation: Suppression of basal plasma cortisol to < 50% of baseline the following morning suggests Cushing's disease. Failure of plasma cortisol to be suppressed indicates an ectopic source of ACTH or an adrenal cortisol-secreting tumor.

Uses: Differential diagnosis of Cushing's disease from other forms of Cushing's syndrome

Standard Low- and High-Dose Dexamethasone Suppression Test (Liddle Test)

Method: The test begins with two baseline 24-hour urine collections for measurement of 17-hydroxycorticosteroids, free cortisol, and creatinine excretion. After the baseline period, dexamethasone is given orally at a dose of 0.5 mg every 6 hours for 2 days (2 mg/day in adults, 30 μg/kg/day in children). This is followed by administration of 2 mg of dexamethasone every 6 hours for 2 more days. (8 mg/day in adults, 120 μg/kg/day in children). Blood for measurement of plamsa cortisol and ACTH is obtained at 8:00 AM before and 24 hours and 48 hours after the low and/or high dexamethasone dose. Daily urine collections for measurements of 17-hydroxycorticosteroids, free cortisol, and creatinine are continued until the end of the test.

Interpretation:

Low-dose: Suppression of urinary 17-hydroxycorticosteroids to < 4 mg per day or to < 2.5 mg/g creatinine during the second day of dexamethasone indicates normal ACTH regulation. Suppression of urine free cortisol to > 50% of baseline or a decrease in plasma cortisol to < 5 μg/dl also suggests normal ACTH regulation.

High-dose: Suppression of urinary 17-hydroxycorticosteroids and cortisol to >50% and 90% of baseline levels, respectively, and suppression of plasma cortisol to < 5μg/dl, suggests Cushing's disease.

Uses: Differential diagnosis of Cushing's disease from ectopic ACTH production or adrenal cortisol-secreting tumors

urements of 24-hour urinary free cortisol excretion should always be performed to ascertain the diagnosis of hypercortisolism.

Overnight 8-mg Dexamethasone Suppression Test. A simple, reliable, and inexpensive high-dose dexamethasone suppression test that has been proposed as an alternative to the Liddle dexamethasone suppression test is the overnight 8-mg dexamethasone suppression test (see Table 5–12). The advantages are its outpatient administration and the avoidance of errors due to incomplete urine collections. The diagnostic accuracy of the overnight 8-mg dexamethasone suppression test may be similar to that of the standard Liddle dexamethasone suppression test.

Liddle Dexamethasone Suppression Test. The Liddle dexamethasone suppression test (see Table 5–12) is regarded as one of the best to discriminate between Cushing's disease and other types of endogenous hypercortisolism. Whereas in normal subjects and patients with pseudo–Cushing's syndrome the "normal" pituitary corticotropes could be suppressed after low-dose administration of dexamethasone (2 mg per day divided every 6 hours for 2 days), in patients with Cushing's disease the abnormal corticotropes in the pituitary adenomas are sensitive to glucocorticoid inhibition only at much higher doses of dexamethasone (8 mg per day divided every 6 hours for 2 days). In contrast, patients with the ectopic ACTH syndrome or Cushing's syndrome due to cortisol-secreting adrenal tumors usually fail to respond to the doses of 8 mg per day. The diagnostic accuracy of this test is approximately 85 percent.

ASSESSMENT OF ADRENAL STATUS BY MEANS OF ADRENAL TESTS

Evaluation of Patients With Hypercortisolism— Cushing's Syndrome

Etiology

Cushing's syndrome results from prolonged exposure to high levels of glucocorticoid hormones and represents a subcategory of hypercortisolism (Table 5–13). The cause of Cushing's syndrome can be exogenous, resulting from the administration of glucocorticoids or ACTH, or endogenous, resulting from the increased secretion of cortisol or ACTH. Spontaneous (endogenous) Cushing's syndrome can result from ACTH excess (ACTH-dependent), which can arise from the pituitary gland or from ectopic ACTH-secreting tumors, or from autonomous secretion of cortisol (ACTH-independent) by a cortisol-secreting adrenal tumor or "micronodular" adrenals (Table 5–14).

ACTH-dependent Cushing's syndrome, which accounts for about 85 percent of endogenous cases, is caused by pituitary ACTH secretion (microadenomas, macroadenomas, corticotrope hyperplasia) in 80 percent of cases and ectopic ACTH secretion in 20 percent. Pituitary ACTH secretion is called Cushing's disease.

TABLE 5–13   Classification of Hypercortisolism

Physiologic states
Stress
Pregnancy
Chronic strenuous exercise
Pathophysiologic states
Cushing's syndrome
Psychiatric states
Depression
Alcoholism
Anorexia nervosa
Panic anxiety
Narcotic withdrawal
Malnutrition
Glucocorticoid resistance

ACTH-independent Cushing's syndrome, which accounts for about 15 percent of endogenous cases, is usually the result of a benign cortisol-secreting adrenal adenoma or an adrenocortical carcinoma. A rare form of Cushing's syndrome, micronodular adrenal disease, is caused by multiple, small, bilateral, cortisol-secreting adenomas. This is mainly a disorder of children and adolescents. Autoantibodies against the ACTH receptor have been suggested as the adrenocortical stimulator in such subjects.

Clinical Presentation

The typical clinical presentation of Cushing's syndrome includes emotional disturbances, truncal obesity, facial rounding (moon facies), plethora, muscle weakness and fatigue, hirsutism, and typical purple skin striae. Hypertension, carbohydrate intolerance or diabetes, amenorrhea, loss of libido, or easy bruising or spontaneous fractures of ribs and vertebrae may be encountered. Although all patients with Cushing's syndrome may exhibit some of these features at the time of diagnosis, few, if any, will have all of them. Pictures of the patient taken over a period of years are particularly helpful in the clinical evaluation.

Diagnosis

Appropriate therapy of patients with Cushing's syndrome depends on accurate diagnosis and classification of the disorder. In addition to the history and clinical

TABLE 5–14   Classification of Cushing's Syndrome and Rate of Occurrence

ACTH-dependent	(85%)
Pituitary (disease)	(80%)
Ectopic ACTH	(20%)
Ectopic CRH	(rare)
ACTH-independent	(15%)
Adrenal adenoma	
Adrenal carcinoma	
Micronodular adrenal disease	(rare)

evaluation, the laboratory evaluation of a patient with cushingoid appearance is necessary to establish the diagnosis and determine the cause of hypercortisolism (Table 5–15).

The first step is the biochemical documentation of endogenous hypercortisolism. This step can usually be accomplished by outpatient tests. These include measurement of 24-hour urinary free cortisol excretion and/or the determination of 24-hour urinary 17-hydroxysteroid excretion (corrected per gram of creatinine). The single-dose dexamethasone suppression test may also be employed as a screening test. Isolated plasma ACTH and cortisol determinations are of limited value since both hormones are secreted episodically and in a circadian fashion and their secretion is influenced by physical or emotional stress. Frequently, patients with hypercortisolism have isolated plasma ACTH and cortisol levels in the normal range.

The determination of 24-hour urinary free cortisol excretion is the best available first-line test for documentation of endogenous hypercortisolism. Assuming complete collections, there are virtually no false-negative results. False-positive results, however, may be obtained in several non-Cushing's hypercortisolemic states (see Table 15–13).

Urinary 24-hour 17-hydroxysteroid excretion corrected for the urinary creatinine excretion gives an indirect measure of the rate of cortisol secretion. It can be used for the establishment of hypercortisolism when assays for urinary free cortisol excretion are not available.

The overnight 1-mg dexamethasone suppression test is a useful screening procedure for hypercortisolism. It is simple and has a low incidence of false normal suppression (less than 3 percent). The same test, however, has a high incidence of false-positive results (approximately 20 to 30 percent) and does not distinguish between hypercortisolism due to Cushing's syndrome and other hypercortisolemic states (see Table 5–13).

If the response to a single-dose dexamethasone suppression test and the 24-hour urinary free cortisol excretion are normal, Cushing's syndrome is excluded. Some patients, however, may have an abnormal cortisol response in a single-dose dexamethasone suppression test but consistently normal urinary free cortisol.

Problems in Diagnosis

The depressed phase of primary affective disorder is frequently associated with sustained hypercortisolism (pseudo–Cushing's state). On the other hand, patients with Cushing's syndrome often have signs of clinical depression. Clinically, patients with depression who are hirsute or obese and who have an inadequate suppression of plasma cortisol after dexamethasone and elevated urinary free cortisol excretion (usually between 90 and 200 μg per day) can be difficult or impossible to distinguish from patients with mild or early Cushing's syndrome.

An ITT and/or a CRH test with measurements of plasma ACTH and cortisol responses could be helpful in the differential diagnosis (see Table 5–15). Most patients with Cushing's syndrome (80 to 90 percent) fail to respond to hypoglycemia, whereas depressed patients have normal cortisol responses. On the other hand, patients with Cushing's disease (85 percent) have a "normal" or exaggerated ACTH response to CRH because of the adenoma resistance to the negative feedback effect of cortisol. In contrast, patients with depression (75 percent) have a blunted ACTH response to oCRH, probably as a result of appropriate pituitary suppression by the elevated levels of cortisol (Fig. 5–2).

In several patients with alcohol-induced pseudo–Cushing's syndrome, the clinical and biochemical picture can closely mimic that of Cushing's disease. The most common characteristics of alcoholic patients are elevated plasma cortisol concentrations at 8:00 AM, insufficient suppression of plasma cortisol in response to 1 mg of dexamethasone, and absence of the diurnal rhythm of plasma cortisol. In contrast to Cushing's syndrome, an increase of plasma ACTH and cortisol response to insulin-induced hypoglycemia is observed. Discontinuation of alcohol consumption is accompanied by correction of hypercortisolism, including normalization of responsiveness to dexamethasone and return of the circadian cortisol rhythm.

Hyperthyroidism, liver disease, and renal failure may cause confusion in the interpretation of adrenal tests. Hyperthyroidism causes elevations of plasma CBG and increased secretion and metabolism of cortisol. Although plasma cortisol levels and urinary cortisol metabolites may be elevated in hyperthyroidism, urinary free cortisol values are generally within the normal range. In patients with liver disease, an altered circadian periodicity of cortisol has been described, whereas a decreased clearance of corticosteroids could at least partly account for the frequently observed excessive response of 11-deoxycortisol to metyrapone. In patients with severe renal failure (creatinine clearance less than 15 ml per minute per 1.73 m²) the urinary values of free cortisol and 17-hydroxysteroids may give falsely low values.

Estrogen may cause a modest increase in plasma cortisol levels because of increases in the concentration of cortisol-binding globulin. The overnight 1 mg dexamethasone suppression test in patients receiving estrogen may show no "suppressibility," but 24-hour urinary free cortisol excretion is usually normal or slightly elevated.

Many drugs, including phenytoin, phenobarbital, and primidone, accelerate the metabolism of dexamethasone and may cause a false-positive "response" in a dexamethasone suppression test owing to the lower plasma dexamethasone levels achieved.

In some patients, such as alcoholics, the gastrointestinal absorption of dexamethasone may be suboptimal. Low plasma dexamethasone concentrations may account for the poor suppression of plasma cortisol in

TABLE 5-15 Diagnostic Testing in Cushing's Syndrome and Pseudo-Cushing States

Type	CRH	Liddle Test (Urinary 17-OHS)	Metyrapone Tests (Urinary 17-OHS)	CT/MRI	BIPSS†	Iodocholesterol Scan	ITT
ACTH-dependent Cushing's syndrome							
Pituitary	ACTH ↑ Cortisol ↑	Low dose — High dose ↓	↑	Pituitary ± Adrenal ↑ (macronodules)	Gradient Lateralization	Bilateral uptake	ACTH — Cortisol —
Ectopic ACTH	ACTH — Cortisol —	Low dose — High dose —	—	Pituitary — Adrenal ↑ (macronodules)	No gradient	Bilateral uptake	ACTH — Cortisol —
Ectopic CRH (rare)	High plasma CRH	(Low dose — High dose ↓)*	? (↑)*	Pituitary — Adrenal ↑	(Gradient)*	(Bilateral uptake)*?	(ACTH —)* (Cortisol —)*
ACTH-independent Cushing's syndrome							
Adrenal adenoma	ACTH ↓ Cortisol —	Low dose — High dose —	—	+	ACTH ↓	Unilateral uptake	—
Adrenal carcinoma	ACTH ↓ Cortisol —	Low dose — High dose —	—	+	ACTH ↓	—	—
Micronodular adrenal disease	ACTH ↓ Cortisol —	Low dose — High dose — (Paradoxical ↑)	—	±	ACTH ↓	± Bilateral uptake	—
Pseudo-Cushing states (depression)	ACTH blunted Cortisol ↑	Low dose ± ↓ High dose ↓	↑	?	?	(Bilateral uptake)*?	ACTH ↑ Cortisol↑

↑ = elevation or enlargement; ↓ = suppression; + = positive test; — = negative test or no change; ± = positive or negative
* Theoretically expected.
† BIPSS = Bilateral Interior Petrosal Sinus Sampling.

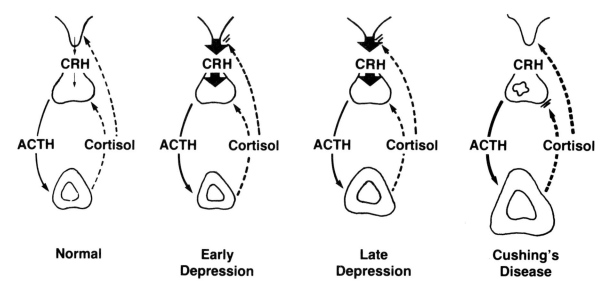

Figure 5-2   Schematic representation of pathophysiologic defects in hypothalamic-pituitary-adrenocortical function in depression and Cushing's disease. (From Gold PW, Chrousos GP. Clinical studies with corticotropin releasing factor: Implications for the diagnosis and pathophysiology of depression, Cushing's disease, and adrenal insufficiency. Psychoneuroendocrinology 1985; 10:401; copyright 1985, Pergamon Press plc; with permission.)

these patients. Delayed clearance of dexamethasone owing to genetic factors may cause apparent cortical suppression in patients with Cushing's syndrome. However, urinary free cortisol excretion is elevated in such patients. Hydrocortisone suppression tests have been developed for such patients and for patients receiving drugs that accelerate metabolism of dexamethasone.

Hypercortisolism without Cushing's syndrome has been found in several families with primary glucocorticoid resistance. In such patients, the dexamethasone suppression tests may show suboptimal suppressibility.

Differential Diagnosis

Once the diagnosis of endogenous Cushing's syndrome has been established, testing should be undertaken to clarify the specific cause. The tests are of two types: those that examine the integrity of the feedback axis and imaging techniques used mainly to examine the size and shape of the pituitary and adrenal glands and to localize ectopic ACTH-secreting tumors (see Table 5–15).

The first category includes the dexamethasone suppression test, the metyrapone test, and the oCRH stimulation test. The standard high-dose dexamethasone test as described by Liddle (1960) (see Table 5–12) is an excellent procedure for differentiating Cushing's disease from the ectopic ACTH syndrome. About 85 percent of patients with Cushing's disease demonstrate a decrease in urinary 17-hydroxysteroid excretion to values less than 50 percent of the baseline values on day 6 of the test, whereas less than 10 percent of patients with the ectopic ACTH syndrome or ACTH-independent Cushing's syndrome respond in this manner (see Table 5–15).

The standard metyrapone test is also useful (see Table 5–9). Eighty percent of patients with Cushing's dis-

ease have normal or increased responses to metyrapone, whereas most patients with the ectopic ACTH syndrome fail to respond in this manner (see Table 5–15).

When a reliable and sensitive ACTH assay is available, determination of plasma ACTH simultaneously with plasma cortisol provides very useful information about the etiology of Cushing's syndrome, as it would distinguish ACTH-dependent from non-ACTH-dependent Cushing's syndrome. Adrenal cortisol-secreting tumors and micronodular adrenal disease are associated with suppressed levels of plasma ACTH. Plasma ACTH concentrations are normal or elevated in Cushing's disease and the ectopic ACTH syndrome. The magnitude of elevation of plasma ACTH also has differential diagnostic value, since frequently patients with the ectopic ACTH syndrome have greater plasma ACTH levels than those with Cushing's disease.

Recently, the oCRH test has been reported to be equal to the standard dexamethasone suppression test in discriminating between Cushing's disease and ectopic ACTH secretion (see Table 5–15). Patients with Cushing's disease respond to oCRH with increases in plasma levels of ACTH and cortisol, whereas patients with ectopic ACTH production do not (Fig. 5–3). The diagnostic power of the dexamethasone suppression test and oCRH test is enhanced when both tests are employed. Negative results from both tests exclude the diagnosis of Cushing's disease with a diagnostic accuracy of more than 98 percent.

Imaging Evaluation

Imaging techniques can help clarify the etiology of hypercortisolism. These include computed tomographic (CT) scanning and MRI of the pituitary gland and CT scan, MRI, and ultrasound imaging of the adrenal glands.

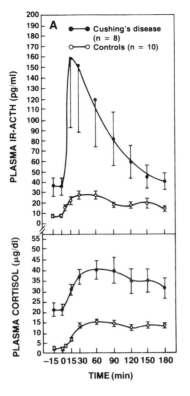
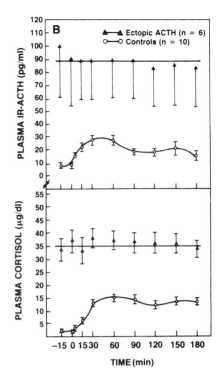

Figure 5-3 Plasma IR-ACTH (*top*) and IR-cortisol (*bottom*) responses to oCRH in eight untreated patients with Cushing's disease (●), six patients with Cushing's syndrome due to ectopic ACTH secretion (▲), and 10 human controls (○). (From Chrousos GP, Schulte HM, Oldfield EH, et al. The corticotropin-releasing factor stimulation test: An aid in the evaluation of patients with Cushing's syndrome. N Engl J Med 1984; 310:622; with permission.)

CT and MRI scans of the chest and abdomen and chest tomography are also employed when tumors secreting ectopic ACTH are sought.

Pituitary ACTH-secreting tumors are mainly microadenomas with a diameter less than 5 mm. Plain sella radiographs and sella tomography are normal in the majority of patients. Less than 10 percent of patients with Cushing's disease have a large enough tumor (macroadenoma) to cause changes in the sella turcica, including sellar enlargement or erosion of the floor.

The most appropriate initial procedure to detect pituitary ACTH-secreting tumors is a CT or an MRI scan of the sella turcica. These have replaced other diagnostic procedures used previously, including tomography, pneumoencephalography, and carotid angiography. The availability of thin-section, high-resolution CT and/or MRI scanners now permits recognition of tumors 3 to 4 mm in diameter, whereas the appropriate use of a contrast material with dynamic scanning has further improved the diagnostic accuracy (Fig 5-4). In spite of these remark-

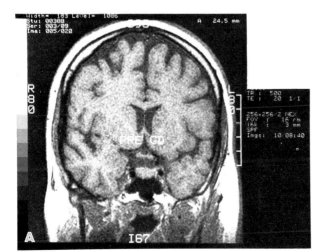
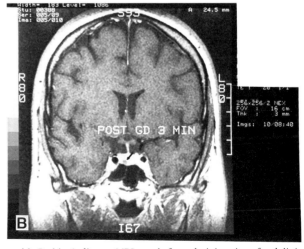

Figure 5-4 *A*, MRI of the pituitary gland in coronal projection in a patient with Cushing's disease. MRI scan before administration of gadolinium shows normal pituitary. *B*, Pituitary MRI after administration of gadolinium demonstrates small adenoma (3 mm in diameter) in the right inferior part of the gland (*arrow*). Note enhancement of the pituitary stalk and gland owing to absence of the blood-brain barrier. (Courtesy of J. Doppman.)

able advances in imaging technology, however, abnormal pituitary CT and MRI scans are found in less than 40 percent of patients with pituitary corticotropinomas. The absence of any radiation exposure and the greater sensitivity on newer MRI scanners provide MRI a great advantage over CT scan for initial or repeated examinations.

CT or MRI of the adrenal glands is useful in the distinction of a cortisol-secreting adrenal adenoma or carcinoma from Cushing's disease and the ectopic ACTH syndrome. Most adrenocortical carcinomas are large in patients with Cushing's syndrome and hence are easily detectable by CT or MRI. Although adrenocortical adenomas are usually smaller (less than 5 cm in diameter) than carcinomas, most can also be demonstrated by CT or MRI. Generally, since most adrenal adenomas causing hypercortisolism are larger than 2 cm in diameter, they can be easily detected because of the excess retroperitoneal periadrenal fat observed in Cushing's syndrome. Although it may be functionally atrophic, the contralateral gland usually appears normal (Fig. 5–5). The appearance on CT or MRI scans of adrenal hyperplasia, diffuse or nodular, includes bilateral enlargement of the adrenal gland, with thickening or subtle nodularity, but with presentation of a relatively normal overall glandular configuration (Fig. 5–6).

The widespread use of abdominal CT or MRI scan has led to increasing discovery of incidental adrenal masses. The majority are nonfunctioning adenomas ("incidentalomas"). The frequency of "incidentalomas" increases with age. After the age of 40 years, approximately 0.5 to 1 percent of the population would have such adrenal masses. Percutaneous aspiration under CT or ultrasound control has been advocated to rule out malignancy or to establish the nature of incidentally discovered

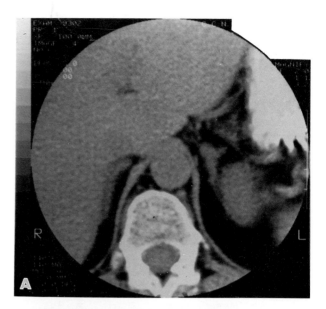

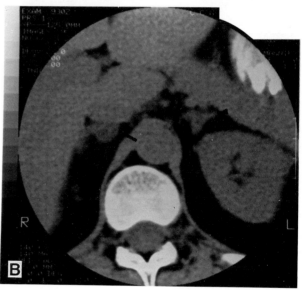

Figure 5–6 *A*, CT shows bilateral hyperplastic adrenal glands in a patient with Cushing's disease. *B*, Focal nodule (*arrow*) in the right adrenal gland in a patient with macronodular adrenal hyperplasia. (Courtesy of J. Doppman.)

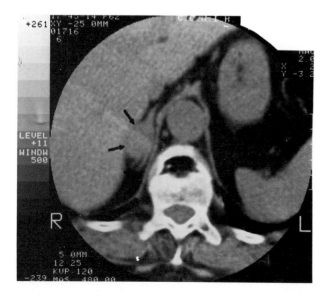

Figure 5–5 Typical cortisol-secreting benign adrenocortical adenoma (*arrows*) involving right adrenal gland. Note atrophy of the rest of the gland (*arrowheads*). (Courtesy of J. Doppman.)

adrenal masses. MRI may be particularly helpful in distinguishing a small adrenal carcinoma from a large adenoma in a patient with Cushing's syndrome. MRI is associated with greater enhancement of the tumoral mass (Fig. 5–7). Also, MRI may help distinguish incidentalomas from small cortical carcinomas or silent adrenal metastases. In the asymptomatic nonhypertensive patient with an "incidentaloma," percutaneous biopsy or adrenalectomy should be seriously considered if the MRI appears suspicious for adrenocortical carcinoma or if the diameter of the adrenal mass exceeds 5 cm. For smaller tumors with nonsuspicious imaging, frequent serial monitoring of the tumor should be undertaken (every 2 to 3 months initially) to ascertain the constancy of size.

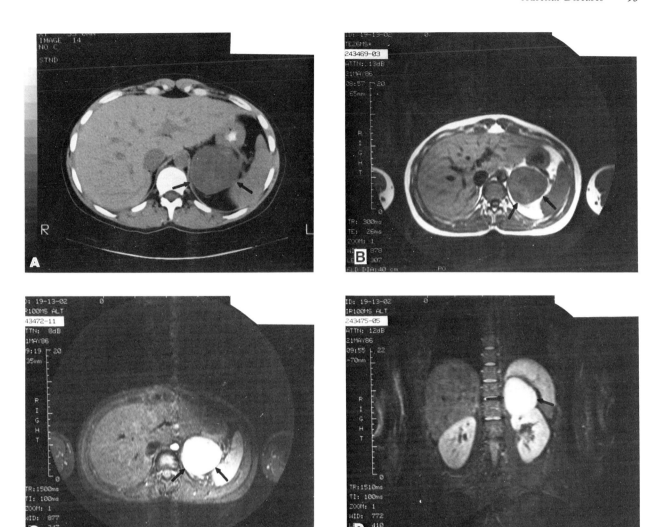

Figure 5-7 *A*, Functioning adrenocortical carcinoma shown on CT. *B*, T₁-weighted MRI showing mass with low signal intensity similar to that of liver tissue. *C*, T₂-weighted MRI showing mass with high signal intensity. *D*, In the coronal projection, one sees the relation of carcinoma of the T₂-weighted MRI (*arrows*) to the upper pole of the kidney. (Courtesy of J. Doppman.)

Ultrasonography provides another noninvasive means for imaging of adrenal lesions, but its sensitivity and accuracy are less than those of the CT or MRI scans. Ultrasound has been useful in thin patients who have little fat to outline structures on CT or MRI. However, considerable technical and diagnostic skill is required for this technique.

The iodocholesterol scan is rarely necessary in the evaluation of patients with Cushing's syndrome (see Table 5-15). This scanning procedure has been largely superseded by CT or MRI scans, which are simpler and faster and involve less radiation. The iodocholesterol scan, however, may on occasion have some advantages over CT or MRI scans. For instance, whereas adrenal carcinomas fail to image with this technique, cortisol-secreting adrenal adenomas and ACTH-dependent nodules concentrate iodocholesterol and, hence, image. Bilateral, symmetrical (adrenocortical hyperplasia), or asymmetrical (macronodular adrenal hyperplasia) adrenal visualization occurs as a result of ACTH-secreting pituitary or ectopic tumors, and unilateral visualization occurs as a result of ACTH-independent macroadenomas.

The iodocholesterol scan is also useful to localize ectopic adrenal tissue (adrenal rest cells in the liver or other sites) or an adrenal remnant that is causing recurrent hypercortisolism after bilateral adrenalectomy. In general, it should be kept in mind that, frequently, 2 days after administration of iodocholesterol may not be sufficient time to allow for visualization of adrenal tissue. Three to seven days may be necessary on occasion.

Catheterization Studies

A major problem in the differential diagnosis of ACTH-dependent Cushing's syndrome is distinguishing Cushing's disease from the ectopic ACTH syndrome. Both entities can have similar clinical and laboratory features. In addition, both pituitary microadenomas and ectopic ACTH-secreting tumors may be radiologically occult. Bilateral inferior petrosal venous sinus and peripheral vein catheterization with simultaneous collection of samples for measurement of ACTH is one of the most specific tests available to localize the source of ACTH production (see Table 5–15).

Venous blood from the anterior pituitary drains into the cavernous sinus and subsequently into the superior and inferior petrosal sinuses (see Fig. 5–8). Catheters are led into each inferior petrosal sinus via the ipsilateral femoral vein. The location of the catheters is confirmed radiologically by injection of radiopaque solution. Samples for measurement of plasma ACTH are collected from each inferior petrosal sinus and a peripheral vein both before and 3, 5, and 10 minutes after injection of 1 μg per kilogram of oCRH. Patients with the ectopic ACTH syndrome have no ACTH concentration gradient between either inferior petrosal sinus and the peripheral sample. On the other hand, an increased gradient (≥ 1.6) of plasma ACTH between any or both of the inferior petrosal sinuses is highly suggestive of Cushing's disease (Figs. 5–9 and 5–10). Petrosal sinus sampling must always be performed bilaterally and simultaneously. Unilateral or nonsimultaneous sampling may provide false results. ACTH levels are often identical to peripheral levels in the inferior petrosal sinus contralateral to a pituitary microadenoma.

Recently, the development of a new transsphenoidal microsurgical approach, hemihypophysectomy, has increased the importance of accurate preoperative localization of the side of pituitary microadenoma. Because in many cases preoperative localization with imaging techniques is impossible and the microadenoma cannot be identified at surgery, the only data on which the surgeon should base the decision to perform hemihypophysectomy are the results of bilateral inferior petrosal sinus sampling (BIPSS).

BIPSS is not indicated in patients with large pituitary adenomas in whom noninvasive tests such as plain radiography or CT and MRI scans suggest unequivocally Cushing's disease. The usefulness of BIPSS in patients with previous transsphenoidal surgery remains to be determined.

Cushing's Syndrome with Unusual Laboratory Behavior

Periodic Cushing's Syndrome.   Occasionally, cortisol production in Cushing's syndrome may not be constantly increased but may range from normal to elevated in a periodic infradian pattern ranging in length from days to months. This rare phenomenon of periodic, cyclic, or episodic hormonogenesis has been described in patients with Cushing's disease, the ectopic ACTH syndrome (bronchial carcinoids were involved in half of the reported cases), and adrenal tumors or micronodular adrenal disease.

Biochemically, patients with periodic hormonogen-

esis may have paradoxically "normal" responses to dexamethasone and poor responsiveness to metyrapone. Discrepancies between the clinical picture and the biochemical pattern are typical. Thus, patients with stigmata of clinical Cushing's syndrome may have consistently normal 24-hour urinary free cortisol levels and normal responses to dexamethasone. In such patients, several weekly 24-hour urinary free cortisol determinations for a period of 3 to 6 months may be necessary to establish the diagnosis.

Adrenocortical Carcinoma with Cushing's Syndrome.   Patients with Cushing's syndrome due to adrenocortical carcinoma frequently also have signs of virilization or feminization. The excretion of urinary 17-ketosteroids is greater in these patients than in patients with cortisol-secreting adrenocortical adenomas. Accordingly, plasma DHEAS levels are usually elevated in patients with adrenocortical carcinomas in contrast to the very low DHEAS levels in patients with cortisol-secreting adrenal adenomas. In the latter, zona reticularis function is suppressed, a result of ACTH suppression.

Occult Ectopic ACTH Syndrome.   The occult ectopic ACTH syndrome has gained increasing recognition. This syndrome can mimic the clinical and biochemical picture of Cushing's disease. Despite extensive localization studies, the tumor frequently eludes detection. The use of the BIPSS test in patients with the occult ectopic ACTH syndrome is the best possible means to ascertain the diagnosis. The absence of a central to peripheral gradient before and after administration of oCRH should rule out Cushing's disease. In the search for the tumor, special emphasis should be placed on the lungs, thymus, pancreas, adrenal medulla, and thyroid, as most described ectopic ACTH-secreting tumors have been found in these organs.

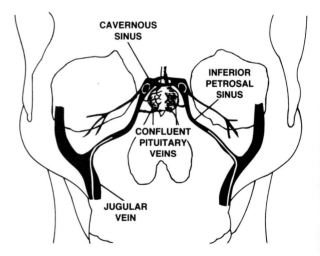

Figure 5–8   Catheter placement for bilateral simultaneous blood sampling of the inferior petrosal sinuses. (From Oldfield EH, Chrousos GP, Schulte HM, et al. Preoperative lateralization of ACTH-secreting pituitary microadenomas by bilateral and simultaneous inferior petrosal venous sinus sampling. N Engl J Med 1985; 312:100. Reprinted with permission from *The New England Journal of Medicine*.)

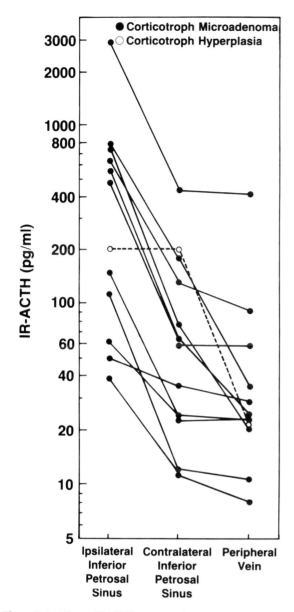

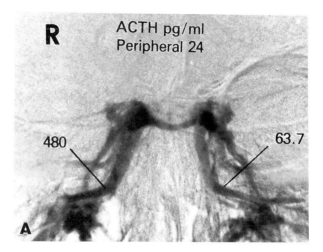

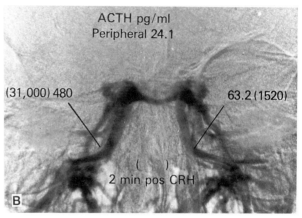

Figure 5-10 *A*, Radiograph of the inferior petrosal sinuses. Numbers indicate plasma IR-ACTH concentrations before oCRH was administered. *B*, Numbers in parentheses indicate plasma IR-ACTH concentrations 2 minutes after administration of 1 μg per kilogram of oCRH.

Figure 5-9 Plasma IR-ACTH concentrations in plasma samples obtained simultaneously from both the inferior petrosal sinuses and a peripheral vein in patients with Cushing's disease who had pituitary microadenomas and in a patient with diffuse corticotrope hyperplasia. (From Oldfield EH, Chrousos GP, Schulte HM, et al. Preoperative lateralization of ACTH-secreting pituitary microadenomas by bilateral and simultaneous inferior petrosal venous sinus sampling. N Engl J Med 1985; 312:100. Reprinted with permission from *The New England Journal of Medicine.*)

Micronodular Adrenal Disease. Micronodular adrenal disease is a rare form of Cushing's syndrome caused by multiple, small, bilateral, autonomous cortisol-secreting adenomas. A disorder of children and adolescents, it can be associated with a family history of similar cases. Pathologically, the adrenal weight is decreased and there is atrophic parenchyma between nodules. These nodules contain a dark brown stain in their cytoplasm. The clinical picture is usually mild, and a long interval between onset of symptoms and diagnosis is not uncom-

mon. On laboratory evaluation, the plasma ACTH value is suppressed and the plasma cortisol moderately elevated. Plasma cortisol is not suppressible by high-dose dexamethasone. In some cases, a paradoxic elevation of plasma or urinary cortisol is observed following administration of dexamethasone. Adrenal CT and MRI scans are usually normal.

Cushing's Syndrome in Pregnancy. In normal pregnancy, a small progressive rise in plasma ACTH and a two- to threefold increase in plasma total and free cortisol occur (see Table 5-13). Urinary free cortisol is also elevated above normal between the 34th and 40th weeks of gestation (90 to 160 μg per day). As noted earlier, in the latter part of pregnancy, IR-CRH of placental origin is detected in plasma, with levels reaching 4,000 pg per milliliter. Since plasma cortisol is poorly suppressed in response to dexamethasone in pregnancy, the diagnosis of mild or early Cushing's syndrome may be difficult to ascertain.

Primary Cortisol Resistance. Glucocorticoid resistance in humans is characterized by spontaneous hypercortisolism without the features of Cushing's syndrome (see Table 5–13). Patients with this rare syndrome have an apparent end-organ insensitivity to cortisol owing to decreased glucocorticoid receptor affinity or concentrations. Despite chronic endogenous biochemical hypercortisolism—increased serum and urinary cortisol, altered excretory profiles of cortisol metabolites, and decreased cortisol suppression by dexamethasone administration—these patients lack the classic features of Cushing's syndrome. Plasma cortisol has a circadian rhythm similar to normal, albeit with elevated concentrations. Radiologic studies of the pituitary and adrenals are normal. Severely affected patients with glucocorticoid resistance can present with hypertension and hypokalemic alkalosis, a result of excessive mineralocorticoid effect of elevated cortisol and other salt-retaining corticoids (11-deoxycorticosterone, corticosterone) on the intact mineralocorticoid receptor.

EVALUATION OF PATIENTS WITH HYPOCORTISOLISM—ADRENAL INSUFFICIENCY

Hypocortisolism results from inadequate adrenocortical function. The disease can be primary, resulting from destruction or dysfunction of the adrenal cortex, or secondary, resulting from ACTH hyposecretion (Table 5–16).

Etiologic Classification

Primary Adrenal Insufficiency

Autoimmune destruction of the adrenal glands is currently the most common cause of primary adrenal insufficiency (Addison's disease) in the industrialized nations of the world, accounting for about 65 percent of cases. Patients with this disorder have a high incidence of hypofunction of other endocrine organ failures (polyglandular autoimmune endocrinopathy). More than 70 percent of addisonian patients have antiadrenal antibodies. A smaller percentage of patients also have antibodies directed at one or more other endocrine glands.

Of the infectious diseases causing primary adrenal insufficiency, tuberculosis used to be the most common. Its frequency has decreased dramatically in recent years, however, and it currently accounts for less than 20 percent of the cases of primary adrenal insufficiency. Fungal infections have also been shown to cause primary adrenal insufficiency. Metastatic tumors and infiltration of the adrenal cortices by tumorous cells are rare causes of primary adrenal insufficiency. Other uncommon causes include sarcoidosis, amyloidosis, injury of both adrenals by trauma, hemorrhage (usually in patients on anticoagulants), sepsis (meningococcemia), and acquired immunodeficiency syndrome. Rare causes of congenital or hereditary adrenal dysfunction include congenital enzyme deficiencies of adrenal steroid biosynthesis (congenital adrenal hyperplasia), adrenal unresponsiveness to ACTH, congenital adrenal hypoplasia, and two demyelinating

TABLE 5–16   Etiologic Classification of Adrenal Insufficiency

Primary
1. Idiopathic (autoimmune) 65%
2. Infectious (tuberculous 17%, fungal, cytomegalovirus)
3. Neoplastic infiltration (metastatic malignancy)
4. Hemorrhage (meningococcemia, anticoagulants, trauma, emboli)
5. Sarcoidosis
6. Amyloidosis
7. Hemochromatosis
8. Congenital—hereditary (congenital adrenal hyperplasia, congenital adrenal hypoplasia, unresponsiveness to ACTH, adrenoleukodystrophy, adrenomyeloneuropathy)
9. Bilateral adrenalectomy
10. Steroid synthesis inhibitors (metyrapone, aminoglutethimide, ketoconazole, etomidate, trilostane)
11. Adrenolytic agents (o,p'-DDD, suramin)
12. Glucocorticoid antagonists (RU 486)

Secondary
1. HPA suppression following endogenous or exogenous hypercortisolism (Cushing's syndrome, exogenous supraphysiologic doses of glucocorticoids, exogenous ACTH)
2. Pituitary and hypothalamic lesions (congenital aplasia, hypoplasia, dysplasia, tumors, hypophysectomy or radiation therapy, autoimmune disease, infarction or hemorrhage, granulomatous disease, vascular malformation)

lipid metabolism disorders, adrenoleukodystrophy (Schilder's disease) and adrenomyeloneuropathy.

Bilateral adrenalectomy, agents that inhibit cortisol biosynthesis (metyrapone, aminoglutethimide, trilostane, ketoconazole), adrenolytic drugs (o,p'-DDD), and glucocorticoid receptor antagonists (RU 486) should also be included as causes of primary adrenal insufficiency.

Secondary Adrenal Insufficiency

Secondary or central adrenal insufficiency has two main causes: first, adrenal suppression resulting from chronic exogenous glucocorticoid administration (iatrogenic hypoadrenalism) or endogenous glucocorticoid overproduction (after surgical cure of Cushing's syndrome) and, second, disorders of the hypothalamic-pituitary unit, resulting in decreased secretion of ACTH.

Transient adrenal insufficiency resulting from chronic suppression of the HPA axis by glucocorticoids is the most common cause of secondary adrenal insufficiency. It can last 6 to 12 months following discontinuation of exposure to glucocorticoids. The degree and duration of suppression depend on both the level and duration of exposure to glucocorticoids.

Hypothalamic-pituitary abnormalities that result in adrenal insufficiency include space-occupying lesions such as tumors (e.g., craniopharyngioma, metastatic lesions) or granulomas (sarcoidosis and tuberculosis), vascular lesions, radiation, head trauma, pituitary apoplexy, lymphoid hypophysitis, massive postpartum hemorrhage (Sheehan's syndrome), and, rarely, isolated ACTH deficiency.

Clinical Presentation

Adrenocortical insufficiency, whether a result of primary disease of the adrenal glands, insufficient pituitary ACTH secretion, or inadequate steroid replacement, can present clinically as an acute state (adrenal crisis) or as a chronic condition.

Acute Adrenal Insufficiency

A history of weight loss, increasing fatigue, anorexia and vomiting, and skin hyperpigmentation is suggestive of the diagnosis of acute adrenal insufficiency. Also, a history of prior glucocorticoid therapy, pituitary surgery or radiation, and acute headache may be important clues to the diagnosis. Patients in adrenal crisis present with hypovolemic shock, fever, an acute abdomen, and occasionally hypoglycemia (primarily in children or young and thin individuals).

Chronic Adrenal Insufficiency

The clinical manifestations of chronic adrenal insufficiency are due to hypocortisolism and/or mineralocorticoid deficiency. Symptoms and signs include weakness and fatigue, anorexia, nausea and vomiting, abdominal pain, diarrhea, muscle and joint pain, postural dizziness, and orthostatic hypotension. Hyperpigmentation (extensor surfaces, creases of the palm, buccal mucosa) and vitiligo are present only in patients with primary adrenal insufficiency. Some patients with primary adrenal insufficiency do not have significant hyperpigmentation.

Diagnosis

Acute Adrenal Insufficiency

The diagnosis of acute adrenal insufficiency is a medical emergency. Therapy should not be delayed by prolonged diagnostic procedures. In patients with acute adrenal insufficiency, the initial laboratory work-up should help establish the diagnosis. A low serum sodium concentration in association with an elevated serum potassium level strongly suggests primary adrenal insufficiency. In contrast, hyponatremia alone is compatible with secondary adrenal insufficiency. The blood glucose may be low or normal. The blood urea nitrogen and calcium may be high. Lymphocytosis and eosinophilia are often found. Blood cultures for bacteria might be positive (usually meningococci). If there are features compatible with pituitary disease or pituitary apoplexy, a pituitary fossa radiograph or CT or MRI scan may be helpful. Adrenal CT or MRI scans may demonstrate enlarged glands of normal configuration. This appearance suggests acute granulomatous adrenalitis, most commonly due to tuberculosis or histoplasmosis.

A specific method for making the diagnosis of acute adrenal insufficiency is to measure plasma cortisol concentrations during the crisis. If the plasma cortisol is greater than or equal to 18 μg per deciliter, the diagnosis of adrenal crisis is ruled out. If the plasma cortisol values in the setting of shock are less than 18 μg per deciliter, adrenal insufficiency is a strong possibility. One should note that in states associated with elevated concentrations of CBG (e.g., pregnancy, drug treatment), total plasma cortisol levels may be artificially elevated within the normal range.

Chronic Adrenal Insufficiency

Normochromic-normocytic anemia and moderate neutropenia with lymphocytosis and eosinophilia are commonly present. Macrocytic anemia can be found in patients with idiopathic adrenal insufficiency, a result of concomitant pernicious anemia. Electrolyte abnormalities (hyponatremia and/or hyperkalemic acidosis) are present in the majority of patients with Addison's disease. Fasting blood glucose may be low, especially in children. Adrenal calcifications may be seen in patients with primary adrenal insufficiency of tuberculous etiology.

If the possibility of adrenal insufficiency has been raised, a rapid ACTH test should be performed (see Table 5–11). Measurements of 24-hour urinary free cortisol or 17-hydroxycorticosteroid excretion are of little value as screening tests for adrenal insufficiency. An abnormal plasma cortisol response to a short ACTH test (plasma cortisol ≤ 18 μg per deciliter) should be followed by the more discriminating long ACTH stimulation test (see Table 5–11). This long test clearly establishes the diagnosis and helps categorize the hypoadrenalism into primary or secondary. Lack of an increase in plasma cortisol or urinary free cortisol and 17-hydroxycorticosteroids confirms adrenal failure. A subnormal response in the first day with an increase in plasma and/or urinary steroids over the next 1 to 2 days is suggestive of central hypoadrenalism. Other tests of adrenal function such as the ITT and the metyrapone test should not be used in patients who are strongly suspected of having adrenocortical insufficiency.

Recently, the oCRH stimulation test has been used as a diagnostic procedure in patients with adrenal insufficiency (Fig. 5–11). As expected, patients with primary adrenal insufficiency show a marked ACTH response to CRH, in association with a diminished cortisol response. Patients with secondary adrenal insufficiency due to pituitary lesions, on the other hand, have diminished ACTH and cortisol responses, whereas patients with hypothalamic lesions have delayed and prolonged ACTH responses.

It is necessary to underscore the importance of the rapid ACTH test in assessing the pituitary-adrenal axis of patients with pituitary or hypothalamic pathology both before and after surgical procedures or radiation of the area. Patients with cortisol values of 18 μg per deciliter or higher require no glucocorticoid replacement. Patients with cortisol values greater than 10 μg per deciliter but

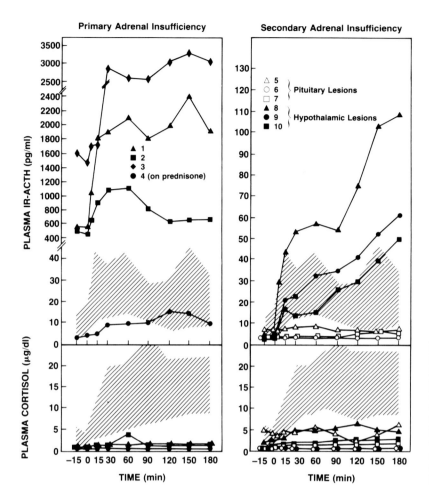

Figure 5-11 Plasma IR-ACTH (*top*) and IR-cortisol (*bottom*) responses to oCRH in patients with primary adrenal insufficiency (*left*) and secondary adrenal insufficiency (*right*). Patients with hypothalamic lesions had IR-ACTH responses to oCRH clearly different from those occurring in two patients with pituitary adrenal insufficiency. (From Schulte H, Chrousos G, Avgerinos P, et al. The corticotropin-releasing hormone stimulation test: A possible aid in the evaluation of patients with adrenal insufficiency. J Clin Endocrinol Metab 1984; 58:1064; with permission.)

less than 18 μg per deciliter should be given glucocorticoids during periods of stress. Patients with cortisol values of 10 μg per deciliter or less should be given glucocorticoid replacement.

INBORN ERRORS OF METABOLISM— CONGENITAL ADRENAL HYPERPLASIA

Congenital adrenal hyperplasia (CAH) results from deficiency of one or more enzymes necessary for the biosynthesis of cortisol and/or aldosterone (Table 5-17; also see Fig. 5-1). The defective cortisol secretion in CAH and the decreased negative feedback effect on the hypothalamic-pituitary unit result in hypersecretion of ACTH and hyperplasia of the adrenal cortex. The clinical presentation of severe CAH includes glucocorticoid deficiency, mineralocorticoid deficiency or excess, and adrenal androgen excess. In rare forms of CAH, sex-steroid deficiency can also be part of the syndrome. Since five enzymatic steps are involved in cortisol biosynthesis, there are five distinct CAH syndromes. All these syndromes are transmitted in an autosomal recessive pattern (see Table 5-17).

21-Hydroxylase Deficiency

21-Hydroxylase deficiency is the most common variant of CAH, accounting for about 95 percent of all cases of CAH. The clinical syndrome is the consequence of defective 21-hydroxylation of progesterone and 17-hydroxyprogesterone, with resulting deficient production of both cortisol and aldosterone (Fig. 5-12A). Cortisol deficiency stimulates increased ACTH release, causing overproduction and accumulation of the enzyme precursors progesterone and 17-hydroxyprogesterone. Increased ACTH stimulation leads to increased biosynthesis of DHEA and androstenedione, which finally can be converted to testosterone (see Fig. 5-1). Patients with 21-hydroxylase deficiency could be divided into two clinical phenotypes: classic 21-hydroxylase deficiency, usually diagnosed at birth or during childhood, and nonclassic or late-onset 21-hydroxylase deficiency manifest during or after puberty.

Classic (Salt-Losing and Simple Virilizing Forms) 21-Hydroxylase Deficiency

Clinical Presentation. Two-thirds of patients with classic 21-hydroxylase deficiency have various degrees of mineralocorticoid deficiency. The remaining one-third

TABLE 5-17 CAH Syndromes

Deficiency	No.	Syndrome	Enzyme	Chromosome	Frequency	Ambiguous Genitalia	Postnatal Virilization	Sexual Infantilism	Salt Metabolism	Steroids Increased	Steroids Decreased
Cholesterol desmolase	1	Lipoid hyperplasia	P450scc	15	Rare	Males	No	Yes	Salt wasting	None	All
3β-OH-steroid dehydrogenase	2	Classic	3β-OH-steroid dehydrogenase	?	Rare	Males and females	Yes	No	± Salt wasting	DHEA, 17OH-pregnenolone	Aldo, cortisol, T
		Nonclassic	3β-OH-steroid dehydrogenase	?	? Frequent	No	Yes	No	Normal	DHEA, 17OH-pregnenolone	—
17α-Hydroxylase	3		P450cl7*	10	Rare	Males	No	Yes	Hypertension	DOC, corticosterone	Cortisol, T, E_2
21α-Hydroxylase	4	Salt wasting	P450c21	6p(HLA)	1/10,000	Females	Yes	No	Salt wasting	17-OHP, Δ^4-androstenedione	Aldo, cortisol
		Simple virilizing	P450c21	6p(HLA)	1/20,000	Females	Yes	No	Normal	17-OHP, Δ^4-androstenedione	Cortisol
		Nonclasic	P450c21	6p(HLA)	0.1% (3% in Ashkenazi Jews)	No	Yes	No	Normal	17-OHP, Δ^4-androstenedione	—
11β-Hydroxylase	5	Classic	P450cl1	8q	1/100,000	Females	Yes	No	Hypertension ± salt wasting	DOC, 11-deoxycortisol	Cortisol ± aldo
		Nonclassic	P450cl1	8q	Rare	No	Yes	No	Normal	11-deoxycortisol, ± DOC	—

DHEA = dehydroepiandrosterone; DOC = 11-deoxycorticosterone; 17-OHP = 17-hydroxyprogesterone; aldo = aldosterone; T = testosterone; E_2 = estradiol.
* P450cl7 and the P450 of 17,20-desmolase are products of the same gene.
Modified from White PL, New MI, Dupont B. Congenital adrenal hyperplasia. N Engl J Med; 316: 1519 (first part) and 316:1580 (second part); with permission.

21-HYDROXYLASE DEFICIENCY

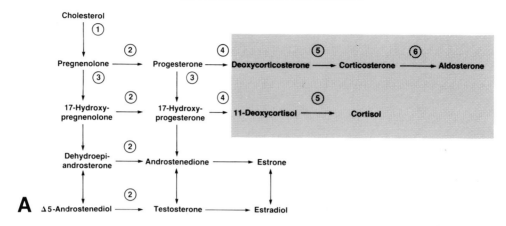

11-HYDROXYLASE DEFICIENCY

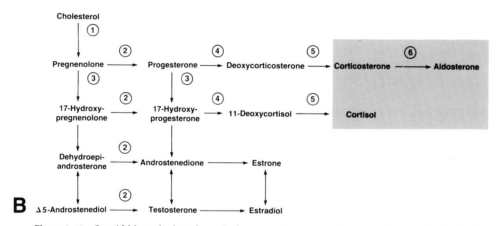

Figure 5–12   Steroid biosynthesis pathway. Each enzyme is represented by a number (see Fig. 1). Shaded area represents deficient steroid compounds after the enzymatic block. *A*, 21-Hydroxylase deficiency; *B*, 11-hydroxylase deficiency.

have the simple virilizing form of the disease. The mechanism of salt loss in the former appears to be decreased aldosterone secretion and increased concentrations of cortisol precursors with mineralocorticoid antagonist activity (progesterone, 17-hydroxyprogesterone). The major reason for symptomatic hypomineralocorticoidism in the salt-losing form appears to be a more profound enzymatic block.

The clinical manifestations of classic 21-hydroxylase deficiency vary between boys and girls. Neonate girls may have masculinization of the genitalia, ranging from clitorimegaly and various degrees of labial fusion to a common urogenital sinus and penile urethra. Neonate boys may have a normal appearance or may exhibit phallic hypertrophy. Both sexes may exhibit a salt-losing tendency with hyponatremia, hyperkalemia, acidosis, dehydration, and hypotension. Adrenal crises usually occur between 7 and 15 days of life. In children from ages 2 to 10 years, classic 21-hydroxylase deficiency presents as isosexual precocious puberty in males and heterosexual precocious puberty in females.

Diagnosis.   In 21-hydroxylase deficiency, the specific

steroids that accumulate in plasma are 17-hydroxyprogesterone and progesterone. The metabolite of the former in urine is pregnanetriol. The most useful measurement for the diagnosis of 21-hydroxylase deficiency is plasma 17-hydroxyprogesterone. There is no overlap between basal normal levels of plasma 17-hydroxyprogesterone (less than 200 ng per deciliter, except on the first day of life) and those found in 21-hydroxylase deficiency. Elevated levels of progesterone, delta[4]-androstenedione, and testosterone in the plasma or increased excretion of 17-ketosteroids in the urine is also helpful. Plasma 17-hydroxyprogesterone levels and urine pregnanetriol or 17-ketosteroids are suppressed by dexamethasone. Hyperreninemia and hypoaldosteronism would be expected in all salt losers and many patients with the simple virilizing form.

Nonclassic Forms of 21-Hydroxylase Deficiency

Late-Onset 21-Hydroxylase Deficiency.   This disorder represents an allelic variant of classic 21-hydroxylase deficiency characterized by a mild enzymatic defect. The syndrome clinically presents around puberty with virilization (primarily hirsutism and acne) and amenorrhea or oligomenorrhea.

Cryptic Form. This form includes subjects without symptoms but with the biochemical abnormalities observed in the late-onset forms. Cryptic forms can be identified in relatives of patients with 21-hydroxylase deficiency. These patients may represent an early asymptomatic phase of late-onset CAH.

Diagnosis. The diagnosis of nonclassic 21-hydroxylase deficiency should be considered in adolescent or adult women with hirsutism and/or menstrual abnormalities. Although morning levels of plasma 17-hydroxyprogesterone may be normal in these patients, they are markedly elevated (> 1,500 ng per deciliter) 30 minutes after administration of synthetic ACTH 1-24 (cosyntropin [Cortrosyn], 250 μg in an intravenous bolus).

Close genetic linkage has been found between the HLA complex and the 21-hydroxylase deficiency gene in both classic and nonclassic forms. Carriers can be defined by a Cortrosyn test (approximately two-thirds of carriers have 17-hydroxyprogesterone responses between 330 and 1,000 ng per deciliter) and by HLA haplotyping. Prenatal diagnosis of 21-hydroxylase deficiency can be based on measuring amniotic fluid levels of 17-hydroxyprogesterone at midgestation and on HLA typing of amniotic cells. Specific oligonucleotide probes could also be used for the prenatal diagnosis of 21-hydroxylase deficiency using biopsy specimens of chorionic villi.

11-Hydroxylase Deficiency

11-Hydroxylase deficiency is the second most common adrenal biosynthetic defect, accounting for about 5 percent of cases of CAH. The abnormality is an inherited deficiency of the 11-beta-hydroxylase enzyme of the adrenal cortex. As a consequence, there is impaired conversion of deoxycortisol to cortisol and of deoxycorticosterone to corticosterone and aldosterone (see Fig. 5–12*B*). The block results also in ACTH hypersecretion, adrenal hyperplasia, and overproduction of 11-deoxycortisol, deoxycorticosterone, and adrenal androgens. The large amounts of deoxycorticosterone secreted can cause hypertension and hypokalemic alkalosis. Overproduction of adrenal androgens causes virilization.

Clinical Presentation. Similar to patients with 21-hydroxylase deficiency, patients with the classic form of 11-hydroxylase deficiency present with virilization, ambiguous genitalia in genetic females, and sexual precocity in both sexes. Unlike patients with 21-hydroxylase deficiency, some patients with 11-hydroxylase deficiency can present with hypertension. Frequently, however, hypertensive manifestations may be delayed until early adulthood. In some cases, hypertension may progress into a malignant phase.

Diagnosis. The diagnosis of 11-hydroxylase deficiency can be confirmed by demonstrating marked accumulation of 11-deoxycortisol in plasma and THS in

urine. Urinary 17-ketosteroids, plasma deoxycorticosterone, delta⁴-androstenedione, and testosterone are also elevated. The elevated steroids are suppressed by dexamethasone. Aldosterone levels are subnormal, and the renin-angiotensin axis is usually suppressed.

3-Beta-Hydroxysteroid Dehydrogenase Deficiency

The enzyme 3-beta-hydroxysteroid dehydrogenase is responsible for transforming 5-steroids into 4-steroids (see Fig. 5–1) and is found in both the adrenals and the gonads. Patients with this biosynthetic defect have deficient production of adrenal glucocorticoids and mineralocorticoids and testicular testosterone. However, they have excessive production of 5-adrenal androgens.

Clinical Presentation. The classic form of this syndrome is rare. The patients present with adrenal insufficiency and ambiguous genitalia in both sexes. Males usually are born with incomplete masculinization of the external genitalia, as a result of defective testosterone biosynthesis by the testis, and females with clitorimegaly, as a result of increased secretion of delta⁵-androgens (DHEA and delta⁵-androstenediol) by the adrenals.

The late-onset form of 3-beta-hydroxysteroid dehydrogenase deficiency is a mild type of the disorder in which partial enzyme deficiency has been suggested. It has been described in women with postpubertal onset of hirsutism and menstrual abnormalities and may be quite common. Diagnostic criteria have not been established as yet, however.

Diagnosis. The diagnosis can be confirmed by demonstrating increased urinary 17-ketosteroid secretion and elevated plasma pregnenolone, 17-hydroxypregnenolone, and DHEA. Elevated steroids are suppressed by dexamethasone. After stimulation with ACTH, pregnenolone and 17-hydroxypregnenolone concentrations increase significantly.

17-Hydroxylase Deficiency

The basic abnormality of 17-hydroxylase deficiency is an inherited deficiency of the 17alpha-hydroxylase enzyme at both the adrenal cortex and gonads (see Fig. 5–1). Patients with this disorder have decreased secretion of cortisol and sex steroid but increased secretion of sodium-retaining corticoids (corticosterone, deoxycorticosterone).

Clinical Presentation. Because these patients cannot convert pregnenolone or progesterone to their 17-hydroxy derivatives, females present with normal external genitalia, failure to develop secondary sex characteristics, and primary amenorrhea. Males frequently fail to develop masculine external genitalia fully (male pseudohermaphroditism). Both sexes have hypertension, hypokalemic alkalosis, and failure to progress into puberty.

Diagnosis. The diagnosis can be established by the demonstration of elevated plasma ACTH, progesterone, deoxycorticosterone, and corticosterone and decreased plasma cortisol and androgen levels. Gonadotropins are elevated at puberty (hypergonadotropic hypogonadism). Aldosterone, renin activity, and angiotension II levels in plasma are low.

20-22 Desmolase Deficiency

The clinical picture of this rare disorder is a result of the inability of steroidogenic tissues (adrenals, gonads) to convert cholesterol to pregnenolone. All five classes of steroids are affected, with resulting hypocortisolism, hypoaldosteronism, and hypogonadism (see Fig. 5–1). Affected patients present with adrenal insufficiency and a female phenotype, regardless of the genotype. Most reported patients have died in infancy.

BIBLIOGRAPHY

Adrenal Physiology

Antoni FA. Hypothalamic control of adrenocorticotropin secretion: Advances since the discovery of 41-residue corticotropin-releasing factor. Endocr Rev 1986; 7:351.

Axelrod J, Reisine TD. Stress hormones: Their interaction and regulation. Science 1984; 224:452.

Brien TG. Free cortisol in human plasma. Horm Metab Res 1980; 12:643.

Chrousos GP, Luger A, Avgerinos PC, et al. Corticotropin releasing hormone: relevance to human physiology and pathophysiology. In: D'Agata R, Chrousos G, eds. Recent advances in adrenal function and regulation. New York: Raven Press, 1987:121.

Coghlan JP, Blair-West JR, Denton DA, et al. Control of aldosterone secretion. J Endocrinol 1979; 81:55.

DeBold CR, Sheldon WR, DeCherney GS, et al. Arginine vasopressin potentiate adrenocorticotropin release induced by ovine corticotropin-releasing factor. J Clin Invest 1984; 73:533.

Drury PL. Disorders of mineralocorticoid activity. Clin Endocrinol Metab 1985; 14:175.

Dunn JF, Nisula BC, Rodbard D. Transport of steroid hormones: Binding of 21 endogenous steroids to both testosterone-binding globulin and corticosteroid-binding globulin in human plasma. J Clin Endocrinol Metab 1981; 53:58.

Follenius M, Brandenberger G. Plasma free cortisol during secretory episodes. J Clin Endocrinol Metab 1986; 62:609.

Guyton AC. The adrenocortical hormones. In: Guyton AC. Textbook of medical physiology. Philadelphia: WB Saunders, 1985:909.

Imura H. ACTH and related peptides: Molecular biology biochemistry and regulation of secretion. Clin Endocrinol Metab 1985; 14:845.

Keller-Wood ME, Dallman MF. Corticosteroid inhibition of ACTH secretion. Endocr Rev 1984; 5:1.

Krieger DT. Physiopathology of Cushing's disease. Endocr Rev 1983; 4:22.

Luger A, Deuster PA, Kyle SB, et al. Acute hypothalamic-pituitary-adrenal responses to the stress of treadmill exercise. N Engl J Med 1987; 316:1309.

McKenna TJ, Cunningham S. Adrenal secretion and ovarian dysfunction. In: D'agata R, Chrousos GP, eds. Recent advances in adrenal function and regulation. New York: Raven Press, 1987: 151.

McKenna TJ, Island DP, Nicholson WE, et al. ACTH stimulates the late steps in cortisol biosynthesis. Acta Endocrinol 1979; 90:122.

Munck A, Guyre PM, Holbrook NJ. Physiological functions of glucocorticoids in stress and their relation to pharmacological actions. Endocr Rev 1984; 5:25.

Neville AM, MacKay AM. The structure of the human adrenal cortex in health and disease. Clin Endocrinol Metab 1972; 1:361.

Neville AM, O'Hare MJ. Histopathology of the human adrenal cortex. Clin Endocrinol Metab 1985; 14:791.

O'Hare MJ, Nice EL, Neville AM. Regulation of androgen secretion and sulfoconjugation in the human adult adrenal cortex: Studies with primary monolayer cell cultures. In: Genazzani AR, ed. Adrenal androgens. New York: Raven Press, 1980:7.

Parker LN, Odell DD. Control of adrenal androgen secretion. Endocr Rev 1980; 1:392.

Rich BH, Rosenfield RL, Lucky AW, et al. Adrenarche: Changing adrenal response to adrenocorticotropin. J Clin Endocrinol Metab 1981; 52:1129.

Rivier C, Rivier J, Mormede P, Vale W. Studies on the nature of the interaction between vasopressin and corticotropin-releasing factor on adrenocorticotropin release in the rat. Endocrinology 1984; 115:882.

Schambelan M, Slaton PE Jr, Biglieri EG. Mineralocorticoid production in hyperadrenocorticism: Role in pathogenesis of hypokalemic alkalosis. Am J Med 1971; 51:299.

Smith EK, Tippit DF. Evaluation of steroid hormone metabolism. In: Kelley VC, ed. Metabolic, endocrine and genetic disorders of children. Hagerstown, MD: Harper & Row, 1974:309.

Streeten DHP, Anderson GH Jr, Dalakos TG. Normal and abnormal function of the hypothalamic-pituitary-adrenocortical system in man. Endocr Rev 1984; 5:371.

Udelsman R, Loriaux DL, Chrousos GP. Surgical stress: The role of glucocorticoids and catecholamines. In: D'Agata R, Chrousos G, eds. Recent advances in adrenal regulation and function. New York: Raven Press, 1987:253.

Weitzman ED, Fukishima D, Nogeire C, et al. Twenty-four hour pattern of the episodic secretion of cortisol in normal subjects. J Clin Endocrinol Metab 1971; 33:14.

West CD, Mahajan DK, Chavre VJ, et al. Simultaneous measurement of multiple plasma steroids by radioimmunoassay demonstrating episodic secretion. J Clin Endocrinol Metab 1973; 36:1230.

Basal Plasma Hormones

Asfeldt VH. Plasma corticosteroids in Cushing's syndrome. Acta Med Scand 1972; 3:17.

Berson SA, Yalow RS. Radioimmunoassay of ACTH in plasma. J Clin Invest 1968; 47:2725.

Caldarella AM, Reardon GE, Canalis E. Analysis for cortisol in serum by liquid chromatography. Clin Chem 1982; 28:538.

Campbell EA, Linton EA, Wolfe CDA, et al. Plasma corticotropin-releasing hormone concentrations during pregnancy and parturition. J Clin Endocrinol Metab 1987; 64:1054.

Cavallo A, Corn C, Bryan GT, Meyer WJ. The use of plasma androstenedione in monitoring therapy of patients with congenital adrenal hyperplasia. J Pediatr 1979; 95:33.

Charlton BG, Leake A, Ferrier IN, et al. Corticotropin releasing factor in plasma of depressed patients and controls. Lancet 1986; 1:161.

Clerico A, Del Chicca MG, Zucchelli G, et al. Free cortisol assay by immunoextraction: Comparison with an equilibrium dialysis procedure. Clin Chem 1982; 28:1343.

Coghlan JP, Scoggins BA, Wintour EM. Aldosterone. In: Gray CH, James VHT, eds. Hormones in blood. Vol 3. 3rd ed., London: Academic Press, 1979:494.

Cotelli GR, Wall JH, Kabra PM, Marton LJ. Fluorometric liquid-chromatographic determination of serum cortisol. Clin Chem 1981; 27:441.

Cunnach D, Jessob DS, Besser GM, Rees LH. Measurement of circulating corticotropin releasing factor in man. J Endocrinol 1987; 113:123.

Doe RP, Lahrenz F, Seal US. Familial decrease in corticosteroid-binding globulin. Metab Clin Exp 1965; 14:940.

Gallagher TF, Yoshida K, Roffwarg HD, et al. ACTH and cortisol secretory patterns in man. J Clin Endocrinol Metab 1973; 36:1058.

Garcia MM. Immunoassay measurement of corticotropin (ACTH) and corticotropin releasing factor (CRF). J Clin Immunoassay 1983; 6:291.

Golden MP, Lippe BM, Kaplan SA, et al. Management of congenital adrenal hyperplasia using serum dehydroepiandrosterone sulfate and 17-hydroxyprogesterone concentrations. Pediatrics 1978; 61:867.

Hansen M, Pedersen AG. Tumor markers in patients with lung cancer. Chest 1986; 89:2195.

Hauffa BP, Kaplan SL, Grumbach MM. Dissociation between plasma adrenal androgens and cortisol in Cushings's disease and ectopic ACTH-producing tumor: regulation to adrenarche. Lancet 1984; 1:1373.

Hiramatsu R. Direct assay of cortisol in human saliva by solid phase radioimmunoassay and its clinical applications. Clin Chim Acta 1981; 117:239.

Jezyk PD, Dauphinais RM. Cortisol specificity by immunoassay and HPLC before and after metyrapone. J Clin Immunoassay 1983; 6:296.

Kao M, Viona S, Nichols A, Horton R. Parallel radioimmunoassay for plasma cortisol and 11-deoxycortisol. Clin Chem 1975; 21:1644.

Kater CE, Biglieri EG. Distinctive plasma aldosterone, 18-hydroxycorticosterone and 18-hydroxydeoxycorticosterone profile in the 21, 17α and 11β-hydroxylase deficiency types of congenital adrenal hyperplasia. Am J Med 1983; 75:43.

Keenan BS, Holcombe JH, Wilson DP, et al. Plasma renin activity and the response to sodium depletion in salt-losing congenital adrenal hyperplasia. Pediatr Res 1982; 16:118.

Krieger DT. Factors influencing the circadian periodicity of adrenal steroid levels. Trans NY Acad Sci 1970; 32:316.

Krieger DT, Allen W. Relationship of bioassayable and immunoassayable plasma ACTH and cortisol concentrations in normal subjects and in patients with Cushing's disease. J Clin Endocrinol Metab 1975; 40:675.

Laudat MH, Cerdas S, Fournier C, et al. Salivary cortisol measurement: A practical approach to assess pituitary-adrenal function. J Clin Endocrinol Metab 1988; 66:343.

Lee PA, Urban MD, Gutai JP, Migeon CS. Plasma progesterone, 17-hydroxyprogesterone, androstenedione and testosterone in prepubertal, pubertal, and adult subjects with congenital virilizing adrenal hyperplasia as indicators of adrenal suppression. Horm Res 1980; 13:347.

Linton EA, McLean C, Nieuwenhuyzen Kruseman AC, et al. Direct measurement of human plasma corticotropin-releasing hormone by "two-site" immunoradiometric assay. J Clin Endocrinol Metab 1987; 64:1047.

Liotta A, Krieger DT. A sensitive bioassay for the determination of human plasma ACTH levels. J Clin Endocrinol Metab 1975; 40:269.

Luisi M, Franchi F, Drafta D, Stroe E. Plasma steroid dynamics in Cushing's syndrome. Ann Endocrinol 1978; 39:107.

McKenna TJ, Miller RB, Liddle GW. Plasma pregnenolone and 17-hydroxypregnenolone in patients with adrenal tumors, ACTH excess, or idiopathic hirsutism. J Clin Endocrinol Metab 1977; 44:231.

Newsome HH Jr, Clements AS, Borum EH. The simultaneous assay of cortisol, corticosterone, 11-deoxycortisol, and cortisone in human plasma. J Clin Endocrinol Metab 1978; 34:473.

Nichols T, Nugent CA, Tyler FH. Steroid laboratory tests in the diagnosis of Cushing's syndrome. Am J Med 1968; 45:116.

Nicholson WE, Davis DR, Sherrell BJ, Orth DN. Rapid radioimmunoassay for corticotropin in unextracted human plasma. Clin Chem 1984; 30:259.

Nicholson WE, DeCherney GS, Jackson RV, et al. Plasma distribution, disappearance half-time, metabolic clearance rate, and degradation of synthetic ovine corticotropin-releasing factor in man. J Clin Endocrinol Metab 1983; 57:1263.

Nolan GE, Smith JB, Chavre VJ, et al. Spurious overestimation of plasma cortisol in patients with chronic renal failure. J Clin Endocrinol Metab 1981; 52:1242.

Ojeifo JO, Winders SJ, Troen P. Basal and adrenocorticotropin hormone-stimulated 17-hydroxyprogesterone in men with idiopathic infertility. Fertil Steril 1984; 42:97.

Orth DN. Adrenocorticotropic hormone (ACTH). In: Jaffe BM, Berman HR, eds. Methods in hormone radioimmunoassay. New York: Academic Press, 1979:245.

Otten BJ, Wellen JJ, Rijken JCW, et al. Salivary and plasma androstenedione and 17-hydroxyprogesterone levels in congenital adrenal hyperplasia. J Clin Endocrinol Metab 1983; 57:1150.

Ratcliffe JG, Podmore J, Stack BHR, et al. Circulating ACTH and related peptides in lung cancer. Br J Cancer 1982; 45:230.

Ratter SJ, Lowry PJ, Besser GM, et al. Chromatographic characterization of adrenocorticotropin in human plasma. J Endocrinol 1980; 85:359.

Robin P, Predine J, Milgram E. Assay of unbound cortisol in plasma. J Clin Endocrinol Metab 1978; 46:277.

Rosman PM, Benn MK, Tito J, et al. Cortisol binding in uremic plasma: II. Decreased cortisol binding to albumin. Nephron 1984; 37:229.

Ruder HJ, Guy RL, Lipsett MB. A radioimmunoassay for cortisol in plasma and urine. J Clin Endocrinol Metab 1972; 35:219.

Rymer JC. Estimation of plasma cortisol by radiocompetition or radioimmunoassay. Use of commercial kits. Ann Biol Clin (Paris) 1978; 36:509.

Sawin CT. Measurement of plasma cortisol in the diagnosis of Cushing's syndrome. Ann Intern Med 1968; 68:624.

Streeten DHP, Stevenson LT, Dalakos TG, et al. The diagnosis of hypercortisolism: Biochemical criteria differentiating patients from lean and obese normal subjects and from females on oral contraceptives. J Clin Endocrinol Metab 1969; 29:1191.

Suda T, Tomori N, Yajima F, et al. Immunoreactive corticotropin-releasing factor in human plasma. J Clin Invest 1985; 76:2026.

Tan SY, Donabedian R, Genel M, et al. False elevation of plasma cortisol in congenital adrenal hyperplasia. J Clin Lab Med 1977; 89:735.

Von Schnakenburg K, Bidlingmaier F, Knorr D. 17α-Hydroxyprogesterone, androstenedione, and testosterone in normal children and in prepubertal patients with congenital adrenal hyperplasia. Eur J Pediatr 1980; 133:259.

Wallace AM, Beastall GH, Cook B, et al. Neonatal screening for congenital adrenal hyperplasia: A programme based on a novel direct radioimmunoassay for 17-hydroxyprogesterone in blood spots. J Endocrinol 1986; 108:299.

Weidmann P, de Myttenaere-Bursztein S, Maxwell MH, et al. Effect of aging of plasma renin and aldosterone in normal man. Kidney Int 1975; 8:325.

White A, Smith H, Hoadley M, et al. Clinical evaluation of a two-site immunoradiometric assay for adrenocorticotrophin in unextracted human plasma using monoclonal antibodies. Clin Endocrinol 1987; 26:41.

Yalow RS, Berson SA. Characteristics of "big ACTH" in human plasma and pituitary extracts. J Clin Endocrinol Metab 1973; 36:415.

Yamaji T, Ishibashi M, Sekihara H, et al. Serum dehydroepiandrosterone sulfate in Cushing's syndrome. J Clin Endocrinol Metab 1984; 59:1164.

Urinary Steroid Measurements

Aranoff G, Rösler A. Urinary tetrahydrocortisone and tetrahydrocortisol glucosiduronates in normal newborns, children and adults. Acta Endocrinol 1980; 94:371.

Bailey CC, Komrower GM, Palmer M. Management of congenital adrenal hyperplasia. Urinary steroid estimations: Review of their value. Arch Dis Child 1978; 53:132.

Beisel WR, Cos JJ, Horton R, et al. Physiology of urinary cortisol excretion. J Clin Endocrinol Metab 1964; 24:887.

Burke CW, Beardwell CG. Cushing's syndrome: An evaluation of the clinical usefulness of urinary free cortisol and other urinary steroid measurements in diagnosis. O J Med 1973; 42:175.

Canalis E, Reardon GE, Caldarella AM. A more specific liquid-chromatographic method for free cortisol in urine. Clin Chem 1982; 28:2418.

Carroll BJ, Curtis GC, Davies BM, et al. Urinary free cortisol excretion in depression. Psychol Med 1976; 6:43.

Contreras LN, Hanes S, Tyrrell JB. Urinary free cortisol in the assessment of pituitary-adrenal function. Utility of 24-hour and spot determinations. J Clin Endocrinol Metab 1986; 62:965.

Dorfman RI. Assay of testosterone and 17-ketosteroids. In: Dorfman RI, ed. Methods in hormone research, 2nd ed. New York: Academic Press, 1968:71.

Eddy RL, Jones AL, Gilliland PF, et al. Cushing's syndrome: A prospective study of diagnostic methods. Am J Med 1973; 55:621.

Espiner EA. Urinary cortisol excretion in stress situations and in patients with Cushing's syndrome. J Endocrinol 1966; 35:29.

Fantl V, Booth M, Gray CH. Urinary pregn-5-ene-3α, 16α, 20α-triol in adrenal dysfunction. J Endocrinol 1973; 57:135.

Finkelstein M. Pregnanetriolone, an abnormal steroid. In: Dorfman RI, ed. Methods in hormone research. 2nd ed. New York: Academic Press, 1968:407.

Forbes AP, Albright F. A comparison of 17-ketosteroid excretion in Cushing's syndrome associated with adrenal tumor and with adrenal hyperplasia. J Clin Endocrinol Metab 1951; 11:926.

Gandy HM, Keutmann EH, Izzo AJ. Characterization of urinary steroids in adrenal hyperplasia: Isolation of metabolites of cortisol, compounds and deoxycorticosterone from a normotensive patient with adrenogenital syndrome. J Clin Invest 1960; 39:364.

Hall FF, Adams HR, Eddy RL, et al. Simultaneous determination of urinary tetrahydro compounds and 17-hydroxycorticosteroids. Clin Chem 1973; 19:678.

Hellman L, Bradlow HL, Zumoff B. Decreased conversion of androgens to normal 17-ketosteroid metabolites as a result of treatment with o,p'-DDD. J Clin Endocrinol Metab 1973; 36:801.

Hendricks SA, Lippe BM, Kaplan SA, et al. Urinary and serum steroid concentrations in the management of congenital adrenal hyperplasia. Am J Dis Child 1982; 136:229.

Honour J, Millar G, Roitman E, Shackleton C. Steroid excretion in urine during suppression and stimulation of adrenals in the 17α-hydroxylase deficiency syndrome. J Clin Endocrinol Metab 1981; 52:1039.

Howanitz JH, Howanitz PJ. Evaluation of endocrine function. In: Henry JB, ed. Clinical diagnosis and management by laboratory methods. 17th ed. Philadelphia: WB Saunders, 1984:322.

Lindsay AE, Migeon CJ, Nugent CA, Brown H. The diagnostic value of plasma and urinary 17-hydroxycorticosteroid determinations in Cushing's syndrome. Am J Med 1956; 20:15.

Murphy BEP, Okouneff LM, Klein GP, et al. Lack of specificity of cortisol determinations in human urine. J Clin Endocrinol Metab 1981; 53:91.

Nakamura J, Yakata M. Age- and sex-related differences in urinary cortisol levels. Clin Chim Acta 1984; 137:77.

Peterson RE, Pierce CE. a) Methodology of urinary 17-ketosteroids. b) Determinations of urinary 17-ketosteroids. In: Sunderman FW, ed. Lipids and the steroid hormones in clinical medicine. Philadelphia: JB Lippincott, 1960:147.

Reddy WJ, Jenkins D, Thorn GW. Estimation of 17-hydroxycorticoids in urine. Metabolism 1952; 1:511.

Schöneshöfer M, Weber B, Oelkers W, et al. Urinary excretion rates of 15 free steroids: Potential utility in differential diagnosis of Cushing's syndrome. Clin Chem 1986; 32:93.

Silber RH, Porter CC. The determination of 17, 21-dihydroxy-20-ketosteroids in urine and plasma. J Biol Chem 1954; 210:923.

Simkin B. Urinary 17-ketosteroid and 17-ketogenic steroid excretion in obese patients. N Engl J Med 1961; 264:974.

Zadik Z, De Lacerda L, De Carmargo LAH, et al. A comparative study of urinary 17-hydroxycorticosteroids, urinary free cortisol, and the integrated concentration of plasma cortisol. J Clin Endocrinol Metab 1980; 51:1099.

Zimmermann W. Eine farbareaktion der sexual hormone unalihre anwendung zur quantitoven colorimetrischen bestimmung. Hoppe Seylers Z Physiol Chem 1935; 233:257.

Dynamic Tests of Adrenal Function

Amsterdam JD, Winokur A, Adelman E, et al. Cosyntropin (ACTH1-24) stimulation test in depressed patients and healthy subjects. Am J Psychiatry 1983; 140:907.

Arana GW, Baldessarini RJ, Ornsteen M. The dexamethasone suppression test for diagnosis and prognosis in psychiatry. Arch Gen Psychiatry 1985; 42:1193.

Aron DC, Findling JW, Tyrrell JB, et al. The overnight high-dose dexamethasone suppression test: A rapid method of differential diagnosis of Cushing's syndrome, abstracted. Horm Res 1980; 13:334.

Ashcraft MW, Van Herle AJ, Vener SL, Geffner DL. Serum cortisol levels in Cushing's syndrome after low- and high-dose dexamethasone suppression. Ann Intern Med 1982; 97:21.

Avgerinos PC, Chrousos GP, Nieman LK, et al. The corticotropin-releasing hormone test in the post-operative evaluation of patients with Cushing's syndrome. J Clin Endocrinol Metab 1987; 65:906.

Bayliss RIS. Adrenal cortex. J Clin Endocrinol Metab 1980; 9:477.

Borst GC, Michenfelder HJ, O'Brian JT. Discordant cortisol response to exogenous ACTH and insulin-induced hypoglycemia in patients with pituitary disease. N Engl J Med 1982; 306:1462.

Brown RD, Van Loon GR, Orth DN, Liddle GW. Cushing's disease with periodic hormonogenesis: One explanation for paradoxical response to dexamethasone. J Clin Endocrinol Metab 1973; 36:445.

Cagliero E, Lorenzi M. The corticotropin-releasing factor test in the diagnosis of ectopic ACTH secretion. West J Med 1987; 146:614.

Carey RM. Suppression of ACTH by cortisol in dexamethasone nonsuppressible Cushing's disease. N Engl J Med 1980; 302:275.

Caro JF, Meikle AW, Check JH, Cohen SN. Normal suppression to dexamethasone in Cushing's disease: An expression of decreased metabolic clearance for dexamethasone. J Clin Endocrinol Metab 1978; 47:667.

Chrousos GP, Schulte HM, Oldfield EH, et al. The corticotropin-releasing factor stimulation test: An aid in the evaluation of patients with Cushing's syndrome. N Engl J Med 1984; 310:622.

Connolly CK, Gore MBR, Stanley N, Willis MR. Single-dose dexamethasone suppression in normal subjects and hospital patients. Br Med J 1968; 2:665.

Crapo L. Cushing's syndrome: A review of diagnostic tests. Metabolism 1979; 28:955.

DeCherney GS, DeBold CR, Jackson RV, et al. Effect of ovine corticotropin-releasing hormone administered during insulin-induced hypoglycemia on plasma adrenocorticotropin and cortisol. J Clin Endocrinol Metab 1987; 64:1211.

de Lange WE, Sluiter WJ, Pratt JJ, Doorenbos H. Plasma 11-deoxycortisol, androstenedione, testosterone and ACTH in comparison with the urinary excretion of tetrahydro-11-deoxycortisol as indices of the pituitary-adrenal response to oral metyrapone. Acta Endocrinol 1980; 93:488.

Donald RA, Espiner EA. The plasma cortisol and corticotropin response to hypoglycemia following adrenal steroid and ACTH administration. J Clin Endocrinol Metab 1975; 41:1.

Feek CM, Bevan JS, Ratcliffe JG, et al. The short metyrapone test: Comparison of the plasma ACTH response to metyrapone with the cortisol response to insulin-induced hypoglycemia in patients with pituitary disease. Clin Endocrinol 1981; 15:75.

Fish HR, Chernow B, O'Brian JT. Endocrine and neurophysiologic responses of the pituitary to insulin-induced hypoglycemia: A review. Metabolism 1986; 35:763.

Gold EM, Kent JR, Forsham P. Clinical use of a new diagnostic agent, methopyrapone (SU-4885) in pituitary and adrenocortical disorders. Ann Intern Med 1961; 54:175.

Gold PW, Chrousos GP. Clinical studies with corticotropin releasing factor: Implications for the diagnosis and pathophysiology of depression, Cushing's disease, and adrenal insufficiency. Psychoneuroendocrinolgy 1985; 10:401.

Jackson IMD, Hassan THA, Prentice CRM, Browning MCK. Insulin-induced hypoglycemia as a test of pituitary-adrenal function in thyrotoxicosis. J Clin Endocrinol Metab 1966; 26:545.

Jubiz W, Meikle AN, Levinson RA, et al. Effect of diphenylhydantoin on the metabolism of dexamethasone: Mechanism of the abnormal dexamethasone suppression in humans. N Engl J Med 1970; 283:11.

Kamilaris TC, DeBold CR, Pavlou SN, et al. Effect of altered thyroid hormone levels on hypothalamic-pituitary-adrenal function. J Clin Endocrinol Metab 1987; 65:995.

Kapcala LP, Hamilton SM, Meikle AW. Cushing's disease with "normal suppression" due to decreased dexamethasone clearance. Arch Intern Med 1984; 144:636.

Kehlet H, Binder C. Validity of an ACTH test in assessing hypothalamic-pituitary-adrenocortical function in glucocorticoid-treated patients. Br Med J 1973; 1:147.

Koletsky RJ, Dluhy RG, Crantz FR, et al. Cortisol suppression test in patients with elevated adrenocorticotropic hormone levels. Ann Intern Med 1982; 96:277.

Kreze A, Veleminshy J, Spirova E. A follow-up of the "low dose suppressible" hypercortisolism. Endocrinol Exp 1983; 17:119.

Liddle GW. Tests of pituitary-adrenal suppressibility in the diagnosis of Cushing's syndrome. J Clin Endocrinol Metab 1960; 20:1539.

Liddle GW, Estep HL, Kendall JW Jr, et al. Clinical application of a new test of pituitary reserve. J Clin Endocrinol Metab 1959; 19:875.

Lindholm J, Kehlet H. Re-evaluation of the clinical value of the 30 min ACTH test in assessing the hypothalamic-pituitary-adrenocortical function. Clin Endocrinol 1987; 26:53.

Linn JE Jr, Bowdoin B, Farmer TA, Meador CK. Observations and comments on failure of dexamethasone suppression. N Engl J Med 1967; 277:403.

Lytras N, Grossman A, Perry L, et al. Corticotropin-releasing factor: Responses in normal subjects and patients with disorders of the hypothalamus and pituitary. Clin Endocrinol 1984; 20:71.

May ME, Carey RM. Rapid adrenocorticotropic hormone test in practice. Am J Med 1985; 79:679.

Meikle AW. Dexamethasone suppression tests. Usefulness of simultaneous measurement of plasma cortisol and dexamethasone. Clin Endocrinol 1982; 16:401.

Meikle AW, Stanchfield JB, West CD, et al. Hydrocortisone suppression test for Cushing's syndrome. Arch Intern Med 1974; 134:1068.

Mills IH, Schedl HP, Chen PS, Bartter FC. The effect of estrogen administration on the metabolism and protein binding of hydrocortisone. J Clin Endocrinol Metab 1960; 20:516.

Nelson JC, Tindall DJ Jr. A comparison of the adrenal responses to hypoglycemia, metyrapone and ACTH. Am J Med 1978; 275:165.

Nieman LK, Chrousos GP, Oldfield EH, et al. The ovine corticotropin-releasing hormone stimulation test and the dexamethasone suppression test in the differential diagnosis of Cushing's syndrome. Ann Intern Med 1986; 105:862.

Orth DN, Jackson RV, DeCherney GS, et al. Effect of synthetic ovine corticotropin-releasing factor: Dose response of plasma adrenocorticotropin and cortisol. J Clin Invest 1983;71:587.

Pavlatos FC, Smilo RP, Forsham PH. A rapid screening test for Cushing's syndrome. JAMA 1965; 193:720.

Rosman PM, Farag A, Peckham R, et al. Pituitary-adrenocortical function in chronic renal failure: Blunted suppression and early escape of plasma cortisol levels after intravenous dexamethasone. J Clin Endocrinol Metab 1982; 54:528.

Sawin CT, Bray GA, Idelson BA. Overnight suppression test with dexamethasone in Cushing's syndrome (letter). J Clin Endocrinol Metab 1968; 28:422.

Sindler BH, Griffing GT, Melby JC. The superiority of the metyrapone test versus the high-dose dexamethasone test in the differential diagnosis of Cushing's syndrome. Am J Med 1983; 74:657.

Spark RF. Simplified assessment of pituitary-adrenal reserve: Measurement of serum 11-deoxycortisol and cortisol after metyrapone. Ann Intern Med 1971; 75:717.

Speckart PF, Nicoloff JT, Bethune JE. Screening for adrenocortical insufficiency with cosyntropin. Arch Intern Med 1971; 128:761.

Spiger M, Jubiz W, Meikle AW, et al. Single-dose metyrapone test: Review of a four-year experience. Arch Intern Med 1975; 135:698.

Staub JJ, Noelpp B, Girard J, et al. The short metyrapone test: Comparison of the plasma ACTH response to metyrapone and insulin-induced hypoglycemia. Clin Endocrinol 1979; 10:595.

Tucci JR, Martin MM. Effect of liver disease upon adrenocortical ACTH and metyrapone responsiveness in men. Gastroenterology 1966; 51:515.

Tyrell JB, Findling JW, Aron DC, et al. An overnight high-dose dexamethasone suppression test for rapid differential diagnosis of Cushing's syndrome. Ann Intern Med 1986; 104:180.

Vale W, Spiess J, Rivier C, Rivier J. Characterization of a 41-residue ovine hypothalamic peptide that stimulates secretion of corticotropin and endorphin. Science 1981; 213:1394.

Watabe T, Tanaka K, Kumagal M, et al. Hormonal responses to insulin-induced hypoglycemia in man. J Clin Endocrinol Metab 1987; 65:1187.

Werk EE Jr. Choi Y, Sholiton L, et al. Interference in the effect of dexamethasone by diphenylhydantoin. N Engl J Med 1969; 281:32.

Hypercortisolism—Cushing's Syndrome

Aron DC, Findling JW, Fitzgerald PA, et al. Cushing's syndrome: Problems in management. Endocr Rev 1982; 3:229.

Aron D, Tyrell J, Fitzgerald P, et al. Cushing's syndrome: Problems in diagnosis. Medicine 1981; 60:25.

Arteaga E, Biglieri EG, Kater CE, et al. Aldosterone-producing adrenocortical carcinoma: Preoperative recognition and course in three cases. Ann Intern Med 1984; 101:316.

Atkinson AB, Chestnutt A, Crothers E, et al. Cyclical Cushing's disease: Two distinct rhythms in a patient with basophil adenoma. J Clin Endocrinol Metab 1985; 60:328.

Asa SL, Kovacs K, Tindall GT, et al. Cushing's disease associated with an intrasellar gangliocytoma producing corticotropin-releasing factor. Ann Intern Med 1984; 101:789.

Axiotis CA, Lipes HA, Merino MJ, et al. Corticotropin cell pituitary adenoma within an ovarian teratoma: A new cause of Cushing's syndrome. Am J Surg Pathol 1987; 11:218.

Becker L, Gold P, Chrousos G. Analogies between Cushing's disease and depression: A case report. Gen Hosp Psychiatry 1983; 5:89.

Belsky JL, Guello B, Swanson LW, et al. Cushing's syndrome due to ectopic production of corticotropin-releasing factor. J Clin Endocrinol Metab 1985; 60:496.

Bergmann P, Ekman H, Håkansson B, Sjogren B. Adrenalectomy during pregnancy with the appearance of pre-eclampsia at term in a case of Cushing's syndrome. Acta Endocrinol 1960; 35:293.

Berkhout FT, Croughs JM, Kater L, et al. Familial Cushing's syndrome due to nodular adrenocortical dysplasia. A putative receptor-antibody disease? Clin Endocrinol 1986; 24:299.

Bertagna C, Orth DN. Clinical and laboratory findings and results of therapy in 58 patients with adrenocortical tumors admitted to a single medical center (1951 to 1978). Am J Med 1981; 71:855.

Besser GM, Edwards CRW. Cushing's syndrome. J Clin Endocrinol Metab 1972; 1:451.

Bilaniuk LT, Zimmerman RA, Wehrli FW, et al. Magnetic resonance imaging of pituitary lesions using 1.0 to 1.5 T field strength. Radiology 1984; 153:415.

Birnholz JC. Ultrasound imaging of adrenal mass lesions. Radiology 1973; 109:163.

Brown LR, Aughenbaugh GL, Wick MR, et al. Roentgenologic diagnosis of primary corticotropin-producing carcinoid tumors of the mediastinum. Radiology 1982; 142:143.

Brown RD, Van Loon GR, Orth DN, Liddle GW. Cushing's disease with periodic hormonogenesis: One explanation for paradoxical response to dexamethasone. J Clin Endocrinol Metab 1973; 36:445.

Bui F, Marci C, Varotto L, et al. Adrenal scintigraphy in the morphological and functional evaluation of Cushing's syndrome. Cardiology 1985; 72:(Suppl 1):76.

Burch WM. Cushing's disease: A review. Arch Intern Med 1985; 145:1106.

Burke CW, Roulet F. Increased exposure of tissues to cortisol in late pregnancy. Br Med J 1970; i:657.

Carey RM, Varna SK, Drake CR, et al. Ectopic secretion of corticotropin-releasing factor as a cause of Cushing's syndrome. N Engl J Med 1984; 311:13.

Carpenter PC. Cushing's syndrome. Update of diagnosis and management. Mayo Clin Proc 1986; 61:49.

Carr BR, Parker CR, Madden JD, et al. Maternal plasma adrenocorticotropin and cortisol relationships throughout human pregnancy. Am J Obstet Gynecol 1981; 139:416.

Case Records of the Massachusetts General Hospital (Case 53-1981). N Engl J Med 1981; 305:1637.

Case Records of the Massachusetts General Hospital (Case 52-1987). N Engl J Med 1987; 317:1648.

Casson IF, Davis JC, Jeffrey RV, et al. Successful management of Cushing's disease during pregnancy by transsphenoidal adenectomy. Clin Endocrinol 1987; 27:423.

Check JH, Caro GF, Kendall B, et al. Cushing's syndrome in pregnancy: Effect of associated diabetes on fetal and neonatal complications. Am J Obstet Gynecol 1979; 133:846.

Chrousos GP, Vingerhoeds A, Brandon D, et al. Primary cortisol resistance in man: A glucocorticoid receptor-mediated disease. J Clin Invest 1982; 69:1261.

Chrousos GP, Vingerhoeds AL, Loriaux DL, Lipsett MB. Primary cortisol resistance: A family study. J Clin Endocrinol Metab 1983; 56:1243.

Clark ES, Carney JA. Pancreatic islet cell tumor associated with Cushing's syndrome. Am J Surg Pathol 1984; 8:917.

Coates PJ, Doniach I, Howlett TA, et al. Immunocytochemical study of 18 tumors causing ectopic Cushing's syndrome. J Clin Pathol 1986; 39:955.

Cook DM, Kendall JW, Jordan R. Cushing's syndrome: Current concepts of diagnosis and therapy. West J Med 1980; 132:111.

Copeland PM. The incidentally discovered adrenal mass. Ann Intern Med 1983; 98:940.

Dixon RM, Lieberman LM, Gould HR, Hafez GR. [^{131}I]-iodocholesterol scintiscan and a rare "functional" black adenoma of the adrenal cortex. J Nucl Med 1983; 24:505.

Donaldson MDC, Grant DB, O'Hare MJ, Shackleton CH. Familial congenital Cushing's syndrome due to bilateral nodular adrenal hyperplasia. Clin Endocrinol 1981; 14:519.

Doppman JL, Miller DL, Dwyer AJ, et al. Macronodular adrenal hyperplasia in Cushing disease. Radiology 1988; 166:347.

Doppman JL, Reinig JW, Dwyer A, et al. Differentiation of adrenal masses by magnetic resonance imaging. Surgery 1987; 102:1018.

Doppman JL, Oldfield E, Krudy AG, et al. Petrosal sinus sampling for Cushing syndrome: Anatomical and technical considerations. Radiology 1984; 150:99.

Dunlap NE, Grizzle WE, Siegel AL. Cushing's syndrome: Screening methods in hospitalized patients. Arch Pathol Lab Med 1985; 109:222.

Dwyer AJ, Frank JA, Doppman JL, et al. Pituitary adenomas in patients with Cushing's disease: Initial experience with Gd-DTPA-enhanced MR imaging. Radiology 1987; 163:421.

Elias AN, Meshkinpout H, Valenta LJ, Grossman MK. Pseudo–Cushing's syndrome: The role of alcohol. J Clin Gastroenterol 1982; 4:137.

Findling JW, Aron DL, Tyrrell JB, et al. Selective venous sampling for ACTH in Cushing's syndrome. Ann Intern Med 1981; 94:647.

Findling JW, Tyrrell JB. Occult ectopic secretion of corticotropin. Arch Intern Med 1986; 146:929.

Freitas JE, Herwing KR, Cerny JC, Beierwaltes WH. Preoperative localization of adrenal remnants. Surg Gynecol Obstet 1977; 145:705.

Gabrilove JL, Freiberg EK, Nicolis GL. Peripheral blood steroid levels in Cushing's syndrome due to adrenocortical carcinoma or adenoma. Urology 1983; 22:576.

Ghali VS, Garcia RL. Prostatic adenocarcinoma with carcinoid features producing adrenocorticotropic syndrome. Immunohistochemical study and review of the literature. Cancer 1984; 54:1043.

Gold DM, Kendall JW, Jordan R. Cushing syndrome: Current concepts of diagnosis and therapy. West J Med 1980; 132:111.

Gold EM. The Cushing syndromes: Changing views of diagnosis and treatment. Ann Intern Med 1979; 90:829.

Gold PW, Loriaux DL, Roy A, et al. Responses to corticotropin-releasing hormone in the hypercortisolism of depression and Cushing's disease. N Engl J Med 1986; 314:1329.

Gold PW, Chrousos G, Kellner L, et al. Psychiatric implications of basic and clinical studies with corticotropin-releasing factor. Am J Psychiatry 1984; 141:619.

Gold PW, Gwirtsman H, Avgerinos PC, et al. Abnormal hypothalamic-pituitary-adrenal function in anorexia nervosa: Pathophysiologic mechanisms in underweight and weight-corrected patients. N Engl J Med 1986; 314:1335.

Gomez-Sanchez CE. Cushing's syndrome and hypertension. Hypertension 1986; 8:258.

Gross MD, Shapiro B, Thrall JH, et al. The scintigraphic imaging of endocrine organs. Endocr Rev 1984; 5:221.

Guerin CK, Wahner HW, Gorman CA, et al. Computed tomographic scanning versus radioisotope imaging in adrenocortical diagnosis. Am J Med 1983; 75:653.

Guilhaume B, Bertagna X, Thomsen M, et al. Transsphenoidal pituitary surgery for the treatment of Cushing's disease: Results in 64 patients and long term follow-up studies. J Clin Endocrinol Metab 1988; 66:1056.

Hale AC, Millar BG, Ratter SJ, et al. A case of pituitary-dependent Cushing's disease with clinical and biochemical features of the ectopic ACTH syndrome. Clin Endocrinol 1985; 22:479.

Hasleton PS, Ali HH, Arfield C, et al. Micronodular adrenal disease: A light and electron microscopic study. J Clin Pathol 1982; 35:1078.

Hiramatsu R, Shimada T, Sato T. A case of dexamethasone-suppressible Cushing's disease hardly differentiated from ectopic ACTH syndrome. Endocrinol Jpn 1983; 30:85.

Howlett TA, Drury PL, Perry L, et al. Diagnosis and management of ACTH-dependent Cushing's syndrome: Comparison of the features in ectopic and pituitary ACTH production. Clin Endocrinol 1986; 24:699.

Howlett TA, Rees LH, Besser GM. Cushing's syndrome. Clin Endocrinol Metab 1985; 14:911.

Huebener K-H, Treugut H. Adrenal cortex dysfunction: CT findings. Radiology 1984; 150:195.

Iatrogenic Cushing's Syndrome-Medical Staff Conference, University of California, San Francisco. West J Med 1974; 120:301.

Kakudo K, Miyauchi A, Ogihara T, et al. Medullary carcinoma of the thyroid with ectopic ACTH syndrome. Acta Pathol Jpn 1982; 32:793.

Katz J. Failure of dexamethasone suppression in adrenal hyperplasia. Arch Intern Med 1966; 118:265.

Katz RL, Shirkhoda A. Diagnostic approach to incidental adrenal nodules in the cancer patient. Cancer 1985; 55:1995.

Kucharczyk W, Davis DO, Kelly WM, et al. Pituitary adenomas: High resolution MR imaging at 1.5T[1]. Radiology 1986; 161:761.

Kuchel O, Bolte E, Chretien M, et al. Cyclical edema and hypokalemia due to occult episodic hypercorticism. J Clin Endocrinol Metab 1987; 64:170.

Lamberts SWJ, Klijn JGM, DeJong FH, Birkenhager JC. Hormone secretion in alcohol-induced pseudo–Cushing's syndrome: Differential diagnosis with Cushing's disease. JAMA 1979; 242:1640.

Larsen JL, Cathey WJ, Odell WD. Primary adrenocortical nodular dysplasia, a distinct subtype of Cushing's syndrome. Am J Med 1986; 80:976.

Leiba S, Shindel B, Weinberger I, et al. Cushing's disease coexisting with a single macronodule simulating adenoma of the adrenal cortex. Acta Endocrinol 1986; 112:323.

Liberman B, Wajchenberg BL, Tambascia MA, Mesquita CH. Periodic remission in Cushing's disease with paradoxical dexamethasone response: An expression of periodic hormonogenesis. J Clin Endocrinol Metab 1976; 43:913.

Lipsett MB, Wilson H. Adrenocortical cancer: Steroid biosynthesis and metabolism evaluated by urinary metabolites. J Clin Endocrinol Metab 1962; 22:906.

MacErlean DP, Doyle FH. The pituitary fossa in Cushing's syndrome: A retrospective analysis of 93 patients. Br J Radiol 1976; 49:820.

McArthur RG, Bahn RC, Hayles AB. Primary adrenocortical nodular dysplasia as a cause of Cushing's syndrome in infants and children. Mayo Clin Proc 1982; 57:58.

Manni A, Latshaw RF, Page R, et al. Simultaneous bilateral venous sampling for adrenocorticotropin in pituitary-dependent Cushing's disease: Evidence for lateralization of pituitary venous drainage. J Clin Endocrinol Metab 1983: 57:1070.

Marieb NJ, Spangler J, Kashgarian M, et al. Cushing's syndrome secondary to ectopic cortisol production by an ovarian carcinoma. J Clin Endocrinol Metab 1983; 57:737.

Maton PN, Gardner JD, Jensen RT. Cushing's syndrome in patients with the Zollinger-Ellison syndrome. N Engl J Med 1986; 315:1.

Meikle AW, Lagerquist LG, Tyler FH. Apparently normal pituitary-adrenal suppressibility in Cushing's syndrome: Dexamethasone metabolism and plasma levels. J Clin Lab Med 1975; 86:472.

Mellinger RL. The conundrum of Cushing's syndrome. Arch Intern Med 1986; 146:858.

Myers EA, Hardman JM, Worsham GF, Eil C. Adenocarcinoma of the lung causing ectopic adrenocorticotropic hormone syndrome. Arch Intern Med 1982; 142:1387.

Oldfield EH, Chrousos GP, Nieman LK, et al: Inferior petrosal venous sinus sampling in lateralization of ACTH-secreting pituitary microadenomas (letter). N Engl J Med 1985; 312:1457.

Oldfield EH, Chrousos GP, Schulte HM, et al. Preoperative lateralization of ACTH-secreting pituitary microadenomas by bilateral and simultaneous inferior petrosal venous sinus sampling. N Engl J Med 1985; 312:100.

Orth DN. The old and the new in Cushing's syndrome. N Engl J Med 1984; 310:649.

Parker MS, Jackson R. Ectopic ACTH syndrome associated with breast carcinoma. South Med J 1984; 77:518.

Petersen P, Hove Jacobsen SE. Cushing's disease presenting with severe osteoporosis. Acta Endocrinol 1986; 111:168.

Powell-Jackson JD, Calin A, Fraser R, et al. Excess deoxycorticosterone secretion from adrenocortical carcinoma. Br Med J 1974; 2:32.

Prunty FTG, Brooks RV, Dupré J, et al. Adrenocortical hyperfunction and potassium metabolism in patients with "nonendocrine" tumors and Cushing's syndrome. J Clin Endocrinol Metab 1963; 23:737.

Rees LH, Besser GM, Jeffcoate WJ, et al. Alcohol-induced pseudo–Cushing's syndrome. Lancet 1977; 1:726.

Reinig JW, Doppman JL, Dwyer AJ, et al. Distinction between adrenal adenomas and metastases using MR imaging. J Comput Assist Tomogr 1985; 9:898.

Reinig JW, Doppman JL, Dwyer AJ, et al. Adrenal masses differentiated by MR. Radiology 1985; 158:81.

Ross EJ, Linch DC. Cushing's syndrome–Killing disease: Discriminatory value of signs and symptoms aiding early diagnosis. Lancet 1982; 2:646.

Ross EJ, Marshall-Jones P, Friedman M. Cushing's syndrome: Diagnostic criteria. Q J Med 1966; 35:149.

Ruder HJ, Loriaux DL, Lipsett MB. Severe osteopenia in young adults associated with Cushing's syndrome due to micronodular adrenal disease. J Clin Endocrinol Metab 1974; 39:1138.

Sample WF. Adrenal ultrasonography. Radiology 1978; 127:461.

Sample WF, Sarti DA. Computed tomography and gray scale ultrasonography of the adrenal gland: A comparative study. Radiology 1978; 114:345.

Saris SC, Patronas NJ, Doppman JL, et al. Cushing syndrome: Pituitary CT scanning. Radiology 1987; 162:775.

Sasaki A, Liotta AS, Luckey MM, et al. Immunoreactive corticotropin-releasing factor is present in human maternal plasma during the third trimester of pregnancy. J Clin Endocrinol Metab 1984; 59:812.

Schteingart DE, Lloyd RV, Akil H, et al. Cushing's syndrome secondary to ectopic corticotropin-releasing hormone-adrenocorticotropin secretion. J Clin Endocrinol Metab 1986; 63:770.

Schteingart DE, Seabold JE, Gross MD, Swanson DP. Iodocholesterol adrenal tissue uptake and imaging in adrenal neoplasms. J Clin Endocrinol Metab 1981; 52:1156.

Schteingart DE, Tsao HS. Coexistence of pituitary adrenocorticotropin-dependent Cushing's syndrome with a solitary adrenal adenoma. J Clin Endocrinol Metab 1980; 50:961.

Scott HW Jr, Abumrad NN, Orth DN. Tumors of the adrenal cortex and Cushing's syndrome. Ann Surg 1985; 201:586.

Sharp N, Devlin JT, Rimmer JM. Renal failure obfuscates the diagnosis of Cushing's disease. JAMA 1986; 256:2564.

Shenoy BV, Carpenter PC, Carney JA. Bilateral primary pigmented nodular adrenocortical disease: Rare cause of the Cushing syndrome. Am J Surg Pathol 1984; 8:335.

Smals A, Kloppenborg P. Alcohol-induced pseudo–Cushing's syndrome (letter). Lancet 1977; 1:1369.

Smals AGH, Pieters GFFM, Van Haelst VJG, Kloppenborg PWC. Macronodular adrenocortical hyperplasia in long-standing Cushing's disease. J Clin Endocrinol Metab 1984; 58:25.

Syversten A, Haughton VM, Williams AL, Cusick JF. The computed tomographic appearance of the normal pituitary gland and pituitary microadenomas. Radiology 1979; 133:385.

Thorner MO, Martin WH, Ragan GE, et al. A case of ectopic ACTH syndrome: Diagnostic difficulties caused by intermittent hormone secretion. Acta Endocrinol 1982; 99:364.

Thrall JH, Freitas JE, Beierwaltes WH. Adrenal scintigraphy. Semin Nucl Med 1978; 8:23.

Vagnucci AH, Evans E. Cushing's disease with intermittent hypercortisolism. Am J Med 1986; 80:83.

Van-Brummelen P, Van-Hooff JP, Van-Seters AP, Giard RW. Ectopic ACTH production by a functioning pheochromocytoma. Neth J Med 1982; 25:237.

Ward PS, Mott MG, Smith J, Hartog M. Cushing's syndrome and bronchial carcinoid tumor. Arch Dis Child 1984; 59:375.

Yamaji I, Iimura O, Mito T, et al. An ectopic ACTH producing oncocytic carcinoid tumor of the thymus: Report of a case. Jpn J Med 1984; 23:62.

Yeh HC, Mitty HA, Rose J, et al. Ultrasonography of adrenal masses: Usual features. Radiology 1978; 127:467.

Yeh HC, Mitty HA, Rose J, et al. Ultrasonography of adrenal masses: Unusual manifestations. Radiology 1978; 127:475.

Zarate A, Kovacs K, Frores M, et al. ACTH and CRH-producing bronchial carcinoid associated with Cushing's syndrome. Clin Endocrinol 1986; 24:523.

Hypocortisolism—Adrenal Insufficiency

Abboud CF. Laboratory diagnosis of hypopituitarism. Mayo Clin Proc 1986; 61:35.

Albert SG, Wolverson MK, Johnson FE. Bilateral adrenal hemorrhage in an adult: Demonstration by computed tomography. JAMA 1982; 247:1737.

Allolio B, Dorr H, Stuttmann R, et al. Effect of a single bolus of etomidate upon eight major corticosteroid hormones and plasma ACTH. Clin Endocrinol 1985; 22:281.

Barnett AH, Donald RA, Espiner EA. High concentrations of thyroid stimulating hormone in untreated glucocorticoid deficiency: Indication of primary hypothyroidism? Br Med J 1982; 285:172.

Burke CW. Adrenocortical insufficiency. Clin Endocrinol Metab 1985; 14:947.

Cardoso ER, Peterson EW. Pituitary apoplexy: A review. Neurosurgery 1984; 14:363.

Carey DC. Isolated ACTH deficiency in childhood: Lack of response to corticotropin-releasing hormone alone and in combination with arginine vasopressin. J Pediatr 1985; 107:925.

Carpenter CGJ, Solomon N, Silverberg SG, et al. Schmidt's syndrome (thyroid and adrenal insufficiency): A review of the literature and a report of fifteen new cases including ten instances of coexistent diabetes mellitus. Medicine 1964; 43:153.

Case Records of the Massachusetts General Hospital (Case 3-1986). N Engl J Med 1986; 314:229.

Chiang R, Marshall ML Jr, Rosmann PM, et al. Empty sella turcica in intracranial sarcoidosis: Pituitary insufficiency, primary polydipsia and changing neuroradiologic findings. Arch Neurol 1984; 41:662.

Cunningham SK, Moore A, McKenna TJ. Normal cortisol response to corticotropin in patients with secondary adrenal failure. Arch Intern Med 1983; 143:2276.

Davis LE, Snyder RD, Orth DN, et al. Adrenoleukodystrophy and adrenomyeloneuropathy associated with partial adrenal insufficiency in three generations of a kindred. Am J Med 1974; 66:342.

Doppman JL, Gill JR Jr, Nienhuis AW, et al. CT findings in Addison's disease. J Comput Assist Tomogr 1982; 6:757.

Dorrington Ward P, Carter G, Banks R, Macgregor G. Trilostane as a cause of addisonian crisis. Lancet 1981; 2:1178.

Elder M, Maclaren N, Riley W. Gonadal autoantibodies in patients with hypogonadism and/or Addison's disease. J Clin Endocrinol Metab 1981; 52:1137.

Feldman D. Ketoconazole and other imidazole derivatives as inhibitors of steroidogenesis. Endocr Rev 1986; 7:409.

Fitzgerald PA, Aron DL, Findling JW, et al. Cushing's disease: Transient secondary adrenal insufficiency after selective removal of pituitary microadenomas: Evidence for a pituitary origin. J Clin Endocrinol Metab 1982; 54:413.

Greene LW, Cole W, Greene JB, et al. Adrenal insufficiency as a complication of the acquired immunodeficiency syndrome. Ann Intern Med 1984; 101:497.

Gwinup G, Johnson B. Clinical testing of the hypothalamic-pituitary-adrenocortical system in states of hypo- and hypercortisolism. Metabolism 1975; 24:777.

Herz KC, Gazze LA, Kirkpatrick LH, et al. Autoimmune vitiligo: Detection of antibodies to melanin producing cells. N Engl J Med 1977; 297:634.

Hjortrup A, Kehlet H, Lindholm J, Stentoft P. Value of the 30-minute adrenocorticotropin (ACTH) test in demonstrating hypothalamic-pituitary-adrenocortical insufficiency after acute ACTH deprivation. J Clin Endocrinol Metab 1983; 57:668.

Irvine WJ, Toft AD, Feek CM. Addison's disease. In: James VHT, ed. The adrenal gland. New York: Raven Press, 1979:131.

Jarvis JL, Jenkins D, Sosman MC, et al. Roentgenologic observations in Addison's disease: A review of 120 cases. Radiology 1954; 62:16.

Jorgensen H. Hypercalcemia in adrenocortical insufficiency. Acta Med Scand 1973; 193:175.

Kehlet H, Lindholm J, Bjerre P. Value of the 30-min ACTH test in assessing hypothalamic-pituitary adrenocortical function after pituitary surgery in Cushing's disease. Clin Endocrinol 1984; 20:349.

Ketchum CH, Riley W, Maclaren N. Adrenal dysfunction in asymptomatic patients with adrenocortical autoantibodies. J Clin Endocrinol Metab 1984; 58:1166.

Loriaux DL. The polyendocrine deficiency syndromes. N Engl J Med 1985; 312:1568.

Major P, Kuchel O, Boucher R, et al. Selective hypopituitarism with severe hyponatremia and secondary hyporeninism. J Clin Endocrinol Metab 1978; 46:15.

Max MB, Deck MDF, Rottenberg DA. Pituitary metastasis: Incidence in cancer patients and clinical differentiation of pituitary adenoma. Neurology 1981; 31:998.

McCante DR, Ritchie CM, Sheridan B, Atkinson AB. Acute hypoadrenalism with associated hepatotoxicity in a patient receiving ketoconazole for Cushing's disease. Lancet 1987; i:573.

McMurray JF Jr, Long D, McClure R, Kotchen T. Addison's disease with adrenal enlargement on computed tomographic scanning. Am J Med 1984; 77:365.

Migeon CJ, Kenny FM, Hung W, Voorhess ML. Study of adrenal function in children with meningitis. Pediatrics 1967; 40:163.

Migeon CLJ, Kenny FM, Kowarski A, et al. The syndrome of congenital adrenocortical unresponsiveness to ACTH: Report of six cases. Pediatr Res 1968; 2:501.

Nerup J. Addison's disease-clinical studies: A report of 108 cases. Acta Endocrinol 1974; 76:127.

Nerup J. Addison's disease—serological studies. Acta Endocrinol 1974; 76:142.

Neufeld M, MacLaren N, Blizzard R. Autoimmune polyglandular syndromes. Pediatr Ann 1980; 9:154.

Neufeld M, MacLaren N, Blizzard RM. Two types of autoimmune Addison's disease associated with different polyglandular syndromes. Medicine 1981; 60:355.

O'Connel TX, Aston SJ. Acute adrenal hemorrage complicating anticoagulant therapy. Surg Gynecol Obstet 1974; 139:355.

Richmond IL, Wilson CB. Paracellar tumors in children: Clinical presentation, preoperative assessment and differential diagnosis. Childs Brain 1980; 7:73.

Richtsmeier AJ, Henry RA, Bloodworth JMB, Ehrlish EN. Lymphoid hypophysitis with selective adrenocorticotropic hormone deficiency. Arch Intern Med 1980; 140:1243.

Riley W, MacLaren N, Neufeld M. Adrenal autoantibodies and Addison's disease in insulin dependent diabetes mellitus. J Pediatr 1980; 97:191.

Sanford JP, Favour CB. The interrelationship between Addison's disease and tuberculosis: A review of 125 cases of Addison's disease. Ann Intern Med 1956; 45:56.

Schambelan M, Sebastian A. Hyporeninemic hypoaldosteronism. Adv Intern Med 1979; 24:385.

Schaumburg HH, Powers JM, Raine CS, et al. Adrenoleukodystrophy: A clinical and pathological study of 17 cases. Arch Neurol 1975; 32:577.

Schulte H, Chrousos G, Avgerinos P, et al. The corticotropin-releasing hormone stimulation test: A possible aid in the evaluation of patients with adrenal insufficiency. J Clin Endocrinol Metab 1984; 58:1064.

Sheeler LR, Myers JH, Eversman JJ, Taylor HC. Adrenal insufficiency secondary to carcinoma metastatic to the adrenal gland. Cancer 1983; 52:1312.

Snyder PJ, Fowble BF, Schatz NJ, et al. Hypopituitarism following radiation therapy of pituitary adenomas. Am J Med 1986; 81:457.

Stuart-Mason A, Meade TW, Lee JAH, Morris JN. Epidemiological and clinical picture of Addison's disease. Lancet 1968; 2:744.

Tapper ML, Rotterdam HZ, Lerner CW, et al. Adrenal necrosis in the acquired immunodeficiency syndrome. Ann Intern Med 1984; 100:239.

Tsukada T, Nakai Y, Koh T, et al. Plasma adrenocorticotropin and cortisol responses to ovine corticotropin-releasing factor in patients with adrenocortical insufficiency due to hypothalamic and pituitary disorders. J Clin Endocrinol Metab 1984; 58:758.

White MC, Kendall-Taylor P. Adrenal hypofunction in patients taking ketoconazole. Lancet 1985; 1:44.

Wilus GE, Baert AL, Kint EJ, et al. Computerized tomographic findings in bilateral adrenal tuberculosis. Radiology 1983; 146:729.

Inborn Errors in Cortisol Biosynthesis— Congenital Adrenal Hyperplasia

Baskin HJ. Screening for late-onset congenital adrenal hyperplasia in hirsutism or amenorrhea. Arch Intern Med 1987; 147:847.

Biglieri EG, Herron MA, Brust N. 17-Hydroxylation deficiency in man. J Clin Invest 1966; 45:1946.

Blankstein J, Fairman C, Ryes FC, et al. Adult-onset familial adrenal 21-hydroxylase deficiency. Am J Med 1980; 68:441.

Bongiovanni AM. Acquired adrenal hyperplasia: With special reference to 3β-hydroxysteroid dehydrogenase. Fertil Steril 1983; 35:599.

Bongiovanni AM. The adrenogenital syndrome with deficiency of 3β-hydroxysteroid dehydrogenase. J Clin Invest 1962; 41:2086.

Brodie BL, Colston Wentz A. Late onset congenital adrenal hyperplasia: A gynecologist's perspective. Fertil Steril 1987; 48:175.

Cacciari E, Balsamo A, Cassio A, et al. Neonatal screening for congenital adrenal hyperplasia using a microfilter paper method for 17α-hydroxyprogesterone radioimmunoassay. Horm Res 1982; 16:4.

Cara JD, Moshang T Jr., Bongiovanni AM, et al. Elevated 17-hydroxyprogesterone and testosterone in a newborn with 3β-hydroxysteroid dehydrogenase deficiency. N Engl J Med 1985; 313:618.

Cathelineau G, Brereult J-l, Fiet J, et al. Adrenocortical 11β-hydroxylation defect in adult women with postmenarchial onset of symptoms. J Clin Endocrinol Metab 1980; 51:287.

Chetkowski RJ, Defazio J, Shamonki I, et al. The incidence of late-onset congenital adrenal hyperplasia due to 21-hydroxylase deficiency among hirsute women. J Clin Endocrinol Metab 1984; 58:595.

Chrousos GP, Loriaux DL, Mann DL, Cutler GB. Late-onset 21-hydroxylase deficiency is an allelic variant of congenital adrenal hyperplasia characterized by attenuated clinical expression and different HLA haplotype associations. Horm Res 1982; 16:193.

Chrousos GP, Loriaux DL, Mann DL, et al. Late-onset 21-hydroxylase deficiency mimicking idiopathic hirsutism or polycystic ovary disease. Ann Intern Med 1982; 96:143.

Chrousos GP, Loriaux DL, Sherins RJ, Cutler GB. Unilateral testicular enlargement resulting from inapparent 21-hydroxylase deficiency. J Urol 1981; 126:127.

Dean HJ, Shackleton CHL, Winter JSD. Diagnosis and natural history of 17α-hydroxylase deficiency in newborn male. J Clin Endocrinol Metab 1984; 59:513.

Degenhart HJ. Prader's syndrome (congenital lipoid adrenal hyperplasia). Pediatr Adolesc Endocrinol 1984; 13:124.

DeWailly D, Vantyghem-Havdiquet M-C, Sainsard C, et al. Clinical and biological phenotype in late-onset 21-hydroxylase deficiency. J Clin Endocrinol Metab 1986; 63:418.

Engel IA, Pang S, New MI. Adrenal sonography and computed tomography in the diagnosis of classical and nonclassical 21-hydroxylase deficiency congenital adrenal hyperplasia (abstract 427). Pediatr Res 1984; 18:167A.

Goldsmith O, Solomon DH, Horton R. Hypogonadism and mineralocorticoid excess: The 17-hydroxylase deficiency syndrome. N Engl J Med 1967; 277:673.

Gourmelen M, Pham-Huu-Trung MT, Bredon MG, Girard F. 17-Hydroxyprogesterone in the cosyntropin test results in normal and hirsute women and in mild congenital adrenal hyperplasia. Acta Endocrinol 1979; 90:481.

Hague WM, Honour JW. Malignant hypertension in congenital adrenal hyperplasia due to 11β-hydroxylase deficiency. Clin Endocrinol 1983; 18:505.

Heremans GF, Moolenaare AJ, Van Gelderan HH. Female phenotype in a male child due to 17-α-hydroxylase deficiency. Arch Dis Child 1976; 51:721.

Hochberg Z, Benderly A, Zadik Z. Salt loss in congenital adrenal hyperplasia due to 11β-hydroxylase deficiency. Arch Dis Child 1984; 59:1092.

Honour JW, Anderson JM, Shackleton CHL. Difficulties in the diagnosis of congenital adrenal hyperplasia in early infancy—the 11-beta hydroxylase defect. Acta Endocrinol 1983; 103:101.

Hughes IA, Winter JSD. The application of a serum 17-OH-progesterone radioimmunoassay to the diagnosis and management of congenial adrenal hyperplasia. J Pediatr 1976; 88:766.

Hurwitz A, Brautbar C, Milwidsky A, et al. Combined 21 and 11β-hydroxylase deficiency in familial congenital adrenal hyperplasia. J Clin Endocrinol Metab 1985; 60:631.

Kirkland RT, Kirklant JL, Johnson CM, et al. Congenital lipoid adrenal hyperplasia in an eight year old phenotype female. J Clin Endocrinol Metab 1973; 36:488.

Kowarski A, Russell A, Migeon CJ. Aldosterone secretion rate in the hypertensive form of congenital adrenal hyperplasia. J Clin Endocrinol Metab 1968; 28:1445.

Kuhnle U, Land M, Ulick S. Evidence for the secretion of an antimineralocorticoid in congenital adrenal hyperplasia. J Clin Endocrinol Metab 1986; 62:934.

Kuttenn F, Cauillin P, Girard F, et al. Late-onset adrenal hyperplasia in hirsutism. N Engl J Med 1985; 313:224.

Lee PA, Rosenwaks Z, Urban MD, et al. Attenuated forms of congenital adrenal hyperplasia due to 21-hydroxylase deficiency. J Clin Endocrinol Metab 1982; 55:866.

Levine LS, Dupont B, Lorenzen F, et al. Cryptic 21-hydroxylase deficiency in families of patients with classical congenital adrenal hyperplasia. J Clin Endocrinol Metab 1980; 51:1316.

Levine LS, Dupont B, Lorenzen F, et al. Genetic and hormonal characterization of cryptic 21-hydroxylase deficiency. J Clin Endocrinol Metab 1981; 53:1193.

Loriaux DL, Cutler GB Jr. Diseases of the adrenal glands. In: Kohler PO, ed. Clinical endocrinology. New York: John Wiley & Sons, 1986:167.

Mallin SR. Congenital adrenal hyperplasia secondary to 17-hydroxylase deficiency: Two sisters with amenorrhea, hypokalemia, hypertension and cystic ovaries. Ann Intern Med 1969; 70:69.

McKenna TJ, Cunningham SK, Loughlin T. The adrenal cortex and virilization. Clin Endocrinol Metab 1985; 14:997.

Midgeon CJ, Rosenwaks Z, Lee PA, et al. The attenuated form on congenital adrenal hyperplasia as an allelic form of 21-hydroxylase deficiency. J Clin Endocrinol Metab 1980; 51:647.

Mitty HA, Yeh H. Virilization and feminization. In: Mitty HA, Yeh H, eds. Radiology of the adrenals with sonography and computed tomography. Philadelphia: WB Saunders, 1982: 173.

Nagamani M, McDonough PG, Ellegood JO, Mahesh VB. Maternal and amniotic fluid 17α-hydroxprogesterone levels during pregnancy: Diagnosis of congenital adrenal hyperplasia in utero. Am J Obstet Gynecol 1978; 130:791.

New MI. Clinical and biochemical spectrum of congenital adrenal hyperplasia: New molecular insights. In: D'Agata R, Chrousos GP, eds. Recent advances in adrenal function and regulation. New York: Raven Press, 1987:171.

New MI, Lorenzen F, Lerner AJ, et al. Genotyping steroid 21-hydroxylase deficiency: Hormonal reference data. J Clin Endocrinol Metab 1983; 57:320.

New MI, Lorenzen F, Pang S, et al. "Acquired" adrenal hyperplasia with 21-hydroxylase deficiency is not the same genetic disorder as congenital adrenal hyperplasia. J Clin Endocrinol Metab 1979; 48:356.

New MI, ed. Congenital adrenal hyperplasia. Ann NY Acad Sci 1985; 458:

New MI, Speiser PW. Genetics of adrenal 21-hydroxylase deficiency. Endocr Rev 1986; 7:331.

New MI, Suvannakul L. Male pseudohermaphroditism due to 17α-hydroxylase deficiency. J Clin Invest 1970; 49:1930.

Pang S, Lerner AJ, Stoner E, et al. Late-onset adrenal steroid 3β-hydroxysteroid dehydrogenase deficiency. I. A cause of hirsutism in pubertal and postpubertal women. J Clin Endocrinol Metab 1985; 60:428.

Rodriguez Portales JA, Artaga E, López Moreno JM, Biglieri EG. Zona glomerulosa function after life-long suppression in two siblings with the hypertensive virilizing form on congenital adrenal hyperplasia. J Clin Endocrinol Metab 1988; 66:349.

Rösler A. The natural history of salt-wasting disorders of adrenal and renal origin. J Clin Endocrinol Metab 1984; 59:689.

Rösler A, Leiberman E. Enzymatic defects of steroidogenesis: 11β-Hydroxylase deficiency congenital adrenal hyperplasia. Pediatr Adolesc Endocrinol 1984; 13:47.

Rösler A, Leiberman E, Rosenmann A, et al. Prenatal diagnosis of 11β-hydroxylase deficiency congenital adrenal hyperplasia. J Clin Endocrinol Metab 1979; 49:546.

Savage MO. Congenital adrenal hyperplasia. Clin Endocrinol Metab 1985; 14:893.

White PL, New MI, Dupont B. Congenital adrenal hyperplasia. N Engl J Med 1987; 316:1519 (first part) and 316:1580 (second part).

Zachmann M, Tassinari D, Prader A. Clinical and biochemical variability of congenital adrenal hyperplasia due to 11β-hydroxylase deficiency: A study of 25 patients. J Clin Endocrinol Metab 1983; 56:222.

6 Diabetes Insipidus and Vasopressin

Daniel G. Bichet, M.D., F.R.C.P.C., F.A.C.P.

Diabetes insipidus is a disorder characterized by the excretion of abnormally large volumes (30 ml per kilogram of body weight per day) of dilute urine (< 250 mmol per kilogram). Three basic defects can be involved. The most common, a deficient secretion of the antidiuretic hormone (ADH) arginine vasopressin (AVP), is referred to as central diabetes insipidus. Diabetes insipidus can also result from renal insensitivity to the antidiuretic effect of AVP which is referred to as nephrogenic diabetes insipidus. Finally, excessive water intake can result in polyuria, which is referred to as primary polydipsia.

ARGININE VASOPRESSIN

Osmotic and Nonosmotic Stimulation

The ADH in humans is AVP, a cyclic nonapeptide. The regulation of ADH release from the posterior pituitary is dependent primarily on two mechanisms involving the osmotic and nonosmotic pathways (Zerbe and Robertson, 1987)(Fig. 6–1).

The osmotic regulation of ADH is dependent on osmoreceptor cells in the anterior hypothalamus. These cells recognize changes in extracellular fluid (ECF) osmolality most likely by altering their volume. Cell volume is decreased most readily by substances that are restricted to the ECF, such as hypertonic saline solution or hypertonic mannitol, which not only enhance osmotic water movement from the cells but also are very effective in stimulating ADH release. In contrast, hypertonic urea that moves rapidly into the cells does not readily alter cell volume nor does it effectively stimulate ADH release (Zerbe and Robertson, 1983). The osmoreceptor cells are very sensitive to changes in ECF osmolality. With fluid deprivation, a 1 percent increase in ECF osmolality stimulates ADH release, whereas with water ingestion, a 1 percent decrease in ECF osmolality suppresses ADH release.

Vasopressin release can also be caused by the nonosmotic stimulation of AVP. Large decrements in blood volume or blood pressure (> 10 percent) stimulate ADH release (see Fig. 6–1).

The osmotic stimulation of AVP release by dehydration or infusion of hypertonic saline solution or both is regularly used to determine the vasopressin secretory capacity of the posterior pituitary. This secretory capacity can be assessed *directly* by comparing the plasma AVP concentrations measured sequentially during the dehydration procedure with the normal values (Zerbe and Robertson, 1981) and then correlating the plasma AVP values with the urinary osmolality measurements obtained simultaneously (Fig. 6–2).

The AVP release can also be assessed *indirectly* by measuring plasma and urine osmolalities at regular intervals during the dehydration test (Miller et al, 1970). The maximal urinary osmolality obtained during dehydration is compared with the maximal urinary osmolality obtained after the administration of vasopressin (Pitressin; 5 units subcutaneously in adults, 1 unit subcutaneously in children) or 1-deamino-(8-D-arginine)-vasopressin (DDAVP) (1 to 4 µg intravenously during 5 to 10 minutes).

The nonosmotic stimulation of AVP release can be used to assess the vasopressin secretory capacity of the posterior pituitary in a rare group of patients with the essential hyponatremia and hypodipsia syndrome (Bichet et al, 1985). Although some of these patients may have partial central diabetes insipidus, they respond normally to nonosmolar AVP release signals such as hypotension, emesis, and hypoglycemia (Bichet et al, 1985). In all other cases of suspected central diabetes insipidus, these nonosmotic stimulation tests will not give additional clinical information (Baylis et al, 1981).

Cellular Actions of Vasopressin

The antidiuretic hormone interacts with two types of receptors: V_1, which mediates the effects of vasopressin on vascular smooth muscle, and V_2 which mediates the antidiuretic effects on renal tubules (Jard, 1985) (Figs. 6–3 and 6–4). Once released from the posterior pituitary, vasopressin exerts its biologic action on water excretion by binding to V_2 receptors on the basolateral membrane of the collecting duct. This binding of AVP to its receptor causes an increase in adenylate cyclase activity, which in turn catalyzes the formation of cyclic adenosine 3', 5'-monophosphate (cyclic AMP) from adenosine triphosphate (ATP). The receptor–adenylate cyclase complex appears to have three components: (1) the receptor that recognizes the hormone, (2) a regulatory subunit,

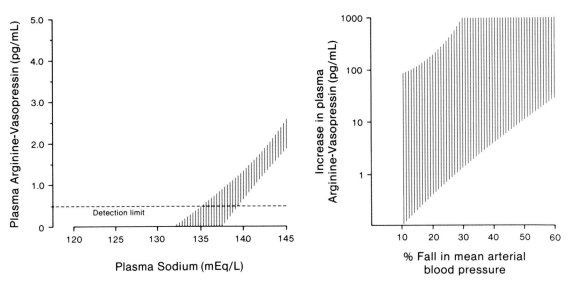

Figure 6-1 Osmotic and nonosmotic stimulation of AVP. *A*, The relationship between plasma AVP and plasma sodium in 19 normal subjects is described by the area with vertical lines, which includes the 99 percent confidence limits of the regression line P_{Na}/P_{AVP}. The osmotic threshold for AVP release is about 280 to 285 mmol per kilogram, or 136 mEq of sodium per liter. AVP secretion should be abolished when plasma sodium is lower than 135 mEq per liter. (From Bichet DG, Kortas C, Mettauer B, et al. Modulation of plasma and platelet vasopressin by cardiac function in patients with heart failure. Kidney Int 1986; 29:1188). *B*, Increase in plasma AVP during hypotension (*vertical lines*). Note that a large diminution in blood pressure in normal humans induces large increments in AVP. (From Vokes T, Robertson GL. Physiology of secretion of vasopressin. In: Czernichow P, Robinson AG, eds: Diabetes insipidus in man. Basel: S. Karger, 1985:127; with permission.)

and (3) the catalytic subunit. All three components are membrane proteins. Considerable evidence indicates that the hormonal activation of adenylate cyclase requires the presence of guanine nucleotides and that the regulatory subunit is a guanine nucleotide–binding protein. The AVP-induced increase in adenylate cyclase activity causes a heightened cyclic AMP formation and ultimately an increase in the permeability of the luminal cell membrane to water.

Unfortunately, although this knowledge of the cellular action of AVP at the collecting duct level would indicate that the measurement of urinary cyclic AMP should

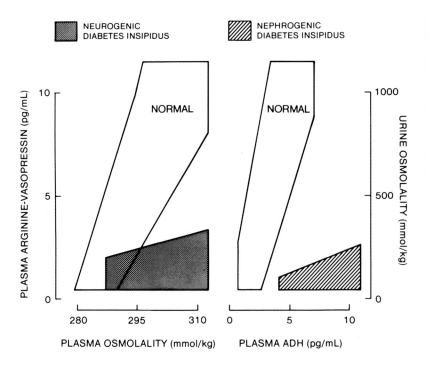

Figure 6-2 *A*, Relationship between plasma AVP and plasma osmolality during infusion of hypertonic saline solution. Patients with primary polydipsia and nephrogenic diabetes insipidus have values within the normal range (*open area*) in contrast to patients with neurogenic diabetes insipidus, who show subnormal plasma ADH responses (*stippled area*). *B*, Relationship between urine osmolality and plasma ADH during dehydration and water loading. Patients with neurogenic diabetes insipidus and primary polydipsia have values within the normal range (*open area*) in contrast to patients with nephrogenic diabetes insipidus, who have hypotonic urine despite high plasma ADH (*cross-hatched area*). (From Zerbe RL, Robertson GL. Disorders of ADH. Medicine North America 1984; 13:1570; with permission.)

help to distinguish between central (neurogenic) and nephrogenic diabetes insipidus, this has not been the case (Uttley et al, 1978).

QUANTITATING RENAL WATER EXCRETION

Osmotic and Nonosmotic Polyuric States

Diabetes insipidus is characterized by the excretion of abnormally large volumes of hypo-osmotic urine (<250 mmol per kilogram). This definition excludes osmotic diuresis, which occurs when excess solute is being excreted, as with glucose in the polyuria of diabetes mellitus. Other agents that produce osmotic diuresis are mannitol, urea, glycerol, contrast media, and loop diuretics. Osmotic diuresis should be considered when solute excretion exceeds 60 mmol per hour.

Osmolar Clearance and Free-Water Clearance

The quantitation of water excretion has been facilitated by the concept that urine flow is divisible into two components (Berl and Schrier, 1986). One component is the urine volume needed to excrete solutes at the concentration of the solutes in the plasma. This isotonic component has been termed osmolar clearance (C_{osm}). The other component is called free-water clearance (C_{H_2O}) and is the theoretic volume of solute-free water

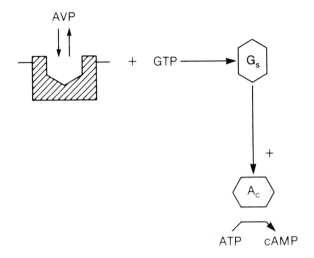

- Kidney tubules
- Amphibian skin and bladder

Figure 6–4   Interaction of AVP with V_2 receptors. The stimulation by vasopressin of the transport of salt and water requires the coupling of the peptide hormone to its V_2 receptor, which results in the activation of adenylate cyclase (A_c) and the generation of cyclic adenosine monophosphate (cAMP) from adenosine triphosphate (ATP). A guanyl nucleotide–binding (G) protein is an intermediary in the activation process. G proteins interconvert between an inactive guanosine diphosphate (GDP) form and an active guanosine triphosphate (GTP) form. The stimulatory G (G_s) protein activates adenylate cyclase.

that has been added to (positive C_{H_2O}) or reabsorbed from (negative C_{H_2O} or $T^c_{H_2O}$) the isotonic portion of the urine (C_{osm}) to create either hypotonic or hypertonic urine, respectively. These terms are calculated as follows:

$$C_{osm} = \frac{\text{Urine osmolality } (U_{osm}) \times \text{Urine flow } (V)}{\text{Plasma osmolality } (P_{osm})}$$

$$V = C_{osm} + C_{H_2O}$$

$$C_{H_2O} = V - C_{osm} \text{ (hypotonic urine)} \quad or$$

$$T^c_{H_2O} \text{ (negative } C_{H_2O}) = C_{osm} - V \text{ (hypertonic urine)}$$

Further inspection of these relationships reveals the following:

1. When U_{osm} equals P_{osm} (isotonic urine), V equals C_{osm}; therefore, C_{H_2O} is zero.
2. When U_{osm} is greater than P_{osm} (hypertonic urine), C_{osm} is greater than V; therefore, C_{H_2O} will be negative (positive $T^c_{H_2O}$).
3. When U_{osm} is less than P_{osm} (hypotonic urine), C_{osm} is less than V, and C_{H_2O} is positive.

This relationship is depicted in Figure 6–5.

To summarize, C_{H_2O} represents the volume of water that would have to be removed from hypotonic urine, and $T^c_{H_2O}$ the volume of water that would have to be

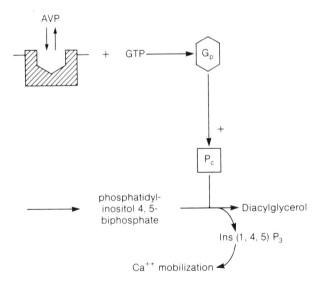

- A large number of vasopressin target cells
- Oxytocin target cells

Figure 6–3   Interaction of AVP with V_1 receptors. Vasopressin produces its functional effects by an activation of phospholipase C (P_c), which promotes the breakdown of phosphatidylinositol 4,5-biphosphate to Ins 1,4,5-P_3 and 1,2-diacylglycerol. This activation of phospholipase C is mediated by a specific pertussis toxin–insensitive receptor-coupled guanyl nucleotide–binding protein (Gp). Ins 1,4,5-P_3 is a calcium-mobilizing second messenger, and 1,2-diacylglycerol activates protein kinase C.

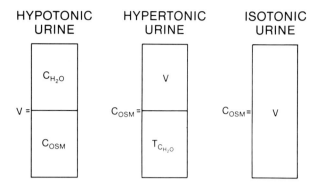

HYPOTONIC URINE **HYPERTONIC URINE** **ISOTONIC URINE**

Figure 6-5 Relationship between urine flow (V), osmolar clearance (C_{osm}), free-water clearance (C_{H_2O}), and negative free-water clearance ($T^c_{H_2O}$), in hypotonic, hypertonic, and isotonic urine.

added to hypertonic urine to make the urine isotonic with the plasma. The excretion of hypertonic urine has the net effect of returning solute-free water to the organism and thereby diluting the body fluids. In contrast, the excretion of hypotonic urine has the net effect of ridding the organism of solute-free water and thus concentrating body fluids. The urinary osmolality value alone does not give the volume of water added to or removed from the organism. The calculation of C_{H_2O} or $T^c_{H_2O}$ allows for a better quantitation of water balance.

Relationship Between Daily Solute Load, Renal Concentrating Capacity, and Daily Urine Volume

A person ingesting a diet containing average amounts of sodium and protein has to dispose of approximately 600 mmol of solute per day. The daily volume of urine in which this solute is excreted will depend on the fluid intake. The 600 mmol of solute can be excreted in 6 L of urine at 100 mmol per kilogram if the daily fluid intake is generous or in 500 ml of urine at 1,200 mmol per kilogram if the fluid intake is limited and the renal concentrating capacity is intact.

This flexibility in daily urine volume for a given solute load is limited if renal concentrating ability is impaired. For example, if the maximal renal concentrating ability is reduced to 300 mmol per kilogram, the 600 mmol of solute will require 2 L of urine per day for excretion. With a more severe concentrating defect, e.g., one that does not allow urine to be concentrated above 60 mmol per kilogram, the 600 mmol of daily solute will require 10 L of urine per day for excretion.

In terms of water conservation, the kidney's ability to increase urinary osmolality from 60 to 300 mmol per kilogram is quantitatively more important than its ability to increase urinary osmolality from 300 to 1,200 mmol per kilogram. For example, with a daily solute load of 600 mmol, a decrease in maximal urinary osmolality from

1,200 to 300 mmol per kilogram increases the obligatory urine flow from 0.5 to 2.0 L per day. Thus, severe polydipsia and polyuria should not be observed even in the absence of the renal capacity to render the urine hypertonic to the plasma. However, a further decrease in maximal urinary concentration from 300 to 60 mmol per kilogram would require 10 L of urine for the daily excretion of 600 mmol of solute. This degree of defect in water conservation obviously is associated with overt polyuria and polydipsia. In the absence of an intact thirst mechanism and a large intake of water, a severe water deficit and hypernatremia would occur.

CLINICAL CHARACTERISTICS OF DIABETES INSIPIDUS DISORDERS

Central Diabetes Insipidus

Common Forms

Failure to synthesize or secrete vasopressin normally limits maximal urinary concentration and, depending on the severity of the disease, causes varying degrees of polyuria and polydipsia. Experimental destruction of the vasopressin-synthesizing areas of the hypothalamus (supraoptic and paraventricular nuclei) causes a permanent form of the disease. Similar results are obtained by sectioning the hypophyseal hypothalamic tract above the median eminence. Sections below the median eminence, however, produce only transient diabetes insipidus. Lesions to the hypothalamic-pituitary tract are frequently associated with a three-stage response both in experimental animals and in humans (Verbalis et al, 1985):

1. An initial diuretic phase lasting from a few hours to 5 to 6 days.
2. A period of antidiuresis unresponsive to fluid administration. This antidiuresis is probably due to vasopressin release from injured axons and may last from a few hours to several days. Since urinary dilution is impaired during this phase, continued water administration can cause severe hyponatremia.
3. A final period of diabetes insipidus. The extent of the injury determines the completeness of the diabetes insipidus, and as already discussed, the site of the lesion determines whether the disease will or will not be permanent.

The etiologies of central diabetes insipidus in adults and in children are listed in Table 6–1 (Czernichow et al, 1985; Greger et al, 1986). No underlying pathologic condition (idiopathic form) could be recognized in 12 to 29 percent of the child and adult cases.

Rare causes of central diabetes insipidus include leukemia, thrombotic thrombocytopenic purpura, pituitary apoplexy, sarcoidosis, and Wegener's granulomatosis (Moses et al, 1985).

TABLE 6-1 Etiology of Central Diabetes Insipidus in Children and Adults*

	Children (%)	Adults (%)
Primary Brain Tumor	49.5	30
Before Surgery	33.5	13
After Surgery	16.0	17
Idiopathic (Isolated or Familial)	29	25
Histiocytosis	16	
Metastatic Cancer	—	8
Trauma	2.2	17
Postinfectious Disease	2.2	—

* Data from Czernichow et al, 1985; Greger et al, 1986; Moses et al, 1985.

Rare Forms: Autosomal Dominant Central Diabetes Insipidus and the DIDMOAD Syndrome

In 1945, Forssman described a "Pituitrin-sensitive" familial polyuric state with X-linked inheritance (1945, 1955). However, no other cases of familial X-linked central diabetes insipidus have been described. Most reported cases of familial central diabetes insipidus were transmitted through an autosomal dominant pattern (Pedersen et al, 1985; Toth et al, 1984). In familial central diabetes insipidus, the polyuria and polydipsia symptoms usually occur after the first year of life, and some limited capacity to release vasopressin can be demonstrated. As a consequence, no severe episodes of dehydration have been described in the affected individuals during their first year of life. The physical and mental development of the affected children are normal. These characteristics are in sharp contrast to those of congenital nephrogenic diabetes insipidus, an X-linked disorder, which can lead to repeated episodes of severe dehydration and eventual mental retardation if left untreated. Familial cases of diabetes insipidus can thus be clearly diagnosed through their mode of inheritance and their clinical characteristics (Table 6-2).

The acronym *DIDMOAD* describes the following clinical features of a syndrome: diabetes insipidus, diabetes mellitus, optic atrophy, sensorineural deafness (Peden et al, 1986). The syndrome is an autosomal recessive trait, the diabetes insipidus is usually partial and of gradual onset (Peden et al, 1986), and the polyuria can be wrongly attributed to poor glycemic control. A severe hyperosmolar state can occur if untreated diabetes mellitus is associated with an unrecognized pituitary deficiency. The dilatation of the urinary tract observed in the DIDMOAD syndrome may be secondary to chronic high urine flow rates and perhaps to some degenerative aspects of the innervation of the urinary tract (Peden et al, 1986).

Syndrome of Hypernatremia and Hypodipsia

As mentioned, some patients with the hypernatremia and hypodipsia syndrome may have partial central diabetes insipidus. These patients also have persistent hypernatremia, which is not due to any apparent extracellular volume loss; absence or attenuation of thirst; and a normal renal response to AVP. In almost all the patients studied to date, the hypodipsia has been associated with cerebral lesions in the vicinity of the hypothalamus. It has been proposed that in these patients there is a "reset-

TABLE 6-2 Inherited Diabetes Insipidus

	Central		Nephrogenic
Inheritance	Autosomal dominant	Autosomal recessive DIDMOAD	X-linked
First clinical manifestations	Variable, usually >1 year	Variable, infancy	First 3 months of life
Mental retardation	Absent	Absent	Severe if repeated unrecognized episodes of dehydration during infancy

ting" of the osmoreceptor, because their urine tends to become concentrated or diluted at inappropriately high levels of plasma osmolality. However, with use of the regression analysis of plasma AVP concentration versus plasma osmolality, it has been shown that in some of these patients the tendency to concentrate and dilute urine at inappropriately high levels of plasma osmolality is due solely to a marked reduction in sensitivity or a gain in the osmoregulatory mechanism (Bichet et al, 1985). This finding is compatible with the diagnosis of partial central diabetes insipidus. In other patients, however, plasma AVP concentrations fluctuate randomly, bearing no apparent relationship to changes in plasma osmolality. Such patients frequently display large swings in serum sodium concentration and frequently exhibit hypodipsia. It appears that most patients with essential hypernatremia fit one of these two patterns (Fig. 6–6). Both of these groups of patients consistently respond normally to nonosmolar AVP release signals, such as hypotension, emesis, hypoglycemia, or all three. These observations suggest that the osmoreceptor may be anatomically as well as functionally separate from the nonosmotic efferent pathways and neurosecretory neurons for vasopressin. Further-

more, a hypothalamic lesion may impair the osmotic release of AVP while the nonosmotic release of AVP remains intact, and the osmoreceptor neurons that regulate vasopressin secretion are not totally synonymous with those that regulate thirst, although they appear to be anatomically close, if not overlapping.

Nephrogenic Diabetes Insipidus

Congenital

Congenital nephrogenic diabetes insipidus is a rare X-linked disorder associated with renal tubular resistance to AVP (Williams and Henry, 1947). In affected families, 50 percent of the males are symptomatic and usually completely unresponsive to vasopressin. Female patients can also be afflicted with variable degrees of polyuria and polydipsia. This variable expression is secondary to the phenomenon of X-chromosome inactivation. The clinical characteristics of patients with congenital nephrogenic diabetes insipidus have been extensively described (Culpepper et al, 1983; Forssman, 1975; Williams and Henry, 1947) and include repeated episodes of dehydration in

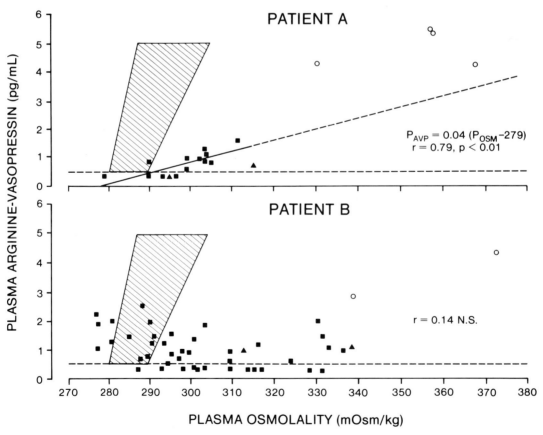

Figure 6–6 Plasma vasopressin as a function of "effective" plasma osmolality in two patients with adipsic hypernatremia. Open circles indicate values obtained on admission; filled squares indicate those obtained during forced hydration; filled triangles indicated those obtained after 1 to 2 weeks of ad libitum water intake. Shaded areas indicate range of normal values. (From Robertson GL. The pathology of ADH secretion. In: Tolis G et al, eds. Clinical neuroendocrinology: A pathophysiological approach. New York:Raven Press, 1979:247; with permission.)

early infancy, hypernatremia, hyperthermia, and mental retardation. Mental retardation, a probable consequence of repeated episodes of dehydration, was prevalent in Bode's and Crawford's study, in which of 44 male patients 39 were classified as mentally retarded (1969). With earlier detection and adequate hydration, it is probable that these catastrophic mental consequences could be entirely prevented (Niaudet et al, 1984).

The physiopathologic basis of the vasopressin resistance in the collecting ducts in congenital nephrogenic diabetes insipidus is unknown. As mentioned the measurement of cyclic AMP excretion is of no value in differentiating between normal individuals and patients resistant to AVP (Uttley et al, 1978). It has been shown that mice with congenital nephrogenic diabetes insipidus have a defect in their cyclic AMP catabolism (Jackson et al, 1980; Kusano et al, 1986). However, this defect is probably not present in humans with congenital nephrogenic diabetes, since in humans the disease is an X-linked inheritance rather than an autosomal semirecessive trait as in mice (Valtin, 1977). The extrarenal defects related to the antidiuretic activity of vasopressin, recently observed in patients with congenital nephrogenic diabetes insipidus and in obligatory transmitters, may be helpful diagnostically (Bichet et al, 1988).

Acquired

The acquired form of nephrogenic diabetes insipidus is much more common than the congenital form of the disease, but it is rarely severe. The ability to elaborate a hypertonic urine is usually preserved despite the impairment of the maximal concentrating ability of the nephrons. Polyuria and polydipsia are therefore moderate (3 to 4 L per day). The more common causes of acquired nephrogenic diabetes insipidus are listed in Table 6-3.

Lithium administration has become the most common cause of nephrogenic diabetes insipidus. A recent review (Boton et al, 1987) reported that this abnormality was estimated to be present in at least 54 percent of 1,105 unselected patients on chronic lithium therapy. Nineteen percent of these patients had polyuria, as defined by a 24-hour urine output exceeding 3 L. The mechanism whereby lithium causes polyuria has been studied extensively. Lithium has been shown to inhibit adenylate cyclase in a number of cell types, including renal epithelia (Christensen et al, 1985; Cogan et al, 1987). The concentration of lithium in the urine of patients on well-controlled lithium therapy (i.e., 10 to 40 mmol per liter) is sufficient to inhibit adenylate cyclase. Recently, measurements of adenylate cyclase activity in membranes isolated from a cultured pig kidney cell line (LLC-PK$_1$) revealed that lithium in the concentration area of 10 mM interfered with the hormone-stimulated guanyl nucleotide regulatory unit (G$_s$) (Goldberg et al, 1988). In patients receiving long-term lithium therapy, amiloride has been proposed to prevent the uptake of lithium in the

TABLE 6-3   Acquired Causes of Nephrogenic Diabetes Insipidus

Chronic Renal Disease
  Polycystic Disease
  Medullary Cystic Disease
  Pyelonephritis
  Ureteral Obstruction
  Far-Advanced Renal Failure

Electrolyte Disorders
  Hypokalemia
  Hypercalcemia

Drugs
  Alcohol
  Phenytoin
  Lithium
  Demeclocycline
  Acetohexamide
  Tolazamide
  Glyburide
  Propoxyphene
  Amphotericin
  Methoxyflurane
  Norepinephrine
  Vinblastine
  Colchicine
  Gentamicin
  Methicillin
  Isophosphamide
  Angiographic Dyes
  Osmotic Diuretics
  Furosemide and Ethacrynic Acid

Sickle Cell Disease

Dietary Abnormalities
  Excessive Water Intake
  Decreased Sodium Chloride Intake
  Decreased Protein Intake

Miscellaneous
  Multiple Myeloma
  Amyloidosis
  Sjögren's Disease
  Sarcoidosis

collecting ducts. Amiloride may thus prevent the inhibitory effect of intracellular lithium on water transport (Battle et al, 1985).

Primary Polydipsia

Primary polydipsia is a state of hypotonic polyuria secondary to excessive fluid intake. Primary polydipsia was extensively studied by Barlow and de Wardener in 1959; however, the understanding of the pathophysiology of this disease has made little progress in the past 30 years. Barlow and de Wardener described seven women and two men who were compulsive water drinkers; their ages ranged from 48 to 59 years except for one patient aged 24. Eight of these patients had histories of psychological disorders, which ranged from delusions, depression, and agitation to frank hysterical behavior. The other patient appeared normal. The consumption of water fluctuated irregularly from hour to hour or from day to day; in some patients there were remissions and relapses lasting several months or longer. In eight patients, the mean plasma osmolality was significantly lower than normal. Vasopressin tannate in oil made most of these patients feel ill; in one, it caused overhydration. In four patients the fluid intake returned to normal after electroconvulsive therapy or a period of continuous narcosis; the improvement in three patients was transient, but in the fourth patient it lasted 2 years. Compulsive water drinking can also occur in infants and leads to a partial nephrogenic diabetes pattern (Moses et al, 1984). At present, there are no clinical or biologic features in these patients that could be used diagnostically. Therefore, the diagnosis of compulsive water drinking must still be made by exclusion.

Diabetes Insipidus and Pregnancy

Pregnancy in a Patient Known to Have Diabetes Insipidus

An isolated deficiency of vasopressin without a concomitant loss of hormones in the anterior pituitary does not result in altered fertility, and with the exception of polyuria and polydipsia, gestation, delivery, and lactation are uncomplicated (Amico, 1985). Treated patients may require increasing dosages of DDAVP. The increased thirst may be due to a resetting of the thirst osmostat (Davison et al, 1984).

Increased polyuria also occurs during pregnancy in patients with partial nephrogenic diabetes insipidus. These patients may be obligatory carriers of the nephrogenic diabetes insipidus gene (Forssman, 1945) or primary polydipsic (one personal observation).

Syndromes of Diabetes Insipidus That Begin During Gestation and Remit After Delivery

Barron and co-workers (1984) described three pregnant women in whom transient diabetes insipidus developed late in gestation and remitted postpartum. In one of these patients dilute urine was present despite high plasma concentrations of AVP. Hyposthenuria in all three patients was resistant to administered aqueous vasopressin. Since excessive vasopressinase activity was not excluded as a cause of this disorder, Barron and colleagues labeled the disease vasopressin resistant rather than nephrogenic diabetes insipidus.

A well-documented case of enhanced activity of vasopressinase involved a woman in the third trimester of a previously uncomplicated pregnancy (Dürr et al, 1987). She had massive polyuria and markedly elevated plasma vasopressinase activity. The polyuria did not respond to large intravenous doses of AVP but responded promptly to DDAVP, a vasopressinase-resistant analogue of AVP. The polyuria vanished with the disappearance of the vasopressinase (Dürr et al, 1987).

The incidence of vasopressinase-mediated, desmopressin-responsive diabetes insipidus is not known. However, another case of transient desmopressin-resistant diabetes insipidus in a pregnant woman has been described (Ford, 1986). It is suggested that pregnancy is associated with several forms of diabetes insipidus, including central, nephrogenic, and vasopressinase mediated.

DIFFERENTIAL DIAGNOSIS OF POLYURIC STATES

Plasma sodium and osmolality are maintained within normal limits (136 to 143 mmol per liter for plasma sodium, 275 to 290 mmol per kilogram for plasma osmolality) by a thirst-ADH-renal axis. Thirst and ADH, both stimulated by increased osmolality, have been termed a "double-negative" feedback system (Leaf, 1979). Thus, even when the ADH limb of this double-negative regulatory feedback system is lost, the thirst mechanism still preserves the plasma sodium and osmolality within the normal range but at the expense of pronounced polydipsia and polyuria. Thus, the plasma sodium concentration or osmolality of an untreated patient with diabetes insipidus may be slightly higher than the mean normal value, but since the values usually remain within the normal range, these small increases have no diagnostic significance.

Theoretically, it should be relatively easy to differentiate between central diabetes insipidus, nephrogenic diabetes insipidus, and primary polydipsia. A comparison of the osmolality of urine obtained during dehydration from patients with central diabetes insipidus or nephrogenic diabetes insipidus with that of urine obtained after the administration of AVP should reveal a rapid increase in osmolality only in the patients with central diabetes insipidus. Urinary osmolality should increase normally in response to moderate dehydration in patients with primary polydipsia.

However, these distinctions may not be as clear as expected because of several factors (Robertson, 1985). First, chronic polyuria of any etiology interferes with the maintenance of the medullary concentration gradient, and this "washout" effect diminished the maximal concentrating ability of the kidney. The extent of the blunting varies in direct proportion to the severity of the polyuria and is independent of its cause. Hence, for any given level of basal urine output, the maximal urinary osmolality achieved in the presence of saturating concentrations of AVP is depressed to the same extent in patients with primary polydipsia, central diabetes insipidus, and nephrogenic diabetes insipidus (Figs. 6–7 and 6–8). Second, most patients with central diabetes insipidus maintain a small, but detectable, capacity to secrete AVP during severe dehydration, and urinary osmolality may then rise above plasma osmolality (Fig. 6–9). Third, many

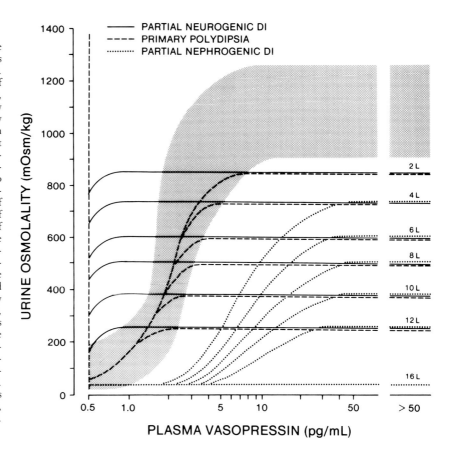

Figure 6-7   The relationship between urine osmolality and plasma vasopressin in patients with polyuria of diverse etiology and severity. Note that for each of the three categories of polyuria—neurogenic diabetes insipidus, nephrogenic diabetes insipidus, and primary polydipsia—the relationship is described by a family of sigmoid curves that differ in height. These differences in height reflect differences in maximal concentrating capacity owing to "washout" of the medullary concentration gradient. They are proportional to the severity of the underlying polyuria (indicated in liters per day at the right end of each plateau) and are largely independent of the etiology. Thus, the three categories of diabetes insipidus differ principally in the submaximal or ascending portion of the dose-response curve. In patients with partial neurogenic diabetes insipidus, this part of the curve lies to the left of normal, reflecting increased sensitivity to the antidiuretic effects of very low concentrations of plasma AVP. In contrast, in patients with partial nephrogenic diabetes insipidus, this part of the curve lies to the right of normal, reflecting decreased sensitivity to the antidiuretic effects of normal concentrations of plasma AVP. In primary polydipsia, this relationship is relatively normal. (From Robertson GL. Diagnosis of diabetes insipidus. In: Czernichow P, Robinson AG, eds. Diabetes insipidus in man. Basel: S. Karger, 1985:176; with permission.)

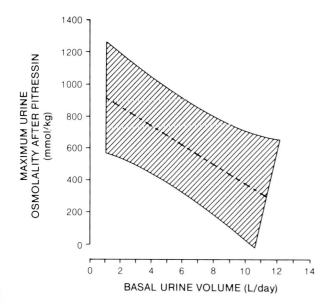

Figure 6-8   Relationship between urinary concentrating capacity and basal urine output. The shaded area depicts the 99 percent confidence limits of data obtained in 24 patients with nonglucosuric polyuria. (From Zerbe RL, Robertson GL. A comparison of plasma vasopressin measurements with a standard indirect test in the differential diagnosis of polyuria. N Engl J Med 1981; 305:1539. Reprinted with permission from *The New England Journal of Medicine*.)

patients with acquired nephrogenic diabetes insipidus have an incomplete deficit in AVP action, and concentrated urine could again be obtained during dehydration testing. Finally, all polyuric states (whether central, nephrogenic, or psychogenic) can induce large dilatations of the urinary tract and bladder (Boyd et al, 1980; Gautier et al, 1981). As a consequence, the urinary bladder of these patients may contain an increased residual capacity, and changes in urinary osmolalities induced by diagnostic maneuvers might be difficult to demonstrate.

Indirect Test

The measurement of urinary osmolality after dehydration or vasopressin administration is usually referred to as indirect testing since vasopressin secretion is indirectly assessed through changes in urinary osmolalities.

The patient is maintained on a complete fluid restriction regimen until urinary osmolality reaches a plateau, as indicated by an hourly increase of less than 30 mmol per kilogram for at least 3 successive hours. After the plasma osmolality is measured, 5 units of aqueous vasopressin are administered subcutaneously. Urinary osmolality is measured 30 and 60 minutes later. The last

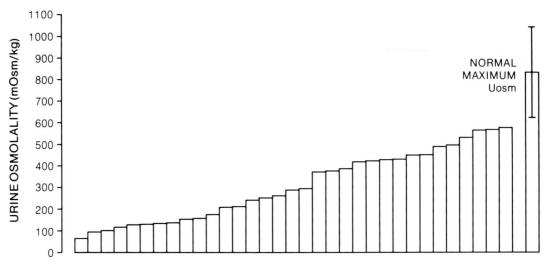

Figure 6-9   Maximum urine osmolality after dehydration in 33 studies of 29 patients with antidiuretic hormone deficiency. (From Miller M, Dalakos T, Moses A, et al. Recognition of partial defects in antidiuretic hormone secretion. Ann Intern Med 1970; 73:721; with permission.)

urinary osmolality value obtained before the vasopressin injection and the highest value obtained after the injection are compared. The patients are then separated into five categories according to previously published criteria (Miller et al, 1970; Table 6-4).

Direct Test

The two approaches of Zerbe and Robertson are used (1981).

First, during the dehydration test, plasma is collected and assayed for vasopressin. The results are plotted on a nomogram depicting the normal relationship between plasma sodium or osmolality and plasma AVP in normal subjects (see Fig. 6-2). If the relationship between plasma vasopressin and osmolality falls below the normal range, the disorder is diagnosed as central diabetes insipidus.

Second, partial nephrogenic diabetes insipidus and primary polydipsia can be differentiated by analyzing the relationship between plasma AVP and urinary osmolality at the end of the dehydration period (see Figs. 6-2 and 6-7). However, a definitive differentiation between these two disorders might be impossible, since a normal or even supranormal AVP response to increased plasma osmolality occurs in polydipsic patients. None of the patients with psychogenic or other forms of severe polydipsia studied by Robertson have ever shown any evidence of pituitary suppression (1985).

Benefits of Direct Test

Zerbe and Robertson (1981) found that in the differential diagnosis of polyuria all seven cases of severe neurogenic diabetes insipidus diagnosed by the standard

TABLE 6-4   Urinary Responses to Fluid Deprivation and Exogenous Vasopressin in Recognition of Partial Defects in Antidiuretic Hormone Secretion

	No. Cases	Maximum U_{osm}* with Dehydration	U_{osm} After Vasopressin	% Change (U_{osm})	U_{osm} Increase After Vasopressin
Normal Subjects	9	1068 ± 69	979 ± 79	−9 ± 3	<9%
Complete Central Diabetes Insipidus	18	168 ± 13	445 ± 52	183 ± 41	>50%
Partial Central Diabetes Insipidus	11	438 ± 34	549 ± 28	28 ± 5	>9% <50%
Nephrogenic Diabetes Insipidus	2	123.5	174.5	42	<50%
Compulsive Water Drinking	7	738 ± 53	780 ± 73	5.0 ± 2.2	<9%

* Urinary osmolality (U_{osm}) in mmol/kg.
Data from Miller M, Dalakos T, Moses A, et al: Recognition of partial defects in antidiuretic hormone secretion. Ann Intern Med 1970; 73:721.

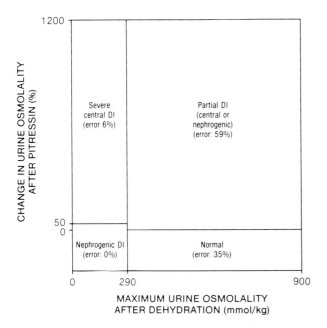

Figure 6-10 The results of direct and indirect tests of AVP function in patients with polyuria of diverse etiology. The indirect tests were performed and interpreted as described by Miller and colleagues (1970). The direct tests, which are based on an immunoassay of plasma AVP, were performed and interpreted as described by Zerbe and Robertson (1981). The error rates indicate the percentage of patients in each of the 4 categories that were misdiagnosed by the indirect tests. (From Robertson GL. Diagnosis of diabetes insipidus. In: Czernichow P, Robinson AG, eds. Diabetes insipidus in man. Basel: S. Karger, 1985:176; with permission.)

indirect test were confirmed when diagnosed by the plasma vasopressin assay. However, two of six patients diagnosed by the indirect test as having partial neurogenic diabetes insipidus had normal vasopressin secretion as measured by the direct assay; one was found to have primary polydipsia and the other nephrogenic diabetes insipidus. Moreover, three of ten patients diagnosed as having primary polydipsia by the indirect test had clear evidence of partial vasopressin deficiency by the direct assay (Zerbe and Robertson, 1981). These patients were thus wrongly diagnosed as being primary polydipsic. The limitations of the indirect test are described in Figure 6-10. A *combined* direct and indirect testing of the AVP function is described in Table 6-5.

TABLE 6-5   Direct and Indirect Tests of AVP Function in Patients With Polyuria

Measurements of AVP cannot be used in isolation but must be interpreted in the light of four other factors:
- Clinical history
- Concurrent measurements of plasma osmolality and of urinary osmolality and maximal urinary response to exogenous vasopressin in reference to the basal urinary flow

Data from Stein P, Valtin H: Verney was right, but ... N Engl J Med 1981; 305:1581.

Therapeutic Trial

In selected patients with an uncertain diagnosis, a closely monitored therapeutic trial of DDAVP (10 μg intranasally twice a day) may be used to distinguish partial nephrogenic diabetes insipidus from partial neurogenic diabetes insipidus and primary polydipsia. If DDAVP at this dosage causes a significant antidiuretic effect, nephrogenic diabetes insipidus is effectively excluded. If polydipsia as well as polyuria is abolished and plasma sodium does not fall below the normal range, the patient probably has central diabetes insipidus. Conversely, if DDAVP causes a reduction in urine output without a reduction in water intake and hyponatremia appears, the patient probably has primary polydipsia. Since fatal water intoxication is a remote possibility, the DDAVP trial should be done with close monitoring.

Recommendations

Table 6-6 lists recommendations for obtaining a differential diagnosis of diabetes insipidus (Robertson, 1987).

New, Potentially Useful Diagnostic Maneuvers in Patients With Congenital Nephrogenic Diabetes Insipidus

The hemodynamic and coagulant-factor–stimulating effects of DDAVP are absent in patients with congenital nephrogenic diabetes insipidus. We recently demonstrated (Bichet et al, 1988; Figs 6–11 and 6–12) that the administration of DDAVP caused a decrease in mean arterial blood pressure (by 10 to 15 percent), an increase in pulse rate (by 20 to 25 percent) and renin activity (by 65 percent), and the release of Factor VIIIc and von Willebrand's factor (two- to threefold) in normal subjects and in patients with central diabetes insipidus. None of these changes were observed in patients with congenital nephrogenic diabetes insipidus, and only minimal responses were observed in the obligatory carriers (the mothers or daughters of the affected male patients). The lack of hemodynamic and coagulation responses to DDAVP confirms the existence of extrarenal vasopressin V$_2$-like receptors (Bichet et al, 1988), which are probably defective in patients with congenital nephrogenic diabetes insipidus.

These new tests might be useful in confirming the diagnosis of congenital nephrogenic diabetes insipidus if in selected cases a dehydration test is difficult to perform, if plasma AVP measurements are not available, or both. DDAVP (0.3 μg per kilogram of body weight) is infused slowly over 20 minutes (to a maximal dose of 24 μg). Mean arterial blood pressure, pulse rate, plasma renin activity, Factor VIIIc, and von Willebrand's factor are monitored or measured at 10- to 30-minute intervals over the next 60 minutes.

TABLE 6-6   Differential Diagnosis of Diabetes Insipidus

1. Measure plasma osmolality and/or sodium concentration under conditions of ad libitum fluid intake. If they are above 295 mmol/kg and 143 mmol/L, the diagnosis of primary polydipsia is excluded and the work-up should proceed directly to step 5 and/or 6 to distinguish between neurogenic and nephrogenic diabetes insipidus. Otherwise,

2. Perform a dehydration test. If urinary concentration does not occur before plasma osmolality and/or sodium reach 295 mmol/kg or 143 mmol/L, the diagnosis of primary polydipsia is again excluded and the work-up should proceed to step 5 and/or 6. Otherwise,

3. Determine the ratio of urine to plasma osmolality at the end of the dehydration test. If it is less than 1.5, the diagnosis of primary polydipsia is again excluded and the work-up should proceed to Step 5 and/or 6. Otherwise,

4. Perform a hypertonic saline infusion with measurements of plasma vasopressin and osmolality at intervals during the procedure. If the relationship between these two variables is subnormal, the diagnosis of diabetes insipidus is established. Otherwise,

5. Perform a vasopressin infusion test. If urine osmolality rises by more than 150 mmol/kg above the value obtained at the end of the dehydration test, nephrogenic diabetes insipidus is excluded. Alternatively,

6. Measure urine osmolality and plasma vasopressin at the end of the dehydration test. If the relationship is normal, the diagnosis of nephrogenic diabetes insipidus is excluded.

Data from Robertson (1987).

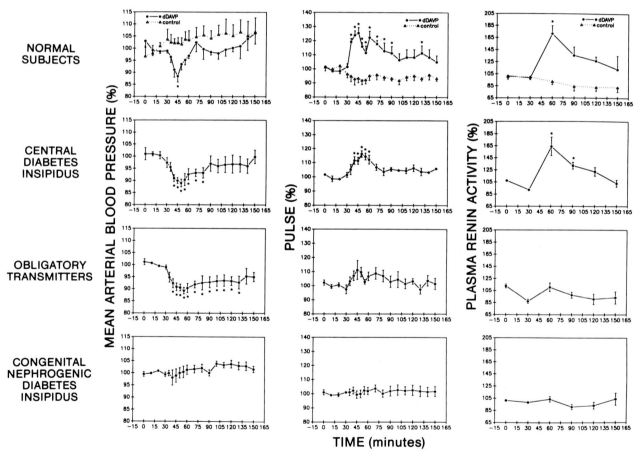

TIME (minutes)

Figure 6–11   Hemodynamic responses to DDAVP infusion. All the subjects received a 20-minute infusion of 0.3 μg of DDAVP per kilogram of body weight during the 30- to 50-minute period. In normal subjects, measurements were obtained without and with the DDAVP infusion (values for the baseline period are represented by triangles, and values for the DDAVP study by circles). Asterisks indicate significant differences from baseline (values at 0 and 30 minutes). (From Bichet DG, Razi M, Lonergan M, et al. Hemodynamic and coagulation responses to 1-deamino[8-D-arginine]vasopressin in patients with congenital nephrogenic diabetes insipidus. N Engl J Med 1988; 318:881. Reprinted with permission from *The New England Journal of Medicine.*)

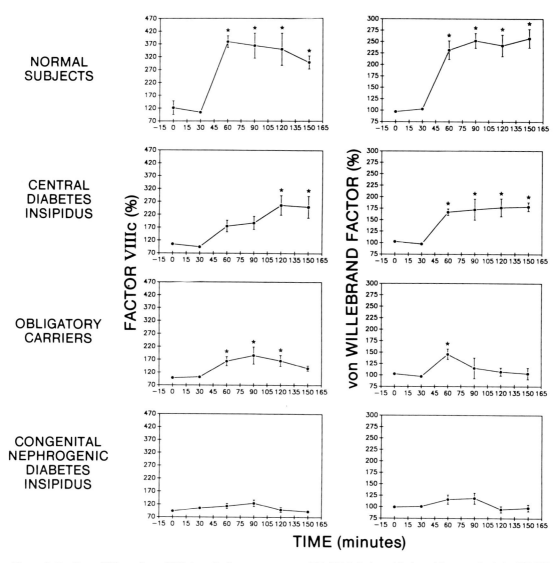

Figure 6–12 Factor VIIIc and von Willebrand's factor responses to DDAVP infusion. All the subjects received the DDAVP infusion during the 30- to 50-minute period. Asterisks indicate significant differences from baseline (values at 0 and 30 minutes). (From Bichet DG, Razi M, Lonergan M, et al Hemodynamic and coagulation responses to 1-deamino[8-D-arginine]vasopressin in patients with congenital nephrogenic diabetes insipidus. N Engl J Med 1988; 318:881. Reprinted with permission from *The New England Journal of Medicine.*)

Female carriers of the nephrogenic diabetes insipidus gene might be detected through linkage studies. Recent studies have localized the nephrogenic diabetes insipidus gene in the Xq28 region (Kambouris et al, 1988; Knoers et al, 1988). This localization could be of considerable importance not only in carrier detection but also in prenatal diagnosis.

RADIOIMMUNOASSAY OF AVP AND OTHER LABORATORY DETERMINATIONS

Radioimmunoassay of AVP

Three developments were basic to the elaboration of a clinically useful radioimmunoassay for plasma AVP (Robertson et al, 1970; 1973): (1) the extraction of AVP

from plasma with petrol-ether and acetone and the subsequent elimination of nonspecific immunoreactivity; (2) the use of highly specific and sensitive rabbit antiserum; and (3) the use of a tracer (^{125}I-AVP) with high specific activity. Almost twenty years later, the same extraction procedures are widely used (Bichet et al, 1987; Davison et al, 1988; Vokes et al, 1987), and commercial tracers (^{125}I-AVP) and antibodies are available. AVP can also be extracted from plasma by using Sep-Pak C18 cartridges (Hartter and Woloszczuk, 1986; Larochelle et al, 1980; Ysewijn-Van Brussel and De Leenheer, 1985).

Blood samples collected in chilled 7-ml lavender stoppered tubes containing EDTA are centrifuged at 4 °C, 1,000 × g (3,000 rpm is a usual laboratory centrifuge), for 20 minutes. This 20-minute centrifugation is mandatory for obtaining platelet-poor plasma samples, since

TABLE 6-7 AVP Measurements—Sample Preparation

4 °C Blood in EDTA tubes
Centrifugation 1,000 g × 20 min
Plasma Frozen -20 °C

Extraction
    2 ml acetone + 1 ml plasma
    1,000 g × 30 min 4 °C
    Supernatant + 5 ml of petrol-ether
    1,000 g × 20 min 4 °C
    Freeze −80 °C
    Throw nonfrozen upper phase
    Evaporate lower phase to dryness
    Store desiccated samples at −20 °C

a large fraction of the circulating vasopressin is associated with the platelets in humans (Bichet et al, 1987; Preibitz et al, 1983). The tubes may be kept for 2 hours on slushed ice prior to centrifugation. Plasma is then separated, frozen at −20 °C, and extracted within 6 weeks of sampling. Details for sample preparation (Table 6–7) and assay procedure (Table 6–8) can be found in writings by Bichet and colleagues (1986; 1987). An AVP radioimmunoassay should be validated by demonstrating (1) a good correlation between plasma sodium or osmolality and plasma AVP during dehydration and infusion of hypertonic saline solution (see Fig. 1) and (2) the inability to obtain detectable values of AVP in patients with severe central diabetes insipidus. It is unlikely that this complicated radioimmunoassay procedure will be replaced by other sensitive methods. A cytochemical assay to measure human plasma AVP was recently published. This assay is based on the stimulation of Na^+-K^+ ATPase activity in the outer medulla of the rat kidney (Baylis et al, 1986). Unfortunately, during an infusion of hypertonic saline solution in six normal volunteers, plasma osmolality increased from 286.8 ± 1.7 to 307.6 ± 7.6 mmol per kilogram, and immunoreactive AVP increased from 1.3 ± 0.2 to 17.7 ± 3.6 pmol per liter, but no change in plasma AVP concentrations was observed (2.1 ± 0.9 and 1.9 ± 1.3 pmol per liter) (Baylis et al, 1986).

In pregnant patients, the blood contains high concentrations of cystine aminopeptidase, which can (in

TABLE 6-8 AVP Measurements, Assay Procedure

Day 1 Assay set-up
    400 μl/tube
      (200-μl sample or standard + 200 μl of
      antiserum or buffer)
    Incubation 80 hours, 4 °C

Day 4 ^{125}I-AVP
    100 μl/tube
      1,000 cpm/tube
    Incubation 72 hours, 4 °C

Day 7 Separation dextran + charcoal

vitro) inactivate enormous quantities (ng × ml^{-1} × min^{-1}) of AVP. However, phenanthrolene effectively inhibits these cystine aminopeptidases (Table 6–9)

Plasma Sodium, Plasma, and Urinary Osmolality Measurements

Measurements of plasma sodium, plasma, and urinary osmolality should be immediately available at various intervals during dehydration procedures. Plasma sodium is easily measured by flame photometry or with a sodium-specific electrode (Maas et al, 1985). Plasma and urinary osmolalities are also reliably measured by freezing-point depression instruments with a coefficient of variation at 290 mmol per kilogram of less than 1 percent.

In our clinical research unit, plasma sodium and plasma and urinary osmolalities are measured at the beginning of each dehydration procedure and at regular intervals (usually hourly) thereafter, depending on the severity of the polyuric syndrome explored.

In one case, an 8-year-old patient (31-kg body weight) with a clinical diagnosis of congenital nephrogenic diabetes insipidus continued to excrete large volumes of urine (300 ml per hour) during a short 4-hour dehydration test. During this time, the patient was suffering from severe thirst; his plasma sodium was 155 mEq per liter, his plasma osmolality was 310 mmol per kilogram, and his urinary osmolality was 85 mmol per kilogram. The patient received 1 μg of DDAVP intravenously and was allowed to drink water. Repeated urinary osmolality measurements demonstrated a complete urinary resistance to DDAVP.

It would have been dangerous and unnecessary to prolong the dehydration further in this young patient. Thus, the usual prescription of overnight dehydration should not be used in patients, and especially children, with severe polyuria and polydipsia (more than 4 L per day). Great care should be taken to avoid any severe hypertonic state arbitrarily defined as a plasma sodium greather than 155 mEq per liter.

At variance with published data (Redetzki et al, 1972; Zerbe and Robertson, 1981), we have found that plasma and serum osmolalities are equivalent (i.e., similar values are obtained). Blood taken in heparinized tubes is easier to handle than blood taken without anticoagulant because the plasma can be more readily re-

TABLE 6-9 Measurements of AVP Levels in Pregnant Patients

1,10-phenanthrolene monohydrate (Sigma)
60 mg/ml—Solubilized with several drops of glacial acetic acid
0.1 ml/10 ml of blood

Data from Davison JM, Gilmore EA, Durr J, et al. Altered osmotic thresholds for vasopressin secretion and thirst in human pregnancy. Am J Physiol 1984; 246:F105.

moved after centrifugation. The green-stopper tube used contains a minuscule concentration of lithium and sodium, which does not interfere with plasma sodium or osmolality measurements. Frozen plasma or urine samples can be kept for further analysis of their osmolalities, since the results obtained are similar to those obtained immediately after blood sampling, except in patients with severe renal failure. In patients with severe renal failure plasma osmolality measurements are increased after freezing and thawing, but the plasma sodium values remain unchanged.

Plasma Sodium Versus Plasma Osmolality

Plasma osmolality measurements can be used to demonstrate the absence of unusual osmotically active substances (e.g. glucose and urea in high concentrations, mannitol, ethanol) (Gennari, 1984). With this information, plasma or serum sodium measurements are sufficient to assess the degree of dehydration and its relationship to plasma AVP. Nomograms describing the normal relationship between plasma sodium and plasma AVP (see Fig. 6–1) are as valuable as "classic"nomograms describing the relationship between plasma osmolality and effective osmolality (i.e., plasma osmolality minus the contribution of "ineffective" solutes—glucose and urea).

BIBLIOGRAPHY

Amico JA. Diabetes insipidus and pregnancy. In: Czernichow P, Robinson AG, eds. Frontiers of hormone research. Vol 13. Diabetes insipidus in man. Basel: S. Karger, 1985:266.

Barlow ED, de Wardener HE. Compulsive water drinking. QJ Med New Series 1959; 28:235.

Barron WM, Cohen LH, Ulland LA, et al. Transient vasopressin resistant diabetes insipidus of pregnancy. N Engl J Med 1984; 310:442.

Battle DC, von Riotte AB, Gaviria M, Grupp M. Amelioration of polyuria by amiloride in patients receiving long-term lithium therapy. N Engl J Med 1985; 312:408.

Baylis PH, Gaskill MG, Robertson GL. Vasopressin secretion in primary polydipsia and cranial diabetes insipidus. Q J Med New Series 1981; 199:345.

Baylis PH, Pippard C, Burd JM. Interference in the cytochemical assay of plasma vasopressin by a circulating factor induced by salt-loading in man. J Endocrinol 1986; 111:495.

Baylis PH, Pippard C, Gill GV, Burd J. Development of a cytochemical assay for plasma vasopressin: Application to studies on water loading normal man. Clin Endocrinol 1986; 24:383.

Berl T, Schrier RW. Disorders of water metabolism. In: Schrier RW, ed. Renal and electrolytic disorders. 3rd ed. Boston: Little, Brown, 1986:1.

Bichet DG, Arthus MF, Barjon JN, et al. Human platelet fraction arginine-vasopressin. Potential physiological role. J Clin Invest 1987; 79:881.

Bichet DG, Kortas C, Mettauer B, et al. Modulation of plasma and platelet vasopressin by cardiac function in patients with heart failure. Kidney Int 1986; 29:1188.

Bichet DG, Levi M, Schrier RW. Polyuria, dehydration, overhydration. In: Seldin DW, Giebisch G, eds. The kidney: physiology and pathophysiology. New York: Raven Press, 1985: 951.

Bichet DG, Razi M, Lonergan M, et al. Hemodynamic and coagulation responses to 1-deamino[8-D-arginine]vasopressin in patients with congenital nephrogenic diabetes insipidus. N Engl J Med 1988; 318:881.

Bode HH, Crawford JD. Nephrogenic diabetes insipidus in North America. The Hopewell hypothesis. N Engl J Med 1969; 280:750.

Boton R, Gaviria M, Battle DC. Prevalence, pathogenesis and treatment of renal dysfuction associated with chronic lithium therapy. Am J Kidney Dis 1987; 10:329.

Boyd SD, Raz S, Ehrlich RM. Diabetes insipidus and nonobstructive dilation of urinary tract. Urology 1980; 26:266.

Christensen S, Kusano E, Yusufi NK, et al. Pathogenesis of nephrogenic diabetes insipidus due to chronic administration of lithium in rates. J Clin Invest 1985; 75:1869.

Cogan E, Svoboda M, Abramow M. Mechanisms of lithium-vasopressin interaction in rabbit cortical collecting tubule. Am J Physiol 1987; 252:F1080.

Culpepper RM, Hebert SC, Andreoli TE. Nephrogenic diabetes insipidus. In: Stanbury JB, Wyngaarden JB, Fredrickson DS, et al, eds. The metabolic basis of inherited disease. 5th ed. New York: McGraw-Hill, 1983:1867.

Czernichow P, Pomarede R, Braumer R, Rappaport R. Neurogenic diabetes insipidus. In: Czernichow P, Robinson AG, eds. Frontiers of hormone research. Vol 13. Diabetes insipidus in man. Basel: S. Karger, 1985:190.

Davison JM, Gilmore EA, Dürr J, et al. Altered osmotic thresholds for vasopressin secretion and thirst in human pregnancy. Am J Physiol 1984; 246:F105.

Davison JM, Shiells EA, Philips PR, Lindheimer MD. Serial evaluation of vasopressin release and thirst in human pregnancy. J Clin Invest 1988; 81:798.

Dürr JA, Hoggard JG, Hunt JM, Schrier RW. Diabetes insipidus in pregnancy associated with abnormally high circulating vasopressinase activity. N Engl J Med 1987; 316:1070.

Ford SM Jr. Transient vasopressin-resistant diabetes insipidus of pregnancy. Obstet Gynecol 1986; 68:288.

Forssman H. On hereditary diabetes insipidus, with special regard to a sex-linked form. Acta Med Scand [Suppl] 1945; 159:1.

Forssman H. The recognition of nephrogenic diabetes insipidus. A very small page from the history of medicine. Acta Med Scand 1975; 197:1.

Forssman H. Two different mutations of the X chromosome causing diabetes insipidus. Am J Hum Genet 1955; 7:21.

Gautier B, Thieblot P, Steg A. Megauretère, mégavessie et diabète insipide familial. Sem Hop Paris 1981; 57:60.

Gennari FJ. Serum osmolality: Uses and limitations. N Engl J Med 1984; 310:102.

Goldberg H, Clayman P, Skorecki KL. Mechanism of inhibition by lithium of vasopressin-sensitive adenylate cyclase (abstract). Kidney Int 1988; 33:265.

Greger NG, Kirkland RT, Clayton GW, Kirkland JL. Central diabetes insipidus. 22 years' experience. Am J Dis Child 1986; 140:551.

Hartter E, Woloszczuk W. Radioimmunological determination of arginine-vasopressin and human atrial natriuretic peptide after simultaneous extraction from plasma. J Clin Chem Clin Biochem 1986; 24:559.

Jackson BA, Edwards RM, Valtin H, Dousa TP. Cellular action of vasopressin in medullary tubules of mice with hereditary nephrogenic diabetes insipidus. J Clin Invest 1980; 66:110.

Jard S. Vasopressin receptors. In: Czernichow P, Robinson AG, eds. Frontiers of hormone research. Vol 13. Diabetes insipidus in man. Basel: S. Karger, 1985:89.

Kambouris M, Dlouhy SR, Trofatter JA, et al. Localization of the gene for X-linked nephrogenic diabetes insipidus to Xq28. Am J Med Genet 1988; 29:239.

Knoers N, v.d. Heyden H, v. Oost BA, et al. Linkage of X-linked nephrogenic diabetes insipidus with DXS52, a polymorphic DNA marker. Nephron 1988; 50:187.

Kusano E, Yusufi ANK, Murayama N, et al. Dynamics of nucleotides in distal nephron of mice with nephrogenic diabetes insipidus. Am J Physiol 1986; 260:F151.

Larochelle T, North G, Stern P. A new extraction of arginine-vasopressin from blood: The use of octadecasilyl-silica. Pflugers Arch 1980; 387:79.

Leaf A. Neurogenic diabetes insipidus. Kidney Int 1979; 15:572.

Maas AHJ, Siggaard-Anderson O, Weisberg HF, Zijistra WG. Ion-selective electrodes for sodium and potassium: A new problem of what is measured and what should be reported. Clin Chem 1985; 31:482.

Miller M, Dalakos T, Moses A, et al. Recognition of partial defects in antidiuretic hormone secretion. Ann Intern Med 1970; 73:721.

Moses AM, Blumenthal SA, Streeten DHP. Acid-base and electrolyte disorders associated with endocrine disease: Pituitary and thyroid. In: Arieff AI, de Fronzo RA, eds. Fluid, electrolyte and acid-base disorders. New York: Churchill Livingstone, 1985:851.

Moses AM, Steinman SJ, Oppenheim A. Marked hypotonic polyuria resulting from nephrogenic diabetes insipidus with partial sensitivity to vasopressin. J Clin Endocrinol Metab 1984; 59:1044.

Niaudet P, Dechaux M, Trivin C, et al. Nephrogenic diabetes insipidus. Clinical and pathophysiological aspects. Adv Nephrol 1984; 13.247.

Peden NR, Gay JDL, Jung RT, Kuwayti K. Wolfram (DIDMOAD) syndrome: A complex long-term problem in management. Q J Med New Series 1986; 58:167.

Pedersen EB, Lamm LV, Albertsen K, et al. Familial cranial diabetes insipidus: A report of five families. Genetic, diagnostic and therapeutic aspects. Q J Med New Series 1985; 57:883.

Preibitz JJ, Sealey JE, Laragh JH, et al. Plasma and platelet vasopressin in essential hypertension and congestive heart failure. Hypertension (Suppl I) 1983; 5:1291.

Redetzki HM, Hughes JR, Redetzki JE. Differences between serum and plasma osmolalities and their relationship to lactic acid values. Proc Soc Exp Biol Med 1972; 139:315

Robertson GL. Diagnosis of diabetes insipidus. In: Czernichow P, Robinson AG, eds. Frontiers of hormone research. Vol 13. Diabetes insipidus in man. Basel: S. Karger 1985:176.

Robertson GL. Posterior pituitary. In: Felig P, Baxter JD, Broadus AE, Frohman LA, eds. Endocrinology and metabolism. 2nd ed. New York: McGraw-Hill, 1987:338.

Robertson GL, Klein LA, Roth J, Gorden P. Immunoassay of plasma vasopressin in man. Proc Natl Acad Sci USA 1970; 66:1298.

Robertson GL, Mahr EA, Athar S, Sinha T. Development and clinical application of a new method for the radioimmunoassay of arginine-vasopressin in human plasma. J Clin Invest 1973; 52:2340.

Toth EL, Bowen PA, Crockford PM. Hereditary central diabetes insipidus: Plasma levels of antidiuretic hormone in a family with a possible osmoreceptor defect. Can Med Assoc J 1984; 131:1237.

Uttley WS, Atkinson B, Adams A. Cyclic adenosine monophosphate excretion in urine of patients and carriers of congenital nephrogenic diabetes insipidus. J Inherited Metab Dis 1978; 1:75.

Valtin H. Genetic models for hypothalamic and nephrogenic diabetes insipidus. In: Andreoli TE, Grantham JJ, Rector FC Jr, eds. Disturbances in body fluid osmolality. Washington: American Physiological Society, 1977:197.

Verbalis JG, Robinson AG, Moses AM. Postoperative and posttraumatic diabetes insipidus. In: Czernichow P, Robinson AG, eds. Frontiers of hormone research. Vol 13. Diabetes insipidus in man. Basel: S. Karger, 1985:247.

Vokes TP, Aycinena PR, Robertson GL. Effect of insulin on osmoregulation of vasopressin. Am J Physiol 1987; 252:E538.

Williams RH, Henry C. Nephrogenic diabetes insipidus: Transmitted by females and appearing during infancy in males. Ann Intern Med 1947; 27:84.

Ysewijn-Van Brussel KARN, De Leenheer AP. Development and evaluation of a radioimmunoassay for Arg^8-vasopressin, after extraction with Sep-Pak C_{18}. Clin Chem 1985; 31:861.

Zerbe RL, Robertson GL. A comparison of plasma vasopressin measurements with a standard indirect test in the differential diagnosis of polyuria. N Engl J Med 1981; 305:1539.

Zerbe RL, Robertson GL. Osmoregulation of thirst and vasopressin secretion in man: The effect of various solutes. Am J Physiol 1983; 244:E607.

Zerbe RL, Robertson GL. Osmotic and nonosmotic regulation of thirst and vasopressin secretion. In: Maxwell MH, Kleeman CR, Narins RG, eds. Clinical disorders of fluid and electrolyte metabolism. 4th ed. New York: McGraw-Hill, 1987:61.

7

Thyroid Diseases

W. Tabb Moore, M.D.
Richard C. Eastman, M.D., F.A.C.P.

Clinical medicine has been revolutionized by developments in the clinical laboratory. This is particularly true of thyroidology, in which many new tests are now available to aid the physician in the clinical assessment of thyroid diseases. In addition, new technologies have improved the precision and the accuracy of some of the older tests so that now they provide much more information for the clinician. As a consequence, the technical interpretation of an increasing number of tests has become an important task of both the internist and endocrinologist.

However, it is important not to accept initial tests at their face value. A careful and thoughtful analysis may be necessary for unraveling a problem. Occasionally, only continued observation, analysis of all medications taken by the patient, or even study of family members may be necessary to arrive at a correct diagnosis.

The purpose of this chapter is to outline those tests most frequently used in current clinical practice and to discuss the methodologies, their clinical utility, and the problems incurred in performing assays and interpreting results.

THYROID PHYSIOLOGY

Thyroid hormone homeostasis is meticulously controlled by the hypothalamus and pituitary. Thyrotrophin-releasing hormone (TRH) is synthesized by the medial basal hypothalamus and secreted into the hypophyseal-portal system from where it travels to the anterior pituitary to bind to receptors on thyrotrophic cells, stimulating both synthesis and release of thyroid-stimulating hormone (TSH). TSH acts to stimulate the thyroid cells and to increase the synthesis and release of thyroxine (T_4) and triiodothyronine (T_3). These hormones, in turn, feed back on the pituitary thyrotroph, where T_4 is converted to T_3 and intracellularly acts to suppress synthesis of TSH. Dopamine and somatostatin also act on the pituitary to inhibit the release of TSH.

TSH is a glycoprotein with a molecular weight of 28,000. It is composed of distinct alpha and beta subunits. The alpha subunit is shared in common with luteinizing hormone (LH), follicle-stimulating hormone (FSH) and human chorionic gonadotropin (hCG). In contrast, assays employing immunoglobulins directed against the beta subunit are specific and are useful clinically.

The two major thyroid hormones are T_4 and T_3. They are secreted by the thyroid in a T_4:T_3 ratio of 10:1. Eighty percent of the T_3 is formed from T_4 by its peripheral deiodination, whereas 20 percent is from direct thyroidal secretion in normals. In pathologic states a greater proportion of T_3 comes from direct thyroidal secretion. Of the two hormones, T_3 is three to four times more potent than T_4. The cellular receptor for the thyroid hormone is within the cell nucleus. The affinity of the receptor for T_3 is about tenfold higher than the affinity for T_4. Nonetheless T_4 is the dominant circulating hormone controlling TSH secretion. In the pituitary, T_4 is rapidly converted to T_3, which then acts locally to regulate the secretion of TSH.

Both T_4 and T_3 are bound in the serum to three distinct proteins, TBG (thyroxine-binding globulin), TBPA (thyroid binding pre-albumin), and albumin. TBG has a high affinity and a low capacity for thyroxine. Albumin has a much lower affinity and a very high capacity for binding of thyroid hormones. TBPA has characteristics that lie between the other two. T_4 and T_3 are very tightly bound—99.97 and 99.7 percent respectively. The bound hormones are in equilibrium with their free circulating hormones. A variety of factors change the quantity or quality of the binding proteins, thus affecting the total measured thyroid hormones while the free hormone level remains normal.

Sex has not been found to have a significant effect on T_4 and T_3 levels. However, age is a different matter. At the time of delivery, the T_4 level is high secondary to an increased level of TBG. In the first 24 hours there is a marked increase in TSH secretion. The T_3 and T_4 both increase and peak at 24 hours (Fig. 7–1). Following the early days of infancy, both T_4 and T_3 gradually decline somewhat until they reach stable adult levels at ages 13 to 15. These changes probably reflect changes in TBG. Previously it was believed that T_3 decreased with increasing age, but this now appears to have been related to disease and not to an aging change.

THYROID FUNCTION TESTS
T_4, T_3, THBR (T_3), Free T_4 Index, Free T_4

To assay T_4, the hormone must first be separated from its binding proteins by adding a deblocker or agent (such as phenytoin [Dilantin]) that competes for T_4 binding sites (Table 7–1). The total amount of T_4 (the T_4 dis-

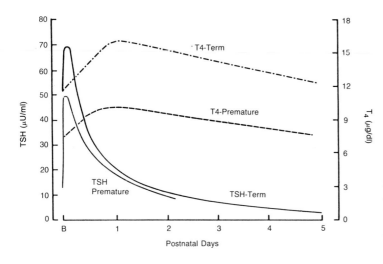

Figure 7–1 Changes in T₄ (*broken lines*) and TSH (*solid lines*) in term and premature infants. (From Fisher DA, Klein AH. Thyroid development and disorders of thyroid function in the newborn. N Engl J Med 1981; 304:702. Reproduced with permission from *The New England Journal of Medicine.*)

sociated from TBGs plus the free T₄) is then quantitated using one of several technologies, e.g., fluorescence polarization or radioimmunoassay (RIA).

Fluorescence polarization assays quantitate the change in fluorescence that occurs when an antibody-fluorescence complex binds a specific ligand such as T₄ (Fig. 7–2). The amount of change in fluorescence is proportional to the T₄ concentrations. The assay (see Fig. 7–2) is a homogeneous one, and there is no separation of free and antibody bonding tracer. When the added fluorescein tracer is not bound, it is freely rotating and polarization is lost. This occurs in the hyperthyroid state. When total T₄ is reduced, then more antibody is bound with reduced rotation in the system and increased net polarization. Fluorescence polarization assays are popular because of their ease of performance, reproducibility, low cost, and lack of potential radiation exposure.

Although widely used in the past, radioimmunoassays have been largely replaced by fluorescence polarization assays. The principles of RIA are well known. A tracer amount of ¹²⁵I(-) T₄ is incubated with a high-affinity specific antibody for T₄. The bound and free hormones are separated by using an inert substance such as char-

coal, or by precipitation of the antigen-antibody complexes by a second antibody against gamma globulin. Increasing concentrations of standard amounts of unlabeled T₄ are added and compete with the labeled hormone for the binding sites. The amount of radioactivity

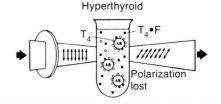

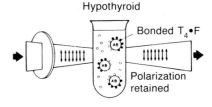

Figure 7–2 The top panel demonstrates the system for doing a fluorescence polarization test for T₄. A light source using a polarized filter is passed through the serum sample to which fluorescein labeled tracer (T₄•F) is added and a detector determines the degree of polarization. The serum sample contains an antibody to T₄ so that the added fluorescein tagged T₄ will be in equilibrium with the patient's T₄. The higher the patient's T₄, the less fluorescein labeled tracer (T₄•F) binds to the antibody. The more unbound tracer, the lower the net polarization. The middle panel demonstrates a high serum T₄, decreased binding of tracer and a low net polarization. The lower panel shows a higher net polarization since more of the T₄•F is bound to the antibody.

TABLE 7–1   Serum Thyroxine (Total T₄)

Method:	Fluorescence polarization Radioimmunoassay (Competitive protein binding)
Normal:	4.5–12.0 μg/dl
Uses:	Screening and follow-up for both hyper- and hypothyroidism
Problems:	1. Changes in TBG affect the value. 2. Antibodies to thyroid hormone may falsely raise or lower the value depending on the assay. 3. Hyperlipidemia may interefere in fluorescence polarization assays

TABLE 7-2   Measuring the Concentration of Serum T₃

Method:	Radioimmunoassay Fluorescence polarization
Normal:	80–200 ng/ml
Uses:	1. Diagnosis and follow-up of hyperthyroidism 2. Diagnosis of T₃ toxicosis
Problems:	1. Recent ingestion of T₃-containing preparations (thyroid extract, liothyronine [Cytomel], liotrix [Thyrolar], Euthyroid) elevates the concentration. 2. Changes in TBG affect the value. 3. Conditions that affect the conversion to T₄ to T₃ affect the value.

TABLE 7-3   THBR (T₃): Indirect Estimate of Thyroxine-Binding Globulin

Method:	Serum incubation with radiolabeled T₃ and binding agent
Normal:	A thyroid hormone–binding ratio 0.83:1.17 T₃ resin uptake 25 to 35% or 35 to 45% depending on method
Uses:	For measurement of binding sites on TBG (NOTE: THIS DOES NOT MEASURE SERUM T₃.) 1. Can be used to calculate free T₄ or T₃ index (see text) 2. Helps to distinguish hyper- and hypothyroidism from increased and decreased TBG, respectively
Problems:	Does not correct for circulating inhibitors of thyroid protein binding such as sometimes seen in severe illness, with Dilantin, or for familial dysalbuminemic hyperthyroxinemia.

bound at each concentration of unlabeled hormone is determined, and a standard curve is plotted. Using this standard curve, the amount of unlabeled hormone in a serum sample can be determined from the amount of radioactivity bound.

The same methodologies can be applied to measuring the concentration of T_3 in serum (Table 7–2). This test is often referred to as the total T_3 or T_3 RIA to distinguish it from the T_3 uptake test, which measures the number of binding sites for thyroid hormones in the sample.

In the T_3 uptake test a known amount of radiolabeled T_3 is added to the patient's serum. The sample is then incubated with a nonspecific binding agent, e.g., a resin. After equilibrium is reached, the resin is separated from the serum, and the amount of labeled T_3 taken up by the binder is measured by gamma counters. The amount of radioactivity bound by the resin is inversely proportional to the number of T_3 binding sites in the serum (Fig. 7–3).

A continuing trap for the unwary is to call the T_3 uptake test the T_3 test, which is then mistaken for the total T_3 test that measures the concentration of T_3 in the serum. This can obviously lead to misdiagnosis or inappropriate treatment. It is the current recommendation that the T_3 uptake test be called the THBR (thyroid hormone–binding resin test) to avoid this pitfall. Designation of which tracer is used in the assay can be expressed as THBR (T_3) or THBR (T_4). In calculating the THBR the counts bound to resin (or other solid matrix) are divided by the residual counts bound to serum proteins to give a ratio (Table 7–3). This ratio is divided by the figure obtained from a serum reference pool and in most assays is normally 1.0. By multiplying this by the total T_4 one obtains an FT₄I (free thyroxine index). The normal range is 4.5 to 12.0 U.

Figure 7–3   T₃ uptake test, or THBR (T₃), schematically shown. The test measures thyroid binding globulin capacity. The patient's serum with an unknown quantity of TBG, T₄, and T₃ is incubated with labeled T₃. The hatchmarked circles represent sites on the TBG which are occupied by serum T₄. The solid circles represent added labeled T₃. This binds to unoccupied sites proportionally. The unbound labeled T₃ is then removed on an added binder and counted on a gamma counter. The THBR (T₃) varies inversely with the number of binding sites available. The normal relationship is shown in the upper panel. The middle two panels contrast hyperthyroidism with hypothyroidism. In the former, the sites on the patient's TBG are occupied with T₄ so that the resin will take up more of the added T₃, thus giving a high THBR (T₃). The situation in hypothyroidism is the converse. In the lower panel, hyper-TBG-emia is contrasted with hypo-TBG-emia. In the former the TBG is increased so that there are increased binding sites for the T₃ tracer and less is taken up on the binder, thus giving a low THBR (T₃). Hypo-TBG-emia is the converse of this.

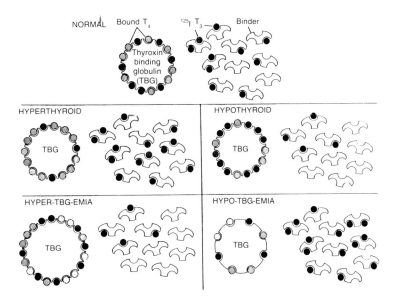

The free T_3 index can be determined in an identical fashion. When using this calculation for the THBR, the FT$_4$I and FT$_3$I show a close correlation with the free T_4 and T_3 measured by equilibrium dialysis (R = 0.77).

The other method for calculating the FT$_4$I is determined by the following equation:

$$FT_4I = \frac{T_4 \times THBR\ (T_3)}{Mean\ THBR\ (T_3)\ or\ control}$$

Unfortunately when the FT$_4$I is determined in this fashion it does not have as good a correlation with the FT$_4$ determined by equilibrium dialysis.

In hyperthyroidism both the total T_4 and the THBR (T_3) are high because the number of free binding sites is reduced, leading to increased uptake by the binding agent (Fig. 7–4). In hypothyroidism the converse is true. Patients with increased TBG show a high T_4 and a low THBR (T_3) (see Fig. 7–4). The THBR (T_3) is low because there is an excess of TBG binding sites competing for the labeled T_3 used in the assay. The T_4 and THBR are altered in the same direction in hyperthyroidism (both high) and hypothyroidism (both low). In contrast the T_4 and THBR diverge in states of TBG excess, or deficiency, while the FT$_4$I remains in the normal range.

Patients have been recognized to have congenital abnormalities of the binding proteins, which affect the THBR test, but less so than in patients with actual increases or decreases in the concentrations of the binding proteins. These patients have increased concentrations of T_4 owing to increased affinity for the hormone, but the THBR is usually normal. The free T_4 index is high, which gives the false impression that the patient is hyperthyroid. In these situations, the free T_4 determined by one of the direct methods is normal.

Free T_4

Of the various methods available for performing direct determinations of the concentration of free T_4 and free T_3, the equilibrium dialysis technique is the "gold standard" (Table 7–4). In this assay a small amount of tracer T_4 and the unknown sample are placed in a dialysis membrane, which limits the diffusion of the bound T_4. The proportion of the hormone that is dialyzable, i.e., free, is determined. The ratio of the dialyzable hormone to total hormone is used with the concentration of T_4 determined in a standard assay to calculate the concentration of free T_4 according to the following formula:

$$\frac{(T_4)(DF)}{D} = Td$$

where T_4 is the concentration of the hormone in the serum, DF is the dialyzable fraction, Td is the concentration of free thyroxine in the dialysis system, and D is the dilution factor. Note that the free T_4 concentration cannot be calculated if the concentration of T_4 is too low to be measured in the standard T_4 assay, although the dialyzable fraction can be determined.

The FT$_4$I has been found to vary in patients with a low total T_4, and in some patients with nonthyroid illness, it can be elevated in the presence of a normal total T_4. The FT$_4$ may not always reflect the true metabolic status of the patient.

The assays developed for free thyroxine can be divided into two general types. The first is the analog or "one step" assay which uses an analog—often an alanine substitution—for T_4 which does not bind to proteins in the serum but does compete for binding with antibody to T_4. These analog assays include Amerex, Coat-a-Count, and one step Gamma Coat. Unfortunately these analogs do bind to albumin, which has a low affinity but high capacity. Thus, while these assays are quite adequate in situations where there are TBG abnormalities they often give spurious results when there are changes in albumin such as in nonthyroid illness and in familial dysalbuminemic hyperthyroxinemia. They are not in general use at the present time. The second type of assay is the two

↑T_4 + ↑THBR (T_3) ⟶ Hyperthyroid

↓T_4 + ↓THBR (T_3) ⟶ Hypothyroid

↑T_4 + ↓THBR (T_3) ⟶ Hyper-TBG-emia

↓T_4 + ↑THBR (T_3) ⟶ Hypo-TBG-emia

Figure 7–4   Serum T_4 and THBR (T_3) values are shown in hyperthyroidism, hypothyroidism, hyper-TBG-emia, and hypo-TBG-emia. Note that the two values move together in hyper- and hypothyroidism but diverge in patients with binding abnormalities.

TABLE 7–4   Free T_4 and Free T_3

Method:	1. Equilibrium dialysis (ultrafiltration) 2. Analog 3. Two step immunoextraction technique using a solid phase antibody.
Normal:	0.8–2.4 ng/ml FT$_4$ 80–350 pg/ml FT$_3$
Uses:	Conditions in which the serum T_4 and T_3 are altered owing to changes in protein binding
Problems:	The equilibrium dialysis method remains the "gold standard" but it is expensive and time consuming. The analog and FT$_4$I are accurate in problems of TBG abnormalities but inaccurate in nonthyroid illness or familial dysalbuminemic hyperthyroxinemia where albumin binding is affected. The two step immunoextraction technique correlates well with equilibrium dialysis and is less expensive.

TABLE 7-4A   Comparison of Free T$_4$ Methods—Including the Free T$_4$ Index

	Expense	Ease of Performance	TBG Abnormalities	NTI	FDH	Correlates With Equilibrium Dialysis
Equilibrium dialysis	Most	Difficult	Normal	Normal	Normal	—
FT$_4$I (T$_3$ resin binding ratio)	Least	Easiest	Normal	High	High	Poor with albumin deficiency
Analog method	Intermediate	Easy	Normal	High	High	Poor
Two step immuno-extraction technique	Intermediate	Easy	Normal	Normal	Normal	Good

NTI = nonthyroid illness; FDH = familial dysalbuminemic hyperthyroxinemia

step radioimmunoassay. The patient's serum is equilibrated with a solid phase antibody to T$_4$. The unoccupied antibody binding sites are then quantitated in a second step in which labeled hormone is added to the solid phase system. Clinical assays two step Gamma Coat and International Immunoassays Laboratories Spiria T$_4$ are examples of this type of assay. A good correlation has been found between these assays and equilibrium dialysis (see Tables 7-4 and 7-4A). They are also easier to perform and less expensive.

Reverse T$_3$

Reverse T$_3$ is formed primarily from the peripheral monodeiodination of T$_4$ (Fig. 7-5, Table 7-5). The inner ring deiodination of T$_4$ by 5′ deiodinase forms reverse

T$_3$. The distinction between formation of T$_3$ and reverse T$_3$ does not appear to be a random event and may be one of the host defense mechanisms against protein deficiency. The metabolic activity of reverse T$_3$ is almost nil. Note that the newborn (see Fig. 7-1) shows markedly elevated levels, but that these values usually decline to normal by the fifth day.

In the euthyroid sick syndrome the reverse T$_3$ is increased owing to two factors (see Fig. 7-5). The activity of the 5′ monodeiodinase enzyme is decreased, and as a result, the production of T$_3$ is decreased. The dominant factor, however, is the decreased conversion of reverse T$_3$ to T$_2$.

Thyroid-Stimulating Hormone

Assays for TSH have changed markedly in recent years. There are now a number of commercially available sensitive assays for TSH, referred to as S-TSH assays. They are based on an immunometric method which uses a "sandwich" method (Fig. 7-6) employing two antibodies. One antibody is attached to a solid phase carrier such as the test tube wall and the other to a signal producer. The sensitivity of the assay is due to the high affinity of the matrix-bound antibody, which produces maximal extraction of TSH. The specificity of the assay is due to the matrix bound antibody for beta TSH subunit. In the past assays performed by RIA (Table 7-6) were inaccurate at the lower range of normal and one was unable to distinguish normals from hyperthyroid patients. With the increased sensitivity of the S-TSH assays this distinction is easily made.

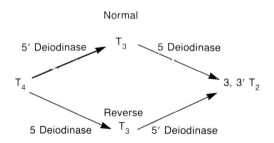

Normal

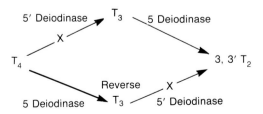

Euthyroid Sick Syndrome

Figure 7-5 The normal pathway for T$_4$ metabolism is demonstrated in the upper panel. In the lower panel is shown the pathway in the euthyroid sick syndrome when reverse T$_3$ is increased and T$_3$ is decreased.

TABLE 7-5   Reverse T$_3$ (3,3′,5′-Triiodothyronine)

Method:	Radioimmunoassay
Normal:	13–50 ng/ml
Use:	Of limited value in differentiating the "euthyroid sick" syndrome from hypothyroidism

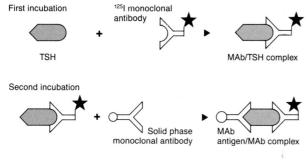

First incubation

TSH   +   ¹²⁵I monoclonal antibody   ▶   MAb/TSH complex

Second incubation

+   Solid phase monoclonal antibody   ▶   MAb antigen/MAb complex

Figure 7-6 Illustration of an S-TSH immunometric assay. "Sandwich method" uses two monoclonal antibodies to TSH—one radiolabeled and the other linked to a solid phase support. Most antibodies now used are to the beta (specific) portion of the molecule. (Reproduced with permission of Celltech Diagnostics, Limited, United Kingdom.)

There are several techniques for the new S-TSH assays. These include immunoradiometric assays (IRMAs) which use ¹²⁵I radiolabeled antibodies and have the disadvantage which goes with the handling of a short-lived radioactive material. IEMAs are immunoenzymometric assays which employ a second antibody labeled with an enzyme such as peroxidase. The most sensitive of all are the chemoluminescent assays (ICMAs) which employ a second antibody labeled with a luminescent compound that generates a light pulse after an appropriate chemi-

cal reaction. The new S-TSH assays offer the advantage of increased speed, sensitivity, and specificity.

Hay and Klee (1988) have proposed five criteria for S-TSH assays:

1. An overlap of less than 1 percent between the variation of the lower normal value limit and the assay detection limit.
2. Subnormal basal TSH values in 95 percent of patients with subnormal TRH responses.
3. Detectable basal TSH values in 95 percent of patients with normal TRH responses.
4. Undetectable TSH values in 95 percent of hyperthyroid patients.
5. Detectable values in 95 percent of clinically euthyroid patients including patients with nonthyroidal illness.

The American Thyroid Association has defined an S-TSH assay as one in which serum from hyperthyroid patients gives results which are more than three log standard deviations below the mean value found in the serum of normal subjects.

There are five areas where the S-TSH assays have proven to be particularly helpful:

1. Thyroid screening in normal populations.
2. Evaluation of thyroid suppression and replacement therapy.
3. Elimination of TRH testing.
4. Detection of subclinical hyperthyroidism.
5. Confirmation of normal thyroid function.

Although expense probably militates against the current use of S-TSH assays for screening normal populations for thyroid disease, this has been proposed by a number of authors. An approach to screening suggested by Caldwell et al (1985) is reproduced here (Fig. 7-7). S-TSH assays do not distinguish patients with hypopituitarism where the S-TSH may be normal despite hypothyroidism. In most clinical settings, however, thyroid failure is not the first manifestation of pituitary insufficiency. Adult patients usually present with gonadotrophic failure, and those in the pediatric group present with growth hormone deficiency. Two other conditions in which the TSH can be misleading are in patients recovering from nonthyroid illness who have an elevated S-TSH or in situations where thyroxine suppression has been discontinued and the thyroid is in a recovery phase. Because of the sensitivity of the pituitary to its feedback hormone, S-TSH (see Fig. 7-2) may show changes before there is a rise or fall in the serum T_4.

In light of this finely tuned feedback response it is reasonable to use the S-TSH as a benchmark for assessing thyroid suppression as well as thyroid replacement. For replacement therapy it is prudent to give only enough thyroid hormone to keep the S-TSH in the normal range. There are several reports in the literature of osteoporosis

---

TABLE 7-6   Thyroid-Stimulating Hormone

Method:	Radioimmunoassay (RIA)
	Immunoenzymometric assay (IEMA)
	Immunoradiometric assay (IRMA)
	Immunochemoluminescent assay (ICMA)
Normal:	RIA UD–6.5 μU/ml
	IEMA 0.6–3.8 μU/ml
	IRMA 0.5–3.8 μU/ml
	ICMA 0.5–3.8 μU/ml
	Many laboratories list 6.5 as the upper normal limit; most patients with levels above 3.8 are hypothyroid.
Uses:	Screening for hypothyroidism—all assays
	Screening for hyperthyroidism—S-TSH assays (IRMA, IEMA, and ICMA)
	Evaluation of metabolic status in patients with acute or chronic nonthyroidal illness—all assays
	Evaluation of T_4 replacement for hypothyroidism or in patients on suppression therapy for carcinoma or thyroid nodule—S-TSH assays (IRMA, IEMA, and ICMA)
	Evaluation of treatment for hyperthyroidism.
Problems:	Some assays currently in use are "non-sensitive" and will detect normal TSH levels in hyperthyroid patients.
	S-TSH assays using antibodies developed in mice may show a false positive TSH elevation. Most commercial assays have eliminated this problem.
	Problems associated with radioactive substance IRMA and IEMA—new instrumentation

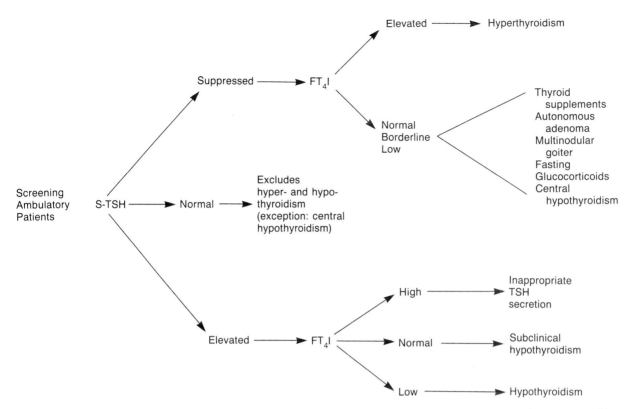

Figure 7-7 An approach to the diagnosis of thyroid function using S-TSH as the initial screening test. Note the significant number of false positives and false negatives for S-TSH assays. (Modified from Caldwell G, Kellett HA, Gow SM, Beckett GJ, Sweeting VM, Seth J, Toft AD. A new strategy for thyroid function testing. Lancet 1985; 1:117–119.)

occurring in patients on thyroid replacement. In these patients it has been assumed that there was a relative hyperthyroid state and consequent bone loss. In addition, levels of liver enzymes including glutathione S-transferase can be increased in patients who receive replacement doses of thyroxine. These values seemed to be higher in those whose S-TSH was suppressed.

A number of studies have shown a close correlation between the basal S-TSH and the TSH response to TRH. Usually there is a tenfold increase in TSH levels following stimulation with TRH. It had been thought that the TRH test would still serve some use in distinguishing patients with undetectable S-TSH who had nonthyroid illness from those with suppressed levels due to hyperthyroidism. The more sensitive ICMAs, however, appear to show that hyperthyroid patients are below 0.005 μU per milliliter whereas those with nonthyroid illness are measurable. As the assays improve there will probably be less need for the TRH test.

One potential difficulty with the S-TSH assay is that a few patients have been described with spuriously high values due to interfering antibodies in the patient's serum. Antimouse immunoglobulins in the serum can cross react with mouse antibodies used in the assay. The antibodies can be removed by treating the sample with mouse serum before running the assay. Another approach is to use the Fab fragment of the mouse anti-TSH anti-

body in the assay. Since the human antibody is directed at the Fac portion of the immunoglobulin, it will not interfere. In situations where the S-TSH level is high in the absence of clinical correlation, one should have a high index of suspicion that one is dealing with an artifact.

Most commercial assays now in use have eliminated this problem.

ASSESSMENT OF THYROID STATUS BY MEANS OF THYROID FUNCTION TESTING

Patients With Increased T_4 and/or T_3

Hyperthyroidism

In over 90 percent of patients with hyperthyroidism, both the T_4 and T_3 are elevated. In 5 percent of patients in this country, T_3 is exclusively elevated (T_3 toxicosis) and the T_4 is normal or even low. Thus failure to obtain a T_3 could result in missing the diagnosis of hyperthyroidism. Initially, it was believed that T_3 toxicosis was most often seen in patients with an autonomous nodule or multinodular goiter. However, this entity is just as often seen in patients with a diffuse goiter. In patients previously treated with drugs, surgical intervention, or radioactive iodine (RAI), T_3 secretion may increase before that of T_4 in recurring hyperthyroidism. Since the serum T_4

is increased in over 90 percent of patients with hyperthyroidism, this test is used initially to screen for the disease. The total T_3 is of value if the T_4 is not elevated. T_3 levels may normalize within several days of initiating therapy with antithyroid therapy.

It has been suggested that the new S-TSH assays may supplant T_4, T_3, and THBR (T_3) as screening tests for hyperthyroidism. Some authors believe that using the new IRMA test, a TSH which is greater than 0.7 μU per milliliter excludes thyroid disease as the primary cause of the hyperthyroidism. It still may be necessary to obtain more than one test to be confident of the diagnosis. When hyperthyroidism is suspected, a serum T_3 should be done to exclude the diagnosis of T_3 toxicosis.

The converse of T_3 toxicosis with elevations of the T_4 and normal levels of T_3 (T_4 toxicosis) is being reported with increasing frequency. The euthyroid sick syndrome may show an elevated serum T_4 with normal or low T_3 indistinguishable from T_4 toxicosis. Those patients with T_4 toxicosis will usually show a rise in T_3 over time into the toxic range, whereas the serum T_4 of the patient with an acute nonthyroidal illness would fall back into the normal range. The RAI uptake does not reliably distinguish between T_4 toxicosis and the euthyroid sick syndrome since it may be normal in hyperthyroidism. Rarely, a normal serum TSH or an absent TSH response to TRH (Fig. 7-8) may also fail to distinguish between these two entities. As a practical matter, it might be necessary to treat such a patient with beta-blockers to provide symptomatic relief.

The absence of a goiter would be strong evidence against the diagnosis of T_4 toxicosis. Painless thyroiditis and exogenous L-thyroxine are notable exceptions. The presence of Graves' ophthalmopathy or a bruit over the gland would be supporting evidence of hyperthyroidism.

TRH Testing. With the advent of the new S-TSH assays TRH testing is used less and less. There are still rare occasions when a TRH test is useful in evaluating patients for hyperthyroidism (Table 7-7). The pituitary secretion of TSH is suppressed in patients with hyperthyroidism and there is no rise in TSH following the administration of TRH (see Fig. 7-7). However, the TSH response to TRH may be suppressed in a variety of conditions in which hyperthyroidism is absent (Table 7-8). This is true of autonomous adenomas, euthyroid Graves' disease, and some patients with multinodular goiter. Therefore, the presence of a flat TSH curve following TRH is not diagnostic of hyperthyroidism, but must be interpreted in light of the patient's clinical signs and symptoms. However, the finding of a normal rise in TSH in a patient suspected of having hyperthyroidism is a compelling argument against that diagnosis.

There is great variability in TSH responses to TRH in patients under treatment with antithyroid drugs for hyperthyroidism. For this reason it is not practical to follow these patients with repeated TRH tests.

The TRH test may also be useful in delineating those patients with exophthalmos due to euthyroid Graves' dis-

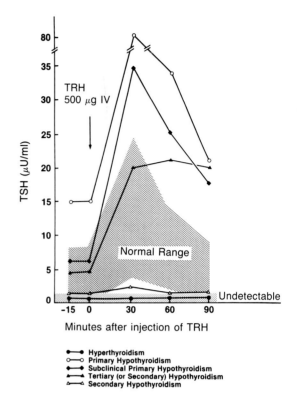

Figure 7-8 Results of TRH stimulation test in normals; in patients with hyperthyroidism; and in cases of primary, secondary, tertiary, and subclinical hypothyroidism. (Reproduced with permission from Kohler, PO. Clinical endocrinology. New York: John Wiley, 1986.)

TABLE 7-7   Thyroid-Releasing Hormone Test

Method:	500 μg of TRH is given intravenously over 1 minute. A serum TSH is drawn at 0, 30, and 60 minutes. Side effects that the patient may experience include nausea, headache, dizziness, and urinary urgency. None of these lasts more than several minutes. Rarely, patients have an increase in blood pressure or hypotension. Administration to patients with underlying cardiovascular disease may precipitate angina.
Normal:	A rapid rise in TSH of 5–30 μU/ml with an average of 15 μU/ml and peak at 30 minutes. In practice it is usually necessary to get only the 30-min specimen (see Fig. 7-8)
Uses:	Diagnosis of hyperthyroidism Evaluation of adequacy of thyroid suppression Assessment of TSH and prolactin reserve in hypothalamic-pituitary disease Post-treatment assessment of patients with acromegaly Differential diagnosis of hypothalamic pituitary hypothyroidism

ease. Many of these patients are unresponsive to TRH. A flat curve and an orbital CT help to distinguish these patients from those with other causes of exophthalmos. The TRH test has replaced the T_3 suppression test that carries with it the small, but definite, hazard of precipitat-

TABLE 7-8   Impaired TSH Response to TRH

Hyperthyroidism
Autonomously functioning thyroid tissue—
    thyroid adenoma
Impaired hypothalamic function
    Cushing's syndrome
    Acromegaly
    Depression
    Systemic illness
Drugs
    Corticosteroids
    Dopamine
    Beta-blockers
Exogenous T_4 or T_3
Pituitary-hypothalamic hypothyroidism
Fasting

TABLE 7-9   Euthyroid Hyperthyroxinemia

Increased protein binding
  1. Inherited TBG increase
  2. Familial dysalbuminemic
      hyperthyroxinemia
  3. TBPA excess
      Inherited
      Ectopic neoplastic
  4. Estrogen-increased TBG
      Pregnancy
      Newborn
      Estrogen-secreting tumors
  5. Liver disease
  6. Acute intermittent porphyria
  7. Hydatidiform mole
  8. Drug-induced increased TBG
      Estrogens administered orally,
        topically, and in the form of oral
        contraceptives
      5-Fluorouracil
      Clofibrate
      Methadone and heroin
Decreased conversion of T_4 to T_3
  1. Acute systemic illness
  2. Acute psychiatric illness
  3. Chronic protein malnutrition
  4. Drugs
      Ipodate (Oragrafin)
      Telepaque
      Amiodarone
Peripheral resistance to thyroid hormone

ing angina or cardiac arrhythmias in older individuals with underlying heart disease.

In most cases of hyperthyroidism, the basal TSH determined by the IRMA and IEMA currently available is less than 0.7 μU per milliliter, and the TRH test is not necessary.

Euthyroid Hyperthyroxinemia

In a variety of situations the concentration of thyroid hormones is found to be elevated in the absence of signs or symptoms of hyperthyroidism (Table 7–9).

Inherited TBG Abnormalities. Congenital TBG excess is inherited in an X-linked pattern. The total T_4 and T_3 are high, whereas the THBR is low. The FT_4I will be normal, indicative of euthyroidism. Although not usually measured, the FT_3I is also normal. The increase in TBG is greater in males than in females. Therefore, the T_4 is usually higher in the male population with this inherited pattern.

Familial Dysalbuminemic Hyperthyroxinemia (FDH). Several groups have reported abnormalities in the albumin-binding sites for T_4 inherited as an autosomal dominant. T_4 levels are elevated while the THBR(T_3) is normal. Consequently, FT_4I is elevated, suggesting a diagnosis of hyperthyroidism. However, levels of free T_4 that are determined by equilibrium dialysis are normal, as is the TRH stimulation test and the basal serum TSH. All of the cases described were metabolically normal. They usually do not have a goiter and their 24-hour RAI uptake is normal. One of the clues in distinguishing these patients from those with Graves' disease has been the finding of a normal total and free serum T_3. Note that the TBG concentration in these patients is normal. In this condition there is an excess of albumin with a very high affinity for thyroxine. Other patients have been described who have albumins with an increased affinity for T_3 or reverse T_3. Appropriate tests to exclude hyperthyroidism will include basal S-TSH, RAI uptakes, and FT_4 and FT_3 by equilibrium dialysis. The abnormal albumin can again be demonstrated by serum electropho-

resis using ^{125}I labeled T_4 or T_3. Patients who are hyperthyroid and have FDH have very high total T_4 levels out of proportion to their degree of hyperthyroidism. In this case the S-TSH will be suppressed. Conversely, when patients with FDH are hypothyroid they have a normal serum T_4 but an elevated S-TSH.

TBPA Abnormalities. A family with increased TBPA has been described by Moses et al (1982). In these patients the serum T_4 was high in the absence of findings of hyperthyroidism or goiter. The T_3, THBR, and FT_4 were normal. The S-TSH in such patients would be in the normal range. The diagnosis can be confirmed with serum electrophoresis using ^{125}I labeled T_4 which will show a peak in the TBPA range. It is felt that there is an increase in affinity of TBPA for T_4 as well as an increased concentration. An abnormality in TBPA has also been reported in two patients with islet cell carcinoma and high serum T_4. These patients were euthyroid with normal T_3, THBR, and free T_4. It has been postulated that the islet cell carcinomas synthesized increased amounts of TBPA.

Increased Binding of T_4 by Antibodies

Many authors have now reported patients with antibodies to T_4 or T_3. Most of these patients have Hashimoto's thyroiditis but the entity has been seen in Waldenstrom's macroglobulinemia, Sjögren's syndrome, and in monoclonal gammopathies. Depending on the method used the values for T_4 may be spuriously high or low. RIA methods based on double antibody techniques will be elevated whereas methods using talc or charcoal to separate bound and free hormone result in low values. It follows that the FT_4 levels will be affected similarly depending on the method used for the T_4 or T_3.

Drug-Induced Elevation of TBG. Perhaps the most common cause of an increased T_4 is drugs that increase the total TBG (see Table 7–9). The most common is estrogen, which can be administered in a variety of forms for an increasing number of indications. Oral contraceptives and oral estrogens for the prevention of osteoporosis and for the treatment of menopausal symptoms often produce TBG excess. Topical creams and vaginal estrogens have been reported to raise serum estrogen levels and consequently may be expected to increase TBG. The change in TBG is due to an increased content of sialic acid which decreases hepatic clearance.

5-Fluorouracil, clofibrate, methadone, and heroin have also been noted to cause an elevated T_4. These drugs cause a high T_4, a low THBR (T_3), and a normal FT_4I.

Drug-Induced Blockage of T_4 to T_3. The other mechanism for the elevation of the serum T_4 by drugs is the blockage of the T_4 to T_3 conversion.

PTU blocks both the 5′ and 5 monodeiodinase steps, while methimazole does not have such an effect in the doses that are usually administered clinically.

Glucocorticoids have a similar effect to that of PTU when given in pharmacologic doses. There is a rise in RT_3 and a fall in T_3; this is in addition to their central effect in suppressing the secretion of TSH.

Propranolol also increases the RT_3 by blocking the T_4 to T_3 conversion. The combination of steroids, PTU, and propranolol acts rapidly to decrease the level of T_3 in severely hyperthyroid patients.

Iopanoic acid (Telepaque), ipodate (Oragrafin), and amiodarone all produce a similar chemical picture. The serum T_3 is reduced, the reverse T_3 is increased, and the serum ratio of $T_3:T_4$ is reduced. Since these agents are often used in clinical settings in which the patient is acutely ill, confusion may arise in the interpretation of the usual tests of thyroid function.

Larsen has pointed out the difficulty of distinguishing elevated T_4 levels from blockade of T_4 to T_3 conversion from T_4 toxicosis. The measurement of the S-TSH usually establishes the diagnosis. In a rare instance, a TRH stimulation test (see Table 7–7) is necessary to separate a truly hyperthyroid patient by showing a flat TSH response. The newer TSH assays, which are discussed later, would distinguish such a condition without the need for a TRH test.

Hyperthyroxinemia in Acute Illness. Patients with acute medical or surgical illnesses may have high concentrations of T_4 with decreased conversion of T_4 to T_3 (see Table 7–9). There is a decreased activity of 5′ deiodinase that results not only in the aforementioned inhibition, but also in the accumulation of reverse T_3 (see Fig. 7–5). The conversion of T_4 to RT_3 and of T_3 to 3,3′

T2 is relatively unaffected. This may represent a protective mechanism so that by reducing the secretion of T_3, the active metabolite of T_4, the body decreases its catabolism of critical protein mass.

Abnormalities in the hypothalamic–pituitary axis have also been found. In cases of prolonged fasting there appears to be a decreased release of TSH.

Peripheral Resistance to Thyroid Hormone. This interesting syndrome was first described in 1968 by Refetoff and Selenkow, who reported three siblings of a consanguineous marriage who showed a high T_4, goiter, deaf-mutism, delayed bone age, and epiphyseal stippling. Their total T_4 concentration was about 20 µg per deciliter with normal TSH levels. There was no clinical evidence of hyperthyroidism.

Subsequent patients with this syndrome have shown findings similar to those of the original family—the hallmark of which has been the finding of an elevated T_4 in the presence of clinical euthyroidism. Patients with this syndrome have had normal basal serum TSH levels and normal responses to TRH. The inheritance pattern has shown both a sporadic and an autosomal dominant pattern. This syndrome is an example of inappropriate TSH secretion as described by Weintraub and associates (1981). It should be noted that a pituitary tumor can mimic just such a chemical picture, which should be excluded by a computed tomography (CT) or magnetic resonance imaging (MRI) scan. The resistance to thyroid hormone should be demonstrated by an absence of metabolic response to exogenous hormone. Tests that could be evaluated include circulatory dynamics, cholesterol levels, creatine metabolism, pulse rate, and urinary excretion of hydroxyproline.

The cellular defect responsible for the peripheral resistance syndrome is not well understood. Nuclear receptor abnormalities have been described in some but not in all cases of this syndrome. Maxon and associates (1982) have described a large kindred with isolated elevations of the serum T_4 without changes in the T_3. They have postulated a defect in the intracellular transport of T_4.

Evaluation of Patients With Decreased T_4 and/or T_3

Hypothyroidism

The sine qua non for the diagnosis of primary hypothyroidism is an elevated serum TSH. With the development of primary thyroid failure, the earliest change is an increase in the pituitary content of TSH. The concentrations of TSH are low or in the normal range in most patients with pituitary or hypothalamic hypothyroidism. However, in some cases the TSH may be elevated owing to the production of biologically inactive hormone. TRH testing distinguishes these patients from those with decreased thyroid reserve attributable to primary thyroid disease.

It has been shown that patients with mild elevations of TSH in the range of 5 to 15 μU per milliliter have evidence of hypothyroidism at the tissue level. This is manifested by an increase in cholesterol levels, decreased sodium and red cell concentrations, and altered circulatory dynamics. It has also been suggested that these patients may have an increased incidence of coronary artery disease, possibly related to changes in the serum lipids. Treatment with thyroid reverses these abnormalities. Early replacement also avoids the development of insidious hypothyroidism, which may occur in this setting. One also prevents the potential development of goiter and thyroid nodules by avoiding the continued stimulation of high levels of TSH.

Patients with hypothyroidism due to abnormalities in pituitary secretion of TSH have low concentrations of the thyroid hormones, low THBR (T_3), and concentrations of TSH that are either in the normal range, low, or occasionally slightly elevated. In the last case, a biologically inactive form of TSH is produced.

It had been hoped that the response to TRH would be able to distinguish patients with hypothalamic hypothyroidism from those with pituitary hypothyroidism. The classic response to TRH in patients with hypothalamic hypothyroidism is a delayed increase in serum TSH following TRH administration (see Fig. 7–6). In pituitary hypothyroidism where the thyrotroph is absent TSH should not increase after the administration of TRH. Unfortunately, there have been many exceptions in both categories. For this reason, one cannot use the TRH test to distinguish hypothalamic from pituitary hypothyroidism. (See Chapter 3 for the use of TRH testing in acromegaly.)

Euthyroid Hypothyroxinemia

There are a number of clinical settings in which the T_4 is low but the patient is clinically euthyroid (Table 7–10). Hypoproteinemia due to malnutrition is common, and because of the deficiency in thyroid-binding proteins, the concentration of total T_4 is low. Severe malnutrition, protein-losing enteropathies, and the nephrotic syndrome may cause TBG deficiency.

An inherited reduction in serum TBG occurs that results in a low serum T_4 and high THBR (T_3). These patients are metabolically euthyroid. The entity is inherited as an X-linked defect with males being more severely affected than females. Qualitative abnormalities in TBG have been reported with an X-linked hereditary pattern. These patients (Table 7–10) have a low total T_4 but are euthyroid. In Aborigines the incidence is reported as 40 percent -TBG-A. In TBG Chicago the T_4 is normal but the TBG differs from normal in that it is heat stable.

TBG deficiency also occurs in patients who are taking androgenic hormones such as testosterone or danazol or who have high circulating cortisol levels, from either exogenous or endogenous sources.

Glucocorticoids produce TBG deficiency not only

TABLE 7–10   Euthyroid Hypothyroxinemia

Decreased TBG production
  Severe systemic illness
  Familial X-linked
  Androgens
  Asparaginase
  Glucocorticoids
Qualitative abnormalities in TBG—X-linked
  TBG-A Aborigines 40%
  TBG-S Blacks, Eskimos, Indonesians, Melanesians,
      Polynesians
  TBG-Quebec
  TBG-Montreal
  TBG-Gary
  TBG-San Diego
Excess loss of TBG
  Protein losing enteropathy
  Nephrosis
  Jejunal-ileal bypass
Inhibition of protein binding
  Systemic illness (free fatty acids)
  Dilantin
  Salicylates
  Furosemide
  Fenclofenac
Exogenous T_3 therapy (factitious or therapeutic)

by decreasing the synthesis of TBG, but also by decreasing the secretion of TSH. Conversion of T_4 to T_3 is also impaired in patients taking glucocorticoids. The net result is a low T_4.

Dilantin, salicylates, and the nonsteroidal anti-inflammatory agent fenclofenac displace the binding of T_4 by its binding proteins and accelerate the metabolism of T_4, thereby tending to lower concentrations of the hormone. Dilantin enhances the degradation of T_4 in the liver. Phenobarbital has similar effects, but in the usual doses employed it does not alter the thyroid tests. Furosemide in large amounts has also been reported to inhibit T_4 binding. In severe systemic illness unsaturated free fatty acids may interfere with T_4 binding.

Finally, suppression of the hypothalamic pituitary axis by the administration of Cytomel (T_3) also lowers the total serum T_4 by inhibiting the production of thyroxine. This is often obvious from the history, but occasionally it is due to the surreptitious use of the drug. The patients may have signs of hyperthyroidism. The diagnosis can be confirmed by obtaining a serum T_3 that is elevated and an RAI uptake that is suppressed.

Euthyroid Sick Syndrome

Patients with severe systemic illnesses may also show a low serum T_4 with or without a low serum T_3. Those patients with a low serum T_4 are usually seriously ill. The lower the serum T_4, the higher the mortality. Several mechanisms may be involved in this. Chopra has reported the presence of a circulating inhibitor of T_4 binding in the serum from sick patients. The serum T_4 is lowered because of an increased metabolic clearance probably secondary to the changes in binding. Because the inhibitor affects the binding of T_3 to the *resin matrix* to a lesser extent than it does the binding to *TBG*, the T_3 uptake is less disturbed than one would expect. For this reason the FT_4I is often low. Note that the free T_4 by dialysis and serum TSH are usually normal in these metabolically euthyroid patients. Reverse T_3 is normal or increased. A difficult diagnostic problem occurs in distinguishing this syndrome from that of hypopituitary patients who develop severe illness. The overall clinical picture, including the previous medical history, CT scan of the pituitary, and serum cortisol level, helps make this distinction.

Jackson and Cobb have pointed out that in very sick patients who are receiving a number of drugs that may affect this clinical and chemical status, it may be impossible to ascertain whether the patient is euthyroid or hypothyroid. In such a situation, it may very rarely be necessary to administer thyroid hormone on a trial basis.

The low T_4, low T_3 syndrome is an extension of the low T_3 syndrome; it is just worse and has a higher mortality. Treatment of the underlying illness is the goal and usually helps to unravel the various permutations of the thyroid hormones that may occur.

EXOGENOUS THYROID HORMONE THERAPY

Administration of thyroid hormone, in the form of either L-thyroxine or triiodothyronine, suppresses the TSH. Suppression can occur with relatively small doses of exogenous thyroid hormone, and concentrations of thyroid hormones in the serum may not be above the normal range.

In patients who are being treated with thyroid suppression for thyroid cancer or nodules, it may be desirable to document the adequacy of TSH suppression by performing a TRH test (see Table 7–7). Spencer (1986) has shown that when using one of the sensitive assays for TSH, 11 percent of the patients with undetectable levels of TSH were responsive to a TRH test. Whether the demonstration of an unresponsive TRH test is a sine qua non for adequate thyroid suppression is currently unclear. In light of the fact that TRH unresponsiveness is the most sensitive indicator of adequate suppression, it seems reasonable to continue to use this as the "gold standard."

EFFECT OF THYROID ILLNESS ON OTHER SERUM TESTS

Thyroid hormones have far-reaching effects on the body (Table 7–11). These effects show up in the blood tests that are frequently ordered on patients. Most of the time these aberrations return to normal as the hyper- or hypothyroidism is treated. Further investigation of these changes is not usually warranted except when improvement does not occur. At times, the presence of one of the abnormalities listed subsequently serves as the clinician's clue to the diagnosis of thyroid disease.

TABLE 7–11   Altered Tests in Hyperthyroidism and Hypothyroidism

Hyperthyroidism
  Increased
    Calcium
    Bilirubin
    SGOT
    Alkaline phosphatase
    Urine calcium
    Ferritin
    Factor VII
    SHBG
  Decreased
    Cholesterol
    K + (rare cases of periodic paralysis)

Hypothyroidism
  Increased
    Cholesterol
    Triglycerides
    Carotene
    CPK–MM isoenzyme
    LDH
    CEA
    SGOT
    Prolactin
  Decreased
    Alkaline phosphatase (active growth phase)

SGOT = serum glutamic oxaloacetic transaminase; SHBG = sex hormone–binding globulin; CPK = creatine phosphokinase; LDH = lactate dehydrogenase; CEA = carcinoembryonic antigen

MISCELLANEOUS THYROID TESTS

Thyroid Antibodies

Thyroid-Stimulating Antibodies

Detection of thyroid-stimulating antibodies (TSAb) has evolved from the initial discovery of long-acting thyroid stimulators (LATS) by Adams and Purves in 1956. This was later identified as an IgG that reacts with the thyrotropin receptor and that, as a consequence, inhibits the binding of ^{125}I–TSH. Two assays have evolved: direct assays, which measure stimulation, and assays measuring inhibition of binding of TSH. Because there are a number of methods for measuring TSH receptor antibodies, it is currently recommended by the American Thyroid Association that such assays be termed TSH receptor antibodies (TRAb) measured by the "designated" assay. One of these is described below and is the prototype for a variety of perturbations that have appeared (Table 7–12).

McKenzie (1980) has pointed out several problems with the tissue assay for TSAb. Nondiseased human thyroid tissue should be used. Failure to do this can result in unresponsive tissue slices. Secondly he feels that the use of frozen tissue can result in discrepancies in the results. Some investigators have used thyroid tissue obtained from tissue culture, thus obviating the need to use human tissue available at the time. The use of human thyroid cells in culture along with a rat cell line (FRTL5) has largely replaced the use of human thyroid slices. There

TABLE 7–12   Assays Measuring Biological Effects of the Interaction of Antibodies With the TSH Receptor

Assay	Method
*LATS—Long-acting thyroid stimulator	^{125}I release from mouse thyroid in vitro Discharge in mice of ^{125}I labeled thyroid components
*Human thyroid slices	Cyclic AMP increase in human thyroid slices or colloid droplet formation
FRTL5 cells in monolayer culture	1) Increase in cellular cyclic AMP 2) Stimulation of iodine uptake 3) Incorporation of thymidine into DNA
Human thyroid cells in monolayer culture	Increase in cyclic AMP in the cells or medium
Assays Measuring Inhibition of TSH-Binding	
Human thyroid particulate membranes	Inhibition of ^{125}I labeled TSH
Solubilized porcine thyroid membranes	Inhibition of ^{125}I labeled TSH
Guinea pig adipocyte membranes	Inhibition of ^{125}I labeled TSH

* Infrequently used assays.
Modified from McKenzie JM. Current concepts of Graves' disease. Fortieth Annual Postgraduate Assembly. The Endocrine Society, 1988.

has been some concern about species specificity in using the FRTL5 line and there are a number of false negatives which occur.

The other assays for thyrotropin-binding inhibitory immunoglobulin (TBII) that have been developed are more readily available than direct assays measuring stimulation. These assays use the inhibition of ^{125}I binding to the receptor by TSAb. Hall and his co-workers have published extensively using such an assay and have found a high correlation of positive responses with Graves' disease activity as well as a correlation with predicting treatment failures with antithyroid drugs. In most assays this TSH-binding inhibition assay has been nonspecific, giving positive results in patients with a variety of other thyroid diseases.

The TBI method which is available commercially measures the degree of inhibition of ^{125}I to solubilized porcine membranes by the patient's serum. Some of the immunoglobulins present in patients with Graves' disease may bind to the receptor without causing stimulation of the gland. Despite this deficiency, the assay is clinically useful and appears to correlate in most cases with a comparable TSAb assay.

There are two clinical situations in which the determination of TSAb can be useful (Table 7–13). In patients who are candidates for treatment with antithyroid drugs, the finding of very high levels of TSAb prior to beginning therapy indicates a high probability of failure. The assay has also been useful at the end of the drug-treatment period in predicting successfully those patients who will relapse. In one series there was a 100 percent correlation with treatment failure within 3 months of withdrawal of the antithyroid drug.

TSAb levels are also useful when looking for newborns who are likely to develop hyperthyroidism because of transplacental transmission of circulating immunoglobulins from a hyperthyroid mother. Such determina-

tions should be carried out in the third trimester since the levels may fluctuate during pregnancy. Levels in these cases have been quite high, greater than 500 percent of basal activity in some laboratories. It has also been pointed out that neonatal hyperthyroidism may occur in the offspring of mothers who have been previously treated successfully and who do not show signs of hyperthyroidism at the time of delivery or during pregnancy. The extrathyroidal manifestations of Graves' disease are present in a high percentage of mothers whose offspring manifest neonatal Graves' disease. TSAb levels in this situation may forewarn the physician.

There is little reason to use the TSAb assays in routine testing for Graves' disease since the other serum hormonal tests are more sensitive and less expensive. TSAb levels are elevated in most patients with euthyroid Graves' disease with ophthalmopathy, but a S-TSH test is preferred in this situation.

Other immunoglobulins that interact with the thyrotropin receptors have been described. These include

TABLE 7–13   TSAb: Human Thyroid Tissue

Method:	Slices of fresh thyroid tissue are incubated with IgG sera from the subject for 2 h. Cyclic AMP production is measured by immunoassay.
Normal:	An increase in cyclic AMP over that of the control serum by 600 to 6,000%.
Uses:	1. Prediction of relapse in patients under drug therapy at onset of therapy as well as at completion. 2. Prediction of neonatal transmission from mother with hyperthyroidism.
Problems:	Test is technically difficult and expensive. A variation in techniques exists from one laboratory to another. There is also lack of a universal standard.

a thyroid growth-stimulating immunoglobulin (TGI), as well as blocking antibodies for both TSI and TGI. TGI in some hands is elevated in patients with both simple diffuse goiter and multinodular goiter. In primary myxedema and congenital hyperthyroidism, blocking antibodies may be found. These blocking antibodies could account for the progressive atrophy that occurs in the face of high titers of TSH. Currently, assays for TGI and blocking antibodies have little role in clinical practice.

Antithyroid Antibodies

A number of thyroid antibodies have been described, but the ones with the greatest clinical usefulness are the antithyroglobulin, microsomal, and TSH receptor and blocking antibodies (Table 7–14). The assays for thyroid microsomal and thyroglobulin include hemagglutination, immunoassay, and ELISA. Normal values are assay dependent.

It is common clinical practice to order both thyroglobulin hemagglutination antibodies (TGHA) and microsomal hemagglutination antibodies (MCHA) in situations in which one suspects Hashimoto's thyroiditis. One may see elevated titers in patients with Graves' disease or multinodular goiter and in relatives of patients with thyroid disease. The presence of a very high titer (1:5,000) in a nontoxic goitrous patient is indicative of Hashimoto's disease. Patients with Hashimoto's thyroiditis are much more likely to have a positive MCHA test than a TGHA. In cases of suspected subacute thyroiditis in which there is a significant titer, one can assume a situation in which there is significant lymphocytic infiltration. Patients with thyroid cancer who have elevated titers generally have evidence of lymphocytic infiltration.

There are a number of factors that influence MCHA and TGHA titers. Treatment of Hashimoto's disease with thyroid replacement results in a decrease in titer. The removal of tissue by subtotal or total thyroidectomy also lowers titers by removing the bulk of thyroid-infiltrating lymphocytes. Corticosteroids decrease antibody levels. Both propylthiouracil and methimazole (Tapazole) decrease the formation of antithyroid antibodies because of an immunosuppressive activity. Young children with Hashimoto's disease usually have lower antibody titers, and in pregnancy the antibody titers decrease with a rebound postpartum. The latter sequence may account for the high incidence of hypothyroidism that occurs in the postpartum period.

RAI, on the other hand, results in a rise in antibody levels that usually peaks 2 to 3 months post-treatment.

Thyroglobulin

The serum thyroglobulin (TG) is a glycoprotein of use in the differential diagnosis of thyroid disease. It is now measured by a double antibody RIA (Table 7–15). The normal level is 0 to 30 ng per milliliter with the mean serum level in the vicinity of 10 ng per milliliter.

TG is released from the gland in a variety of states (Table 7–16). TG levels are most useful in following patients with thyroid cancer. It is not generally useful in the initial evaluation of the patient with thyroid cancer since it does not always correlate with metastatic disease, and it may be elevated in patients with benign adenomas. It does seem to have a correlation with the type of tumor, tending to be much higher in follicular cancer than in pure papillary cancer. Interestingly, it is not elevated in patients with medullary cancer of the thyroid. It is most useful in monitoring cases after ablation of the gland. In thyroid cancer patients with consistently low TG levels there is less need for frequent withdrawal of thyroxine suppression and administration of repetitive doses of RAI for scanning purposes. When metastases do occur, the serum levels are almost always elevated. A survey of the literature by Van Herle (1981) shows that less than 3.2 percent of all patients with metastatic disease

TABLE 7–14 Antithyroid Antibodies

Antithyroglobulin Antibodies

Method:	Tanned red cell hemagglutination Radioimmunoassay
Normal:	< 1:100
Uses:	Primarily useful in making a diagnosis of Hashimoto's thyroiditis
Problems:	Insensitivity: 50% of patients with Hashimoto's thyroiditis have a negative TGHA assay. Treatment with steroid, antithyroid drugs, surgery, thyroid, and pregnancy lower titers; RAI increases them.

Antithyroid Microsomal Antibodies

Method:	MCHA Radioimmunoassay Enzyme immunoassay
Normal:	< 1:100
Uses:	More sensitive in diagnosing Hashimoto's 90% positive.
Problems:	Similar to TGHA

TABLE 7–15 Thyroglobulin

Normal value:	0–30 ng/ml (elevated cord blood – 29.3 ng/ml ± 4.7)
Uses:	1. In thyroid cancer: follow-up of patients who have had gland ablation 2. In subacute thyroiditis: indicator of disease activity 3. In distinguishing thyrotoxicosis factitia from silent thyroiditis 4. In Graves' disease: follow-up of treated patients 5. In identification of unknown metastatic thyroid carcinoma by thyroglobulin immunoperoxidase staining 6. Diagnosis of congenital athyrogenesis

TABLE 7-16   Thyroglobulin Concentrations in Different Disease States

Condition	Mean ± SEM (ng/ml)	No. of subjects
Controls	5.1 ± 0.49	95
Cord blood	29.3 ± 4.7	23
Pregnancy	10.1 ± 1.3	23
Active Graves' disease	176.0 ± 30.0	33
Euthyroid Graves' disease	6.8 ± 1.25	10
Non–Graves' thyrotoxicosis	145.0 ± 27.0	7
Subacute thyroiditis	136.8 ± 74.5	12
Differentiated thyroid cancer	103.4 ± 125.6	32
Metastatic thyroid cancer	464.9 ± 155.6	6
Medullary thyroid cancer	4.9 ± 1.6	6
Thyroid adenoma	424.6 ± 189.4	27
Endemic goiter	208.1 ± 19.8	77

Van Herle AJ. Serum thyroglobulin measurement in the diagnosis and management of thyroid disease. Thyroid Today 1981; 4(2):1; with permission.

have a normal serum TG level while still on suppressive doses of thyroid.

In patients with thyroid cancer who have had ablation, serial determinations of TG at 6-month intervals following the initial ablation and scan for metastatic disease is a reasonable approach to follow-up. If the serum TG is less than 1.0 ng per milliliter, then T_4 withdrawal for the purposes of scanning should be done at 3-year intervals to pick up the small percentage of patients with metastatic disease who do not demonstrate increased levels of TG. Thyroglobulin level should be monitored at 6-month intervals for the first 2 years and thereafter at yearly intervals. Patients who are found to have detectable TG levels at any time should have withdrawal of thyroid suppression and whole body imaging should be done. Some patients with elevated levels will prove to have metastases that do not concentrate radioiodine.

As many as 57 percent of hyperthyroid patients are found to have high levels of circulating thyroglobulin. The administration of TSH and TRH raises the level of thyroglobulin in the serum. However, thyroxine and T_3 have been shown to suppress the levels of thyroglobulin. In patients with Graves' disease who have been treated, thyroglobulin levels have been useful. In those patients receiving surgical or radioactive iodine treatment, the level of TG rises and then falls to normal in patients who are becoming euthyroid. In those who have been treated long term with antithyroidal drugs the levels fall toward normal. An elevated level at the end of the treatment period may be predictive of those who will relapse following the withdrawal of the drug. It is important to note that the presence of thyroid antibodies prevents the determination of TG in many cases. In such a situation, the determination of thyroid-stimulating immunoglobulins may be helpful in predicting which patients will have recurrent disease after discontinuation of their antithyroid drugs.

In subacute thyroiditis, TG levels are elevated and fall rapidly to normal when the inflammation is subsiding. Painless thyroiditis is characterized by persistently high levels of TG that have been shown to be high for periods of more than 8 months after the onset of initial symptoms. In cases in which the possibility of factitious T_4 ingestion has to be distinguished from silent thyroiditis, the TG levels may be particularly useful. They would be expected to remain in the low range in cases of exogenous thyroid ingestion.

Immunoperoxidase staining for TG has been useful in determining the source of metastatic adenocarcinoma of unknown etiology. Staining for TG can be performed on tissue obtained by needle biopsy and, when positive, would be diagnostic for metastatic thyroid carcinoma. This could change treatment plans, and thus it should be included in the work-up of such lesions.

The failure to detect measurable levels of TG in the newborn is usually indicative of athyrogenesis.

Radioactive Iodine Uptake

Currently, three isotopes are most commonly employed in determining the radioactive iodine uptake (Table 7-17). The most commonly used is ^{131}I. It has a relatively long shelf life and is inexpensive. Although ^{123}I has the potential advantage of a lower radiation dose to the thyroid, it is expensive, has a short shelf life, and must be used on the day of delivery to avoid a considerably higher radiation dose from long-lived radiocontaminants, which would negate any advantage. Production and distribution are a problem with commercially available ^{123}I. To administer an uptake dose (20 μCi) of ^{123}I, the less convenient liquid form must be used since the smallest available capsule is 200 μCi (adult scan dose). The radiation dose to the thyroid for an ^{123}I uptake and scan versus an ^{131}I uptake and ^{99m}Tc scan is similar for adults and most children, although ^{123}I would have an advantage for very young children.

The patient is usually given the dose of RAI in the morning while fasting. The dose can be given either in a capsular or in a liquid form. Currently, the former is often used in departments of nuclear medicine in the

TABLE 7–17   Radionuclides Used in Thyroid Uptake Tests

Isotope	Half-Life	Rad to Thyroid	Comments
^{131}I	8 days	6.6	5–10 µCi dose readily available
^{99m}Tc	6 h	0.06	Does not measure organification Done in one visit Given intravenously
^{123}I	13 h 20 µCi for uptake, 200 µCi for scan	0.6–1.1 6.0–11.0	Expensive, little irradiation Shipping problems Scheduling problems

form of capsules obtained from pharmaceutical firms. At times the dissolution and subsequent absorption of the RAI will be incomplete, thus falsely lowering the uptake. This factor should be kept in mind when assessing the test.

Once the RAI has been administered, one determines the uptake using a scintillation counter. The uptake is compared with a dose standard inserted in a neck phantom. For the usual uptake done after 24 hours, a correction is made for extrathyroidal uptake by counting over the thigh so that:

$$\text{Percent of thyroid uptake} = \frac{\text{Neck counts–Thigh counts}}{\text{Dose—Standard counts (background)}}$$

This count is usually done at 24 hours when the uptake has reached a plateau. In a small percentage of cases of hyperthyroidism the uptake peaks much earlier so that by 24 hours the value returns to normal. Many laboratories do a 2- to 6-hour uptake when the hyperthyroidism appears severe clinically. The 2- to 6-hour uptake is also useful in picking up organification defects. A major effect on the RAI uptake is iodine intake. In this country an increase in the content of iodide in bread has resulted in a significant decrease in the normal uptake. This change has made the RAI uptake much less useful in detecting cases of hypothyroidism. Because of such environmental changes it is important to determine the normal values for each individual laboratory. In areas of iodine deficiency there is a marked increase in the avidity of the gland's uptake of a standard dose. Those factors which will decrease the uptake of iodine in the gland are listed in Table 7–19. The usual normal 24-hour uptake in our laboratory is 8 to 32 percent. Elderly patients with hyperthyroidism may exhibit a normal uptake.

The radioactive isotope uptake does not accurately reflect a patient's thyroid status. The uptake simply de-

TABLE 7–18   Factors That Increase Radioactive Iodine Uptake

Hyperthyroidism
  a. Graves'
  b. Plummer's (multinodular goiter)
  c. Toxic adenoma
  d. Metastatic trophoblastic tumors
  e. Excessive TSH
     TSH-producing adenoma
     Selective pituitary resistance to thyroid
  f. "Hashitoxicosis"
Thyroid avidity for iodine
  a. Iodine deficiency
  b. Excessive loss of iodine (pregnancy or dehalogenase defect)
Inherited biosynthetic defects
Excessive hormone losses
  a. Nephrosis
  b. Chronic diarrhea
  c. Soybean ingestion
Rebound following antithyroid drugs
Rebound following thyroid medication
Recovery from subacute or silent thyroiditis
Hashimoto's thyroiditis—early phase

TABLE 7–19   Factors That Decrease Radioactive Iodine Uptake

Primary and secondary hypothyroidism
Hyperthyroidism
  Factitious hyperthyroidism
  Subacute thyroiditis
  Silent thyroiditis
  Jodbasedow (excess iodides)
  Ectopic thyroid tissue
    Lingual thyroid
    Substernal thyroid
    Struma ovarii
Excess iodine
  Drugs
  Foods
  Radiographic media (CT scans with contrast)
Hormones
  Thyroid
  Glucocorticoids
Inhibitors of organification
  Propylthiouracil
  Methimazole (Tapazole)
  Aminosalicylic acid
  PABA
  Sulfonylureas
  Phenylbutazone (Butazolidin)
Iodide transport inhibitors
  Perchlorate
  Thiocyanate
Impaired renal iodide clearance
  Renal failure
  Severe cardiac failure
Hashimoto's thyroiditis
Subacute thyroiditis

PABA = para-aminobenzoic acid

TABLE 7–20   T₃ Suppression Test

Method:	RAI uptake is measured, and T₃ 75 μg per day is given orally for 1 week. The uptake is measured again on the completion of the week.
Normal:	50% or greater fall in uptake. Failure to suppress indicates thyroid autonomy.
Uses:	In the detection of hyperthyroidism in cases in which the laboratory work is not diagnostic
Problems:	Elderly patients or patients with underlying ischemic heart disease may not tolerate the T₃. Abnormal tests are often found in patients who are euthyroid after treatment for hyperthyroidism.

THIS TEST HAS BEEN SUPPLANTED BY THE TRH TEST AND HAS LITTLE CLINICAL USE TODAY

TABLE 7–22   TSH Stimulation Test

Method:	Give bovine TSH, 10 units per day IM for 3 days. Uptake and scan are repeated at completion of the series of injections.
Normal:	Increase in uptake by 10%. No change is exhibited on the scan.
Uses:	1. Of use in determination of whether there is thyroid tissue that is being suppressed by an autonomous nodule. 2. This test is used on rare occasions to increase uptake in patients with known thyroid cancer in whom one is interested in looking for metastatic disease or for developing a treatment regimen.
Problems:	Allergic responses to bovine TSH.

termines the turnover of iodine in the gland. This particular function can be low in the face of hyperthyroidism or high in the face of hypothyroidism (Tables 7–18 and 7–19). It is most useful in the differential diagnosis of hyperthyroidism. With the exception of classical cases of Graves' disease, in which ophthalmopathy and/or clubbing and pretibial myxedema are present, the physician should do a RAI uptake before definitive therapy is carried out. A low uptake may pick up a case of "silent thyroiditis," thyrotoxicosis factitia, struma ovarii, or subacute thyroiditis. The finding of a low uptake may lead to a different course of management as well as a prognosis.

In the case of low values for the T₄ and T₃, the RAI uptake may show a normal uptake in those patients who have a severe systemic illness, which strongly suggests that hypothyroidism is an unlikely diagnosis.

Three tests are occasionally performed in conjunction with the radioactive iodine uptake test. These are the T₃ suppression test (Table 7–20), the perchlorate discharge test (Table 7–21), and the TSH stimulation test (Table 7–22).

OTHER TESTS

The basal metabolism test is mentioned here for the sake of completeness. The details of its proper performance are covered in other reviews, and the reader is referred to these sources for details. The test is no longer of clinical value in the management or diagnosis of thyroid disease.

The Achilles reflex test is another test that the authors believe has little value in the current evaluation and treatment of thyroid disorders. However, other sources cover this in detail.

The systolic time interval test, however, is of interest, not as a diagnostic test, but sometimes for following patients with hyperthyroidism or hypothyroidism.

Acknowledgment.   The authors are grateful to Dr. Bruce Weintraub and Dr. Paul Ladenson for their critical review and helpful suggestions.

BIBLIOGRAPHY

Thyroid Physiology

Abuid J, Larsen PR. Triiodothyronine and thyroxine in thyrotoxicosis: acute response to therapy with antithyroid agents. J Clin Invest 1974; 54:201.

Cornell JS, Pierce JG. The subunits of human pituitary thyroid-stimulating hormone. J Biol Chem 1973; 248:4327.

Escobar Del Rey F, Garcia MD, Bernal J, et al. Concomitant decrease of the effects of thyroxine on TRH-induced TSH release, and of the pituitary content of triiodothyronine in animals on propylthiouracil. Endocrinology 1974; 95:916.

Fisher DA. Thyroid physiology in the perinatal period and during childhood. Chapter 62. In: Ingbar SH, Braverman LE, eds. Werner's: the thyroid: a fundamental and clinical text. Philadelphia: JB Lippincott, 1986:1393.

Fisher DA, Klein AH. Thyroid development and disorders of thyroid function in the newborn. N Engl J Med 1981; 304:702.

Fisher DA, Sack J, Odie TH, et al. Serum T4, TBG, T3 uptake, T3, reverse T3, and TSH concentrations in children 1–15 years of age. J Clin Endocrinol Metab 1977; 45:191.

Geffner DD, Azukizawa M, Hershman JM. Propylthiouracil blocks extrathyroidal conversion of thyroxine to triiodothyronine and augments thyrotropin secretion in man. J Clin Invest 1975; 55:224.

Kourides IA, Landon MB, Hoffman BJ, et al. Excess free alpha relative to beta subunits of the glycoprotein hormones in normal and abnormal human pituitary glands. Clin Endocrinol 1980; 12:407.

Larsen PR. Thyroid pituitary interaction. N Engl J Med 1982; 306:23.

Larsen PR, Dick TE, Markovitz MM, et al. Inhibition of intrapituitary thyroxine to 3,5,3′-triiodothyronine conversion prevents the acute suppression of thyrotropin release by thyroxine in hypothyroid rats. J Clin Invest 1979; 64:117.

TABLE 7–21   Perchlorate Discharge Test

Method:	RAI uptake is measured at 2 h, 1 g of potassium perchlorate is given, and the uptake is measured 30 and 60 min later.
Normal:	A normal response shows no change in uptake, whereas a patient with an organification defect shows a 10% decrease or more in uptake.
Uses:	Demonstrates inability of the gland to organify in: 1. Congenital goiter 2. Hashimoto's disease 3. Post-RAI and postsurgical hyperthyroidism
Problems:	If the 2 h uptake is low, the test loses its reliability.

Larsen PR, Silva JE. Intrapituitary mechanisms in the control of TSH secretion. In: Oppenheimer JH, Samuels HH, eds. Molecular basis of thyroid hormone action. New York: Academic Press, 1983:352.

Larsen PR, Silva JE, Kaplan MM. Relationships between circulating and intracellular thyroid hormones: physiological and clinical implications. Endocr Rev 1981; 2:87.

Manjunath P, Sairam MR. Biochemical, biological, and immunological properties of chemically deglycosylated human choriogonadotropin. J Biol Chem 1982; 257:7109.

Martin JB, Reichlin S. Clinical neuroendocrinology. 2nd ed. Philadelphia: FA Davis, 1985.

Oppenheimer JH, Schwartz HL, Surks MI. Propylthiouracil inhibits the conversion of L thyroxine to L-triiodothyronine: an explanation of the antithyroxine effect of propylthiouracil and evidence supporting the concept that triiodothyronine is the active thyroid hormone. J Clin Invest 1972; 51:2493.

Pierce JG. Eli Lilly lecture: the subunits of pituitary thyrotropin—their relationship to other glycoprotein hormones. Endocrinology 1971; 89:1331.

Pierce JG, Parsons TF. Glycoprotein hormones: structure and function. Ann Rev Biochem 1981; 50:465.

Reichlin S. Control of thyrotropic hormone secretion. In: Martini L, Ganong WF, eds. Neuroendocrinology. Vol 1, New York: Academic Press, 1966:455.

Vale W, Brazeau P, Rivier C, et al. Somatostatin. Recent Prog Horm Res 1975; 31:365.

Thyroid Function Tests

Beckers C, Corvette C, Thalasso M. Evaluation of serum thyroxine by radioimmunoassay. J Nucl Med 1973; 14:317.

Berson SA, Yalow RS. General principles of radioimmunoassay. Clin Chim Acta 1968; 22:51.

Cavalieri RR. Peripheral metabolism of thyroid hormones. Thyroid Today 1980; 3:7.

Chopra IJ. A radioimmunoassay for measurement of thyroxine in unextracted serum. J Clin Endocrinol Metab 1972; 34:938.

Chopra IJ. A radioimmunoassay for measurement of a 3,3',5' -triiodothyronine (reverse T3). J Clin Invest 1974; 54:583.

Chopra IJ, Solomon DH, Beale GN. Radioimmunoassay for measurement of triiodothyronine in human serum. J Clin Invest 1971; 50:2033.

Chopra IJ, Solomon DH, Chopra U, et al. Reciprocal changes in serum reverse T3 (RT3) and T3 in systemic illnesses: evidence for independent pathways of T4 metabolism in adults. J Clin Endocrinol Metab 1975; 41:1043.

Clark F, Horn DB. Assessment of thyroid function by combined use of serum protein bound iodine and resin uptake of I-131 triiodothyronine. J Clin Endocrinol Metab 1965; 25:39.

Cobb WE, Lamberton RP, Jackson IMD. Use of a rapid sensitive immunoradiometric assay for thyrotropin to distinguish normal from hyperthyroid subjects. Clin Chem 1984; 1930:1558.

Green BJ, Volper NJ, Cross EG, et al. A comparison of the fluorescent polarization method for free thyroxine index vs other conventional methods. Abstract presented at the International Symposium on Thyroid Function Tests. Il Debendre, France, May 9–10, 1985.

Hamburger JI. Factitious elevations of thyrotropin in euthyroid patients (letter to the editor). N Engl J Med 1985; 314:521.

Hay ID, Klee GG, et al. Thyroid dysfunction. Endocr Metab Clin North Am 1988; 17:473.

Homata S, Nakagawa T, Mori T, et al. Reevaluation of thyroxine binding and free thyroxine in human serum by paper electrophoresis and equilibrium dialysis in a new free thyroxine index. J Clin Endocrinol Metab 1970; 31:166.

Howarth PJN, Maclagan NF. Clinical application of serum-total-thyroxine estimation, resin uptake and free thyroxine index. Lancet 1969; 1:224.

Ingbar SH. The thyroid gland. In: Wilson and Foster, eds. Williams' textbook of endocrinology. Philadelphia: WB Saunders, 1985:718.

Ingbar SH, Braverman LE, Dauber NA, et al. A new method for measuring the free thyroid hormone in human serum and analysis of the factors that influence its concentration. J Clin Invest 1965; 44:1679.

Jackson IMD, Cobb WE. Disorders of the thyroid. In: Kohler PO, ed. Clinical endocrinology. New York: John Wiley & Sons, 1986:82.

Kaptein EM, MacIntyre SS, Weiner JM, et al. Free thyroxine estimates in nonthyroidal illness comparison of eight methods. J Clin Endocrinol Metab 1981; 52:1073.

Ladenson PW. Diseases of the thyroid gland. Endocr Metab Clin North Am 1985; 14:145.

Larsen PR, Dockalover J, Sipula D, et al. Immunoassay of thyroxine in unextracted human serum. J Clin Endocrinol Metab 1973; 37:177.

Lieblich J, Utiger RD. Triiodothyronine radioimmunoassay. J Clin Invest 1972; 51:157.

McBride JH, Thibeault RV, Rodgerson DO. Thyrotropin as measured by (a) sensitive immunoradiometric assay. Clin Chem 1985; 31:1865.

Oppenheimer JH, Squef R, Surks MI, et al. Binding of thyroxine by serum proteins evaluated by equilibrium dialysis and electrophoretic techniques alterations in nonthyroidal illness. J Clin Invest 1963; 42:1769.

Pekary AE, Hirshman JM, Parlo AF. A sensitive and precise radioimmunoassay for human thyroid stimulating hormone. J Clin Endocrinol Metab 1975; 41:676.

Robin NI, Hagen SR, Collaco F, Refetoff S, Swelenkow HA. Serum tests for measurement of thyroid function. Hormones 1971; 2:266.

Smith EM, Phan M, Kreger TE, et al. Human lymphocyte production of immunoreactive thyrotropin. Proc Natl Acad Sci USA 1983; 80:6010.

Spring T, Hofler J, Meyer J, et al. The development of fluorescence polarization assays for serum thyroxine and unsaturated thyroxine binding proteins. Abstract presented at the European Thyroid Association Meeting, July, 1983, Madrid, Spain.

Sterling K, Brenner MA. Free thyroxine in human serum simplified measurement with the aid of magnesium precipitation. J Clin Invest 1966; 45:153.

Weeks I, Sturgess M, Siddle K, et al. A high sensitivity immunochemiluminometric assay for human thyrotropin. Clin Endocrinol 1984; 20:489.

Free Thyroxine

Czako G, Zweig MH, Benson C, et al. On the albumin dependence of measurements of free thyroxin. I. Technical performance of serum methods. Clin Chem 1986; 32:108.

Czako G, Zweig MH, Benson C, et al. On the albumin dependence of measurements of free thyroxine. II. Patients with nonthyroidal illness. Clin Chem 1987; 33:87.

Ekins R. Validity of analog free thyroxine immunoassays. Clin Chem 1987; 33:2137.

Ekins R, Filetti S, Kurtz AB, et al. A simple general method for the assay of free hormones (and drugs): Its application to the measurement of serum free thyroxine levels and the bearing of assay results on the free 'thyroxine' concept. J Endocrinol 1980; 85:29.

Ekins RP, Jackson T, Sinha A, et al. Principles of free hormone measurement. J Endocrinol Invest 1986; 9(Suppl 4):3.

Gruhn JG, Barsano CP, Kumar Y. The development of tests of thyroid function. Arch Pathol Lab Med 1987; 111:84.

Ingbar SH. The thyroid gland. In: Williams RH, Wilson JD, Foster DW (eds). Williams textbook of endocrinology. 7th ed. Philadelphia WB Saunders, 1985:682.

Kaptein EM, MacIntyre SS, Weiner JM, et al. Free thyroxine estimate in non-thyroidal illness: Comparison of eight methods. J Clin Endocrinol Metab 1981; 52:1073.

Lalloz MRA, Byfield PGH, Goel KM, et al. Hyperthyroxinaemia due to the coexistence of two raised affinity thyroxine-binding protein (albumin and prealbumin) in one family. J Clin Endocrinol Metab 1987; 64:346.

Moses AC, Lawlor J, Haddow J, et al. Familial euthyroid hyperthyroxinemic resulting from increased thyroxine binding to thyroxine binding prealbumin. N Engl J Med 1982; 306:966.

Ruiz M, Rajatanavin R, Young RA, et al. Familial dysalbuminemic hyperthyroxinemia: A syndrome that can be confused with thyrotoxicosis. N Engl J Med 1982; 306:635.

Spencer CA. Clinical evaluation of free T4 techniques. J Endocrinol Invest 1986; 9 (Suppl 4):47.

Wartofsky L, Burman KD. Alterations in thyroid function in patien with systemic illness: The "euthyroid sick syndrome." Endocr Rev 1982; 3:164.

Witherspoon LR, Said El Shami A, Shuler SE, et al. Chemically blocked analog assays for free thyronines. II. Use of equilibrium dialysis to optimize the displacement by chemical blockers of T$_4$ analog and T$_3$ analog from albumin while avoiding displacement of T$_4$ and T$_3$ from thyroxine-binding globulin. Clin Chem 1988; 34:17.

TSH

Alexander NM. Free thyroxine in serum: Labeled thyroxin-analog methods fall short of their mark. Clin Chem 1986; 32:417.

Bassett F, Eastman CJ, Ma G, Maberly GF, Smith HC. Diagnostic value of thyrotropin concentrations in serum as measured by a sensitive immunoradiometric assay. Clin Chem 1986; 32:461.

Bounaud MP, Bounaud JY, Bouin-Pineau MH, et al. Chemilumines-cence immunoassay of thyrotropin with acridinium-ester-labeled antibody evaluated and compared with two other immunoassays. Clin Chem 1987; 33:2096.

Caldwell G, Kellett HA, Gow SM, et al. A new strategy for thyroid function testing. Lancet 1985; 1:1117.

Dubuis JM, Burger AG. Thyroid-stimulating hormone measurements by immunoradiometric assay in severely ill patients [Letter]. Lancet 1986; 2:1036.

Ehrmann DA, Sarne DH, Weinberg M. A suppressed serum thyrotropin measured by a sensitive assay may not be diagnostic of thyrotoxico-sis. Arch Intern Med 1989; 149(in press).

Gorman CA. Thyroid function testing: A new era. Mayo Clin Proc 1988; 63:1026.

Gow SM, Kellett HA, Seth J, Sweeting VM, Toft AD, Beckett GJ. Limi-tations of new thyroid function tests in pregnancy. Clin Chim Acta 1985; 152:325.

Haigler ED, Pittman JA, Hershman JM, et al. Direct evaluation on pituitary thyrotropin reserve utilizing synthetic thyrotropin releas-ing hormone. J Clin Endocrinol Metab 1971; 33:573.

Hamblin PS, Dyer SA, Mohr VS, et al. Relationship between thyrotropin and thyroxine changes during recovery from severe hypothyroxine-mia of critical illness. J Clin Endocrinol Metab 1986; 62:717.

Hay ID, Klee GG. Thyroid dysfunction. Endocrinol Metab Clin N Am 1988; 17:473.

Hennessey JV, Evaul JE, Tseng VC, Burman KD, Wartofsky L. L-thyroxine dosage: a reevaluation of therapy with contemporary preparations. Ann Intern Med 1986; 105:11.

Kahn BB, Weintraub BD, Csako G, Zweig MH. Factitious elevation of thyrotropin in a new ultrasensitive assay: Implications for the use of monoclonal antibodies in "sandwich" immunoassay. J Clin En-docrinol Metab 1988; 66:526.

Klee GG, Hay ID. Assessment of sensitive thyrotropin assays for an ex-panded role in thyroid function testing: Proposed criteria for ana-lytic performance and clinical utility. J Clin Endocrinol Metab 1987; 64:461.

Krenning EP, Doctor R, van Toor H, et al. Strategy of thyroid-function testing: A comparative study using TT$_4$, various FT$_4$ and IRMA-TSH kits. J Endocrinol Invest 1986; 9(Suppl 4):95.

Larsen PR, Alexander NM, Chopra IJ, et al. Revised nomenclature for tests of thyroid hormones and thyroid-related proteins in serum. J Clin Endocrinol Metab 1987; 64:1089.

Martino E, Bambini G, Bartalena L, et al. Human serum thyrotrophin measurement by ultrasensitive immunoradiometric assay as a first-line test in the evaluation of thyroid function. Clin Endocrinol (Oxf) 1986; 24:141.

McBride JH, Thibeault RV, Rodgerson DO. Thyrotropin as measured by a sensitive immunoradiometric assay. Clin Chem 1985; 31:1865.

Pekary AE, Turner LF, Hershman JM. New immunoenzymetric assay for human thyrotropin compared with two radioimmunoassays. Clin Chem 1986; 32:511.

Piketty ML, Talbot JN, Askienazy S, Milhaud G. Clinical significance of a low concentration of thyrotropin: five immunometric "kit" assays compared. Clin Chem 1987; 33:1237.

Ridgway EC. Thyrotropin radioimmunoassays: birth, life, and demise. Mayo Clin Proc 1988; 63:1028.

Ross DS. New sensitive immunoradiometric assays for thyrotropin. Ann Intern Med 1986; 104:718.

Schlumberger M, DeVathaire F, Wu-Ahouju G, et al. Post-operative surveillance of differentiated thyroid carcinoma: Contribution of the ultra-sensitive TSH assay. Presse Med 1987; 16:1791.

Semple CG, Slater SD, Reid AM, Glen AC. A sensitive immunoradio-metric assay for serum thyroid stimulating hormone [Letter]. Br Med J [Clin Res] 1985; 290:69.

Seth J, Kellett HA, Caldwell G, et al. A sensitive immunoradiometric assay for serum thyroid stimulating hormone: a replacement for the thyrotrophin releasing hormone test? Br Med J 1984; 289:1334.

Spencer CA, Eigen A, Shen D, et al. Specificity of sensitivity assays of thyrotropin (TSH) used to screen for thyroid disease in hospital-ized patients. Clin Chem 1987; 33:1341.

Spencer CA, Lai-Rosenfeld AO, Guttler RB, et al. Thyrotropin secre-tion in thyrotoxic and thyroxine-treated patients: assessment by a sensitive immunoenzymometric assay. J Clin Endocrinol Metab 1986; 63:349.

Spencer CA, Nicoloff JT. Heterogeneity of circulating TSH in nonthyroi-dal illness (NTI) revealed by comparison of sensitive TSH (S-TSH) assays (abstract). Endocrinology 1988; 122(Suppl):278.

Toft AD. Use of sensitive immunoradiometric assay for thyrotropin in clinical practice. Mayo Clin Proc 1988; 63:1035.

Utiger RD. Thyrotropin-releasing hormone and thyrotropin secretion. J Lab Clin Med 1987; 109:327.

Weeks I, Sturgess M, Siddle K, et al. A high sensitivity im-munochemiluminometric assay for human thyrotropin. Clin En-docrinol 1984; 20:489.

Wehmann RE, Gregerman RI, Burns WH, Saral R, Santos GW. Sup-pression of thyrotropin in the low-thyroxine state of severe nonthyroi-dal illness. N Engl J Med 1985; 312:546.

Wenzel KW. Thyroxine analogue assay kits in clinical medicine. Lan-cet 1985; 2:781.

Assessment of Thyroid Status Using Thyroid Function Testing

Bantle JP, Seeling S, Mariash CN, et al. Resistance to thyroid hormone: a disorder frequently confused with Graves' disease. Arch Intern Med 1982; 142:1867.

Birkhauser M, Busset R, Burer TH, et al. Diagnosis of hyperthyroidism when serum thyroxine alone is raised. Lancet 1977; 2:53.

Britton KE, Ellis SM, Miralles JM, et al. Is T4 toxicosis a normal biochemical finding in elderly women? Lancet 1975; 2:141.

Brooks MH, Barbato AT, Collins S, et al. Familial thyroid hormone resistance. Ann J Med 1981; 71:414.

Brugi H, Wimpfheimer C, Burger A, et al. Changes of circulating thyrox-ine triiodothyronine and reverse triiodothyronine after radiographic contrast agents. J Clin Endocrinol Metab 1976; 43:1203.

Chopra IJ, Solomon DH. Latent Graves' disease. In: Ingbar SH, Braver-man LE, eds. Werner's: the thyroid: a fundamental and clinical text. Philadelphia: JB Lippincott, 1986.

Chopra IJ, Williams DE, Orgiazi J, et al. Opposite effects of dexametha-sone on serum concentrations of 3,3',5'-triiodothyronine (reverse T3) and 3, 3',5'-triiodothyronine (T3). J Clin Endocrinol Metab 1975; 41:911.

Cooper DS, Ladenson PW, Nasula BC, et al. Familial thyroid hormone resistance. Metabolism 1982; 31:504.

Gavin LA, Rosenthal M, Cavalieri RR. The diagnosis dilemma of iso-lated hyperthyroxinemia in acute illness. JAMA 1979; 242:251.

Gomez-Pan A, Alvarez-Ude F, Yeo PPB, et al. Function of the hypothalamo-hypophyseal-thyroid axis in chronic renal failure. Clin Endocrinol 1979; 11:567.

Hamburger JI. Factitious elevations of thyrotropin in euthyroid patients (letter to the editor). N Engl J Med 1986; 314:521.

Hodgson SF, Wahner HW. Hereditary increased thyroxine binding globulin capacity. Proc Mayo Clin 1972; 47:720.

Hollander CS, Mitsuma T, Kastin AJ, et al. Hypertriiodothyroniaemia as a premonitory manifestation of thyrotoxicosis. Lancet 1971; 2:731.

Hollander CS, Mitsuma T, Shankman L, et al. T3 toxicosis in an io-dine deficient area. Lancet 1972; 2:1276.

Jackson IMD. Thyrotropin-releasing hormone. N Engl J Med 1982; 306:145.

Jones JE, Seal US. X chromosome linked inheritance of elevated thyroxine-binding globulin. J Clin Endocrinol Metab 1967; 27:1521.

Kaplan MM. Interactions between drugs and thyroid hormones. Thyroid Today 1981; 4:1.

Kourides IA. Pituitary thyrotropin secretion in thyroid disorders. Thyroid Today 1980; 3:2.

Larsen PR. Thyroid hormone concentrations. In: Ingbar SH, Braverman LE, eds. Werner's: the thyroid: a fundamental and clinical text. Philadelphia: JB Lippincott, 1986:486.

Lee WNP, Golden MP, Van Herle AJ, et al. Inherited abnormal thyroid hormone-binding protein causing selective increase in total serum thyroxine. J Clin Endocrinol Metab 1979; 49:292.

Maxon HR, Burman KD, Premachandra BN, et al. Familial elevation of total and free thyroxine in healthy euthyroid subjects without detectable binding protein abnormalities. Acta Endocrinol 1982; 100:224.

Naeije R, Goldstein J, Clumeck N, et al. A low T3 syndrome in diabetic ketoacidosis. Clin Endocrinol 1978; 8:467.

Refetoff S, Dewind LT, Degroot LJ. Familial syndrome combining deaf-mutism, stippled epiphyses, goiter, and abnormally high PBI: possible target organ refractoriness to thyroid hormone. J Clin Endocrinol Metab 1967; 27:279.

Ruiz M, Rajatanabin R, Young RA, et al. Familial dysalbuminemic hyperthyroxinemia. N Engl J Med 1982; 206:635.

Stockigt JR. Euthyroid hyperthyroxinemia. Thyroid Today 1984; 7:3.

Stockigt JR, Topliss DJ, Barlow JW, et al. Familial euthyroid thyroxine excess: an appropriate response to abnormal thyroxine binding associated with albumin. J Clin Endocrinol Metab 1981; 53:353–359.

Vagenakis AJ, Fang SL, Ransil B, et al. Effect of starvation on the production and peripheral metabolism of 3,3',5' -triiodothyronine in euthyroid obese subjects. J Clin Endocrinol Metab 1978; 47:889.

Weintraub BD, Gershengorn MC, Kourides IA, et al. Inappropriate secretion of thyroid stimulating hormone. Ann Intern Med 1981; 95:349.

Euthyroid Hyperthyroxinemia

Burr WA, Evans SE, Lee J, et al. The ratio of thyroxine thyroxine-binding globulin in the assessment of thyroid function. Clin Endocrinol 1979; 11:333.

Davis PJ, Gregerman RI. Separation of thyroxine-binding proteins in human serum at pH 7.4. II. Effect of pH and temperature on the binding capacities of thyroxine-binding globulin (TBG) and thyroxine-binding prealbumin (TBPA). J Clin Endocrinol Metab 1971; 33:699.

Geola FL, Hershman JM, Reed AW, et al. Circulating thyroid hormone autoantibodies in a hypothyroid patient: Effect on thyroxine metabolic clearance rate. J Clin Endocrinol Metab 1981; 53:580.

Gershengorn MC, Larsen PR, Robbins J. Radioimmunoassay for serum thyroxine-binding globulin: Results in normal subjects and in patients with hepatocellular carcinoma. J Clin Endocrinol Metab 1976; 42:907.

Hesch RD, Gatz J, McIntosh CHS, et al. Radioimmunoassay of thyroxine-binding globulin in human plasma. Clin Chim Acta 1976; 70:33.

Lalloz MRA, Byfield PGH, Himsworth RL. Hyperthyroxinaemia: Abnormal binding of T4 by an inherited albumin variant. Clin Endocrinol 1983; 18:11.

Lee WNP, Golden MP, Van Herle AJ, et al. Inherited abnormal thyroid hormone-binding protein causing selective increase of total serum thyroxine. J Clin Endocrinol Metab 1979; 49:292.

Litherland PGH, Bromage NR, Hall RA. Thyroxine binding globulin (TBG) and thyroxine binding prealbumin (TBPA) measurement, compared with the conventional T3 uptake in the diagnosis of thyroid disease. Clin Chim Acta 1982; 122:345.

Meek RL, Klee GG, Preissner CM, et al. Development of a solid-phase, monoclonal, enzyme immunoassay for TBG. Clin Chem 1985; 31:951.

Neild JE, Byfield PGH, Lalloz MRA, et al. Familial abnormalities of thyroxine binding proteins: Some problems of recognition and interpretation. J Clin Pathol 1985; 38:327.

Premachandra BN, Blumenthal HT. Abnormal binding of thyroid hormone in sera from patients with Hashimoto's disease. J Clin Endocrinol 1967; 27:931.

Rajatanavin R, Braverman LE. Euthyroid hyperthyroxinemia. J Endocrinol Invest 1983; 6:493.

Refetoff S. Resistance to thyroid hormone. Thyroid Today 1980; 3:6.

Roberts RC, Nikolai TF. Determination of thyroxin-binding globulin. A simplified procedure utilizing dextran-coated charcoal. Clin Chem 1969; 15:1132.

Safran M, Braverman LE. Euthyroid hyperthyroxinemia in hormone resistance and other endocrine paradoxes. In: Cohen MP, Foa PP, eds. New York: Springer Verlag 1987:62.

Silverberg JDH, Premanchandra BN. Familial hyperthyroxinemia due to abnormal thyroid hormone binding. Ann Intern Med 1982; 96:183.

Stockigt JR, Topliss DJ, Barlow JW, et al. Familial euthyroid thyroxine excess: An appropriate response to abnormal thyroxine binding associated with albumin. J Clin Endocrinol Metab 1981; 53:353.

Evaluation of Patients with Decreased T_4 and/or T_3

Hypothyroidism

Barbosa J, Seal US, Doe RP. Effects of anabolic steroids on hormone-binding proteins, serum cortisol, and serum nonprotein bound cortisol. J Clin Endocrinol Metab 1970; 32:232.

Beck-Peccoz P, Iran MR, Meneguz-Ferrerira MM, et al. Decreased receptor binding of biological inactive thyrotropin in central hypothyroidism. Effective treatment with TRH. N Engl J Med 1985; 312:1085.

Cavalieri RR, Gavin LA, Wallace A, et al. Serum thyroxine, free T4, triiodothyronine, and reverse T3 in diphenylhydantoin treated patients. Metabolism 1979; 28:1161.

Chen JJS, Ladenson PW. Discordant hypothyroxinemia and hypertriiodothyroninemia in treated patients with hyperthyroid Graves' disease. J Clin Endocrinol Metab 1986; 63:102.

Chopra IJ, Chuateco GN, Nguyen AH, et al. In search of an inhibitor of thyroid hormone binding to serum proteins in nonthyroid illnesses. J Clin Endocrinol Metab 1969; 49:63.

Faglia G, Beck-Peccoz P, Ambrosi B, et al. Prolonged and exaggerated elevations in plasma thyrotropin (hTSH) after thyrotropin-releasing factor (TRF) in patients with pituitary tumor. J Clin Endocrinol Metab 1971; 33:99.

Faglia G, Beck-Peccoz P, Ferari C, et al. Plasma thyrotropin response to thyrotropin-releasing hormone in patients with pituitary and hypothalamic disorders. J Clin Endocrinol Metab 1973; 37:595.

Hanson J. Increased fecal thyroxine losses: with protein losing enteropathy. NY State J Med 1974; 74:1993.

Heyma P, Larksin RG, Perry-Keene D, et al. Thyroid hormone levels and protein binding in patients on long term diphenylhydantoin treatment. Clin Endocrinol 1977; 6:369.

Ingbar SH, Freinkel N. Regulation of the peripheral metabolism of the thyroid hormones. Recent Prog Horm Res 1960; 16:353.

Krieger DT. Glandular and organ deficiency associated with secretion of biologically inactive pituitary peptides. J Clin Endocrinol Metab 1974; 38:964.

Nusynowitz ML, Clark RF, Strater WJ, et al. Thyroxine-binding globulin deficiency in 3 families and total deficiency in a normal woman. Am J Med 1971; 50:458.

Oppenheimer JH, Fisher LV, Nelson KM, et al. Depression of the serum protein bound iodine level by diphenylhydantoin. J Clin Endocrinol Metab 1961; 21:252.

Oppenheimer JH, Werner SC. Effect of prednisone on thyroxine-binding proteins. J Clin Endocrinol Metab 1966; 26:715.

Ratcliff WA, Hazelton RA, Thomson JA. Effect of fenclofenac on thyroid-function tests. Lancet 1980; 1:432.

Refetoff S, Selenkow HA. Familial thyroxine binding globulin deficiency in a patient with Turner's syndrome (XO): genetic study of a kindred. N Engl J Med 1968; 278:1081.

Ridgway CG, Walker H, Rodbard D, et al. Peripheral response to thyroid hormone before and after L-thyroxine therapy in patients with some subclinical hypothyroidism. J Clin Endocrinol Metab 1981; 53:1238.

Schussler GC. Thyroid function tests in patients with nonthyroidal disease. Thyroid Today 1980; 3:3.

Snyder PJ, Jacobs LS, Rubello MM, et al. Diagnostic value of thyrotropin-releasing hormone in pituitary and hypothalamic diseases: assessment of thyrotropin and prolactin secretion in 100 patients. Ann Intern Med 1974; 81:751.

Spencer CA, Lai-Rosenfeld AO, Guttler RB, et al. Thyrotropin secretion in thyrotoxic and thyroxine-treated patients: assessment by a sensitive immunoenzymometric assay. J Clin Endocrinol Metab 1986; 63:349.

Wartofsky L, Burman KD. Alterations in thyroid function in patients with systemic illness: the "euthyroid sick syndrome." Endocr Rev 1982; 3:164.

Euthyroid Hypothyroxinemia

Bellabarba D, Inada M, Varsano-Aharon N, Sterling K. Thyroxine transport and turnover in major nonthyroidal illness. J Clin Endocrinol Metab 1968; 28:1023.

Burr WA, Ramsden DB, Hoffenberg R. Hereditary abnormalities of thyroxine-binding globulin concentration. QJ Med 1980; 49:295.

Chopra IJ, Solomon DH, Teco GNC, Eisenberg JB. An inhibitor of binding of thyroid hormones to serum proteins is present in extrathyroidal tissues. Science 1982; 215:407.

Hansen J. Increased fecal thyroxine losses: with protein-losing enteropathy. NY State J Med 1974; 74:1993.

Isaacs AJ, Monk BE. Fenclofenac interferes with thyroid-function tests. Lancet 1980; i:267.

Larsen PR. Salicylate-induced increases in the triiodothyronine in human serum: evidence of inhibition of triiodothyronine binding to thyroxine-binding globulin and thyroxine-binding prealbumin. J Clin Invest 1972; 51:1125.

Murata Y, Refetoff S, Sarne DH, Dick M, Watson F. Variant thyroxine-binding globulin in serum of Australian Aborigines: its physical, chemical and biological properties. J Endocrinol Invest 1985; 8:225.

Murata Y, Takamatsu J, Refetoff S. Inherited abnormality of thyroxine-binding globulin with no demonstrable thyroxine-binding activity and high serum levels of denatured thyroxine-binding globulin. N Engl J Med 1986; 314:694.

Oppenheimer JH, Tavernetti RR. Displacement of thyroxine from human thyroxine-binding globulin by analogues of hydantoin. Steric aspects of the thyroxine-binding site. J Clin Invest 1962; 41:2213.

Refetoff S, Murata Y. X-Chromosome-linked inheritance of the variant thyroxine-binding globulin in Australian Aborigines. J Clin Endocrinol Metab 1985; 60:356.

Refetoff S, Murata Y, Vassart G, Chandramouli V, Marshall JS. Radioimmunoassays specific for the tertiary and primary structures of thyroxine-binding globulin (TBG): Measurement of denatured TBG in serum. J Clin Endocrinol Metab 1984; 59:269.

Robbins J, Rall JE, Petermann ML. Thyroxine-binding in serum and urine proteins in nephrosis. Qualitative aspects. J Clin Invest 1957; 36:1333.

Robin NI, Hagen SR, Collaco F, Refetoff S, Selenkow HA. Serum tests for measurement of thyroid function. Hormones 1971; 2:266.

Sarne DH, Refetoff S, Nelson JC, Linarelli LG. A new inherited abnormality of thyroxine-binding globulin (TBG-San Diego) with decreased affinity for thyroxine and triiodothyronine. J Clin Endocrinol Metab 1989; 68:114.

Takamatsu J, Ando M, Weinberg M, Refetoff S. Isoelectric focusing of variant thyroxine-binding globulin in American blacks: increased heat lability and reduced serum concentration. J Clin Endocrinol Metab 1986; 63:80.

Takamatsu J, Refetoff S. Inherited heat-stable variant thyroxine-binding globulin (TBG-Chicago). J Clin Endocrinol Metab 1986;63:1140.

Takamatsu J, Refetoff S, Charbonneau M, Dussault JH. Two new inherited defects of the thyroxine-binding globulin (TBG) molecule presenting as partial TBG deficiency. J Clin Invest 1987; 7:833.

Thyroid-Stimulating Antibodies

Adams DD, Purves HD. Abnormal responses in the assay of thyrotrophin. Univ Otago Med School Proc 1956; 34:11.

Ambesi-Impiombato FS, Parks LAM, Coon HF. Culture of hormone-dependent epithelial cells from rat thyroids. Proc Natl Acad Sci USA 1980; 77:3455.

Amino N. Thyroid directed antibodies. In: Ingbar SH, Braverman LE, eds. Werner's: the thyroid: a fundamental and clinical text. Philadelphia: JB Lippincott, 1986.

Amino N, Hagan SR, Yamada N, et al. Measurement of circulating thyroid microsomal antibodies by the tanned red cell haemagglutination technique: its usefulness in the diagnosis of autoimmune thyroid diseases. Clin Endocrinol 1976; 5:115.

Amino N, Kuro R, Tanizawa O, et al. Changes of serum antithyroid antibodies during and after pregnancy and autoimmune thyroid diseases. Clin Exp Immunol 1978; 31:30.

Beck K, Feldt-Rasmussen U, Bliddal H, et al. The acute changes in thyroid stimulating immunoglobulins, thyroglobulin, and thyroglobulin antibodies following subtotal thyroidectomy. Clin Endocrinol 1982; 16:235.

Beck K, Madsen SN. Influence of treatment with radioiodine and propylthiouracil on thyroid stimulating immunoglobulins in Graves' disease. Clin Endocrinol 1980; 13:417.

Davies TF, Evered DC, Rees Smith B, et al. Value of thyroid stimulating antibody determinations in predicting short term thyrotoxic relapse in Graves' disease. Lancet 1977; 1:1181.

Doniach D, Marshall NJ. Autoantibodies to the thyrotropin receptors on thyroid epithelium and other tissues. In: Talal N, ed. Autoimmunity. New York: Academic Press, 1977:621.

Doniach D. Humoral and genetic aspects of thyroid autoimmunity. Clin Endocrinol Metab 1975; 4:267.

Ito S, Tamura T, Nishikawa M. Effects of desiccated thyroid, prednisolone and chloroquine on goiter and antibody titer and chronic thyroiditis. Metabolism 1968; 17:317.

Matsuura N, Yamato Y, Nohara Y, et al. Familial neonatal transient hypothyroidism due to maternal TSH-binding inhibitor immunoglobulins. N Engl J Med 1980; 303:738.

McGregor AM, Peterson MM, McLachlan SM, et al. Carbimazole and the autoimmune response in Graves' disease. N Engl J Med 1980; 303:302.

McGregor AM, Rees-Smith B, Hall R, et al. prediction of relapse in hyperthyroid Graves' disease. Lancet 1980; 1:1101.

McKenzie JM. Neonatal Graves' disease. J Clin Endocrinol Metab 1964; 24:660.

McKenzie JM. Thyroid stimulating antibody (TSAb) in Graves' disease. Thyroid Today 1980; 3:5.

McMullan NM, Smyth PPA. In vitro generation of NADPH as an index of thyroid stimulating immunoglobulins (TGI) in goitrous disease. Clin Endocrinol 1984; 20:269.

Orgiazzi J, Williams DE, Chopra IJ, et al. Human thyroid adenyl-cyclase stimulating activity in immunoglobulin G of patients with Graves' disease. J Clin Endocrinol Metab 1976; 42:778.

Pinchera A, Liberti P, Martino E, et al. Effective antithyroid drug therapy on the long-acting thyroid stimulator and the anti-thyroglobulin antibodies. J Clin Endocrinol Metab 1969; 29:231.

Smith BR, McLachlin SM, Furmaniak J. Autoantibodies to the thyrotropin receptor. Endocr Rev 1988; 9:106.

Strakosch CR, Wenzel BE, Row VV, Volpe R. Immunology of autoimmune thyroid diseases. N E J Med (Seminars in Medicine of the Beth Israel Hospital, Boston) 1982; (24):1499.

Stutter H. A fresh look at an old thyroid disease: euthyroid and hyperthyroid nodular goiter. J Endocrinol Invest 1982; 5:57.

Weetman AP, McGregor AM. Autoimmune thyroid disease; development in our understanding. Endocr Rev 1984; 5:309.

Weiss M, Ingbar SH, Winblad S, Kaspar DL. Demonstration of a saturable binding site for thyrotrophin in Yersinia enterocolitica. Science 1983; 219:1331.

Zakarija M, McKenzie JM. Absorption of thyroid stimulating antibody of Graves' disease by homologous and heterologous thyroid tissue. J Clin Endocrinol Metab 1978; 47:906.

Zarkarija M, McKenzie JM. The spectrum and significance of autoantibodies reacting with the thyrotropin receptor. Endocrinol Metab Clin North Am 1987; 16:343.

Thyroid Antibodies

Delespesse G, Hubert C, Gausset P, et al. Radioimmunoassay for human antithyroglobulin antibodies of different immunoglobulin classes. Horm Metab Res 1976; 118:293.

McLachlan SM, Pegg CAS, Atherton MC, et al. In vitro studies of human thyroid autoantibody synthesis. Mt Sinai J Med 1986; 53:38.

Parkes AB, Machlan SM, Bird P, et al. The distribution of microsomal and thyroglobulin antibody activity among the IgG subclasses. Clin Exp Immunol 1984; 57:239.

Pinchera A, Fenzi GF, Barttalena I, et al. Thyroid antigens involved in autoimmune thyroid disorders. In: Klein E, Horster FA, eds. Autoimmunity in thyroid diseases. Stuttgart: Schattauer, 1979:49.

Volpe R. Autoimmunity in thyroid disease. In: Volpe R, ed. Autoimmunity in endocrine diseases. New York, Marcel Dekker, 1985:109.

Volpe R. Pathogenesis of autoimmune thyroid diseases. In: Ingbar SH, Braverman LE, eds. Werner's the thyroid. JB Lippincott, 1986.

Thyroglobulin

Ashcraft MW, Van Herle AJ. The comparative value of serum thyroglobulin measurements and iodine 131 total body scans in the follow-up study of patients with treated differentiated thyroid cancer. Am J Med 1981; 71:806.

Czernichow P, Schlumberger M, Pomarede R, et al. Plasma thyroglobulin measurements help determine type of thyroid defect in congenital hypothyroidism. J Clin Endocrinol Metab 1983; 56:242.

Gardner DF, Rothman J, Utiger RD. Serum thyroglobulin in normal subjects and patients with hyperthyroidism due to Graves' disease: effects of T3, iodide, 131 iodide, and anti-thyroid drugs. Clin Endocrinol 1979; 11:585.

Glinoer D, Puttemans N, Van Herle AJ, et al. Sequential study of impairment of thyroid function in the early stages of subacute thyroiditis. Acta Endocrinol 1974; 77:26.

Izumi M, Larson PR. Correlation of sequential changes in serum thyroglobulin, triiodothyronine, and thyroxine in patients with Graves' disease and subacute thyroiditis. Metabolism 1978; 27:449.

Meyers FJ, Goodnight JE. Identification of unsuspected thyroid carcinoma using immunoperoxidase for thyroglobulin. Am J Med 1986; 81:177.

Solomon DH, Chopra IJ, Chopra U, et al. Identification of subgroups of euthyroid Graves' opthalmopathy. N Engl J Med 1971; 296:181.

Uller RP, Van Herle AJ. Effective therapy on serum thyroglobulin levels in patients with Graves' disease. J Clin Endocrinol Metab 1978; 46:747.

Van Herle AJ. Serum thyroglobulin measurement in the diagnosis and management of thyroid disease. Thyroid Today 1981; 4(2):1.

Van Herle AJ, Vassart G, Dumont JE. Control of thyroglobulin synthesis and secretion. N Engl J Med 1979; 301:307.

Van Herle AJ, Uller RP, Matthews NL, et al. Radioimmunoassay for measurements of thyroglobulin in human serum. J Clin Invest 1973; 52:1320.

Radioactive Iodine Uptake

Cavalieri RR. Quantitative in vivo tests. In: Ingbar SH, Braverman LE, eds. Werner's: the thyroid: a fundamental and clinical text. Philadelphia: JB Lippincott, 1986.

Keyes JW Jr, Thrall JH, Carey JE. Technical considerations in in vivo thyroid studies. Semin Nucl Med 1978; 8:43.

Pittman JA Jr, Dailey GE, Beschir J. Changing normal values for thyroidal radioiodine uptake. N Engl J Med 1969; 280:1431.

8 Fine-Needle Aspiration of the Thyroid

Yolanda C. Oertel, M.D.

Fine-needle aspiration of the thyroid is a diagnostic tool being used increasingly; it should not be confused with needle biopsies of the thyroid, which require a Tru-cut or Vim-Silverman needle and yield tissue fragments for histologic diagnosis (Vickery, 1981).

Solitary thyroid nodules are one of the most common clinical problems encountered by endocrinologists. Palpation, radionuclide imaging, and sonography do not determine whether a thyroid nodule is benign or malignant. Although firm nodules raise the suspicion of carcinoma, some benign cystic lesions under tension may be quite firm. Likewise, nonfunctioning solid nodules are not necessarily malignant. Although not a panacea, fine-needle aspiration is the easiest, least expensive, fastest, and most accurate way to make a diagnosis. We believe it should be one of the first steps in diagnosing thyroid disease and in helping the endocrinologist decide which patients might benefit from suppression and which patients need surgical treatment.

Since 1984, thyroid aspirates have exceeded the number of breast aspirations performed yearly at The George Washington University Medical Center, making it the most common type of aspiration (1,036 thyroid aspirates in 1986).

FINE-NEEDLE ASPIRATION TECHNIQUE

Although the aspiration technique has been covered in previous publications (Oertel, 1982; 1987), for the sake of completeness it is summarized here, emphasizing the particular aspects related to the thyroid.

Equipment Required

Equipment is simple and relatively inexpensive (Fig. 8–1). It includes:

1. Disposable plastic syringe (10 ml) with Luer-Lok tip.
2. Syringe holder to fit the 10-ml syringe. The only holder of this size is the Cameco syringe pistol.
3. Disposable needles with clear plastic hubs: 22-gauge, 1 inch and 1.5 inches long. Also 23- and 25-gauge, 1 inch long.
4. Glass slides with one frosted end on which identification can be written with a pencil.
5. Hemacytometer coverglass, to make the smears.
6. Alcohol wipes or cotton swabs soaked in alcohol.
7. Gauze sponges (4 inches by 4 inches).

Twenty-milliliter syringes are rarely used because little suction is needed when thyroid lesions are aspirated. The thyroid is a vascular gland, and cells from benign and malignant lesions are dislodged easily. Only when it is already known that the mass is cystic and quite large (as in lesions that have been aspirated previously and the fluid has reaccumulated) is the procedure started with a 1-inch, 22-gauge needle attached to a 20-ml syringe and the Cameco handle.

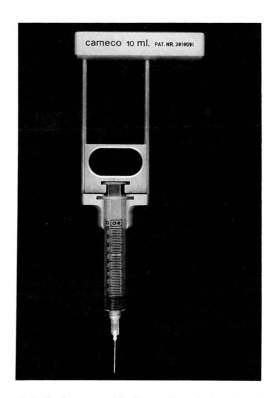

Figure 8–1 Equipment used for fine-needle aspiration of the thyroid.

Obtaining the Sample

We believe that obtaining the sample is the crucial part of the entire process. A correct diagnosis depends on an adequate and representative sample of the lesion. For more than 30 years, the Scandinavians have advocated having the pathologist do the aspirations (Zajicek, 1974). It has been our experience that better results are obtained when the pathologist who interprets the slides is the one who performs the aspiration (Oertel, 1987). However, some institutions have reported large series in which endocrinologists and surgeons perform the aspirations with great success (Hamburger et al, 1979; Hamberger et al, 1982).

After a brief clinical history is taken, the patient's neck is examined and the lesion located. Before taking the sample, it is important to discuss three matters with the patient.

1. The needle used is thinner than that used for venipuncture. Hence the procedure is less painful than having blood drawn.
2. There is no need for anesthesia. The prick of the needle for the anesthetic hurts as much as the aspiration.
3. The lesion usually must be aspirated at least twice to obtain both a representative and an adequate sample.

The procedure can be performed with the patient lying down or sitting up. It is easier to start the procedure with the patient lying down, unless he or she is obese or has emphysema and cannot tolerate a supine position.

The patient should be told to expect some coldness on the neck from the alcohol swab used to clean the skin (Fig. 8-2A). The skin can be dried with a piece of gauze or the alcohol can be allowed to evaporate (to avoid stinging when the needle is inserted). The patient should be warned that when the prick from the needle is felt, no talking, moving, or swallowing is allowed. Then the cytotechnologist gives the pathologist the aspiration device and holds the patient's hand. (Frequently, a patient will mention how helpful and reassuring it is to have somebody hold his or her hand.) The patient is asked to swallow. After swallowing, the needle is introduced through the skin (Fig. 8-2B) and into the gland (Fig. 8-2C). Once the lesion is reached, suction is applied very gently. At the same time, the clear needle hub should be watched. If fluid appears in the needle hub, more suction is applied until the syringe is filled up or until no more fluid is aspirated. If blood appears in the needle hub, suction must be stopped immediately (Fig. 8-2D), whether the plunger of the syringe is at the 1-cc mark or at the 3- or 4-cc mark. The needle is moved back and forth several times, suction released, and then the needle withdrawn. If no blood appears, suction is increased until the plunger reaches the 10-cc mark on the syringe. The plunger of the syringe is held in place while moving the needle in the lesion until aspirated material just begins to fill the needle hub. The angle of the needle should not be changed or directed into different parts of the lesion, as frequently advised in the literature. In our experience, this excessive movement of the needle creates a hematoma and renders subsequent samples of poor quality. Suction should be released before withdrawal of the needle (Fig. 8-2E). Once the smears have been prepared and the technologist has started drying and staining one slide, the patient should be helped to sit up (to improve the venous return and prevent a hematoma) and pressure applied at the site of aspiration. Pressure is applied until the technologist has finished staining one slide. The patient should continue applying pressure while the pathologist reviews the slide. This simple precaution of applying steady pressure at the puncture site prevents the formation of hematomas.

After checking the wet smear and deciding (in most instances) on the nature of the entity, the pathologist takes a second sample. As a general rule, a minimum of two aspirations per lesion should be done (even if the lesion is 4 or 5 mm in diameter). If the lesion is more than 1 cm, three samples should be taken: the first from the center of the lesion, the second from the upper portion, and the third from the lower portion of the lesion. A new needle and syringe for each aspiration should be used.

When a thyroid nodule bleeds easily on aspiration, a 22-gauge needle should be switched to a 23-gauge needle and less suction applied. If the lesion still bleeds, a 25-gauge needle should be used. In between aspirations it is essential to apply pressure to the site. Sometimes it is necessary to apply cold to the area. A supply of ice cubes should be kept in individual plastic bags to use when needed. This is also useful when the patient complains of slight pain or discomfort. The application of the ice cube to the area to be aspirated causes numbness as well.

It cannot be overemphasized that judicious sampling and good-quality samples are a must. Every possible effort should be made to improve one's technique.

Making the Smears

The cytotechnologist assists in the preparation of the smears. Because the aspirate tends to clot rapidly, prompt preparation of the smears is extremely important. The following procedure is used:

1. The needle is detached from the syringe.
2. The syringe is filled with air.
3. The needle is reattached to the syringe.
4. The bevel of the needle is placed against the glass slide and the contents of the needle squirted on the plain glass slide (one drop on each slide).
5. Using a hemacytometer coverglass, the cytotechnologist then smears the cellular material as if it were a blood smear.
6. Smears are allowed to air-dry.
7. The air-dried smears are then ready for staining and interpretation.

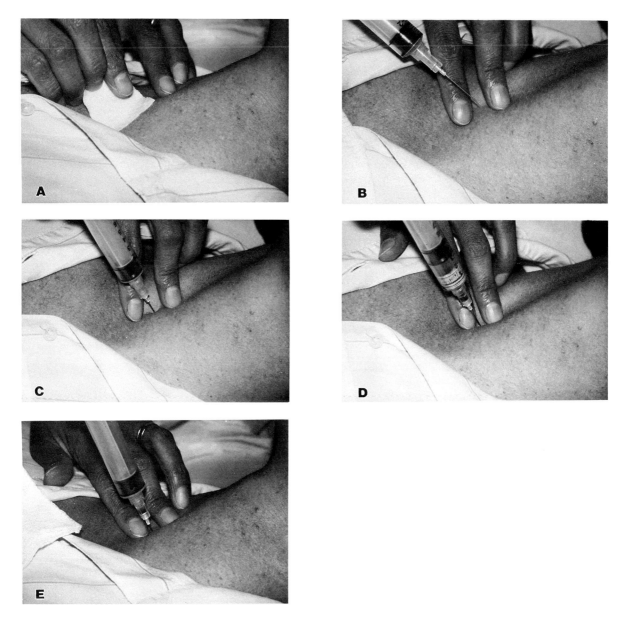

Figure 8-2 Performance of fine-needle aspirations. *A*, The skin is cleansed with an alcohol-soaked cotton swab. *B*, The needle is inserted through the skin. Notice that the syringe plunger is at the "0-cc" mark. *C*, The needle is introduced into the lesion. Again, notice that the syringe plunger is at the "0-cc" mark. *D*, Suction is applied very gently until aspirated material is visible in the clear plastic needle hub (in this particular case the plunger is at the "3-cc" mark). *E*, The suction is released before withdrawal of the needle.

Staining Techniques

We stain all aspirates with Diff-Quik (Dade Diagnostics). The staining procedure is simple and provides consistently good results. After 12 years and more than 18,000 fine-needle aspirates from all sites, we find hematologic stains most desirable.

Abele and Miller (1985), Frable (1986), and Lowhagen and colleagues (1981) provide additional information on fine-needle aspiration. Although our technique of performing aspirations and preparing and staining smears works very well for us, it may not be ideal for everyone. The best approach for both the physician and the patient must be decided individually.

ADVANTAGES OF FINE-NEEDLE ASPIRATION

Fine-needle aspiration is a simple, relatively inexpensive diagnostic procedure essentially free of complications that allows a prompt decision regarding management of a patient's thyroid nodule.

Papillary carcinoma of the thyroid, for example, can present initially as a cervical node metastasis. In our own practice, we have had several cases in which the thyroid was normal to palpation. On one occasion, even the thyroid scan showed no abnormalities. If a diagnosis of metastatic papillary carcinoma in a cervical lymph node is made by aspiration, time, expense, and potential complications are reduced.

Many patients are followed for several years with a thyroid nodule that "has remained unchanged." Subsequently, fine-needle aspiration reveals a carcinoma of the thyroid, and by the time of surgery the tumor has already metastasized.

Fine-needle aspiration can be used to avoid the indiscriminate suppression of thyroid nodules. For example, a clinician may suppress a nodule for several months, and when it does not respond to the medication, he or she sends the patient for fine-needle aspiration. At that point, a diagnosis of carcinoma is made. Suppression of a carcinoma is therefore questionable in these cases.

PROBLEMS AND POSSIBLE COMPLICATIONS

For those physicians who want to perform fine-needle aspirations of the thyroid, we advise first mastering aspirations of breast or other superficial lesions; once that is learned, one can proceed to aspirate thyroids.

In our opinion, thyroid aspirates are the most stressful procedures. The patients are extremely nervous, as a rule, because they have no experience with needles in their necks. Also, they fear a diagnosis of cancer, so reassurance must be given.

The thyroid is a vascular organ, and it is easy to create hematomas. Vials of ammonia are kept in the aspiration room in case a patient faints or feels faint.

CYTOLOGIC DIAGNOSTIC CRITERIA

An outline of diagnostic entities is presented in Table 8-1.

Normal Thyroid

Smears show small epithelial cells arranged in sheets or singly. Their nuclei are round to ovoid, uniform in size, and slightly larger than an erythrocyte. The nucleoli are inconspicuous. The cytoplasm is delicate and pale and has fine blue paravacuolar granules, which represent lipofuscin granules or phagolysosomes (Plate 1, A). The colloid stains blue with Diff-Quik and orange-green with Papanicolaou's stain. It has a variable appearance. Frequently, calcium oxalate crystals are observed.

Goiter

The term *goiter* denotes any diffuse or nodular enlargement of the thyroid gland regardless of etiology. It is a clinical, not a cytologic, diagnosis. We make this diagnosis only when we have seen the patient and aspirated the lesion(s). The cytopathology report is phrased as follows: adenomatoid nodules, consistent with multinodular goiter. If we would be interpreting the same smears, but submitted by another physician, the

TABLE 8-1   Diagnostic Entities

Normal thyroid
Goiter
Nonneoplastic lesions
  Cystic lesions
  Inflammatory processes
    Acute suppurative thyroiditis
    Subacute thyroiditis
    Lymphocytic thyroiditis
  Adenomatoid nodule(s)
  Graves' disease (toxic goiter)
Cellular adenomatoid nodule
Follicular neoplasia
  Follicular adenoma versus follicular carcinoma
  Follicular neoplasia of Hürthle cell type
Papillary carcinoma
Follicular carcinoma
Medullary carcinoma
Anaplastic carcinoma
Small cell carcinoma
Malignant lymphoma
Metastatic carcinoma

cytopathology report would read "adenomatoid nodule(s)."

Nonneoplastic Lesions

Cystic Lesions

We believe that there are no "true cysts" in the thyroid except for rare intraglandular thyroglossal duct cysts and the extremely rare cystic ultimobranchial remnants. The cystic lesions commonly observed are most frequently the result of cystic degeneration of adenomatoid nodules and follicular adenomas. However, papillary and/or follicular carcinomas also undergo cystic changes. Rather than referring to "papillary carcinoma in a cyst" or "papillary carcinoma associated with a cyst," one should diagnose papillary carcinoma with cystic degeneration. Vickery (1981) has reported, "It is doubtful if there is such an entity as a primary thyroid cyst, although it is common practice for both clinicians and pathologists to make this diagnosis."

Aspirates of cystic lesions yield a variable amount of fluid (from a few drops to 20 ml or more), ranging from pale yellow to tan, green, or brown and also varying in consistency from thin and watery to very viscid. If the lesion collapses, aspiration should not be repeated; this induces bleeding and refilling of the collapsed cavity. If there is a residual nodule, this should be reaspirated. Direct smears from the fluid and smears prepared from the spun-down sediment show colloid (Fig. 8-3), many foamy and hemosiderin-laden macrophages (Figs. 8-4 and 8-5), and sheets of follicular epithelial cells with scant cytoplasm and small nuclei. Cholesterol crystals are seen frequently.

The patient should be warned that the lesion might recur and that one cannot predict when that will take place.

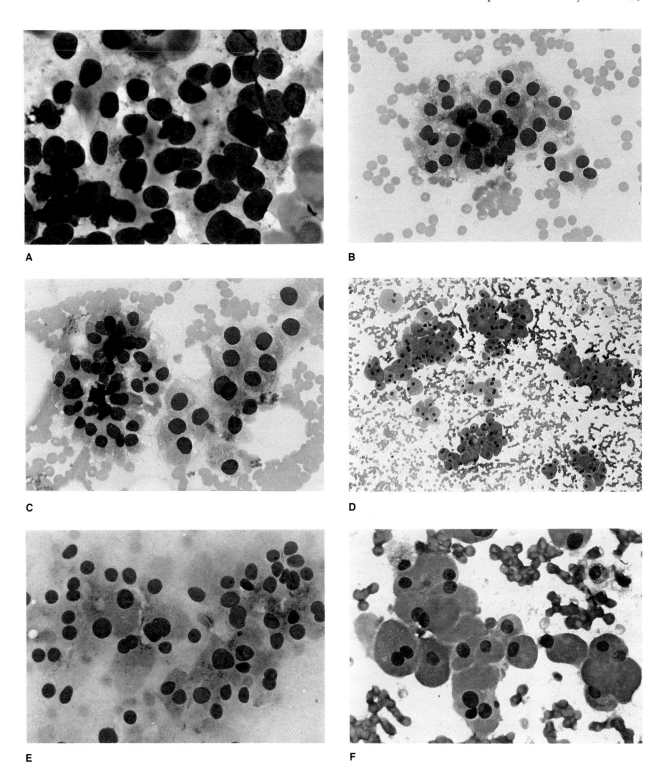

Plate 1   *A*, Follicular cells with blue paravacuolar granules in the cytoplasm. *B*, Follicular neoplasia. Note the inspissated colloid in the center of the neoplastic follicles. *C*, Follicular neoplasia. Dense colloid molds the neoplastic nuclei. *D*, Follicular neoplasia of Hürthle cell type. Tumor cellularity is seen at low magnification. *E*, Follicular neoplasia of Hürthle cell type. Follicular cells with abundant bluish pink cytoplasm, enlarged nuclei, and prominent nucleoli are seen. *F*, Follicular neoplasia of Hürthle cell type. Note binucleation.

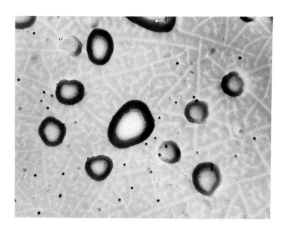

Figure 8-3   Colloid. Thick rings of colloid are seen. Thinner (cracked) colloid is visible in the background (Diff-Quik, × 200).

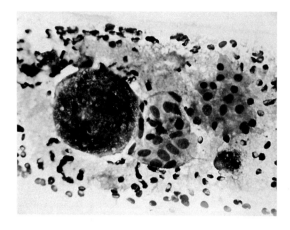

Figure 8-5   Cystic lesion. Two groups of follicular epithelial cells and a large multinucleated histiocyte (the nuclei are obscured by the hemosiderin pigment) are seen. Red blood cells are present in the background. (Diff-Quik, × 400.)

Inflammatory Processes

Acute suppurative thyroiditis is extremely rare. We have not had a case in more than 5,000 thyroid aspirates.

Subacute thyroiditis is also known as de Quervain's thyroiditis, granulomatous thyroiditis, and viral thyroiditis. We have not seen many of these cases in our practice. We saw more cases of granulomatous thyroiditis in 3 weeks in Sweden than in 10 years in Washington, D.C. There is no explanation for this marked difference in our observed incidence. The follicular epithelial cells are usually small, and some appear degenerated. Paravacuolar granules are present in the cytoplasm of the better preserved cells. Macrophages, lymphocytes, polymorphonuclear leukocytes, and epithelioid cells are common. Multinucleated histiocytes are readily seen (Persson, 1968). The amount of colloid varies. Usually it appears dense and in small fragments in close proximity to multinucleated histiocytes and macrophages (Fig. 8-6). This is virtually the only instance in which fine-needle aspiration can be painful.

Lymphocytic thyroiditis is also referred to as Hashimoto's thyroiditis, autoimmune thyroiditis, chronic nonspecific thyroiditis, and struma lymphomatosa. The smears are extremely cellular, causing the appearance of "tumor cellularity." A constant artifact is the presence of crushed cells that have been called lymphoid tangles (Fig. 8-7). At higher magnification these cells are hyperchromatic lymphoid cells and some follicular cells with marked nuclear fragility. The lymphocytes vary in size; some are quite large and have abundant deep blue cytoplasm. Collections of lymphocytes (Fig. 8-8)—and even entire lymphoid follicles—as well as macrophages containing tingible bodies in their cytoplasm may be seen. The number of plasma cells varies markedly from case to case. Another common feature we describe as clearing of the leukocytes. The nuclei of white blood cells, predominantly lymphocytes, have a clear center, and the chromatin appears marginated and stains darkly (Fig. 8-9). These should not be confused with the intranuclear inclusions observed in papillary carcinoma and other tumors; there, the intranuclear inclusions are seen in the

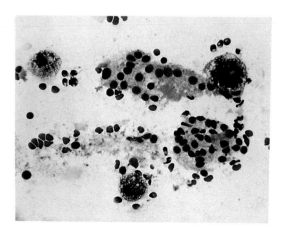

Figure 8-4   Cystic lesion. Sheets of follicular epithelial cells and three hemosiderin-laden macrophages are seen (Diff-Quik, × 400.)

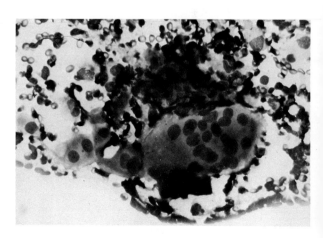

Figure 8-6   Subacute thyroiditis. Dense colloid adjacent to multinucleated histiocyte is seen. (Diff-Quik, × 400.)

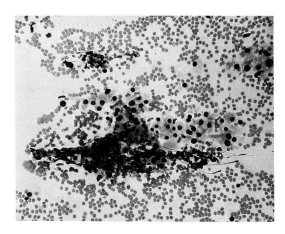

Figure 8-7   Lymphocytic thyroiditis. Crushed lymphoid cells, "lymphoid tangles," and sheets of follicular cells with some variation in nuclear size are seen. Many red blood cells are in the background. (Diff-Quik, × 200.)

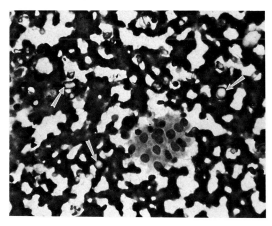

Figure 8-9   Lymphocytic thyroiditis. Lymphoid cells with clear centers and marginated chromatin *(arrows)* are seen. (Diff-Quik, × 400.)

epithelial cells and represent cytoplasmic evaginations (this has been confirmed by electron microscopy). The clearing effect is seen only in the leukocytes.

The epithelial cells may be seen singly or in clusters. Many have thin cytoplasm. Others have dense, grayish pink, and finely granular cytoplasm and are the so-called Hürthle cells, Askanazy cells, oncocytes, or mitochondrion-rich cells (Fig. 8–10). Some of these oxyphilic cell clusters have poorly defined cellular borders and are reminiscent of a syncytium. Nucleoli are present, but they are not as prominent or as common as in Hürthle cell tumors. Groups of epithelioid cells are common. Multinucleated giant cells also are seen frequently. Generally, very little colloid is present, but occasionally one can find a moderate amount of it. The amount of fibrocollagenous tissue varies.

Usually these patients present with a symmetrically enlarged and firm gland, but some may have a single

nodule mimicking a tumor. In the latter cases, if the "nodule" shows cytologic changes consistent with Hashimoto's disease, we proceed to aspirate the contralateral lobe even though it may appear uninvolved clinically.

Sometimes, Hashimoto's disease can be a source of false-positive diagnosis of papillary carcinoma. If intranuclear inclusions, psammoma bodies, and "bubble-gum" colloid are present, the diagnosis of papillary carcinoma can be made (Table 8–2). At other times these criteria are lacking, but the smears are extremely cellular and the cells show nuclear enlargement. When we are faced with this problem, we communicate our uncertainty to the referring physician. Usually, if the antibodies are negative, we will reaspirate the thyroid 2 or 3 months later. Also, reaspiration after 4 to 6 months of suppression may yield smears that are easier to interpret. We favor this conservative approach.

Adenomatoid Nodule(s)

The smears show sheets of follicular cells with regular nuclei and delicate cytoplasm, a "mosaic" arrangement (Fig. 8–11). Most of these cells do not show paravacuolar granules in the cytoplasm. They have small, round, dark, regular nuclei, about 7 to 9 μ in diameter. Generally nucleoli are not conspicuous. Sometimes the cells are arranged in tight clusters called spherules, and on other occasions they can be found singly. Usually the cytoplasm is very delicate, and some single cells appear as naked nuclei, which can be confused with lymphocytes. Some groups of cells may show oxyphilic changes (Hürthle cells), and others may show squamous metaplasia. The amount of colloid varies from scant to abundant. There will be many macrophages if the lesion has undergone cystic degeneration.

When the adenomatoid nodule is composed mostly of colloid, the smears show abundant colloid. Microscopic examination reveals that the colloid may have

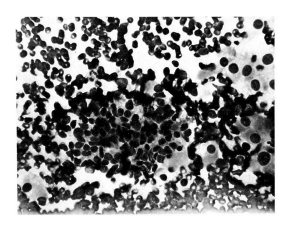

Figure 8-8   Lymphocytic thyroiditis. Small, crowded lymphoid cells with small, dark nuclei and scant cytoplasm contrast with follicular cells (to the right), showing some variation in nuclear size and variable amounts of delicate to dense cytoplasm. Many red blood cells are in the background. (Diff-Quik, × 400.)

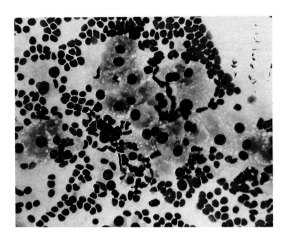

Figure 8-10 Lymphocytic thyroiditis. Follicular epithelial cells with abundant, dense cytoplasm are seen. Some nucleoli are visible. (Diff-Quik, × 400.)

TABLE 8-2 Differential Diagnosis of Papillary Carcinoma and Hashimoto's Thyroiditis

Diagnostic Criteria	Papillary Carcinoma	Hashimoto's Thyroiditis
Follicular cells arranged in:	Sheets, papillary fragments, singly	Sheets
Intranuclear inclusions	+ + +	−
Multinucleated histiocytes	+ + +	+ +
Colloid	Ropy Bubble gum	Scant to moderate, in background
Oxyphilic cells	+	+ +
Psammoma bodies	+ +	−
Lymphocytes and plasma cells	±	+ + + Lymphoid tangles
Lymphoid follicles	−	+
Epithelioid cells	−	+ +
Histiocytes (foamy and/or with hemosiderin granules)	+ + + when cystic	±

−, absent; ±, sometimes present; +, few present; + +, some present; + + +, many present

a homogeneous appearance, or it may adopt quite variable patterns: ribbon-like, mosaic, and others that are best demonstrated in Figures 8-12 to 8-14. Sometimes, when the colloid is very thick, the slides must be left overnight in the fixative solution. This allows the colloid to attach firmly to the slides, and it will not wash off during staining and rinsing. A few small, uniform follicular cells are mixed with the colloid. They are arranged in groups or clusters; some will be forming spherules. The nuclei of these cells are round, dark, and small (less than 7 μ) and appear uniform (Fig. 8-15). No nucleoli are observed. Some foamy histiocytes can be seen. When the nodules have undergone cystic degeneration, the macrophages (mononucleated and multinucleated) will be much more numerous and will have bluish granules in the cytoplasm. The size of these granules is extremely variable, from very fine to quite coarse. The color will vary from deep blue to yellowish green. They represent hemosiderin pigment and as such stain positive for iron.

Graves' Disease (Toxic Goiter)

We believe this is a clinical and chemical diagnosis and not a cytologic one. A bubbly appearance of the cytoplasm or "fire-flare–like vacuoles" in the periphery of the cells has been described as diagnostic of this entity. We have observed these cytoplasmic changes in adenomatoid nodules of euthyroid patients.

Cellular Adenomatoid Nodule

We reserve the category of cellular adenomatoid nodules for lesions that are fairly cellular but do not meet the criteria of follicular neoplasia. The number of follicular cells is striking. Their arrangement varies from sheets to rosettes to single cells scattered throughout the smears. The nuclei are enlarged and vary in size and shape. The colloid is usually scant (Table 8-3). These are the cases in which we request that the thyroid be suppressed and the aspiration repeated after 4 to 6 months of suppression. In our experience, when these patients have undergone surgery, some of them have had follicular neoplasias (adenomas) and others have had adenomatoid nodules. We have become more conservative lately and do not send

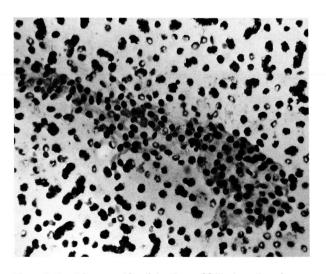

Figure 8-11 Adenomatoid nodule. Sheet of follicular cells and many red blood cells are in the background. (Diff-Quik, × 400.)

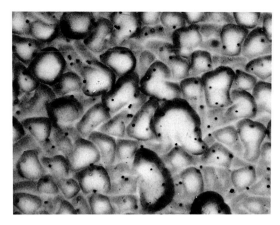

Figure 8-12 "Cobblestone" colloid. (Diff-Quik, × 200.)

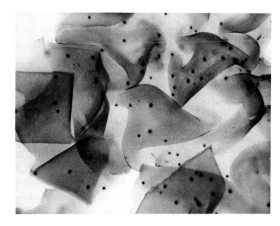

Figure 8-14 "Triangles and squares" colloid. (Diff-Quik, × 200.)

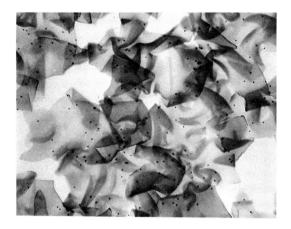

Figure 8-13 "Crumpled" colloid. (Diff-Quik, × 100.)

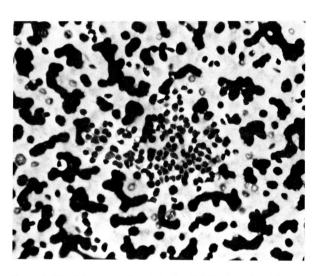

Figure 8-15 Adenomatoid nodule. Small follicular cells with scant cytoplasm and dark, round nuclei are present. (Diff-Quik, × 400.)

these patients to surgery unless their thyroids have been suppressed for at least 6 months, as none of them has had a follicular carcinoma.

Follicular Neoplasia

Cytologically, we cannot differentiate between a follicular adenoma and a follicular carcinoma. Diagnosing carcinoma requires a tissue diagnosis based on evidence of vascular or capsular invasion. Hence, in aspirated material we make the diagnosis of follicular neoplasia.

Follicular Adenoma Versus Follicular Carcinoma

These lesions bleed easily on aspiration, and the cellular sample usually is diluted with blood. However, abundant cellularity is observed if the procedure is performed with extra care. The smears show follicular cells, with enlarged nuclei, arranged in sheets and rosettes. Many single cells and naked nuclei are present. The nuclear borders are irregular, the chromatin is not as dense as in papillary carcinoma, and nucleoli are seen often. Neoplastic follicles are observed. Some show the

TABLE 8-3 Differential Diagnosis Between Cellular Adenomatoid Nodule and Follicular Neoplasia

Cytologic Criteria	Cellular Adenomatoid Nodule	Follicular Neoplasia
Nuclear enlargement	Present	Present and more evident
Follicular cells arranged in:		
Sheets	+ + +	+
Rosettes	+ + +	+
Cords	+	+ +
Follicles	+	+ + +
Colloid:		
In background	+ +	−
Inspissated	+	+ + +
Cystic changes	Frequent	Rare

−, absent; +, few or scant; ++, some; +++, many

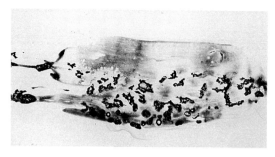

Figure 8-16 Follicular neoplasia. Tissue fragments, and some colloid in the background, that have been crushed (too thick to be smeared) on the glass slide. (Diff-Quik, × 2.7.)

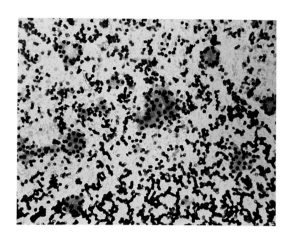

Figure 8-18 Follicular neoplasia. Small follicular (and tubular) structures are scattered through the entire field. (Diff-Quik, × 200.)

enlarged follicular cells surrounding bluish globules of dense colloid (inspissated colloid, "toothpaste" colloid) (Plate 1, B). Frequently, the dense colloid molds the nuclei of the follicular cells (Plate 1, C). Other follicles appear empty.

In some instances, fine-needle aspirates yield solid plugs of tissue that instead of being smeared have to be crushed on the slides (Fig. 8-16). Microscopic examination reveals very cellular smears with innumerable small follicles (Figs. 8-17 and 8-18), some of which have inspissated colloid (Fig. 8-19). When these lesions are excised, the histologic pattern usually is that of the so-called trabecular adenomas or microfollicular adenomas.

Follicular Neoplasia of Hürthle Cell Type

The smears are extremely cellular (Plate 1, D). Many large cells with abundant, grayish pink granular cytoplasm and well demarcated cell borders are observed. They have enlarged, round, eccentric nuclei and prominent nucleoli (Plate 1, E). Binucleation is seen frequently (Plate 1, F). The cells are arranged in irregular tissue fragments, sheets, clusters, and neoplastic follicles (either empty or with inspissated colloid) (see Plate 1, E).

We reiterate that we cannot differentiate cytologically between a follicular adenoma and a follicular carcinoma of Hürthle cell type. Also, some hyperplastic nodules in multinodular goiters may consist almost entirely of oxyphilic cells (Kini et al, 1981) and can lead to a false diagnosis of Hürthle cell neoplasia.

Papillary Carcinoma

Papillary carcinoma is the most common thyroid carcinoma. On physical examination, the majority of these lesions are small and quite firm. There is a gritty sensation upon introduction of the needle, similar to piercing an apple with a hypodermic needle. When a papillary carcinoma is aspirated, it is necessary to apply maximum suction and to move the needle in the mass several times. Even then a drop of blood is barely visible coming into the needle hub. Papillary carcinomas and Hashimoto's thyroiditis are the only lesions that will give a "dry tap."

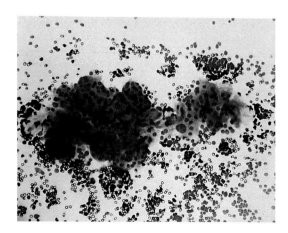

Figure 8-17 Follicular neoplasia. There is a fragment of tissue with numerous small, overlapping follicles. Note the large nucleus to the right of center. (Diff-Quik, × 200.)

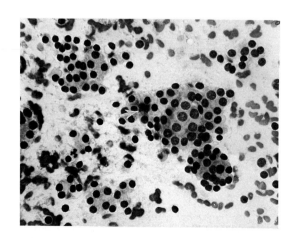

Figure 8-19 Follicular neoplasia. Inspissated colloid (*arrow*) is molded by the nuclei of neoplastic follicular cells. (Diff-Quik, × 400.)

TABLE 8–4   Summary of Cytologic Criteria for the Diagnosis of Papillary Carcinoma

1. Smears are rich in cells: "tumor cellularity"
2. Neoplastic cells
   Size: Much larger than normal follicular cells
   Nuclei: Enlarged and of variable shape; frequent intranuclear inclusions
   Cytoplasm: Abundant, dense, well-defined borders
   Arrangement: Single cells and as sheets, clumps, and papillary fronds
3. "Intranuclear inclusions"
   Occupy over 30% of nuclear area
   Have a pale center (evaginated cytoplasm)
   Dark, thick, continuous rim of chromatin
   Typically one inclusion per nucleus
4. Multinucleated histiocytes
   Delicate to dense irregular cytoplasm
   Multiple round to ovoid nuclei
5. Colloid
   "Bubblegum" or "ropy" appearance
   In close contact with neoplastic cells
6. Psammoma bodies
   Concentric lamellated bodies
   Yellowish to brown-black with Diff-Quik stain
   Not birefringent

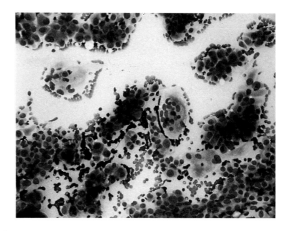

Figure 8–21 Papillary carcinoma. Many neoplastic cells with thick cytoplasm are seen. Note the multinucleated histiocyte in the center. (Diff-Quik, × 200.)

The larger lesions, as a rule, feel soft on palpation and are cystic on aspiration. The amount of fluid varies from 1 to 20 ml or more. The color and consistency vary from pale yellow and thin to dark brown and thick (similar to chocolate syrup). Fluid reaccumulates rapidly in cases of papillary carcinoma. After evacuating the fluid and feeling no residual mass, in the short time that it takes to stain and look at one smear, sometimes we find that the nodule has reappeared when we reexamine the patient's neck. In general, if a cystic nodule recurs within a week, we are always concerned about the possibility of a papillary carcinoma, even though no diagnostic cells may be present. Cytologic criteria for diagnosis of papillary carcinoma are listed in Table 8–4.

If a residual mass is felt after evacuating the fluid, it always should be reaspirated. Occasionally, the fluid may show only hemosiderin-laden macrophages, but smears from the residual mass may reveal papillary carcinoma.

At low magnification the smears show many cells: "tumor cellularity" (Fig. 8–20 and Plate 2, A). The cells are in groups of variable sizes and shapes, some in papillary fragments, others in sheets, or they may be found singly. The amount of colloid varies from scanty to abundant. Hence, its presence or absence is not a useful diagnostic criterion. However, its consistency and its intimate relationship to the cells is quite different from those seen in benign processes. The Swedes refer to it as ropy colloid. It also has been called bubble-gum colloid, (Abele and Miller, 1985), which is the term I find most descriptive. Multinucleated histiocytes are seen frequently (Fig. 8–21 and Plate 2, A and B). Psammoma bodies are sometimes present (Figs. 8–22 and 8–23).

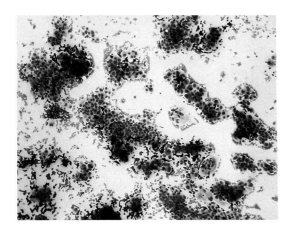

Figure 8–20 Papillary carcinoma. Tumor cellularity is seen. (Diff-Quik, × 100.)

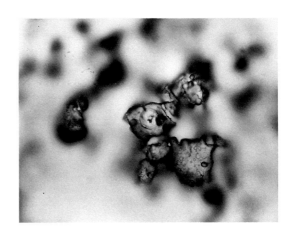

Figure 8–22 Papillary carcinoma. Psammoma bodies are seen. (Diff-Quik, × 400.)

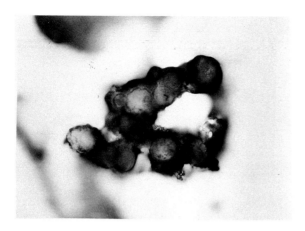

Figure 8–23 Papillary carcinoma. Psammoma bodies are seen. (Diff-Quik, × 400.)

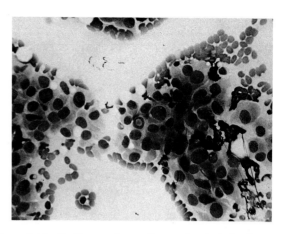

Figure 8–25 Papillary carcinoma. Intranuclear inclusion is present. (Diff-Quik, × 400.)

At higher magnification the cells are much larger than normal follicular cells (Fig. 8–24). The nuclei are enlarged, and the cytoplasm is more abundant and denser. The shape of the nucleus varies from round and regular to ovoid or triangular, depending on the degree of differentiation of the tumor.

We would like to emphasize that the pale nuclei with ground-glass appearance or "Orphan Annie nuclei" are a fixation artifact observed in tissue sections but not in cytologic smears. Also, nuclear grooves have been described as a reliable diagnostic criterion. This is true when the smears are stained with Papanicolaou's stain, but they are not common or obvious in air-dried smears stained with Diff-Quik.

Intranuclear inclusions are a common finding in smears stained with both Papanicolaou (Kini et al, 1980) and Diff-Quik (Fig. 8–25 and Plate 2, C and D) and also in tissue sections. They represent cytoplasmic evaginations into the nucleus. Although originally believed to be

pathognomonic of papillary carcinoma, they also may be observed in other entities, such as medullary carcinoma.

Histologically, the presence of psammoma bodies is one of the more reliable diagnostic criteria of papillary carcinoma. This is not so in fine-needle aspirations. If psammoma bodies can be considered pathognomonic of papillary carcinoma in tissue sections, it is our experience that they can be a source of false-positive diagnosis in aspirates.

Follicular Carcinoma

This category is covered in the section on follicular neoplasia.

Medullary Carcinoma

Medullary carcinomas originate from C cells and produce calcitonin. The smears show abundant cellularity, or "tumor cellularity." The epithelial cells are enlarged

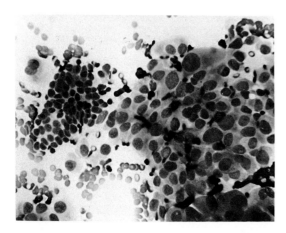

Figure 8–24 Papillary carcinoma. On the left is a cluster of benign follicular epithelial cells to compare with neoplastic cells on the right. (Diff-Quik, × 400.)

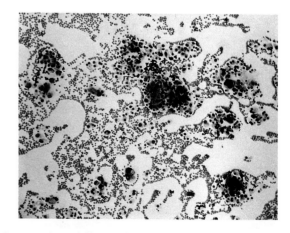

Figure 8–26 Medullary carcinoma. Tumor cellularity is seen. (Diff-Quik, × 100.) Compare with papillary carcinoma (in Figure 8–20) at same magnification.

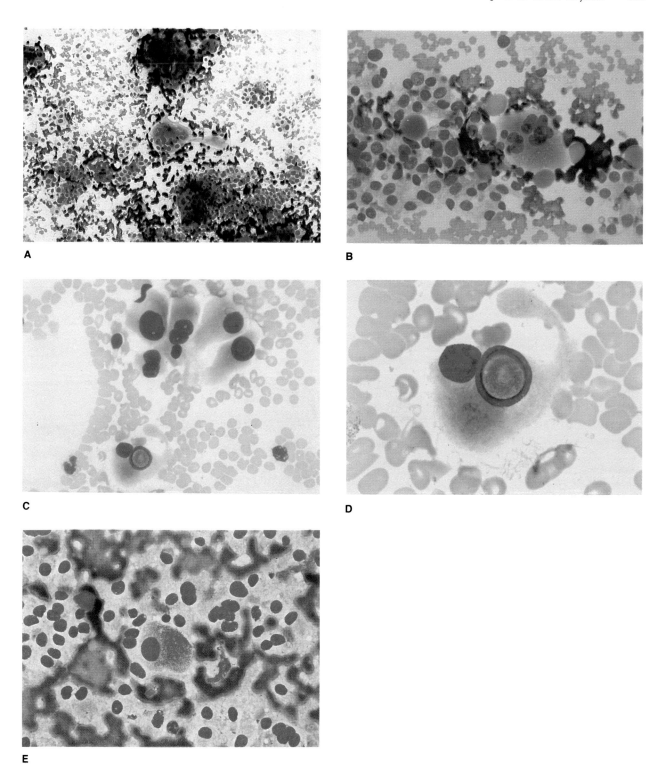

Plate 2 *A*, Papillary carcinoma. Tumor cellularity is seen at low magnification. Note the multinucleated histiocyte in the center. *B*, Papillary carcinoma. Neoplastic cells and a multinucleated histiocyte are seen. *C*, Papillary carcinoma. Neoplastic cells with intranuclear inclusions are present. *D*, Papillary carcinoma. Higher magnification (of one of the cells seen in Plate 2, *C*) of intranuclear inclusion is seen. *E*, Medullary carcinoma. Neoplastic cell with red cytoplasmic granules is seen.

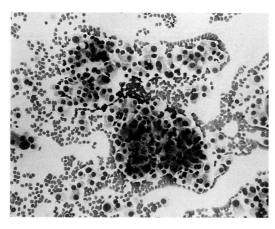

Figure 8-27 Medullary carcinoma. Same field as in Figure 8-26 but at higher magnification. Neoplastic cells are loosely cohesive. (Diff-Quik, × 200.)

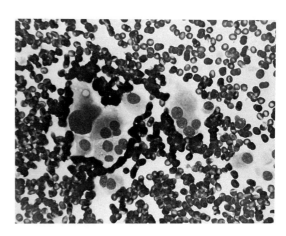

Figure 8-29 Medullary carcinoma. One markedly atypical cell is seen. (Diff-Quik, × 400.)

in comparison with normal follicular cells, and their shape and appearance are variable (polygonal, round, spindled, plasmacytoid). They may appear singly or in small, loose clusters (Figs. 8-26 and 8-27) and less frequently in large sheets or clusters. The nuclei have moderate to marked variation in size and are eccentrically situated (Fig. 8-28); binucleation is common. However, nucleoli are not conspicuous in most cases. Intranuclear inclusions are present sometimes. Scattered bizarre mononucleated or multinucleated neoplastic cells are observed (Fig. 8-29). Multinucleated histiocytes are seen rarely, except in those cases in which amyloid is abundant.

The cytoplasm varies from scant and pale to more abundant and pink. When hematologic stains are used, reddish pink cytoplasmic granules can be seen. In some cases tedious search is required to find the granules in a few cells, but in other cases many cells display easily recognizable granules (Plate 2, E). Amyloid (which stains

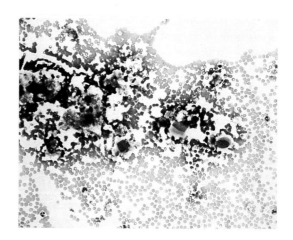

Figure 8-30 Anaplastic carcinoma. Necrotic debris (*left*) and markedly atypical epithelial cells (*right*) are seen. (Diff-Quik, × 200.)

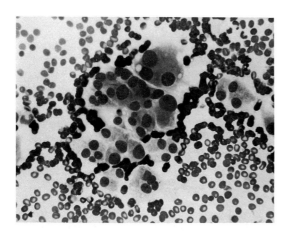

Figure 8-28 Medullary carcinoma. Note the variation in nuclear size and eccentric nuclei. (Diff-Quik, × 400.)

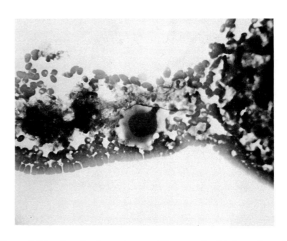

Figure 8-31 Anaplastic carcinoma. Bizarre cell with large irregular nucleus and scant cytoplasm is seen. (Diff-Quik, × 400.)

pink with Diff-Quik) is present in variable amounts. It can be distinguished from colloid, which stains blue.

Anaplastic Carcinoma

The smears show abundant blood, necrotic debris, fragments of fibrocollagenous tissue, and markedly atypical epithelial cells that have variable shapes and high nuclear-cytoplasmic ratios (Figs. 8–30 and 8–31). Some cells are very large and polygonal, and others are spindled. Mitotic figures are observed (Fig. 8–32). Sometimes the smears may show only fibrous tissue, and multiple aspirations have to be performed until a diagnostic focus is sampled.

These tumors are believed to represent an anaplastic transformation of papillary or follicular carcinomas.

Fine-needle aspiration is helpful in the management of patients with anaplastic carcinoma by obtaining a diagnosis without surgery on the rapidly enlarging mass.

Small Cell Carcinoma

Most of the so-called small cell carcinomas of the thyroid have been identified as non-Hodgkin's malignant lymphomas or, rarely, medullary carcinomas. We have not had any small cell carcinomas in more than 5,000 thyroid aspirates.

Malignant Lymphoma

Usually the patient with malignant lymphoma is a woman over 40 years of age with a long history of Hashimoto's disease who presents with an enlargement of one lobe of the thyroid of a few weeks' duration.

Some of the aspirates will show chronic lymphocytic thyroiditis. However, because of the aforementioned presentation, multiple aspirates have to be performed until the abnormal lymphoreticular cells are obtained.

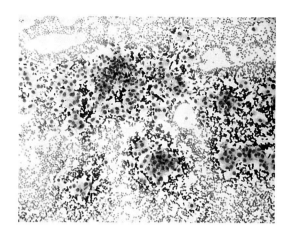

Figure 8-33   Metastatic renal cell carcinoma. Tumor cellularity and innumerable red blood cells are in the background. (Diff-Quik, × 100.) Compare with papillary carcinoma (Fig. 8–20) and medullary carcinoma (Fig. 8–26) at same magnification.

Sometimes this requires as many as 10 needle insertions in a thyroidal mass to obtain diagnostic material.

Usually the lymphoid infiltrate is monotonous, mitotic figures are present, and the follicular epithelial cells are rare, as many of them have been destroyed by the lymphoid proliferation. In some instances it is extremely difficult to determine whether the changes observed in the smears represent a long-standing lymphocytic thyroiditis or a malignant lymphoma.

Most thyroidal lymphomas are B-cell types, probably follicular center-cell lymphomas and lymphoplasmacytic lymphomas (Oertel and Heffess, 1987).

Metastatic Carcinoma

Renal cell carcinoma has been reported as the most common metastasis to the thyroid gland (Figs. 8–33 and 8–34). We occasionally have seen metastases from pul-

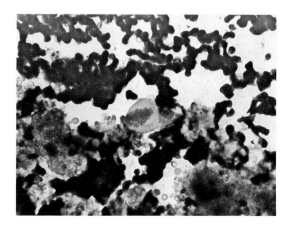

Figure 8-32   Anaplastic carcinoma. Abnormal mitotic figure is seen. (Diff-Quik, × 400.)

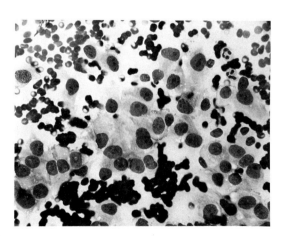

Figure 8-34   Metastatic renal cell carcinoma. Neoplastic cells with clear cytoplasm, large nuclei, and prominent nucleoli are seen. (Diff-Quik, × 400.)

monary and breast carcinomas. Colonic and uterine carcinomas may also metastasize to the thyroid.

Parathyroid Lesions

We have had no cases of parathyroid adenoma or parathyroid carcinoma in our cytologic practice. However, we have seen 11 parathyroid cysts. Clear, colorless, watery fluid aspirated from an anterior neck mass with subsequent collapse of the mass is pathognomonic of a parathyroid cyst. Microscopic examination of smears and/or Cytospin preparations show occasional erythrocytes, histiocytes, and rarely a cluster of small, uniform epithelial cells. We believe that a parathyroid hormone assay of the cyst fluid may be of academic interest but is not necessary for the diagnosis of the lesion or management of the patient (Oertel and Wargotz, 1987).

SAMPLING DIFFICULTIES

In our experience the most common problem is the inadequate sample. Physicians fail to recognize that the technique is deceptively simple and that it must be mastered.

Causes of Inadequate Sample

Missing the Lesion

The lesion could be missed because of the following:

1. Not enlisting the patient's cooperation. It is very important to establish a rapport with the patient, and this will have to be accomplished in a relatively short time if the pathologist is performing the aspiration. The physician should be reassuring and try to relieve the patient's anxiety.
2. Incorrect positioning of the patient. The physician should take time before inserting a needle and make sure that the patient is in the best position to reach the lesion easily. Sometimes the patient must be asked to slide up on the bed and hyperextend his or her neck (chin up). Other times a pillow might be needed under the patient's shoulders. In other instances, it is easier to palpate the nodule when the neck muscles are not hyperextended, so the patient should be asked to slide down on the examining bed and bring his or her chin down. At other times it is easier to aspirate when the patient is sitting upright. Usually we warn the patients that positioning them takes longer than the procedure itself.
3. Uncomfortable positioning of the operator. It has been recommended that if the patient is lying down, the operator should stand on the opposite side of the lesion. I perform the aspirations standing on the same side of the lesion and find this more comfortable for me. The physician must decide which is more comfortable for him or her.

Poor Quality of the Sample

1. The most common mistake when aspirating thyroid lesions is applying too much suction, which dilutes the specimen with blood and interferes with further sampling by causing a hematoma. It is indispensable to be extremely gentle.
2. Inadequate sampling of the lesion. The larger the lesion, the more needles one has to use to sample different areas and obtain a representative specimen.
3. Delay in making the smears. This causes the specimen to clot.
4. Forgetting to release the suction before withdrawing the needle from the lesion. This causes the specimen to go into the syringe, and the only way to recover it is by rinsing the syringe with saline solution or a balanced salt solution and making a Millipore filter or a Cytospin preparation.
5. Poor smearing technique with crushing of the cells.

PITFALLS

The most common error made by pathologists is attempting to diagnose unsatisfactory samples.

A source of concern is false-positive and false-negative diagnoses, with their medicolegal implications. As no test is 100 percent accurate, some of these mistakes are unavoidable. In a preliminary analysis of our first 4,000 cases, we have 0.1 percent false-positive and 7 percent false-negative results. If we would include those cases in which the diagnosis of carcinoma was made or suspected on reaspiration, then our false-negative rate would be 4.5 percent. However, we do not have follow-up information on every case, and as papillary carcinomas can be very indolent lesions, our false-negative rate most likely is between these two figures. In most large series, the false-positive diagnoses have occurred in the early stages and can be attributed to the inexperience of the pathologist. There is no substitute for good judgment and for close communication between the physician taking care of the patient and the pathologist performing the aspiration. Very good results, although not perfect, may be attained by improving the aspiration technique, by being self-critical, and by constantly reviewing material in the light of follow-up information.

BIBLIOGRAPHY

Abele JS, Miller TR. Fine needle aspiration of the thyroid nodule: Clinical applications. In: Clark OH, ed. Endocrine surgery of the thyroid and parathyroid glands. St. Louis: CV Mosby, 1985: 293.

Frable WJ. The treatment of thyroid cancer. The role of fine-needle aspiration cytology. Arch Otolaryngol 1986; 112:1200.

Hamberger B, Gharib H, Melton LJ, et al. Fine-needle aspiration biopsy of thyroid nodules. Impact on thyroid practice and cost of care. Am J Med 1982; 73:381.

Hamburger JI, Miller JM, Kini SR. Clinical-pathological evaluation of thyroid nodules: Handbook and atlas. Limited edition. Private publication, Southfield, MI:1979.

Kini SR, Miller JM, Hamburger JI. Cytopathology of Hürthle cell lesions of the thyroid gland by fine needle aspiration. Acta Cytol 1981; 25:647.

Kini SR, Miller JM, Hamburger JI, Smith MJ. Cytopathology of papillary carcinoma of the thyroid by fine needle aspiration. Acta Cytol 1980; 24:511.

Lowhagen T, Willems JS, Lundell G, et al. Aspiration biopsy cytology in diagnosis of thyroid cancer. World J Surg 1981; 5:61.

Oertel YC. Fine-needle aspiration: A personal view. Lab Med 1982; 13:343.

Oertel YC. Fine needle aspiration of the breast. Boston: Butterworths, 1987.

Oertel JE, Heffess CS. Lymphoma of the thyroid and related disorders. Semin Oncol 1987; 14:333.

Oertel YC, Heffess CS. Diagnosis of parathyroid cysts (letter to the editor). Am J Clin Pathol 1987; 88:252.

Persson PS. Cytodiagnosis of thyroiditis. A comparative study of cytological, histological, immunological and clinical findings in thyroiditis, particularly in diffuse lymphoid thyroiditis. Acta Med Scand Suppl 1968; 483:7.

Vickery AL. Needle biopsy pathology. Clin Endocrinol Metab 1981; 10:275.

Zajicek J. Aspiration biopsy cytology. Part 1. Cytology of supradiaphragmatic organs vol 4. Basel: S Karger AG, 1974:24.

9

Diabetes Mellitus

Robert J. Tanenberg, M.D., F.A.C.P.
David K. Alster, M.D.
Marilyn Tuttleman, B.S., M.T.(ASCP)

The evaluation and treatment of the patient with diabetes mellitus is one of the most common and challenging problems confronting physicians. Although diabetes mellitus has been recognized for thousands of years, the physician could offer little help until the discovery of insulin in 1921. Our understanding of this disease has progressed rapidly since that time. It is now appreciated that diabetes mellitus is actually a group of disorders that are heterogenous in their genetics, pathogenesis, and clinical presentations and may require different approaches to treatment.

In 1979 the National Diabetes Data Group (NDDG) of the National Institutes of Health published a new classification of diabetes and other categories of glucose intolerance. Type I diabetes, or insulin-dependent diabetes mellitus (IDDM), encompasses about 20 percent of cases and is usually characterized by severe insulinopenia in children and young adults. These patients present with sudden onset of polyuria, polydipsia and weight loss, and often ketoacidosis. There is a strong association with certain histocompatibility antigen (HLA) types and with autoimmune phenomena in IDDM. In contradistinction, Type II diabetes, or non-insulin-dependent diabetes mellitus (NIDDM), is characterized by insulin resistance with decreased tissue responsiveness to both endogenous and exogenous insulin. The disease usually occurs after the age of 40, and 60 to 90 percent of the patients are obese. The onset of the disease is often difficult to ascertain, and patients are often asymptomatic at the time of diagnosis. This disease may be noted for the first time during pregnancy, stress, or infection or with the use of drug therapy (e.g., steroids). A third subclass known as "other types" of diabetes mellitus includes a small number of patients whose diabetes is secondary to pancreatic disease, endocrinopathies, or chemical agents or is associated with uncommon genetic syndromes or insulin receptor abnormalities. Impaired glucose tolerance (IGT) and gestational diabetes mellitus (GDM) are common and important clinical entities that are discussed later. In addition to the preceding clinical classes, statistical risk classes are included in the current NDDG classification (Table 9–1).

It has been estimated that more than 6 million people in the United States have diagnosed cases of diabetes mellitus and an additional 4 to 6 million cases are currently undiagnosed. The incidence of this disease is increasing, and diabetes has become a significant cause of mortality. In 1987 there were 40,078 deaths directly attributed to diabetes and an additional 40,261 deaths in which diabetes was a contributing factor. Renal failure, debilitating neuropathy, blindness, gangrene, and ischemic heart disease are among the major causes of morbidity from diabetes. However, the sobering statistics for this disease must be balanced by the benefits of diabetes research over the past two decades. Recent advances in clinical diabetes care include self–blood glucose monitoring and the measurement of glycosylated hemoglobins to monitor control. Therapeutic advances include recombinant DNA human insulin, external insulin pumps, and the use of multiple daily injections to achieve tighter control of blood glucose.

Although therapy is the greatest challenge in the management of patients with diabetes, knowledge of diagnostic testing for diabetes is essential for the practicing physician. This chapter reviews methodologies for testing blood glucose, the indication for and proper interpretation of the oral glucose tolerance test (OGTT), and the newest diagnostic criteria for diabetes mellitus and IGT. In addition, measurement of C-peptide, glycosylated hemoglobins, and fructosamine is reviewed, as these tests have become important adjuncts in the evaluation and management of patients with diabetes. Newer tests for islet cell antibodies (ICA) are reviewed since they help define the etiology of diabetes and may predict the likelihood of patients with prediabetes developing overt disease.

GLUCOSE AND GLUCOSE TOLERANCE TESTING

Currently, most laboratories prefer to measure glucose as serum or plasma rather than whole blood. Plasma and serum glucose values are approximately 15 percent higher than whole blood values. Capillary whole blood has become the method of choice for self–blood glucose monitoring but has little role in diagnostic testing for diabetes mellitus. In addition, capillary whole blood may be 30 mg per deciliter higher than venous whole blood in the postprandial state, although there is no difference

TABLE 9–1 Classification of Diabetes Mellitus and Other Categories of Glucose Intolerance*

Clinical Classes	Distinguishing Characteristics
Diabetes mellitus (DM) Type I, insulin-dependent diabetes mellitus (IDDM)	Patients may be of any age, are usually thin, and usually have abrupt onset of signs and symptoms with insulinopenia before age 40. They are dependent on insulin to prevent ketoacidosis and weight loss.
Type II, Non-insulin-dependent diabetes mellitus (NIDDM) (obese or nonobese)	Patients usually are older than 40 years at diagnosis, are obese, and may be asymptomatic. They are not prone to ketoacidosis except during periods of stress. Although not dependent on exogenous insulin for survival, they may require it for stress-induced hyperglycemia and hyperglycemia that persists in spite of other therapy.
Impaired glucose tolerance (IGT) (obese or nonobese)	Patients with IGT have plasma glucose levels that are higher than normal but not diagnostic for diabetes mellitus.
Gestational diabetes mellitus (GDM)	Patients with GDM have onset or diagnosis of glucose intolerance *during* pregnancy.
Statistical Risk Classes†	*Distinguishing Characteristics*
Previous abnormality of glucose tolerance (PrevAGT)	Persons in this category have normal glucose tolerance and a history of transient diabetes mellitus or IGT.
Potential abnormality of glucose tolerance (PotAGT)	Persons in this category have never had abnormal glucose tolerance but have a greater than normal risk of developing diabetes mellitus or IGT.

* Table excludes "other types" of diabetes mellitus and IGT categories (e.g., secondary diabetes or IGT resulting from hemachromatosis or Cushing's syndrome).
† Used for epidemiologic and research purposes.
Adapted from The physician's guide to Type II diabetes (NIDDM): Diagnosis and treatment. Alexandria, VA: American Diabetes Association, 1984. Reproduced with permission of the American Diabetes Association, Inc.

in the fasting state. When serum is desired, a red-top tube is filled, and the technician should separate the serum from the clot within 15 to 30 minutes after collection.

Enzymatic assays have become the method of choice for measuring glucose because of the high degree of specificity. Glucose oxidase is an older and still widely used method. The hexokinase procedure was proposed as a national glucose reference method by the Centers for Disease Control in 1976 because of its greater precision (Table 9–2).

Prior to 1979, the indications for and interpretations of the glucose tolerance test (GTT) were highly controversial. Different criteria for interpretation of the GTT were proposed by Fajans, Wilkerson, the Joslin Clinic, and the U.S. Public Health Service. Terms such as *latent, chemical*, and *borderline diabetes* added to the confusion over whether certain patients were "diabetic." To address these problems, a meeting of the NDDG of the National Institutes of Health was convened in 1978. The recommendations of the NDDG were published in 1979, and a new abbreviated and somewhat different version was published by the World Health Organization (WHO) Expert Committee in 1980 (Tables 9–3 and 9–4). According to the NDDG, "The diagnosis of diabetes should be

based on (1) unequivocal elevation of plasma glucose (PG) concentration, together with the classic symptoms of diabetes, or (2) elevated fasting plasma glucose (FPG) on more than one occasion, or (3) elevated PG concentration after an oral glucose challenge on more than one occasion." It is important to note that acute illness, trauma, burns, pregnancy, endocrinopathies, and various drugs induce hyperglycemia, elevating the fasting plasma glucose level as well as impairing glucose tolerance. Furthermore, physical inactivity and a restricted diet (with less than 150 g of carbohydrate per day) preceding a GTT may produce abnormal glucose tolerance. In addition, studies have demonstrated individual variability with repeated GTTs. For this reason, the NDDG recommended that an elevated FPG or GTT be demonstrated on at least two occasions before a diagnosis of diabetes is made in any patient.

When patients present with symptoms of polyuria, polydipsia, weight loss, and a plasma glucose level of over 200 mg%, the diagnosis of diabetes is made and does not need confirmation. Patients with or without symptoms having an FPG of more than 140 mg% on two or more occasions are also diagnosed as having diabetes by the NDDG criteria. When there is a strong suspicion that diabetes may be present and the FPG is less than

TABLE 9-2 Glucose Assays

Method	Glucose oxidase Hexokinase O-toluidine Somogyi-Nelson Autoanalyzer ferricyanide Autoanalyzer neocuproine
Normal	Fasting plasma glucose* < 115 mg/dl
	Plasma glucose values following 75-g oral glucose dose* 30 min < 200 mg/dl 60 min < 200 mg/dl 90 min < 200 mg/dl 120 min < 140 mg/dl
	Venous whole blood and capillary whole blood concentrations are 15% less than plasma glucose levels in fasting samples.
Sample Collection	Venous plasma glucose is the preferred measurement. Samples should be analyzed immediately or collected in tubes containing 30 mg of sodium fluoride for each 5 ml of whole blood, separated within 4 h of collection, and the plasma frozen until analysis.
Uses	Diagnosis of hyperglycemia and hypoglycemia.
Problems	Drug interference with the assays (see Fischbach FT. A Manual of Laboratory Diagnostic Tests. 2nd ed. Philadelphia: JB Lippincott, 1984:834). Glucose utilization by formed elements of blood may lower results if samples are not handled properly.

* Nonpregnant adults
Normal values adapted from The physician's guide to Type II diabetes (NIDDM): Diagnosis and treatment. Alexandria, VA: American Diabetes Association, 1984. Reproduced with permission of the American Diabetes Association, Inc.

TABLE 9-3 Diagnostic Criteria for Impaired Glucose Tolerance and Diabetes Mellitus in Nonpregnant Adults

Impaired Glucose Tolerance

Fasting plasma glucose of less than 140 mg%
and
2-hour OGTT plasma glucose of 140–200 mg%
and
Intervening OGTT plasma glucose of 200 mg% or greater

Diabetes Mellitus

Random plasma glucose of 200 mg% or greater plus classic signs and symptoms of diabetes mellitus, including polydipsia, polyphagia, polyuria, and weight loss
or
Fasting plasma glucose of 140 mg% or greater on at least two occasions
or
Fasting plasma glucose of less than 140 mg% plus sustained elevation of plasma glucose levels during at least two OGTTs. Both the 2-h sample and at least one other glucose sample between 0 and 2 h should be 200 mg% or greater.

Adapted from the National Diabetes Data Group. Classification and diagnosis of diabetes mellitus and other categories of glucose intolerance. Diabetes 1979; 28:1039. Reproduced with permission of the American Diabetes Association, Inc.

TABLE 9-4 Criteria for Diagnosis of Gestational Diabetes*

Time	Venous Plasma (mg/dl)	Capillary or Venous Whole Blood (mg/dl)
Fasting (0)	105	90
1 h	190	170
2 h	165	145
3 h	145	125

* Two or more of the above values after a 100-g oral glucose challenge must be met or exceeded.
Adapted from the National Diabetes Data Group. Classification and diagnosis of diabetes mellitus and other categories of glucose intolerance. Diabetes 1979; 28:1039. Reproduced with permission of the American Diabetes Association, Inc.

140 mg% but more than 110 mg%, a 2- or 3-hour OGTT may be ordered to establish a diagnosis. Davidson (1986) has published a 12-point checklist to be certain that a GTT is valid (Table 9–5). After the test is completed, the NDDG criteria should be used to determine if the patient has diabetes mellitus or IGT or is normal. Some patients have a nondiagnostic test if one or two but not all three criteria for IGT are met. It is important to identify patients with IGT since they have an increased prevalence and susceptibility to cardiovascular disease. It is the experience of these authors that these patients often have diabetic polyneuropathy if they are examined very carefully. Clinically significant diabetic retinopathy and nephropathy are usually not seen in this group.

Bennett conducted a 14-year survey of the Pima Indians, who have a very high incidence of diabetes. He administered a glucose load and divided the study popu-

TABLE 9-5   Routine for a Valid Glucose Tolerance Test

Do only on those whose fasting venous plasma glucose (FPG) level is less than 140 mg%.

Before a glucose load is given, measure FPG.

If it is greater than 140 mg%, cancel the GTT.

Do on ambulatory patients only.

Do not do on patients who are hospitalized or on patients who have an acute or chronic illness that can affect the test.

Discontinue all drug therapy that can affect the test for at least 3 days prior to the test (see Table 9-6).

Have patient eat a carbohydrate intake of at least 150 g/day for 3 days prior to the test.

Fast 14 to 15 hours (from 6 PM of the day preceding the test to 8 or 9 AM of the day of the test).

Give 75 g of orange or lemon-flavored pure glucose as 25% solution (400 ml). Have the patient drink it within 5 min. The first swallow is time zero. Nausea and vomiting rarely occur. Should they occur, the test should be terminated.

Collect samples at ½, 1, 2, and 3 h.

Have patient abstain from tobacco, coffee, tea, food, and alcohol during the test

Have patient sit upright and quietly during the test. Slow walking is permitted, but vigorous exercise should be avoided.

Venous blood is preferable, collected in a gray-top tube containing fluoride and an anticoagulant.

Analyses should be done by a method specific for glucose, such as glucose oxidase or hexokinase.

The test should be interpreted using the NDDG criteria (see Table 9-3).

Reprinted by permission from Davidson JK. Clinical diabetes mellitus: A problem-oriented approach. 1st ed. New York: Thieme Medical Publishers, 1986.

TABLE 9-6   Drugs That May Impair Glucose Tolerance

Diuretics* and Antihypertensives

Chlorthalidone, furosemide, thiazides, diazoxide, metalozone, propranolol, bumetanide, ethacrynic acid, clonidine, calcium channel blockers

Hormones

Corticosteroids, adrenocorticotropic hormone, glucagon, oral contraceptives, thyroid hormones (Thyrotoxic doses)

Psychoactive Agents

Haloperidol, lithium carbonate, tricyclic antidepressants (amitriptyline, desipramine, doxepin, imipramine, nortriptyline), phenothiazines, marijuana

Catecholamines and Other Neurologically Active Agents

Phenytoin, epinephrine, isoproterenol, levodopa, norepinephrine

Antineoplastic Agents

Alloxan, streptozotocin, L-asparaginase, cyclophosphamide

Miscellaneous

Caffeine, indomethacin, isoniazid, nicotinic acid, acetaminophen, morphine, cimetidine, encainide, pentamidine

* Hyperglycemia response may be independent of fluctuations in serum potassium.
Adapted from the National Diabetes Data Group Report. Classification and diagnosis of diabetes mellitus and other categories of glucose intolerance. Diabetes 1979; 28:1039. Reproduced with permission of the American Diabetes Association, Inc.

lation into two groups: those whose 2-hour values were below 200 mg% and those whose values were above 240 mg%. He found that retinopathy and nephropathy were confined to those subjects in the above 240 mg% group. The absence of these complications in Bennett's group of Pima Indians whose 2-hour values were below 200 mg% was responsible for the abandonment of the term *chemical diabetes* in favor of *impaired glucose tolerance* by the NDDG. It is estimated that patients with IGT progress to overt diabetes at a rate of 1 to 5 percent per year, varying with the patient's age and country of origin. To diagnose IGT, the full 2- or 3-hour OGTT is usually performed. However, the NDDG recommended a modification for epidemiologic studies whereby only

a fasting and 2-hour value is obtained. If the FPG is
less than 140 mg% and the 2-hour value falls between
140 and 200 mg%, the individual may be classified as
having IGT for epidemiologic purposes.

The diagnosis of diabetes mellitus in children is
usually made when the patient presents with polyuria,
polydipsia, ketonuria, and rapid weight loss together with
a random plasma glucose level greater than 200 mg%.
On occasion, an asymptomatic child (with or without a
family history of diabetes) will be found to have glycosuria. Since diabetes may be present without symptoms,
a GTT may be indicated to exclude the diagnosis. The
test is performed in the same manner as with adults
except that the dose of glucose administered should be
1.75 g per kilogram of ideal body weight (up to a maximum of 75 g). In addition, the criteria for diabetes in
children defined by the NDDG include both an FPG
equal to or greater than 140 mg% (capillary whole blood
equal to or greater than 120 mg%) *and* two or more
values equal to or greater than 200 mg% during the test.
IGT may be diagnosed in children with an FPG below
140 mg% and a 2-hour postload value above 140 mg%.
If either the 2-hour or an intermediate value is greater
than 200 mg% but the fasting value is less than 140
mg%, the diagnosis is IGT, not diabetes mellitus. This
is in contradistinction to adults, in whom the latter situation would meet the criteria for diabetes mellitus.

Gestational diabetes mellitus, or GDM, develops in
up to 3 percent of all pregnancies, and the correct diagnosis of this condition is important because it requires
intervention with diet with or without insulin, meticulous
self–blood glucose monitoring, and special obstetric testing such as non–stress testing, ultrasound, and am-

niocentesis. This aggressive intervention with a team
approach by the endocrinologist and obstetrician should
lessen the increased risk for perinatal loss or morbidity.
It has also been estimated that 10 to 30 percent of women
who are diagnosed as having GDM will eventually develop nonpregnant diabetes. At increased risk for developing GDM are women who develop glycosuria, have a
positive family history of diabetes, have a history of large-
for-gestational-age infants, have had a stillbirth or a parity
of five or more, and are obese or over age 35. Since recognition of this entity is so important for both mother and
offspring and since GDM is usually asymptomatic, the
diagnosis should be considered not only in women with
the preceding risk factors but in all pregnancies. In fact,
in 1980 the first American Diabetes Association (ADA)
Workshop-Conference on Gestational Diabetes recommended that all pregnant women be screened for diabetes between the 24th and 28th weeks of pregnancy.
Patients fast overnight, and a 50-g oral glucose load is
administered. A plasma glucose is drawn 1 hour later and
is positive if greater than 150 mg%. Tests below 150 mg%
are negative, but if the obstetrician has a high index of
suspicion, the screen may be repeated at 32 weeks of
gestation (Table 9-7). A positive screen is an indicator
for a 3-hour OGTT.

The NDDG recommended that the criteria originally established by O'Sullivan and Mahan in 1964 be
used to diagnose GDM. In pregnancy, a 100-g glucose
load must be used, and plasma or whole blood is measured while the patient is fasting and at 1, 2, and 3 hours
after the glucose challenge. Patients should be prepared
and the test conducted as in the nongravid state with the
preceding exceptions noted. It is very important that these
women fast overnight after consuming a daily intake of
at least 250 g of carbohydrate for 3 days prior to the test
and also that they be ketosis-free at the time of the GTT.

The diagnostic criteria for GDM are as follows: The
upper limits for plasma values are 105 mg% fasting,
190 mg% at 1 hour, 165 mg% at 2 hours, and 145 mg%
at 3 hours. In contradistinction to the nongravid state,
the test must be done for the full 3 hours since the diagnosis of GDM is made when two of the four values equal
or exceed these upper limits (see Table 9-4). If, for
example, a patient's FPG is 110 mg% and her 2-hour
value is 175 mg%, GDM may be diagnosed even if her
1- and 3-hour values are normal. It is vital that the test be
accomplished exactly as per the protocol to be sure to
avoid both false-positives and false-negatives. If there is
any doubt as to the accuracy of the test, we recommend
either repeating the test or treating the patient as if GDM
were present. Assuming a normal patient has GDM
should cause no harm because it is the usual practice to
closely monitor asymptomatic patients on an ADA diet
(at least 35 kcal per kilogram of prepregnancy weight)
for several days prior to instituting insulin therapy. On
the other hand, failure to monitor and treat a patient
with GDM may lead to stillbirth or to the birth of an
infant with a greater likelihood of significant morbidity.

GLYCOHEMOGLOBINS

Over the past two decades there has been an increased understanding of the nature and clinical importance of nonenzymatic carbohydrate-protein linkage or glycation. Measurement of glycated or glycosylated hemoglobins (GHb) has become the most important tool in monitoring glycemic control in diabetes.

The red blood cell (RBC) membrane is freely permeable to glucose. The amount of glucose that enters the RBC will depend on the ambient concentration of glucose over the 120-day life span of the RBC. Glucose within the RBC combines with hemoglobin A in a two-step nonenzymatic process. The first step is reversible and involves a rapid reaction between glucose and the terminal valine of one or both beta chains to form an aldimine or Schiff base. This product is also known as pre-A_{1c} or the labile component. The second step involves a slow and irreversible Amadori rearrangement to form the stable ketoamine (Fig. 9–1).

Separation of hemoglobin components is based on electrical charge. The less negatively charged "fast" hemoglobins migrate, and therefore elute, more rapidly than the slow-moving hemoglobin A_0. "Fast" hemoglobins comprise hemoglobin A_1 and can be further divided into four components: HbA_{1a1}, HbA_{1a2}, HbA_{1b}, and HbA_{1c} (Fig. 9–2). Hemoglobins A_{1a1} and HbA_{1a2} are formed by the interaction of fructose diphosphate and glucose-6-phosphate, respectively, with the beta terminal amine, and each comprises about 0.2 percent of total hemoglobin in normoglycemic individuals. Hemoglobin A_{1b} comprises approximately 0.4 percent total hemoglobin and probably occurs as a deamination product of HbA_0. HbA_{1c} comprises 3 to 6 percent of total hemoglobin, and because it represents an adduct of glucose, it is the most specific GHb reflecting average glucose concentration over the preceding 4 to 8 weeks. In 1984 the NDDG published a list of standardized definitions of hemoglobin nomenclature (Table 9–9).

Many methods have been developed to provide a reliable test to determine glycohemoglobin values. These

TABLE 9–8   Glycohemoglobin (GHb) (Hemoglobin A_1 and A_{1c})

Method	Cation-exchange chromatography Agar gel electrophoresis Colorimetry (thiobarbituric acid) Affinity chromatography (isoelectric focusing)
Normal	3.0–6.0% of total hemoglobin (HbA_{1c}) 5.1–7.8% of total hemoglobin (HbA_1)
Uses	Assessment of glycemic control in patients with diabetes over the preceding 4–8 weeks. Screening for diabetes (highly specific but not as sensitive as OGTT).
Problems	Affected by states altering RBC survival, hemoglobinopathies, uremia, and other factors (see Table 9–10)

include cation-exchange chromatography, agar gel electrophoresis, colorimetry, and affinity chromatography. Methods may measure either HbA_1 (total fast hemoglobin) or HbA_{1c}.

The cation-exchange method is the most widely used. The less negatively charged HbA_1 fraction elutes first, followed by the more negatively charged HbA_0. HbA_1 or HbA_{1c} is expressed as a percentage of the total hemoglobin A. High-pressure liquid chromatography (HPLC) and commercial columns are based on this principle. HPLC has the advantages of greater precision and the ability to separate HbA_{1c} from the other minor hemoglobins. Its disadvantages are that it is costly and more time-consuming. The commercial kits use prefilled disposable columns containing cation-exchange resin. These kits have the advantages of a lower cost, faster turnaround time, and greater simplicity. All cation-exchange techniques are subject to the same problems with respect to conditions that can impair performance and reliability. Strict maintenance of temperature, ionic strength, and pH is critical. Another important consideration concerns the presence of abnormal hemoglobins. Hemoglobins S and C will falsely lower the HbA_{1c}

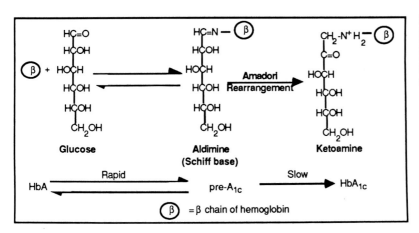

Figure 9–1 Nonenzymatic glycosylation of hemoglobin. (From Bunn HF, Gabbay KH, Gallop PM. The glycosylation of hemoglobin: Relevance to diabetes mellitus. Science 1978; 200:21. Copyright 1978 by the American Association for the Advancement of Science.)

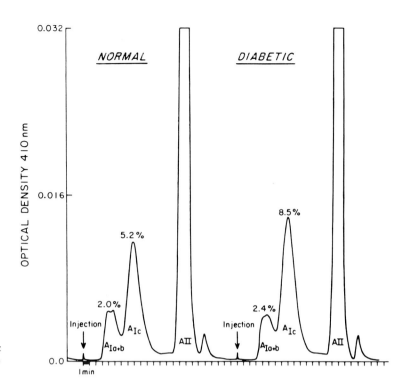

Figure 9-2 Representative chromatographs of diabetic and nondiabetic samples for hemoglobins $A_{1a+b}\%$ and $A_{1c}\%$ (Soeldner 1979; with permission.)

results, whereas hemoglobin F will give falsely elevated results as it coelutes with the "fast" hemoglobins. There are now available, however, newer HPLC systems that are not affected by hemoglobins S, C, and F.

Agar gel electrophoresis offers an alternative to cation-exchange methods and is of comparable accuracy. The technique also separates the various hemoglobin components on the basis of their electrical charge characteristics. GHb percentages are obtained using a scanning densitometer. The test measures HbA_1. This method is not affected by the presence of HbS, elevated triglyceride concentrations, and variations in temperature.

Both cation-exchange chromatography and agar gel electrophoresis require the removal of the labile fraction when the sample is prepared to ensure accurate determination of GHb. Failure to do so may result in spuriously high GHb values since this fraction is proportional to the PG at the time of blood sampling.

Colorimetry measures total GHb using the thiobarbituric acid (TBA) method. This method is not subject to interference by hemoglobinopathies or uremia and has been demonstrated to be reproducible on frozen hemolysates or packed RBCs stored up to 5 months. However, the main problem with this method is lack of a reference standard, and values obtained cannot be directly compared among different laboratories. The method is not commercially available in kit form.

The affinity chromatography method measures total glycohemoglobin using the principle of differential adherence to a ligand of glucose-conjugated

hemoglobin compared to unconjugated hemoglobin. The method has advantages for long-term storage and low cost. The assay is not subject to interference by hemoglobinopathies, nonglucose adducts, and lactescent plasma. The results of affinity chromatography correlate well with cation-exchange and colorimetric methods.

Clinical conditions that shorten RBC survival, such as hemolytic anemias, decrease GHb values. Conversely, splenectomy may lengthen RBC survival and increase GHb measurements. These conditions are summarized in Table 9-10.

The measurement of GHb has become accepted as an important tool in the assessment of glucose control in the patient with diabetes. It provides objective information not obtainable from other sources, including historical data, 24-hour urine glucose measurements, random urine glucose testing, and frequent self–blood glucose monitoring. GHb values reflect the mean glucose during the preceding 4 to 8 weeks and are most useful to the clinician in the assessment of long-term blood glucose control. Measurements of GHb also provide an invaluable retrospective index of glucose control in patients enrolled in clinical trials such as the Diabetes Control and Complications Trial (DCCT). GHb values rise with the loss of endogenous C-peptide and decrease following improved glycemic control. Knowledge of GHb values may also enhance patient compliance.

In a recent review, Goldstein and colleagues (1986) noted that several studies indicate a linear correlation between a particular GHb value and the plasma glucose

TABLE 9-9   Hemoglobin Nomenclature

HbA	The major form of hemoglobin, a native, unmodified tetramer consisting of two alpha and two beta chains.
HbA_0	The major component of HbA, identified by its chromatographic and electrophoretic properties. Post-translational modifications, including glucosylation, do exist in this fraction but do not significantly affect the charge properties of the protein.
HbA_1	Post-translationally modified, more negatively charged forms of HbA, as detected by chromatographic and electrophoretic methods.
HbA_{1a1}, HbA_{1a2}, HbA_{1b}, HbA_{1c}	Chromatographically distinct components of HbA_1.
HbA_{1c}	Adduct of glucose attached to the beta-chain terminal valine residue by a keto-amine linkage.
pre-HbA_{1c}	A labile form of glucosylated hemoglobin containing glucose attached by aldimine linkage at the beta-chain terminal valine residue.
"Fast" hemoglobin(s)	The total HbA_1 fraction, which, because of a more negative charge, migrates more rapidly toward the anode in electrophoresis and elutes earlier in cation-exchange chromatography than does HbA_0.
Glucosylated hemoglobin(s)	Hemoglobin modified by glucose at alpha- and beta-chain terminal valine residues and epsilon-amino groups of lysine residues.
Glycated (glycosylated) hemoglobin(s)	A generic term for hemoglobin containing glucose and (or) other carbohydrate.

Adapted from National Diabetes Data Group. Report of the expert committee on glucosylated hemoglobin. Diabetes Care 1984; 7:602 (reproduced with permission of the American Diabetes Association, Inc.); and Goldstein DE, Little RR, Wiedmeyer H, et al. Glycated hemoglobin: Methodologies and clinical applications. Clin Chem 1986; 32:B64.

TABLE 9-10   Clinical Conditions That Affect GHb Measurements

Conditions That Elevate Glycohemoglobin Values
    Splenectomy
    Thalassemias[*]
    Hemoglobin Wayne[*]
    Hemoglobin F[*,†]
    Iron deficiency[*]
    Uremia[*]
    Hyperbilirubinemia[*]
    Hypertriglyceridemia[*]
    Alcoholism[*]
    Lead poisoning[*]
    Large doses of salicylates[*,†]
    Opiate addiction[*]

Conditions That Decrease Glycohemoglobin Values
    Hemolytic anemias
    Acute blood loss and phlebotomy
    Hemoglobin C[*]
    Hemoglobin S[*]
    Pregnancy

[*] Ion-exchange method
[†] Electrophoretic method
Conditions not coded affect GHb using all four methods discussed in text.

level. They correlate each 1 percent change in GHb with a 25 to 35 mg% change in average plasma glucose and state that regardless of the methodology employed, GHb values greater than 3 percent above the upper limits of normal indicate a mean plasma glucose value greater than 200 mg%. Alternatively, a single GHb value falling in the normal range suggests that the average plasma glucose for that individual was within normal limits over the preceding weeks to months. These correlations are most clearly demonstrated from data comparing mean HbA_{1c} values and mean quarterly blood glucose profiles in a cohort of 278 IDDM patients entering the DCCT (Fig. 9-3).

Nathan and associates (1984) studied 21 IDDM diabetic patients performing multiple reflectance meter capillary blood glucose samples over a 2-month period.

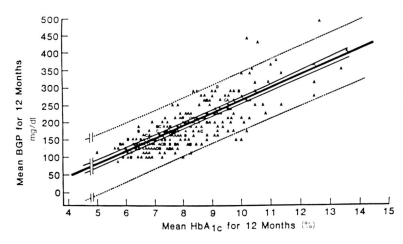

Figure 9-3   Comparison of mean quarterly blood glucose profiles (BGP) by laboratory determination with mean of all quarterly HbA_{1c} results. Dark lines represent mean regression line ± 2 SD. Dotted line represents 95 percent confidence interval for individual values. A = 1 point, B = 2 points, and C = 3 or more points. r = .80, P < .0001. (From DCCT Research Group. The DCCT Feasibility Study. Diabetes Care 1987; 10:10. Reproduced with permission of the American Diabetes Association, Inc.)

Patients performed at least four tests per day and the data generated were used to calculate a mean blood glucose concentration (MBG) for each patient during this period. Hemoglobin A_{1c} values were measured at the end of the 2-month period in these subjects, and a linear regression equation was derived. The equation may be stated as follows:

$$\text{MBG estimate} = 33.3\,(\text{HbA}_{1c}) - 86$$
$$(r = 0.958)$$

With this equation one may convert the patient's HbA_{1c} value to an estimated MBG over the preceding 60 days. For example, an HbA_{1c} of 6.0 percent is equivalent to an MBG of 114 mg per deciliter, and an HbA_{1c} of 10.0 percent is equivalent to 247 mg per deciliter.

The Health and Public Policy Committee of the American College of Physicians recommends measuring GHb four times per year in patients with Type I diabetes and two times per year in patients with Type II diabetes. An exception may be patients who are pregnant, those on intensive therapy (multiple daily injections or external insulin pump), or those who have undergone a major change in therapy. A more difficult question to answer is, What are desirable GHb levels for individual patients with diabetes? Many studies suggest that the degree of chronic hyperglycemia is an important risk factor for the development of the microvascular complications (retinopathy, nephropathy, and neuropathy) and that normalization of the GHb value would be a desirable goal. However, the clinician must realize that although a normal GHb in a patient with diet-controlled Type II diabetes represents glucose values falling in the normal range, a similar normal GHb in a patient with insulin-treated Type I diabetes may indicate glucose values in both the hypoglycemic and hyperglycemic ranges. Our experience is that normalization of GHb in both Type II and C-peptide-positive Type I patients with diabetes is generally not an unreasonable goal. With proper self-blood glucose monitoring and patient education, normalization of GHb should also be a safe undertaking in these patients. However, in C-peptide-negative patients who are often characterized as "brittle diabetics," normalization of GHb may lead to hazardous hypoglycemia. For this reason, we strive for "excellent" ($A_{1c} \leq 7$ percent) or "good" ($A_{1c} = 7$ to 8.5 percent) control in lieu of normalization of GHb in patients with Type I diabetes. Furthermore, normalization of GHb is contraindicated in diabetic patients with coronary artery disease, those with proliferative retinopathy, and those who do not counterregulate in response to hypoglycemia and in the elderly patient on insulin therapy.

The exact course of glycosylation of hemoglobin during pregnancy is not entirely understood. Pregnancy affects RBC mass and survival time, iron stores, and glucose tolerance. In normal pregnancy there is a progressive fall in the FPG, although postprandial glucose levels are relatively high in late gestation. The combined effects of these changes on GHb seem to result in an initial fall in HbA_{1c} from 10 to 24 weeks of gestation and then in a rise during the third trimester. In addition, postpartum values are significantly higher than those in pregnant and nonpregnant controls. Unfortunately, there have been no large series of normal pregnant patients so as to establish pregnancy-specific normal ranges. Nonetheless, HbA_{1c} has been demonstrated to be a useful parameter to measure in diabetic pregnancy.

Miller and co-workers (1981) from the Joslin Diabetes Center studied records of 116 pregnant women with IDDM (pregestational diabetes) to determine if there was a correlation between GHb and the incidence of congenital anomalies. They, in fact, found a strong correlation between the HbA_{1c} (HPLC method, including the labile component) measured in the first trimester and the incidence of congenital anomalies. None of these women with an HbA_{1c} less than 6.9 percent (n = 19) and only 3.4 percent of the women with an HbA_{1c} less than 8.5 percent (n = 58) gave birth to infants with major congenital anomalies. In contrast, 22.4 percent of the women whose initial HbA_{1c} was greater than 8.5 percent (n = 58) had infants with congenital anomalies (e.g., anencephaly, ventricular septal defect). This study demonstrated the value of GHb as an important tool to retrospectively determine glycemic control. The study used GHb to confirm the role of hyperglycemia in congenital malformations and to lead to the concept that good metabolic control is a desirable goal prior to conception and in the early weeks of pregnancy.

A potential use for the GHb assay is for the diagnosis of diabetes. This test would have advantages over fasting, postprandial glucose values, and GTT in that it can be performed without patient preparation and in the nonfasting state. When children are tested, venipuncture can be substituted with a capillary blood sample. Unfortunately, although an elevated GHb is indicative of hyperglycemia, a normal GHb does not exclude mild diabetes or IGT. The American College of Physicians, in a position paper, notes that GHb "may be useful as a diagnostic test for diabetes mellitus in patients with fasting plasma glucose levels greater than 115 mg per deciliter who are not obviously diabetic."

In a recent report, Little and associates (1988) studied 381 Pima Indians, performing simultaneous HbA_{1c} (HPLC method) and modified OGTT (WHO criteria). Of 159 subjects with normal GTTs, 14 (9 percent) had modestly elevated HbA_{1c} values (Fig. 9–4). Of 131 subjects with a diabetic GTT, 85 percent had an elevated HbA_{1c} and 15 percent had a normal HbA_{1c}. This latter group of patients was characterized by much lower fasting and 2-hour plasma glucose values than the subjects with high HbA_{1c} values. HbA_{1c} determinations were relatively insensitive for detecting people with IGT. The authors concluded that HbA_{1c} was a highly specific and moderately sensitive test for the diagnosis of diabetes mellitus. These investigators speculate that if GHb is even-

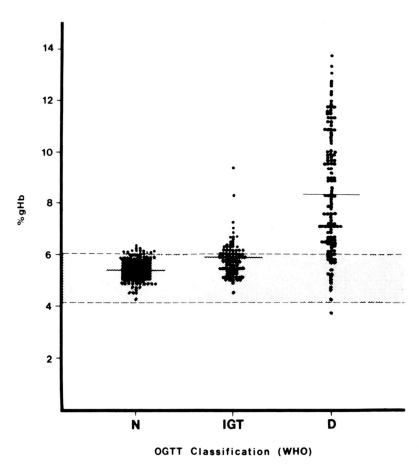

Figure 9-4 GHb (specifically HbA$_{1c}$) levels in 381 subjects with normal glucose tolerance (N; n = 159), impaired glucose tolerance (IGT; n = 91), and diabetes (D; n = 131). Shaded area represents normal range (mean ± 1.96 SD) of HbA$_{1c}$. (From Little RR, England JD, Wiedmeyer H, et al. Relationship of glycosylated hemoglobin to oral glucose tolerance. Diabetes 1988; 37:6. Reproduced with permission of the American Diabetes Association, Inc.)

tually found to be a better predictor of diabetic complications than the OGTT, it would then become the preferred screening test for diabetes.

FRUCTOSAMINE

In addition to the nonenzymatic glycation of hemoglobin, nonenzymatic glycation of serum proteins represents an avenue to measure time-integrated mean blood glucose. The mechanism of the glycation of serum proteins is similar to that of hemoglobin: the formation of an aldimine configuration followed by an Amadori rearrangement. The rearranged product, a ketoamine linkage, is referred to as fructosamine. Johnson and co-workers devised a method to measure the amount of ketoamine-linked glucose on serum proteins. The principle of their method utilizes the property of ketoamines to act as reducing agents under appropriate conditions. Furthermore, the premise of this assay is that the metabolism of albumin, the predominant serum protein, is not affected by glycation, so that the circulating half-life of glycoalbumin is the same as that of serum albumin, i.e., approximately 20 days. The fructosamine assay is not as technically demanding as measurements of GHb by chromatographic and electrophoretic methods. In addition, currently available automated systems may

be applied to the measurement of fructosamine. Intra-assay variation of 2 percent has been reported. Unlike methodologies used to determine glycation of other proteins, fructosamine is not affected by fluctuations in the ambient glucose concentration (Table 9–11).

Normal values for fructosamine have been reported in different studies. One study from New Zealand reports fructosamine measured in 30 healthy volunteers and 42 subjects with Type I diabetes. In the control population, fructosamine levels range from 1.28 to 1.76 mmol per liter with a median value of 1.52 mmol per liter. In the diabetic population, fructosamine ranged from 1.62 to 2.79 mmol per liter with a median value of 2.28 mmol per liter. The investigators also found a highly significant correlation (r = 0.82; $P < 0.001$) between fructosamine and HbA$_{1c}$ values in these groups.

In a more recent report, these same investigators modified their assay, which resulted in a 0.8 mmol per liter increase in the average fructosamine level. They report a range of 1.87 to 2.87 mmol per liter with a median value of 2.37 mmol per liter in a group of 502 control subjects (Fig. 9–5). In a group of 115 subjects with Type II diabetes, fructosamine levels ranged from 2.20 to 5.22 mmol per liter with a median value of 3.02 mmol per liter with this assay. The procedure was modified to reduce batch-to-batch variation in the reducing activity

TABLE 9–11 Glycosylated Serum Protein (Fructosamine)

Method	Glycosylated protein is isolated from serum or plasma by affinity chromatography. It is then eluted with sorbitol and quantitated by nephelometry.
Normal	1.5–2.6% of total serum albumin 1.87–2.87 mmol/L
Uses	Assessment of glycemic control in patients with diabetes over the preceding 1–3 weeks. May be particularly helpful in pregnant patients, patients with diabetes and hemoglobinopathies, patients with Type I diabetes on intensive insulin therapy regimens, and patients with uremia.
Problems	Assay is not valid if total serum albumin is ≤3.0 g/L*. The test is also subject to interference by the presence of heparin, hyperbilirubinemia, and hyperuricemia.

* A fructosamine/albumin index (FAI) has been proposed (McCance et al 1987):

$$FAI = \frac{fructosamine\ mmol/L\ \times\ 100}{albumin\ g/L}$$

of different human albumin preparations. In addition, the pH was modified to minimize interference from glucose and other analytes.

A very recent study from the U.S. (Negoro et al, 1988) compared fructosamine to HbA_{1c} in 145 normal and diabetic subjects who were 20 to 86 years old. The mean fructosamine in the normal group was 2.22 ± 0.02 mmol per liter versus a mean of 3.09 ± 0.08 mmol per liter in the diabetic group ($P < 0.001$). Fructosamine

levels also correlated well with other measures: r = 0.73 with FPG, r = 0.76 with GHb, and r = 0.80 with glycosylated albumin (Fig. 9–6). They found fructosamine measurements were not affected by hyperlipidemia, opiates, or aging and were minimally affected by chronic illness.

Since fructosamine is highly sensitive to acute metabolic deterioration (periods of 1 to 3 weeks), it may have advantages over GHb in certain clinical situations. This would include pregnancy and possibly the monitoring of patients on intensive insulin therapy regimens. Fructosamine may also be preferred over GHb in patients with sickle cell trait or other hemoglobinopathies. Further studies will be needed to determine the ultimate value of this test in the clinical management of patients with diabetes.

C-PEPTIDE TESTING

Evidence accumulated over the past two decades has revealed that human pancreatic beta cells secrete an 86-amino-acid prohormone known as proinsulin. Proinsulin is rapidly cleaved intracellularly into insulin (51 amino acids) and a biologically inactive fragment of 31 amino acids known as C-peptide. Insulin and C-peptide are secreted in equimolar quantities directly into the portal vein. Although 50 to 70 percent of insulin is extracted by the liver, only negligible amounts of C-peptide are subject to hepatic extraction. The half-life of C-peptide is about 33 minutes (versus a 9-minute half-life for insulin), resulting in a molar ratio of C-peptide to insulin of 5 in normal fasting subjects. It has been demonstrated that about 70 percent of C-peptide is extracted by the kidney, and in normal subjects, urinary C-peptide ranges from 36 to 65 μg per 24 hours.

Figure 9–5 Histogram of fructosamine concentrations of 502 nondiabetic volunteer blood donors. (From Baker JR, Metcalf PA, Johnson RN, et al. Use of protein-based standards in automated colorimetric determinations of fructosamine in serum. Reprinted with permission from *Clinical Chemistry* (1985), volume 31, no. 9, page 1553, Figure 3. Copyright American Association for Clinical Chemistry, Inc.)

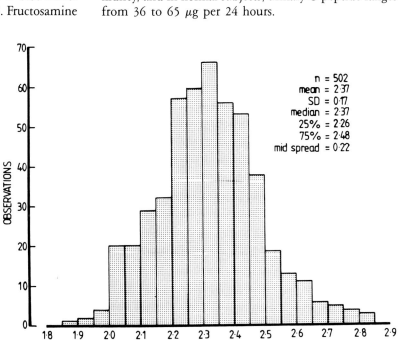

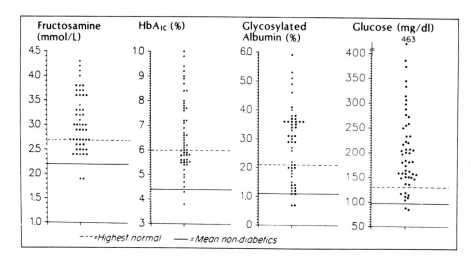

Figure 9-6 Comparison of fructosamine, HbA₁c, glycosylated albumin, and fasting plasma glucose (FPG) values in 53 diabetic subjects. A group of 92 nondiabetic subjects were also studied and their mean and maximum values for each of the four tests are also depicted. (From Negoro H, Morley JE, Rosenthal MJ. Utility of serum fructosamine as a measure of glycemia in young and old diabetic and non-diabetic subjects. Am J Med 1988; 85:360; with permission.)

Since antibodies to exogenous insulin may interfere with the radioimmunoassay for insulin, measurement of C-peptide has become the method of choice for determining endogenous insulin secretion in patients with diabetes. Measurement of baseline and stimulated C-peptide is a useful test to differentiate between Type I and Type II diabetes and to categorize Type I patients as those with (C-peptide-positive) and those without (C-peptide-negative) any insulin reserve. Studies have correlated the presence of C-peptide with metabolic stability in patients with Type I diabetes. Measurement of C-peptide in Type II diabetes may help the clinician differentiate those patients who are good candidates for treatment with diet and/or sulfonylureas from those who require insulin to maintain acceptable control (Table 9–12).

The classic stimulus for C-peptide has been the intravenous injection of glucagon. Studies have demonstrated that 1-mg injections administered to a group of patients with diabetes result in peak C-peptide concentrations 6 minutes later. Normal subjects have a peak response at 8.7 minutes (range 4 to 15 minutes). Although this test correlates well with C-peptide response to a meal, we prefer the use of Sustacal as a stimulus. This test is easier to perform, eliminates the need to inject a drug, is less expensive, and is well tolerated by patients.

Investigators of the DCCT Research Group reported the successful use of Sustacal to stimulate C-peptide in more than 600 patients with Type I diabetes. They measured C-peptide and serum glucose after an overnight fast. Patients were given 6 ml per kilogram (to a maximum of 360 ml) of Sustacal over a period not exceeding 10 minutes. After 90 minutes another sample was obtained for determination of glucose and C-peptide. In 239 patients with IDDM under 5 years' duration, the basal C-peptide levels were 0.11 pmol per milliliter and rose to 0.24 pmol per milliliter after administration of Sustacal. Not surprisingly, 371 patients with IDDM over

5 years' duration were found to have basal C-peptide levels of 0.04 pmol per milliliter rising to just 0.06 pmol per milliliter after Sustacal challenge. The investigators also noted that a subgroup of adolescents with IDDM had a much sharper decline in C-peptide than did the adult patients with IDDM. Comparable to similar studies, the DCCT study confirmed a close correlation between fasting and stimulated C-peptide levels. However, 19 percent of patients with very low C-peptide values (0.05 pmol per milliliter) did have a substantial increase in C-peptide after taking Sustacal (Fig. 9–7). The protocol for C-peptide testing used by the DCCT is reproduced in Table 9–13.

When the C-peptide test became available, it was assumed that it would be a useful tool to distinguish between those patients with Type II diabetes requiring insulin and those who could successfully be treated with

TABLE 9–12   C-Peptide Testing

Method	Polyethylene glycol is used to remove endogenous antibody to insulin from serum by precipitation. C-peptide is then quantitated by radioimmunoassay. Stimulated values may be obtained 6 min after 1 mg of glucagon is given by intravenous injection or 90 minutes after oral ingestion of Sustacal (Table 9–13).
Normal	Basal 0.5–3.0 ng/ml Stimulated 150–300% increase over basal level
Uses	Determines endogenous insulin reserve. May be helpful in differentiating between Type I and Type II diabetes. May be helpful in determining the proper pharmacologic therapy in the adult with diabetes.
Problems	The test may fail to discriminate between those patients who require insulin for acceptable control and those who may be treated with diet and/or sulfonylureas.

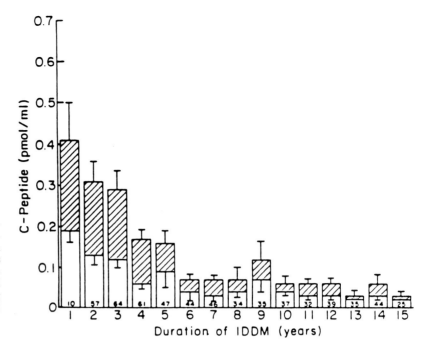

Figure 9-7 Mean (±SEM) basal (*open rectangles*) and stimulated serum C-peptide (*crosshatched rectangles*) levels in relation to duration of IDDM. (From DCCT Research Group. Effects of age, duration and treatment of insulin-dependent diabetes mellitus on residual beta-cell function: Observations during eligibility testing for the diabetes control and complications trial [DCCT]. J Clin Endocrinol Metab 1987; 65(1):30. Copyright by The Endocrine Society.)

diet and sulfonylureas. However, the overlap of C-peptide levels between sulfonylurea-treated patients and insulin-treated Type II patients has led to uncertainty and debate over the usefulness of this test. A recent study by Osei (1986) found that patients with fasting C-peptide levels of 2.46 ± 0.23 ng per milliliter or more responded to oral agents. Patients with lower C-peptide levels required insulin to achieve the same degree of glycemic control. Further predictive value was obtained using a C-peptide/glucose score. The score is defined as fasting C peptide ÷ fasting glucose × 100. The mean score of the control group was 2.22 ± 0.32. Patients with diabetes responding to oral agents had scores greater than 1.0, whereas nonresponders had scores less than 1.0 (Table 9–14).

ISLET CELL ANTIBODIES

Over 20 years ago it was demonstrated that IDDM had features of an autoimmune disease. The presence of inflammatory cells and insulitis in the pancreatic islets resembled similar features of autoimmune thyroid disease. It was not until 1974, however, that pancreatic ICA were described independently by Bottazzo and MacCuish and their co-workers. The patients described in these reports had insulin-dependent diabetes and coexistent polyendocrine diseases. Associations between Type I diabetes mellitus and Hashimoto's thyroiditis, Addison's disease, pernicious anemia, and other autoimmune diseases are well documented and support an autoimmune pathogenesis of IDDM. Although the exact role of ICA in beta-cell destruction is not clear, the test has become an important marker for recent-onset Type I diabetes and prediabetes. Other immunologically mediated measures of islet cell destruction distinct from ICA such as islet

TABLE 9-13 Protocol for Sustacal-Stimulated C-Peptide Test

The patient should receive nothing by mouth on the night before testing in order to be fasting for 8 h.

On the morning of the scheduled C-peptide test, the patient should not take his or her usual insulin injection.

As soon as the patient arrives, blood glucose should be checked by reflectance meter. If the blood glucose value is <250, proceed with the test. If the blood glucose value is >250 but <400, proceed only if urine ketones are negative. If the blood glucose value is >400 or if the blood glucose value is <240 and moderate or greater ketonuria is present, the test should be rescheduled.

A blood sample should be obtained by venipuncture for measurement of C-peptide and glucose. The sample should consist of 10 ml and be placed in a red-topped tube and the separated serum frozen.

Immediately following the collection of the blood sample, the patient should ingest the test meal, which is to be consumed within 10 min. The test meal consists of a commercial mixed meal, Sustacal. The amount to be ingested should be calculated as follows:

Amount required = 20% of total daily caloric requirement of 30 cal per kilogram body weight with a maximum of 360 cal (12 oz or 360 ml of Sustacal).

The test meal consists of 1 cal per milliliter.

A second blood sample is obtained by venipuncture 90 min after the ingestion of the test meal. It should consist of 10 ml of blood placed in a red-topped tube and handled as above.

Immediately following the second blood sample, the patient takes his or her usual morning insulin dosage and returns to his or her usual diabetes care regimen.

Adapted from Diabetes Control and Complications Trial (DCCT). Manual of operations. Accession no. PB8 142161/AS. Springfield, VA: U.S. Department of Commerce, National Technical Information Service; with permission.

TABLE 9-14 Clinical Characteristics and Glucose and C-Peptide Indexes in Type II Diabetic Patients (Mean ± SEM)

	Group A: Oral Agent Alone (n = 16)		Group B: Insulin Alone (n = 16)		Group C: Combined Insulin and Oral Agent[†] (n = 8)	Normal[‡] (n = 10)
	Responders (HbA$_1$,* < 10.5%)	Nonresponders (HbA$_1$, > 10.5%)	Responders (HbA$_1$, < 10.5%)	Nonresponders (HbA$_1$, > 10.5%)	Nonresponders (HbA$_1$, > 10.5%)	
Age (yr)	64.6±4.7	57.1±4.8	62.0±5.7	58.6±2.4	60.50±3	40.30±4.5
Sex (F/M ratio)	7/2	6/1	6/2	6/2	8/0	7/3
BMI* (kg/sq m)	32.5±2.7	30.2±3.3	30.3±2.7	27.1±2.5	30.6±6.1	26.85±1.10
Duration of diabetes (yr)	12.7±3.7	11.8±2.7	11.4±3.6	12.4±2.9	11.9±2.0	—
Daily dosage						
Insulin (units)	—	—	31.5±5.6	41.4±8.3[§]	37.6±4.5	—
Oral agent (mg)	550±25	600±50	—	—	607±196	—
C-peptide (ng/ml)						
Fasting	2.46±0.23	1.93±0.47[||]	1.60±0.28[¶||]	1.50±0.30	1.37±0.25[**††]	1.75±0.20
Random	2.48±0.42	1.93±0.20[||]	1.99±0.41[¶||]	1.58±0.29	1.75±0.46	7.30±1.10
Serum glucose (mg/dl)						
Fasting	151±11	290±31[††]	147±21	333±40[††]	285±29[‡‡]	78±2
Random	158±15	315±30[††]	176±32	326±13[††]	340±30[‡‡]	100±9
HbA$_1$ (%)	8.59±0.54	12.34±0.34[||]	8.13±0.32	12.80±0.90[||]	11.98±0.77[§§]	5.20±0.80
C-peptide/BMI score*	7.4±1.0	8.14±1.2	5.91±0.91	6.01±0.82	6.36±1.67	6.5±0.7
C-peptide/glucose score*	1.73±0.27	0.81±0.12[||]	1.40±0.33	0.71±0.18[||]	0.68±0.19[§§]	2.22±0.32
Glucose/BMI score*	493±54	1,082±168[§]	535±84	1,300±79[§]	1,062±103[||||]	298±17

* HbA$_1$ indicates glycosylated hemoglobin; BMI, body mass index; C-peptide/BMI score, (C-peptide/BMI) × 100; C-peptide/glucose score, (C-peptide/glucose) × 100; and glucose/BMI score, (glucose/BMI) × 100.
† Patients were treated with combined therapy for 6±2 months without improvement in metabolic control.
‡ Values for nondiabetic population are shown for comparison.
§ $P<.001$ (responders versus nonresponders).
|| $P<.05$ (responders versus nonresponders).
¶| $P<.05$ (responders in group A versus group B).
** $P<.02$ (group C versus group A responders).
†† $P<.05$ (group C versus group B responders).
‡‡ $P<.001$ (responders versus nonresponders)
§§ $P<.05$ (group C versus responders in groups A and B).
|| || $P<.001$ (group C versus responders in groups A and B).
(From Osei KO. Clinical evaluation of determinants of glycemic control: A new approach using serum glucose, C-peptide, and body mass indexes in Type II diabetic patients. Arch Intern Med 1986; 146:281.)

cell surface antibodies, cytotoxic ICA, antibody-dependent cytotoxicity, and insulin autoantibodies have been described but will not be discussed.

Pancreatic ICA are of the IgG class directed against cytoplasmic components of islet cells. ICA are not specific and are directed against alpha and delta as well as beta cells. The standard technique to detect ICA employs indirect immunofluorescence (Table 9–15). Serum from the individual being tested is added to snapfrozen cadaver pancreas tissue. Sections are cut and dried onto slides and incubated in antibody-containing serum. The slide is then washed, and a fluorescent dye-labeled reagent is added that will bind the ICA. The preparation is then examined with a fluorescence microscope for the presence of a characteristic pattern of the immunostaining islet cells. Fluorescence may be semiquantitative based on the highest dilution of serum capable of showing fluorescence over background controls. Although Type O pancreases are routinely used, other sources of antigen are from a Syrian hamster cell line, rat islet cells, and human insulinoma cell lines.

The prevalence of ICA in the normal population is 0.5 percent or less. The prevalence and titer of ICA are highest among newly diagnosed patients with Type I

TABLE 9-15 Pancreatic Islet Cell Antibodies (ICA)

Method	Patient serum is applied to sections of human pancreas. IgG antibodies directed against cytoplasmic components of islet cells are then detected by indirect immunofluorescence.
Normal	None detected.
Uses	The test may help distinguish between Type I and Type II diabetes in newly diagnosed patients. Positive ICA suggest a much greater risk of insulin dependence. First-degree relatives of patients with Type I diabetes mellitus who are ICA positive are at increased risk of developing Type I diabetes.
Problems	Assay problems include interlaboratory variability, absence of defined units to quantitate positive findings, and lack of knowledge regarding the nature of the antigen. Although 50–80% of recently diagnosed Type I diabetes patients are ICA positive, the percentage of positivity decreases rapidly over time. False-positive results occur in 1% or less of the general population.

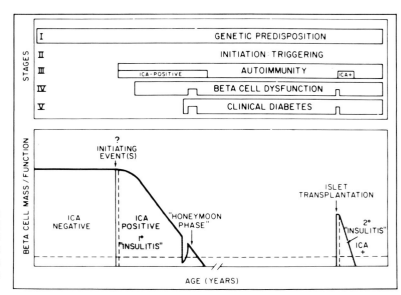

Figure 9-8 Pathogenic scheme for autoimmune beta cell destruction with islet cell antibody (ICA) activity in IDDM. The five stages of IDDM as described by Eisenbarth are also depicted. (From Hale PM, Pasquarello TJ, Vardi P. State of the art: Islet cell antibody tests. Diabetes Educator 1987; 13:381; with permission.)

diabetes and decrease with increasing duration of the disease. Titers are often higher among patients with polyglandular endocrinopathies. Although 50 to 80 percent of recently diagnosed patients with IDDM are ICA positive, at 20 years' duration only 3 percent remain positive. In one study of Type I diabetic patients, high titers and persistence of ICA were associated with lower C-peptide levels and a greater insulin requirement at 30 months' duration.

ICA antibodies are more prevalent among first-degree relatives of patients with Type I diabetes than normal control populations. These nondiabetic relatives with ICA positivity are more likely to have impairment of their insulin-secreting capacity.

ICA may be present for several years prior to the clinical diagnosis of Type I diabetes. Eisenbarth (1986) has described five stages of Type I diabetes. Stage I, called genetic susceptibility, is characterized by a normal beta-cell mass and ICA negativity. Stage II, known as triggering, refers to a time when environmental factors trigger autoimmune mechanism. Stage III, known as active immunity, is the time at which ICA are positive and insulitis is present. In Stage IV there is progressive loss of glucose-stimulated insulin secretion as measured by an intravenous GTT. As progressive beta-cell mass is lost, these subjects develop overt diabetes (Stage V) (Fig. 9-8). These stages were best illustrated by studies of discordant monozygotic diabetic twins who developed clinical diabetes up to 8 years after they were found to have ICA. In a 2-year study of first-degree relatives of Type I patients, 0.9 percent were ICA positive. Of those who were positive, 2 of 16 developed IDDM in contrast to 1 of 1,700 ICA-negative relatives who also developed IDDM. On the basis of actuarial analysis, one group has calculated an incidence of 8 percent per year of IDDM in nondiabetic ICA-positive subjects. Although ICA-negative

Type I diabetes exists, subjects who are ICA negative are highly unlikely to develop Type I diabetes.

Some patients with NIDDM (Type II) will progress to insulin dependency. Studies have found that ICA may be useful in predicting which of these patients ultimately become insulin dependent. In a 60-month study of non-insulin-dependent patients, beta-cell function, as assessed by C-peptide and OGTT testing, deteriorated in persistently ICA-positive patients. Similar patients who are ICA negative had no deterioration in C peptide or OGTT. The group that progressed to insulin dependency and was ICA positive tended to be younger and less obese at the time of diagnosis.

At this time the presence of ICA positivity alone does not predict the development of IDDM with sufficient certainty to permit clinical use of immunosuppressive therapy to prevent loss of beta-cell function. The major problems with ICA assays are the lack of knowledge about the exact nature of the antigen, the absence of defined units to quantitate positive findings, and inter-laboratory variability. The ultimate identification of the ICA antigen should result in a more useful assay.

BIBLIOGRAPHY

General

American Diabetes Association. Direct and indirect costs of diabetes in the United States in 1987. Reston, VA: Center for Economic Studies in Medicine, 1988.

Bennett PH, Rushforth NB, Miller N, LeCompte PM. Epidemiologic studies of diabetes in the Pima Indians. Recent Prog Horm Res 1976; 32:333.

Cooper GR. Methods for determining the amount of glucose in blood. CRC Crit Rev Clin Lab Sci 1974; 4:101.

Davidson JK. Clinical diabetes mellitus: a problem oriented approach. New York: Thieme, 1986.

DCCT Research Group. Diabetes Control and Complications Trial (DCCT): Results of feasibility study. Diabetes Care 1987; 10:1.

Drury TF, Harris M, Lipsett L. National Center for Health Statistics: prevalence and management of diabetes. In: Health US—1981. Department of Health and Human Services (DHHS) Publication No. [Public Health Service 82–1232. Washington, DC: Government Printing Office, 1981.

Fischbach FT. A manual of laboratory diagnostic tests. 2nd ed. Philadelphia: JB Lippincott, 1984.

Marble A, Krall LP, Bradley RF, et al. Joslin's diabetes mellitus. 12th ed. Philadelphia: Lea & Febiger, 1985.

National Diabetes Data Group. Classification and diagnosis of diabetes mellitus and other categories of glucose intolerance. Diabetes 1979; 28:1039.

Nelson RL. Oral glucose tolerance test: Indications and limitations. Mayo Clin Proc 1988; 63:263.

O'Sullivan JB, Mahan CM. Criteria for the oral glucose tolerance test in pregnancy. Diabetes 1964; 13:278.

Pirart J. Diabetes mellitus and its degenerative complications: A prospective study of 4400 patients observed between 1947 and 1973. Diabetes Care 1978; 1:168.

Service FJ, O'Brien PC, Rizza RA. Measurements of glucose control. Diabetes Care 1987; 10:225.

Singer DE, Samet JH, Coley CM, Nathan DM. Screening for diabetes mellitus. Ann Intern Med 1988; 109:639.

SmithKline Bio-Science Laboratories. The SmithKline bio-science laboratories handbook. 14th ed. King of Prussia, PA: SmithKline, 1987.

Summary and Recommendations of the Second International Workshop—Conference on Gestational Diabetes. Diabetes 1985; 34(Suppl 2):123.

Workshop Conference on Gestational Diabetes. Diabetes Care 1980; 3:399.

Glycohemoglobins

Bunn HF, Gabbay KH, Gallop PM. The glycosylation of hemoglobin: Relevance to diabetes mellitus. Science 1978; 200:21.

Dunn PJ, Cole RA, Soeldner JS. Further development and automation of a high pressure liquid chromatography method for the determination of glycosylated hemoglobins. Metabolism 1979; 28:777.

Goldstein DE, Little RR, Wiedmeyer H, et al. Glycated hemoglobin: methodologies and clinical applications. Clin Chem 1986; 32:B64.

Health and Public Policy Committee, American College of Physicians. Position paper. Glycosylated hemoglobin assays in the management and diagnosis of diabetes mellitus. Ann Intern Med 1984; 101:710.

Little RR, England JD, Wiedmeyer H, et al. Relationship of glycosylated hemoglobin to oral glucose tolerance. Diabetes 1988; 37:60.

Mayer TK, Freedman ZR. Protein glycosylation in diabetes mellitus: a review of laboratory measurements and of their clinical utility. Clin Chim Acta 1983; 127:147.

Menard L, Dempsey ME, Blankstein L, et al. Quantitative determination of glycosylated hemoglobin A₁ by agar gel electrophoresis. Clin Chem 1980; 26:1598.

Miller E, Hare JW, Cloherty JP, et al. Elevated maternal hemoglobin A₁c in early pregnancy and major congenital anomalies in infants of diabetic mothers. N Engl J Med 1981; 304:1331.

Nathan DM, Singer DE, Hurxthal K, et al. The clinical information value of the glycosylated hemoglobin assay. N Engl J Med 1984; 310:341.

National Diabetes Data Group: Report of the expert committee on glucosylated hemoglobin. Diabetes Care 1984; 7:602.

Peterson CM, Jovanovic L, Raskin P, et al. A comparative evaluation of glycosylated haemoglobin assays: feasibility of references and standards. Diabetologia 1984; 26:214.

Wacks MT, Starkman HS, Soeldner JS. Hemoglobin A₁c by high pressure liquid chromatography (HPLC). In: Kabra PM, Marton LJ, eds. Clinical liquid chromatography. Vol. II. Boca Raton: CRC Press, 1984:131.

Worth R, Potter JM, Drury J, et al. Glycosylated haemoglobin in normal pregnancy: a longitudinal study with two independent methods. Diabetologia 1985; 28:76.

Fructosamine

Baker JR, Metcalf PA, Holdaway IM, et al. Serum fructosamine concentration as measure of blood glucose control in Type I (insulin dependent) diabetes mellitus. Br Med J 1985; 290:352.

Baker JR, Metcalf PA, Johnson RN, et al. Use of protein-based standards in automated colorimetric determinations of fructosamine in serum. Clin Chem 1985; 31:1550.

Dolhofer R, Wieland OH. Increased glycosylation of serum albumin in diabetes mellitus. Diabetes 1980; 29:417.

Dominiczak MH, Smith LA, McNaught J, et al. Assessment of past glycemic control: Measure fructosamine, hemoglobin A₁ or both? Diabetes Care 1988; 11:359.

Flückiger R, Woodtli T, Berger W. Evaluation of the fructosamine test for the measurement of plasma protein glycation. Diabetologia 1987; 30:648.

Johnson RN, Metcalf PA, Baker JR. Fructosamine: A new approach to the estimation of serum glycosylprotein. An index of diabetic control. Clin Chim Acta 1982; 127:87.

McCance DR, Coulter D, Smye M, et al. Effect of fluctuations in albumin on serum fructosamine assay. Diabetic Medicine 1987; 4:434.

Negoro H, Morley JE, Rosenthal MJ. Utility of serum fructosamine as a measure of glycemia in young and old diabetic and non-diabetic subjects. Am J Med 1988; 85:360.

C-Peptide

Bonser AM, Garcia-Webb P. C-peptide measurement: Methods and clinical utility. Crit Rev Clin Lab Sci 1984; 19:297.

DCCT Research Group. Effects of age, duration and treatment of insulin-dependent diabetes mellitus on residual β-cell function: Observations during eligibility testing for the Diabetes Control and Complications Trial (DCCT). J Clin Endocrinol Metab 1987; 65:30.

DCCT Research Group. Manual of operations. Accession No. PB8 142161/AS. Springfield, VA: U.S. Department of Commerce, National Technical Information Service.

Faber OK, Binder C. C-peptide response to glucagon. Diabetes 1977; 26:605.

Frazier LM, Mulrow CD, Alexander JR LT, et al. Need for insulin therapy in Type II diabetes mellitus: A randomized trial. Arch Intern Med 1987; 147:1085.

Hoekstra JBL, van Rijn HJM, Erkelens DW, et al. C-peptide. Diabetes Care 1982; 5:438.

Laaksa M, Rönnemaa T, Sarlund H, et al. Factors associated with fasting and postglucagon plasma C-peptide levels in middle-aged insulin-treated diabetic patients. Diabetes Care 1989; 12:83.

Osei KO. Clinical evaluation of determinants of glycemic control: A new approach using serum glucose, C-peptide, and body mass indexes in Type II diabetic patients. Arch Intern Med 1986; 146:281.

Islet Cell Antibodies

Bottazzo GF, Florin-Christensen A, Doniach D. Islet-cell antibodies in diabetes mellitus with autoimmune polyendocrine deficiencies. Lancet 1974; ii:1279.

Eisenbarth GS. Type I diabetes mellitus. A chronic autoimmune disease. N Engl J Med 1986; 314:1360.

Gleichmann H, Bottazzo GF. Progress toward standardization of cytoplasmic islet cell—antibody assay. Diabetes 1987; 36:578.

Groop L, Bottazzo GF, Doniach D. Islet cell antibodies identify latent type I diabetes in patients 35–75 years at diagnosis. Diabetes 1986; 35:237.

Hale PM, Pasquarello TJ, Vardi P. State of the art: Islet cell antibody tests. The Diabetes Educator 1987; 13:381.

Lernmark A. Islet cell antibodies. Diabetic Med 1987; 4:285.

MacCuish AC, Irvine WJ, Barnes EW, Duncan LJP. Antibodies to islet-cell insulin-dependent diabetics with coexistent autoimmune disease. Lancet 1974; ii:1529.

Marner B, Agner T, Binder C, et al. Increased reduction in fasting C-peptide is associated with islet cell antibodies in Type I (insulin-dependent) diabetic patients. Diabetologia 1985; 28:875.

Riley WJ, Winter WE, Maclaren NK. Identification of insulin-dependent diabetes mellitus before the onset of clinical symptoms. J Pediatr 1988; 112:314.

Srikanta S, Ganda OP, Eisenbarth GS, et al. Islet-cell antibodies and beta-cell function in monozygotic triplets and twins initially discordant for Type I diabetes mellitus. N Engl J Med 1983; 308:322.

10

Hypoglycemia

Richard C. Eastman, M.D., F.A.C.P.
C. Ronald Kahn, M.D.

Abnormally low levels of blood glucose, or hypoglycemia, may occur in a spectrum of disorders affecting the absorption of glucose and other nutrients from the gastrointestinal tract, the hormonal responses to the ingested glucose load, the utilization of glucose by peripheral tissues, and the production of glucose from endogenous substrates during periods of fasting (Table 10–1). In the adult it is useful to distinguish reactive hypoglycemia, which occurs after food ingestion, from hypoglycemia which occurs in the fasting state. With rare exceptions, patients with postprandial hypoglycemia have a benign, self-limiting condition. In contrast, patients with fasting hypoglycemia are more likely to have a serious underlying process, and they need detailed evaluation and specific treatment.

POSTPRANDIAL (REACTIVE) HYPOGLYCEMIA

Pathophysiology

In normal humans, ingestion of carbohydrate initiates secretion of insulin and other gastrointestinal tract hormones that control the metabolic fate of glucose. Insulin levels reach a maximum within 30 minutes after carbohydrate ingestion, and by stimulating an increase in glucose utilization by the liver, fat, and skeletal muscle, as well as inhibiting glycogenolysis and gluconeogenesis, gradually returns blood glucose to the preprandial level. The gastrointestinal hormones increase the insulin response to oral carbohydrate, promoting more rapid clearance of glucose.

Patients with reactive hypoglycemia have a functional abnormality in glucose utilization that leads to exaggeration of the glucose changes that normally occur after a carbohydrate load. Several factors may play a role in producing this abnormality. Rapid gastric emptying, either functional or secondary to surgery, may lead to rapid glucose absorption and abnormal stimulation of insulin release (Veverbrants et al, 1967). Such an exaggerated insulin release is characteristic of patients with alimentary hypoglycemia (Yalow and Berson, 1965; Anderson and Herman, 1969; Shultz et al, 1971; Breuer et al, 1972; Johnson et al, 1980; Zaloga and Chernow, 1983). A similar mechanism may apply in some patients with idiopathic hypoglycemia, although more often the release

TABLE 10–1 Hypoglycemia in Adults

Postprandial Hypoglycemia
Alimentary hypoglycemia
Impaired glucose tolerance
Idiopathic hypoglycemia
Insulinoma
Factitious Hypoglycemia
Autoimmune Syndromes
Insulin
Insulin receptor
Non–Islet Cell Tumors
Hormonal Deficiencies
Adrenal, pituitary, thyroid,
glucagon
Liver Disease—Severe
Inadequate Substrate for Gluconeogenesis
Uremia
Inanition
Alcohol
Drugs
Glucose Utilization in Vitro
Red blood cells
White blood cells
Rapid Discontinuation of Dextrose
Infusions (Especially Hyperalimentation)

of insulin does not appear excessive and the etiology is less clear (Groen et al, 1952; Sussman et al, 1966; Luyckx and Lefebvre, 1971).

In individuals with impaired glucose tolerance, the patients tend to have not only an exaggerated but also a delayed response of insulin to a glucose load (Seltzer et al, 1956; Arky and Arons, 1971; Ensick and Williams, 1974). Insulin levels reach a peak at a time when absorption of the glucose from the intestine has already declined. However, other factors must play a role since all patients with delayed insulin secretion do not develop reactive hypoglycemia (Luyckx, 1971; Hoefeldt, 1972).

In many cases patients will have significant, symptomatic hypoglycemia without a history of surgery for ulcer disease and without impaired glucose tolerance (Conn and Seltzer, 1955; Zieve et al, 1964; Anderson and Herman, 1969; Freinkel and Metzgher, 1969; Permutt et al, 1973). Additionally, patients may have postprandial symptoms without clear-cut evidence of low blood glucose, an entity that has been termed the idiopathic postprandial syndrome (Charles et al, 1981). Increases in sympathetic activity may contribute to the postprandial symptoms of autonomic excess experienced by patients during glucose tolerance testing or during ingestion of foods with a high sucrose content (Welle et al, 1980; Rowe et al, 1981; Landsberg and Young, 1983).

Recent studies have increased our understanding of the hormonal mechanisms that augment insulin release in response to an oral carbohydrate load. Two hormones that may play a role in reactive hypoglycemia are gastric inhibitory peptide (GIP) and enteroglucagon. GIP increases the insulin response to ingested carbohydrate and other nutrients. The response is greater than normal in patients with duodenal ulcer disease (Creutzfeldt et al, 1977), after vagotomy (Becker et al, 1978), and in non-obese patients with Type II diabetes (Ross and Dupre, 1977). GIP has been implicated in the hyperinsulinemia of mild non-insulin-dependent diabetes (May and Williams, 1978). These data suggest a possible etiologic role for GIP in reactive hypoglycemia in certain patients with impaired glucose tolerance and in patients with alimentary hypoglycemia.

Enteroglucagon is distributed widely throughout the mucosa of the intestinal tract. The concentration increases following oral glucose administration and is higher following vagotomy and pyloroplasty. A particularly exaggerated response is seen in patients with the dumping syndrome (Bloom et al, 1972). The increased enteroglucagon response seen in patients with reactive hypoglycemia may contribute to the fall in blood glucose following oral glucose challenge by competing for glucagon receptors in the liver. This action thereby impairs the glycogenolytic effect of pancreatic glucagon, leading to an exaggerated hypoglycemic phase (Walsh, 1978).

Diagnosis

Physicians frequently evaluate patients with symptoms that occur in the postprandial state. Often the patient is self-referred and suspects, on the basis of writings in the lay literature or hearsay that the symptoms are due to hypoglycemia. Although many patients with postprandial symptoms have "nonhypoglycemia," or a psychiatric disorder (Cahill and Soeldner, 1974; Yager and Young 1974; Gastineau, 1983), a minority of these patients have disorders of glucose homeostasis that can be recognized through appropriate testing. Within this group are patients with self-limited, functional abnormalities of glucose homeostasis that lead to postprandial symptoms of sympathoadrenal activity and, less commonly, to symptoms of neuroglycopenia. These patients may have reactive hypoglycemia induced by low carbohydrate diets, due to impaired glucose tolerance or mild diabetes, or due to alimentary hypoglycemia. Less common causes of reactive hypoglycemia are hypothyroidism, adrenal insufficiency, or insulinomas. Patients with these disorders may experience postprandial symptoms of hypoglycemia, as well as fasting hypoglycemia, and should not be overlooked because of

the high prevalence of nonhypoglycemia in patients with similar complaints. Correct interpretation of properly performed diagnostic tests is the only way to reliably diagnose or rule out these causes of reactive hypoglycemia.

In 1973 the American Diabetes Association, the Endocrine Society, and the American Medical Association issued a joint statement concerning the diagnosis and treatment of hypoglycemia (Statement on Hypoglycemia, 1973). It recommended that before any patient is treated for hypoglycemia, the following conditions should be met: the occurrence of hypoglycemia should be documented; the patient's symptoms should be shown to be due to low blood glucose; the symptoms should be relieved by ingestion of food or sugar; and the particular kind of hypoglycemia that is producing the symptoms should be established. The application of these principles to the evaluation of patients with postprandial symptoms will be discussed in this section.

Documenting the Occurrence of Low Levels of Blood Glucose

The diagnosis of all forms of hypoglycemia is based on the concentration of glucose in whole blood or plasma. Both stimulatory and suppressive tests are used under controlled conditions to establish the diagnosis. For reactive hypoglycemia, the oral glucose tolerance test and the mixed meal challenge test are used. Hypoglycemia occurring during spontaneous symptoms is diagnostic but difficult to document in practice. Unfortunately, neither the mixed meal challenge test nor the glucose tolerance test is an ideal diagnostic tool.

Mixed meal challenge tests performed in patients with postprandial symptoms rarely lead to hypoglycemia (Charles et al, 1981; Buss et al, 1982; Hogan et al, 1983). However, the absence of hypoglycemia after a mixed meal does not necessarily rule out hypoglycemia, and some patients with bona fide hypoglycemia may be overlooked by this approach. The glycemic index of different foods varies significantly, and for many foods the blood glucose response is flat, particularly if they are consumed with a mixed meal. Peak insulin concentrations may be lower after certain meals compared with the standard glucose tolerance test (Buss et al, 1982). Additionally, data on glucose and insulin values after different mixed meals in patients with bona fide hypoglycemia are not available. Two patients with insulinomas had hypoglycemia after a mixed meal in one study, but the true false-negative rate of this test in patients with bona fide hypoglycemia is unknown (Hogan et al, 1983). Until such data are available, the absence of hypoglycemia after a mixed meal challenge test should be interpreted with caution. The oral glucose tolerance test remains the test of choice for establishing the diagnosis of reactive hypoglycemia.

The glucose tolerance test is also an imperfect test for the evaluation of hypoglycemia. There is a high frequency of low blood glucose concentrations in normal, asymptomatic individuals during the test (Table 10–2) (Sisk et al, 1970; Jung et al, 1971; Lev-Ran and Anderson, 1981). From 10 to 38 percent of asymptomatic individuals have glucose nadirs below 50 mg per deciliter, a level that is often considered diagnostic for reactive hypoglycemia. In contrast, patients with bona fide hypoglycemia may have glucose nadirs between 50 and 65 mg per deciliter. For these reasons the diagnosis of hypoglycemia should be based not on the glucose concentration per se, but rather on the occurrence of symptoms of hypoglycemia that are temporally related to the glucose concentration and are relieved by food.

The widespread availability of self–blood glucose monitoring has made it feasible for patients to monitor their blood glucose levels when symptoms occur. This application of self–blood glucose monitoring makes it possible to obtain glucose concentrations at the time of spontaneous symptoms occurring during daily activities, rather than during a mixed meal or oral glucose challenge in an artificial surrounding. Unfortunately, there are no published data evaluating this approach to diagnosis at this time. Furthermore, the error of these methods varies from 10 to 15 percent, and some of the strip methods are inaccurate in the low range. Despite these limitations, it is likely that glucose values of less than 50 mg per deciliter occurring after meals and associated with symptoms of hypoglycemia indicate true hypoglycemia. Conversely, if the glucose is repeatedly normal at the time of symptoms, true hypoglycemia is unlikely.

Performing and Interpreting the Oral Glucose Tolerance Test

Restriction of dietary carbohydrate, especially if the fat content of the diet is increased, can lead to exaggeration of the hypoglycemic phase of the postprandial glucose profile in normals (Conn, 1940; Anderson and Herman, 1975; Permutt et al, 1976). Therefore, knowledge of the patient's dietary composition is required to interpret the glucose tolerance test correctly. One approach to this effect of dietary composition is to have the patient follow a high carbohydrate diet for several days prior to the test. In fact, most patients do not require any special dietary preparation. However, some patients with postprandial symptoms are following restrictive diets that are self-imposed or prescribed to treat the symptoms. These patients may have dietary-induced postprandial hypoglycemia. Preparing the patient with a high carbohydrate diet for several days prior to the test corrects the abnormality, thereby missing the diagnosis. A diagnosis of nonhypoglycemia or psychiatric illness may be made incorrectly. For this reason, performing the glucose tolerance test without dietary preparation may help establish the correct diagnosis. If the test is consistent with reactive hypoglycemia and the patient is on a highly restrictive diet, and if other causes of reactive hypoglycemia are excluded, the information is used to promote more rational dietary habits. If impaired glucose tolerance or diabetes is present during a test performed without dietary preparation, the test is repeated at a later date after a period of more normal intake, with a minimum of 150 g of carbohydrate consumed daily for 3 to 5 days.

The 100-g glucose tolerance test has traditionally been performed in patients with suspected hypoglycemia. This dose is most likely to lead to a low glucose value during the test, since the frequency of low blood glucose concentrations increases as the dose of glucose is increased (Sisk et al, 1970). The American Diabetes Association recommends a glucose dose of 1.75 g per kilogram up to 75 g for the diagnosis of hyperglycemic disorders (National Diabetes Data Group, 1979). No recommendations are made regarding the performance or interpretation of the test when it is applied to the diagnosis of hypoglycemia. Although minimal differences in postprandial glucose values are obtained when comparing 75-g with 100-g oral glucose loads, values obtained after a 100-g glucose load should be interpreted cautiously with respect to the diagnosis of diabetes and impaired glucose tolerance.

TABLE 10–2   Nadir Glucose Concentrations During Oral Glucose Tolerance Tests (OGTT) in Normal Subjects

Duration of OGTT	% of Normal Subjects with Glucose Nadir Less Than Value Indicated			Glucose Determination
	40 mg/dl	50 mg/dl	60 mg/dl	
5 h (Lev-Ran and Anderson, 1981)	2.3	16	—	Plasma
3 h (Sisk et al, 1970) (male subjects)	4	17	37	Plasma
5 h (Jung et al, 1971) (female subjects)				Whole blood
Weight < 145 lb				
Age 20–45	—	—	19	
Age 46–50	—	—	2	
Weight > 145 lb				
Age 20–45	—	—	31	
Age 46–50	—	—	11	

Interpretation

If the plasma glucose reaches a nadir below 45 mg% (whole blood glucose < 40 mg per deciliter) during the test associated with the patient's specific symptoms of hypoglycemia, the diagnosis of reactive hypoglycemia is justified (Table 10–3). The diagnosis of reactive hypoglycemia should not be made in patients who remain asymptomatic during the glucose tolerance test, even when the plasma glucose nadir is below 45 mg%, since glucose nadirs in this range occur in healthy, asymptomatic controls (see Table 10–2). If the plasma glucose nadir is above 65 mg per deciliter, the diagnosis is excluded.

In normals during experimental hypoglycemia, the counterregulatory hormone responses and the symptoms experienced by the patient are influenced by the rate of fall of the glucose concentration as well as the absolute concentration of glucose. Counterregulatory hormone responses and symptoms of sympathoadrenal activity are likely to be greater if the fall in glucose concentration is abrupt. Therefore, the rate of fall of the blood glucose should be taken into account when evaluating patients for symptoms of hypoglycemia. Calculation of the hypoglycemic index has been proposed to take this factor into account (Cole et al, 1976).

The hypoglycemic index relates the glucose nadir to the fall of the glucose during the preceding 90 minutes (see Table 10–3) (Cole et al, 1976; Hadji-Georgopoulos et al,1981). The index correlates with the insulin concentration 90 minutes prior to the nadir. The upper limit of normal is 0.8 if intermittent blood sampling is used (sampling every half hour and at the time of symptoms) and is 1.0 if continuous blood sampling is used during the test. The index is elevated in most patients with symptoms of hypoglycemia that occur during the test and also in a significant proportion of the asymptomatic normals. During glucose tolerance tests performed on asymptomatic patients, calculated indexes were greater than 0.8 in 146 of 325 patients tested (Lev-Ran and Anderson, 1981). This index, like the absolute concentration of glucose reached during the test, has a high false-positive rate in asymptomatic individuals.

A significant number of patients with postprandial symptoms that are reproduced during the glucose tolerance test have nondiagnostic glucose values. The diagnosis of idiopathic postprandial syndrome (IPS) has been suggested for such patients (Charles et al, 1981). The hypoglycemic index was normal in 50 percent of patients with IPS in one series (Chalew et al, 1984). Symptoms in these cases are not due to neuroglycopenia but are nevertheless related to the ingestion of glucose. Measurements of the concentrations of counterregulatory hormones during the test may identify these patients. Concentrations of plasma cortisol are elevated in some patients at the time of the glucose nadir, although the overlap with the normal range is great (Hoefeldt et al, 1972, 1975b; Anthony et al, 1973). Measurement of the concentrations of epinephrine at the time of the glucose nadir appears to provide the clearest separation between symptomatic and asymptomatic individuals (Chalew et al, 1984). Mean values were 458 pg per milliliter in symptomatic patients with IPS, compared with 72 pg per milliliter in normal controls. Clear separation was seen

---

TABLE 10–3   Diagnostic Criteria for Reactive Hypoglycemia

Reactive Hypoglycemia
  Plasma glucose nadir < 45 mg/dl (whole blood glucose < 40 ml/dl)
                              AND
  The patient's symptoms of hypoglycemia (e.g., confusion, drowsiness, sweating, hunger) occur during the test.

Possible Reactive Hypoglycemia
  Plasma glucose nadir between 45 and 55 mg/dl (whole blood glucose 40 to 50 mg/dl)
                              AND
  The patient's symptoms of hypoglycemia occur during the test.
                              AND
  Hypoglycemia index > 0.8 (intermittent blood glucose sampling during the glucose tolerance test). The hypoglycemic index is calculated using the following formula (Cole et al, 1976):

$$\text{Hypoglycemic index} = \frac{\text{Glucose 90 min prior to glucose nadir in mg/dl} - \text{Glucose at the nadir in mg/dl}}{\text{Glucose at nadir in mg/dl}}$$

Hypoglycemia Unlikely
  Plasma glucose nadir greater than 55 mg/dl
                              OR
  Patient asymptomatic, regardless of glucose nadir

between the symptomatic and the asymptomatic groups. In each case the symptomatic patients had peak values in excess of 250 pg per milliliter.

Establishing the Cause of the Patient's Hypoglycemia (Figure 1)

Patients with reactive hypoglycemia induced by low-carbohydrate diets are recognized by the worsening of their symptoms with low-carbohydrate, high-protein diets (often prescribed for the same condition they induce). In some cases, impaired glucose tolerance develops and is reversible with normalization of the diet (Anderson and Herman, 1975).

Alimentary hypoglycemia is a form of reactive hypoglycemia due to exaggerated insulin responses to oral carbohydrate. Insulin concentrations are typically in excess of 300 µU per milliliter during the glucose tolerance test, and symptoms occur within 3 hours of the glucose load (Table 10-4) (Yalow and Berson, 1965; Veverbrants, 1969; Anderson and Herman, 1969; Shultz et al, 1971; Breuer et al, 1972; Zaloga and Chernow, 1983; Zaloga and Dons, 1984) A history of or surgery for ulcer disease is usually but not invariably present.

Individuals with impaired glucose tolerance accompanied by late hypoglycemia are recognized by elevated blood glucose concentrations during the test. The insu-

TABLE 10-4   Insulin Assays

Method:	Radioimmunoassay To measure free insulin, samples are treated with polyethylene glycol to remove antibody-bound material prior to radioimmunoassay.
Uses:	Differential diagnosis of hypoglycemias.
Normal:	Fasting 5–20 µU/ml Postprandial < 180 µU/ml
Problems:	1. Patients with insulin resistance due to obesity or other causes have elevated fasting and post-prandial concentrations of insulin. 2. Antibodies to insulin that develop as a result of insulin injection, or occasionally in spontaneous autoimmune syndromes, interfere with the assay. Spuriously high concentrations are seen with assays using double-antibody or solid-phase techniques to separate bound and free hormone, and spuriously low levels are seen when adsorptive techniques (talc, charcoal) are utilized.

lin responses are greater than in thin normal controls, and insulin release is delayed(Seltzer et al, 1956; Arky and Arons, 1971; Ensick and Williams, 1974; Hoefeldt 1972, 1974). In addition to diets low in carbohydrate, stress due to illness, underlying endocrine diseases, and a number of drugs may induce transient carbohydrate in-

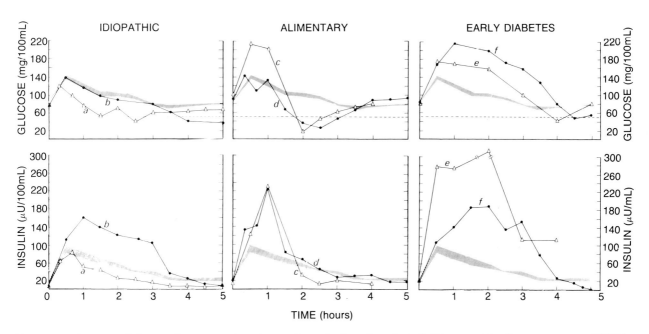

Figure 10-1   Spectrum of glucose tolerance tests in patients with reactive hypoglycemia. *Left*: Glucose and insulin responses to an OGTT in two patients with idiopathic reactive hypoglycemia. Patient A demonstrates normal insulin response with relatively early reactive hypoglycemia, while patient B represents an exaggerated insulin response with late reactive hypoglycemia. (Data for patient A are redrawn from Sussman and Stimmler, 1966.) *Middle*: Glucose and insulin responses to an OGTT in two patients with alimentary hypoglycemia. Both have had gastric surgery and both show early excessive insulin responses and early reactive hypoglycemia. Patient C demonstrates early hyperglycemia, while patient D has normal glucose tolerance during the first hour. (Data for both patients are redrawn from Anderson and Herman, 1969.) *Right*: Glucose and insulin responses in patients with NIDDM with late reactive hypoglycemia. These patients (E and F) show early glucose intolerance with exaggerated and delayed insulin peaks. (Data for patient E are redrawn from Sussman and Stimmler, 1966.) (Reproduced from Eastman RC, et al. Hypoglycemia. In: Kohler PO, ed. Basic clinical endocrinology. New York: John Wiley & Sons, 1986:466; with permission.)

tolerance and should be considered in the differential diagnosis (National Diabetes Data Group, 1979).

Finally, some patients have significant, symptomatic hypoglycemia without a history of surgery for ulcer disease and without impaired glucose tolerance (Conn and Seltzer, 1955; Zieve et al, 1964; Anderson and Herman, 1969; Freinkel and Metzgher, 1969; Permutt et al, 1973). The etiology of the abnormality in the patients remains to be discovered.

Occasionally, patients with hypothyroidism or adrenal insufficiency present with symptoms of postprandial hypoglycemia. Appropriate tests of end-organ function will establish the diagnosis in these cases. Patients with insulinoma may also have reactive hypoglycemia; therefore, patients with reactive hypoglycemia should be evaluated for the possibility of insulinoma. The laboratory evaluation of fasting hypoglycemia is discussed subsequently.

FASTING HYPOGLYCEMIA

Fasting hypoglycemia occurs when there is excessive utilization of glucose by tissues or when there is limitation of the endogenous production of glucose, primarily by the liver. Hepatic glucose production may be impaired by humoral mechanisms (insulinoma, exogenous insulin administration), hepatic parenchymal disease, counterregulatory hormone deficiencies (adrenal insufficiency), and deficiencies in the substrates required for gluconeogenesis (inanition, renal failure). Patients with malignant tumors may in addition experience hypoglycemia due to production of insulin-like substances or, in some cases, due to massive glucose utilization by the neoplasms (see Table 10-1). Additionally, a variety of drugs used in clinical practice will produce hypoglycemia, particularly if other predisposing factors are present (Table 10-5). Rarely do autoantibodies to insulin or to the insulin receptor cause hypoglycemia. Distinguishing among the various etiologies of hypoglycemia is a diagnostic challenge, and it depends heavily on the interpretation of laboratory values. The characteristic laboratory findings in patients with various causes of hypoglycemia are discussed as follows.

Insulinoma

Stimulatory and suppressive tests of insulin secretion have been developed to aid in the differential diagnosis of fasting hypoglycemia (Table 10-6). Of these tests, the demonstration of normal suppression of insulin secretion during fasting is the most important in the evaluation of any patient suspected of having an insulinoma.

Supervised Fasting

During supervised fasting, most patients with insulinoma develop diagnostic levels of glucose and insulin (Khurana et al, 1971; Fajans and Floyd, 1976; Kahn,

TABLE 10-5   Drugs and Combinations of Drugs that Produce Hypoglycemia

Single Hypoglycemia Drugs
  Sulfonylureas
  Alcohol
  Salicylates
Combined Hypoglycemia Drugs
  Insulin and sulfonylureas
  Insulin and alcohol
  Sulfonylurea and alcohol
  Sulfonylurea and salicylate
Hypoglycemia Drugs with Potentiating Drug
  Sulfonylureas with
    Sulfisoxazole or related agents
    Anticoagulants (bishydroxycoumarin, dicumarol)
    Phenylbutazone
    Chloramphenicol
    Azapropazone
  Insulin with
    Propranolol
    Oxytetracycline
    EDTA
    Monoamine oxidase inhibitors (tranylcypromine, mebanazine)
    Manganese
  Miscellaneous drugs
    Para-aminobenzoic acid (PABA)
    Haloperidol
    Propoxyphene
    Chlorpromazine and orphenadrine
    Quinine

Modified from Seltzer HS. Drug-induced hypoglycemia. A review based on 473 cases. Diabetics 1972; 21:955.

1978). However, in occasional patients it is necessary to extend the fast until 72 hours, and even then the level may not be diagnostic. Since insulin levels in as many as 50 percent of patients with insulinoma are within the normal range, it is helpful to calculate the ratio of immunoreactive insulin (in microunits per milliliter) to plasma glucose (in mg per deciliter) (IRI:G ratio) once fasting hypoglycemia with plasma glucose less than 60 mg per deciliter is attained (Table 10-7; Fig. 10-2). Ninety-five percent of patients with insulinomas will have abnormal IRI:G ratios after 14 hours of fasting (Fajans and Floyd, 1976).

TABLE 10-6   Tests Used in Evaluation of Fasting Hypoglycemia

Suppressive
  Fasting insulin/glucose
  C-peptide suppression during insulin tolerance test
  Diazoxide therapeutic trial
  Fish insulin suppression test

Stimulatory
  Leucine
  Glucagon
  Tolbutamide
  Calcium

TABLE 10-7   Fasting Insulin to Glucose Ratio for the Diagnosis of Hyperinsulinism

Uses: Evaluation of suspected fasting hypoglycemia.

Patient Preparation: Patients who are unable to fast overnight should be admitted to the hospital. Outpatients should take precautions against the development of hypoglycemia (including carrying food to treat symptoms if they occur and being accompanied by a responsible party). In most cases the test can be performed safely on an outpatient basis. The patient should not eat or drink after midnight on the day of the test. Medications should be discontinued for 3 days prior to testing, if possible.

Procedure: In an inpatient or outpatient setting, samples for glucose and insulin are obtained at intervals of 4 h, unless the glucose is less than 50 mg/dl on any sample or if the patient has symptoms of hypoglycemia, in which case samples should be obtained at least hourly. The patient should be carefully observed for hypoglycemia during the fast, and intravenous dextrose should be available for resuscitation if hypoglycemia occurs. Provisions should be made to obtain blood glucose results quickly. (A glucometer with good sensitivity below 50 mg/dl is adequate for following the blood glucose but should not be used for diagnosis.) A physician should be available at all times during the procedure, and nursing personnel should monitor the patient during the test. Fasting of inpatients can be continued for up to 72 h. Fasting of outpatients is terminated in the afternoon of the fasting day. Patients with nondiagnostic insulin to glucose ratios return on a separate occasion, having fasted from 6 PM on the previous day, and are studied in an identical manner.

Calculation of Insulin to Glucose Ratios:

$$IRI:G = \frac{Insulin\ \mu U/ml}{Glucose\ mg/dl}$$

Normal: < 0.30 (nonobese)*

In obese individuals the ratio is valid only if the blood glucose is below 60 mg/dl.

$$Amended\ IRI:G = \frac{Insulin\ \mu U/ml \times 100}{Glucose\ mg/dl - 30}$$

Normal: < 50[†]

* Fajans and Floyd, 1976.
† Turner et al, 1971.

In normal males and females, plasma insulin levels decline steadily throughout fasting and by 60 to 70 hours of fasting are below 7 μU per milliliter (Fajans and Floyd, 1976). In normals, the fall in insulin is more rapid than the fall in glucose; thus, after an overnight fast, the IRI:G ratio will be less than 0.30 (Fajans and Floyd, 1976). In contrast, in patients with insulinoma, basal insulin levels are usually increased and the IRI:G ratio is above 0.30. Furthermore, with continued fasting, the glucose falls faster than insulin and the ratio increases.

The ratio of insulin to glucose is potentially misleading in patients with insulin resistance due to obesity or other causes. In obesity, insulin levels may be elevated, leading to a false-positive increase in the basal insulin to glucose ratio. However, if the patient fasts until the glucose concentration is less than 60 mg per deciliter, the ratio will decrease to below 0.30 in most cases. False-positive elevations in the IRI:G ratio may occasionally be seen in normal individuals fasting for 72 hours. Calcula-

tion of an amended IRI:G ratio, which takes into account that in normals (if glucose concentration was lowered to 30 mg per deciliter) plasma insulin would be below 1 μU per milliliter, will help in most cases (Turner et al, 1971). Application of the amended ratio to normal individuals with elevated IRI:G ratios during fasting does appear to normalize the ratio in most cases.

Glucose levels below 60 mg per deciliter may occur in healthy individuals without insulinoma (Table 10–8). Although blood glucose usually does not fall below this level in healthy males during 24 hours of fasting, blood glucose may decline to below 60 mg per deciliter and rarely below 50 mg per deciliter when the fast is extended to 72 hours (Merimee and Tyson, 1974; Fajans and Floyd, 1976). However, low blood glucose levels may occur during vigorous exercise in healthy males. One study reported that 37 percent of males exercising to exhaustion developed hypoglycemia in the range of 25 to 48 mg per deciliter (Felig et al, 1982).

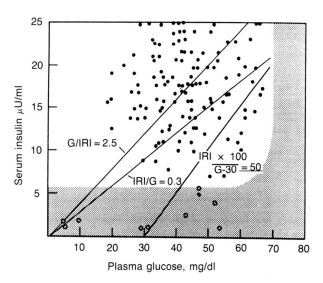

Figure 10-2 Simultaneously measured serum insulin and plasma glucose concentrations in patients with insulinoma (*closed circles*) and noninsulin-mediated hypoglycemia (*open circles*). The lines are the upper limits of normal for each ratio shown: glucose:insulin (G/IRI); insulin:glucose (IRI/G); and the amended ratio (IRI × 100/G−30). Points from patients with insulinoma (*closed circles*) falling below each line are false negatives. It is apparent that false-negative ratios occur most commonly with the G/IRI method and least commonly with the amended ratio. (Reproduced with permission from Service FT. Hypoglycemic disorders. Boston: GK Hall, 1983.)

During prolonged fasting, glucose concentrations in premenopausal females may fall to levels between 22 and 47 mg per deciliter (see Table 10-8) (Merimee and Tyson, 1974). Since insulin secretion is suppressed, the insulin to glucose ratio is less than 0.30 even when the plasma glucose falls as low as 22 mg per deciliter. If there is any question about the diagnosis, the patient may be told to exercise between 70 and 72 hours of fasting. This will lead to a rise in plasma glucose in healthy females with blood sugar levels below 50 mg per deciliter, presum-

ably as a result of increased hepatic conversion of lactate derived from muscle glycogen to glucose during exercise.

Although IRI:G ratios obtained during supervised fasting will distinguish normals from patients with hyperinsulinemia in most cases, there are exceptions worth noting (Dons et al, 1984). In one case the IRI:G ratio remained normal during 72 hours of fasting, and in a second case the ratio became elevated and then subsequently returned to normal after a catecholamine surge.

Monitoring the patient for the development of ketonuria during fasting is of value. In contrast to normals during fasting, patients with insulinomas often do not develop ketonuria (Wolfsdorf et al, 1984). Insulin levels do not suppress as hypoglycemia occurs, and there is continued inhibition of lipolysis in adipose tissue. Free fatty acid levels remain low, and there is insufficient substrate for fatty acid oxidation to occur. An exception occurs in hyperinsulinemic children in whom, despite lower free fatty acid and ketone body levels, ketonuria is frequently seen.

Other Suppressive Tests

Other suppressive tests of insulin secretion have been devised to permit the more rapid diagnosis of fasting hypoglycemia and to avoid prolonged fasting of patients in the hospital setting. Suppression of endogenous C-peptide secretion during hypoglycemia induced by exogenous insulin is one approach (Table 10-9) (Service et al, 1977). C-peptide is excreted along with insulin in excessive amounts in patients with insulinomas, even when hypoglycemia is present. In contrast, pancreatic insulin secretion is suppressed in normals during the insulin tolerance test, and C-peptide levels should be less than 1.2 ng per milliliter. Another approach is to suppress endogenous insulin secretion by administering fish insulin, which is biologically active but is not detected in radioimmunoassays for human insulin (Turner and Heding, 1977).

A trial of diazoxide may be useful if the preceding tests are equivocal (Table 10–10). About half of the patients with insulin-secreting carcinomas and almost all patients with benign adenomas show a fall in insulin levels and improvement in hypoglycemia (Schein et al, 1973). Patients with insulinomas that secrete large amounts of proinsulin may be less likely to respond to diazoxide. Since the primary action of the diazoxide is to inhibit insulin secretion, one would expect a response only in patients with hypoglycemia due to overproduction of insulin. Currently, however, there are not enough studies of other diseases to ensure the diagnostic accuracy of this test.

Stimulatory Tests

A number of provocative tests of insulin secretion have been developed to facilitate the diagnosis of insulinoma and to help distinguish patients with equivocal glu-

TABLE 10-8 Glucose Concentrations During Fasting in Normal Subjects

Duration of Fasting	Mean ± SD Plasma Glucose (mg/dl)
24 h	
Men	79 ± 13
Women	58 ± 13
48 h	
Men	75 ± 12
Women	41 ± 6
72 h	
Men	68 ± 9
Women	41 ± 13

Adapted from Merimee TJ, Tyson JE. Stabilization of plasma glucose during fasting. Normal variations in two separate studies. N Engl J Med 1974; 291:1275.

TABLE 10-9   C-Peptide Suppression Test

Uses:	Evaluation of hyperinsulinism and factitious hypoglycemia.
Patient Preparation:	The patient should be NPO after midnight on the day of the test. Patients who are unable to fast overnight should be admitted to the hospital for study. The development of hypoglycemia during the procedure may provoke angina or arrhythmias; therefore, the test should not be performed in patients with known or suspected cardiovascular disease.
Procedure:	An indwelling intravenous catheter is placed in a suitable arm vein. Regular insulin (0.1 U/kg/h ideal body weight) is administered as an intravenous infusion. Samples for glucose and C-peptide are obtained every 10 min. Intravenous dextrose for infusion should be available during the test, and a physician should be in attendance. The infusion is continued for 60 min or until signs of hypoglycemia necessitate earlier termination.
Interpretation:	Normal: Suppression of C-peptide below 1.2 ng/ml during the test, when blood glucose is <40 mg/dl Abnormal: C-peptide > 1.7 ng/ml
Problems:	1. The normal range of suppressibility of C-peptide should be established for each assay. 2. Antibodies that prolong the half-life of proinsulin increase the apparent C-peptide immunoreactivity. 3. Close monitoring by medical personnel, intravenous infusion, and frequent blood monitoring are required. 4. There is risk of hypoglycemia. 5. Normal results may be obtained in patients with neoplasms secreting predominantly proinsulin.

Adapted from Service et al, 1977.

TABLE 10-10   Therapeutic Trial of Diazoxide

Uses:	As a diagnostic test for insulinoma As a therapeutic trial.
Initial Dosage:	50 mg b.i.d.
Subsequent Doses:	3-8 mg/kg/day (400-600 mg total dose) in 2 or 3 divided doses. Since the drug has a long half-life of 30 h, the dosage should be increased gradually.
Evaluation of Effect:	Once the maximum tolerable dose has been reached, and after at least 4 days at a stable dose, fasting is repeated to determine whether the duration of fasting is increased by the medication.
Adverse Effects:	Fluid retention, gastrointestinal irritation, thrombocytopenia, neutropenia, postural hypotension, hyperuricemia, and hirsutism (particularly in children). The fluid retention responds to the administration of thiazide diuretics, which also may increase the therapeutic efficacy of the drug.

cose and insulin levels during fasting (see Table 10-6). Unfortunately, although these tests may occasionally be diagnostic, the responses often overlap with the normal range, producing frequent false-positive and false-negative results. None of the provocative tests obviate the need to perform fasting, nor has the diagnostic precision of fasting. These tests are not required for diagnosis in most patients but may occasionally be used in patients in whom other studies are borderline and to follow the response to treatment in certain patients with malignant insulinomas.

Oral leucine was suggested as a diagnostic test for insulinoma since it was believed that only the neoplastic beta cell would respond, yielding qualitative rather than simply quantitative differences between patients and controls (Table 10-11). In fact, this was not the case. It is the finding of hypoglycemia during the leucine tolerance test that is most suggestive of the presence of insulinoma since the plasma insulin responses are not markedly exaggerated in most patients with insulinomas (Khurana et al, 1971) (Fig. 10-3). Fewer false-negative blood glucose responses are seen after testing with oral leucine (Fajans et al, 1963). Plasma glucose responses are rarely below 55 mg per deciliter in normal subjects following an oral leucine load. However, children and adults who have received sulfonylureas (including tolbutamide for

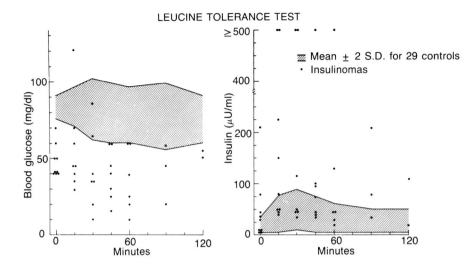

Figure 10-3 Leucine tolerance test. (Reproduced from Eastman RC, et al. Hypoglycemia. In: Kohler PO, ed. Basic clinical endocrinology. New York: John Wiley & Sons, 1986:476; with permission.)

diagnostic studies) may be unusually sensitive to leucine.

Stimulation of insulin secretion by glucagon has also been used for the diagnosis of insulinoma (Table 10–12; Fig. 10–4). Glucagon stimulates insulin secretion from both normal and hyperplastic islet cell tissue (Khurana et al, 1971). Exaggerated insulin responses are seen in patients with insulinomas, and hypoglycemia is less likely to occur than after taking tolbutamide. However, patients with elevated insulin levels for other reasons, such as obesity or acromegaly, may show exaggerated responses.

Intravenous administration of tolbutamide may provoke insulin secretion from both normal and neoplastic beta cells, leading to a marked increase in plasma insulin levels during the first 15 minutes following the administration of the drug (Table 10–13; Fig. 10–5). Most patients with insulinomas have higher plasma insulin levels than thin, young normal subjects given tolbutamide infusions, and as a result, they have more severe and prolonged hypoglycemia (Fajans et al, 1961). Prior to widespread availability of the insulin radioimmunoassay, hypoglycemia was the diagnostic feature of the test. However, reliable insulin assays are now generally available; therefore, the test may be terminated after 30 minutes by intravenous glucose or feeding, while still yielding the important values of immunoreactive insulin. Obese subjects or subjects taking a variety of medications may have exaggerated responses, leading to difficulty in interpretation. False-negative responses are frequently seen in patients with insulinomas.

There is also limited experience with the use of calcium as a secretagogue for insulin. Abnormal responses may be seen in patients with insulinoma (Kaplan et al, 1979).

In summary, stimulation tests with tolbutamide, leucine, calcium, and glucagon may be helpful in selected cases but alone are inadequate for the diagnosis of an insulinoma in most patients. These tests must be performed when the 72-hour fast has been equivocal, when additional information may be useful in following the patient (for example, the patient with a malignant tumor receiving chemotherapy), or for research purposes.

Miscellaneous Tests

The determination of the proinsulin-like components of plasma insulin has been shown to be of value in identifying patients with islet cell neoplasms (Table 10–14). In the normal individual in the basal state, approximately 20 percent of the immunoreactive insulin in blood is proinsulin-like (Gorden et al, 1972). In approximately 90 percent of patients with islet cell adenomas and almost all cases of islet cell carcinoma, greater than 30 percent of the immunoreactive insulin is in the higher-molecular-weight, proinsulin-like components (Gutman

TABLE 10–11   Leucine Tolerance Test

Uses:	Diagnosis of insulinoma and leucine-sensitive hypoglycemia. Following the response to treatment of malignant insulinoma.
Patient Preparation:	The patient should consume a normal diet for at least 3 days prior to the test and should be fasting for 8 h (if possible).
Procedure:	Leucine (oral or intravenous preparation, 150 mg/kg) is given orally, and samples for glucose are obtained at 0, 10, 20, 30, 60, 75, and 90 min. The test is terminated by intravenous infusion of glucose if the patient becomes symptomatic.
Normal:	Blood glucose >55 mg/dl
Problems:	1. Physician attendance is required during the test. 2. Hypoglycemia. 3. False-positives in children and subjects taking oral hypoglycemic agents.

TABLE 10–12 Glucagon Stimulation Test

Uses:	Diagnosis of insulinoma. Following the response to treatment of malignant insulinoma.
Patient Preparation:	The patient should consume a normal diet for at least 3 days prior to the test and should be fasting for 8 h (if possible).
Procedure:	Glucagon (1 mg intravenous preparation in 10 ml of saline solution for injection) is administered as an intravenous bolus over 30 min. Blood samples for insulin and glucose are obtained at 0, 1, 3, 5, 10, 20, and 30 min after the infusion. The test is terminated by intravenous injection of 25 g of dextrose.
Normal:	Peak insulin concentration <130 µU/ml.
Problems:	1. Physician attendance is required during the test. 2. Sudden hypoglycemia may occur in patients with insulinoma. 3. Nausea and vomiting may occur. 4. Hypersensitivity reactions. 5. False-negative and false-positives.

TABLE 10–13 Tolbutamide Test

Uses:	Diagnosis of insulinoma. Following the response to treatment of malignant insulinoma.
Patient Preparation:	The patient should consume a normal diet for at least 3 days prior to the test and should be fasting for 8 h (if possible) before the procedure.
Procedure:	Diagnostic tolbutamide (1 g) is given as a bolus injection over no less than 2–3 min. Samples for glucose and insulin are obtained at 0, 1, 3, 5, 10, 15, and 30 min. The test is terminated after 30 min by the administration of 25 g of intravenous glucose.
Normal:	Peak plasma insulin concentration <130 µU/ml (thin normals).
Problems:	1. Physician attendance is required during the test. 2. Hypoglycemia. 3. High false-negative rate (40%–60%) in patients with insulinoma. 4. High false-positive rate in patients with obesity or other causes of insulin resistance. 5. Dicumarol, salicylates, sulfonamides, phenylbutazone, chloramphenicol, probenecid, and monoamine oxidase inhibitors may potentiate the action of tolbutamide. 6. Venospasm or thrombosis (0.8%–2.4%) may develop at the site of infusion. 7. Hypersensitivity reactions.

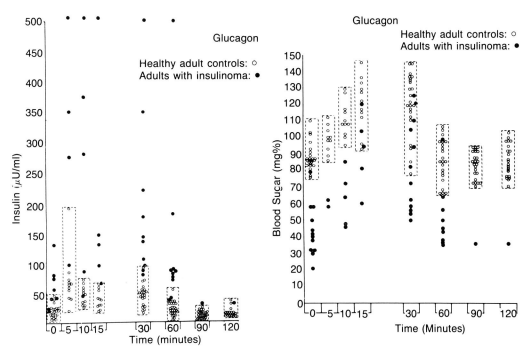

Figure 10–4   Stimulation of insulin secretion by glucagon. (Reproduced with permission from Khurana et al, 1971.)

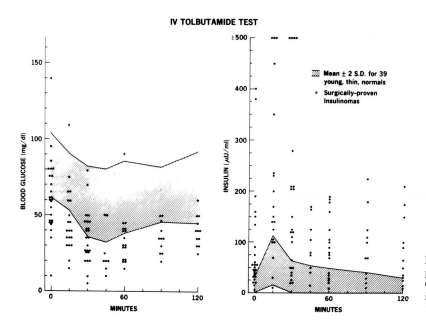

Figure 10-5 Tolbutamide test. (Reproduced with permission from Eastman RC, Rittmaster RS, Kahn CR. Hypoglycemia. In: Kohler PO, ed. Basic clinical endocrinology. New York: John Wiley & Sons, 1986:474.)

et al, 1971; Schein et al, 1973). The finding of an increased proportion of proinsulin-like components is consistent with an islet cell neoplasm, but it does not distinguish between benign and malignant insulinomas.

Recently, radioimmunoassays for proinsulin have been developed which are specific for the junctions between the a and c chains or the b and c chains of proinsulin (Cohen et al, 1985). Twenty patients with surgically proven insulinomas had proinsulin concentrations in these assays that were more than 3 standard deviations above the mean in lean and obese controls. Further studies of the specificity and sensitivity of these assays for the diagnosis of insulinoma are needed (Cohen and Camus, 1988).

The measurement of human chorionic gonadotropin (hCG) and the alpha and beta subunits of hCG may also be helpful in evaluating patients with islet cell tumors (Kahn et al, 1977). Elevated levels of hCG alpha and hCG beta were present, respectively, in 8 and 3 of 14 patients with malignant insulinomas. Intact hCG was also detected in two cases. In contrast, hCG and its subunits were normal in 41 patients with islet cell adenomas. Since it is difficult to diagnose malignant islet cell tumors on histologic grounds before extrapancreatic invasion of tumor or metastases has occurred, an elevated hCG or subunit level may aid in the diagnosis of malignancy preoperatively and provide a tumor marker that can be followed through subsequent therapy (Kahn et al, 1977).

Factitious Hypoglycemia

Surreptitious injection of insulin or ingestion of oral hypoglycemic agents may simulate the other etiologies of hypoglycemia. The patients may or may not be diabetic themselves, and deny insulin or oral hypoglycemic agent abuse, presenting as diagnostic dilemmas (Grunberger et al, 1988). Significant psychopathology is invariably present.

The diagnosis of factitious hypoglycemia is often suspected from the patient's inappropriate affect and the irregular and bizarre pattern of hypoglycemia. The most useful test to distinguish endogenous hyperinsulinism due to insulinoma from exogenous hyperinsulinism is to measure the concentration of C-peptide during hypoglycemia (Table 10–15) (Scarlett et al, 1977). C-peptide is not present in commercial insulins, and endogenous C-peptide and insulin secretion are suppressed during hypoglycemia in patients without islet cell tumors (Table 10–16, case 1). In contrast, patients with insulinoma have elevated levels of both C-peptide and insulin (Table 10–16, case 3).

TABLE   10-14   Proinsulin and Proinsulin-Like Components

Uses:	Differential diagnosis of hypoglycemia.
Methods:	Insulin radioimmunoassay of column fractions after gel filtration. Immunoreactivity of higher-molecular-weight material (proinsulin-like material) is expressed as a percentage of the total immunoreactivity in all of the column fractions. Proinsulin radioimmunoassay
Normal:	Less than 25% proinsulin-like components (gel filtration method). Variable proinsulin assay
Problems:	1. Gel filtration of plasma samples is not routinely available 2. Proinsulin assays have not been fully validated for diagnostic accuracy. Levels in normals and insulinoma patients vary with specificity of antisera

TABLE 10-15 C-Peptide Assays

Method:	Radioimmunoassay To determine free C-peptide concentration, samples are treated with polyethylene glycol to remove antibody-bound material prior to radioimmunoassay.
Normal:	Fasting 1.2–1.7 ng/ml
Problems:	1. Antibodies to proinsulin increase the half-life of proinsulin. This elevates the proinsulin concentration which cross-reacts in the C-peptide assay, leading to falsely high C-peptide concentrations. 2. Normal ranges must be established for each assay.

TABLE 10-17 Insulin Antibody Assays

Uses:	Diagnosis of factitious hypoglycemia. Diagnosis of insulin resistance.
Methods:	Modifications of radioimmunoassay using the patient's plasma as the source of antibody. Enzyme-linked immunosorbent assay (ELISA)
Normal:	Not present
Problems:	1. Low titers of antibody may not be detected in screening procedures but may nevertheless interfere in radioimmunoassays. 2. Differences in species specificity of the antibodies may limit the detection of antibodies unless multiple tracers (beef, pork, human) are used in the assay. 3. Saturation of antibodies by insulin may prevent detection by radioimmunoassay techniques. ELISA assays may detect antibodies in the presence of insulin.

Interpretation of C-peptide levels may, however, pose some problems (Horwitz et al, 1976). Although insulin does not cross-react in the C-peptide assays, proinsulin may be detected as C-peptide immunoreactivity due to cross-reactivity in the assay. Insulin antibodies, usually present in patients who have used insulin for several months, bind proinsulin and prolong its half-life; in insulin-dependent diabetic individuals and patients with factitious hypoglycemia, as much as 80 percent of the circulating C-peptide immunoreactivity may be proinsulin. In these cases, determination of the concentration of free C-peptide should be low (Table 10–16, case 2).

Extremely high circulating levels of insulin are frequently encountered in patients with factitious hypoglycemia and should be a clue to the diagnosis (Table 10–16, cases 1 and 2). High levels may result from the injection of a bolus of insulin or from interference of anti-insulin antibodies in the insulin assay (see Table 10–4). Insulin levels of 1000 μU per milliliter or more are frequently encountered, whereas patients with insulinomas rarely have insulin levels in excess of 200 μU per milliliter.

The detection of anti-insulin antibodies in a patient who claims never to have received insulin should suggest the possibility of surreptitious insulin use (Table 10–17). However, antibodies may develop spontaneously. Conversely, the absence of antibodies to insulin does not exclude the diagnosis of factitious hypoglycemia, since antibodies may not develop in the first 2 months of in-

sulin use and are less likely to develop in patients using pure pork or human insulin.

Determination of the binding specificity of anti-insulin antibodies, available in research laboratories, may aid in distinguishing insulin autoimmune antibodies (IAA) from insulin antibodies (IA) due to exogenous insulin (Table 10–18) (Wilkin and Nicholson, 1984; Wilkin et al, 1985; Diaz and Wilkin, 1987). Sera from patients with insulin autoimmunity bind only with human insulin in half of the cases.

Factitious hypoglycemia due to ingestion of oral hypoglycemic agents may also occur. Insulin and C-peptide are elevated. A white precipitate of carboxytolbutamide may appear following acidification of the urine of patients who have ingested tolbutamide. Blood levels of the oral hypoglycemic agents will confirm the diagnosis.

AUTOIMMUNE SYNDROMES AND HYPOGLYCEMIA

Hypoglycemia has been reported in patients with autoimmune syndromes associated with the development of antibodies to insulin (IAA) and to the insulin receptor (AIRA) (see Table 10–18) (Hirata et al, 1974; Hirata, 1983; Anderson et al, 1978; Blackshear et al, 1983). The

TABLE 10-16 Insulin Glucose and C-Peptide Levels in Patients with Factitious Hypoglycemia and Insulinoma

Case	Glucose (mg/dl)	Insulin (μU/ml)	Total CPR (ng/ml)	Free CPR (ng/ml)	AB
1. Factitious	39	5,067	0.56	—	Negative
2. Factitious	25	4,600	4.41	0.65	Positive
3. Insulinoma	40	97	12.0	—	Negative

CPR = C-Peptide immunoreactivity ng/ml (<1.0–2.5 ng/ml normal)
AB = Anti-insulin antibodies
Adapted from Scarlett JA, Mako ME, Rubenstein AH, et al: Factitious hypoglycemia. Diagnosis by measurement of serum C-peptide immunoreactivity and insulin binding antibodies. N Engl J Med 1977; 297:1029.

TABLE 10–18   Antibody Types in Patients with Hypoglycemia

Type	Specificity		
	H	B	P
IA—Antibodies to exogenous insulin	+	+	+
IAA—Insulin autoimmune antibodies	+	v	v
AIRA—Anti-insulin receptor antibodies	−	−	−

H = Human insulin   + = Cross-reactivity
B = Beef insulin   − = No cross-reactivity
P = Pork insulin   v = Variable cross-reactivity

spontaneous development of anti-insulin antibodies has been reported primarily in Japanese patients who are taking methimazole for the control of hyperthyroidism, although other drugs have been implicated. Antibodies may lead to reactive hypoglycemia by delaying the onset of action of insulin after ingestion of a meal. Fasting hypoglycemia may also occur because of prolongation of the duration of insulin action or because of potentiation of the action of insulin at the tissue level (Kahn et al, 1978).

It may be extremely difficult to distinguish patients with spontaneous anti-insulin antibodies from patients with antibodies due to surreptitious insulin use. In both situations, insulin levels may be either very high or undetectable in insulin assays, depending on the technique used to separate bound from free hormone in the particular assay (see Table 10–4). In addition, antibodies that cross-react with proinsulin may lead to apparently elevated concentrations of C-peptide, owing to the cross-reactivity of proinsulin in C-peptide assays.

Patients with the syndrome of insulin resistance and acanthosis nigricans, Type B, typically present with extreme insulin resistance due to antibodies to the insulin receptor (AIRA) (Kahn et al, 1976; Taylor et al, 1982). The patients have evidence of a generalized autoimmune process, manifested by abnormal serum tests and proteinuria. Hypergammaglobulinemia, increased erythrocyte sedimentation rates, positive rheumatoid factor, and antinuclear or anti-DNA antibodies are variably present. In several patients, fasting or reactive hypoglycemia has occurred during the evolution of the patients' autoimmune syndrome, and in one case hypoglycemia was the only manifestation of the antireceptor antibodies (Flier et al, 1978). The antireceptor antibodies may block the binding of insulin to its receptor, producing insulin resistance, or in some cases may activate the insulin receptors and produce the metabolic effects of insulin. Tests for insulin receptor antibodies, available through research laboratories, are necessary to establish the diagnosis.

NON–ISLET CELL TUMOR HYPOGLYCEMIA

Hypoglycemia may occur in patients with extrapancreatic neoplasms by a variety of mechanisms (Kreisberg and Pennington, 1970; Kahn, 1980). Endogenous glucose production may be suppressed by the production of insulin-like substances or rarely by the production of insulin itself. Hepatic glucose production may also be impaired if there is massive hepatic replacement by tumor or if hypopituitarism or adrenal insufficiency occurs through direct extension or metastatic spread of tumor. Glucose consumption by the neoplasms has been proposed as a mechanism for hypoglycemia in patients with large neoplasms but has rarely been documented. An alternative mechanism has been suggested recently by the finding of proliferation of insulin receptors in one case of extrapancreatic neoplasm and hypoglycemia (Stuart et al, 1986).

Most commonly, hypoglycemia is associated with mesenchymal tumors, including fibromas, fibrosarcomas, rhabdomyosarcomas, leiomyosarcomas, and mesotheliomas (Gorden et al, 1981). Hepatomas and adrenal cortical carcinomas are also frequently implicated. The tumors are usually large, greater than 0.5 kg in weight and 5 cm in diameter, and are located in the mediastinum or abdomen, often in the retroperitoneum. Detection is usually easy, and most of the tumors are obvious on physical examination and routine chest radiographs, although occult tumors have been reported.

Assays of sera from patients with non–islet cell tumors with hypoglycemia have yielded conflicting results (Table 10–19). Elevated concentrations of insulin-like activity were demonstrated in approximately 40 percent of the cases described by Gorden and co-workers (Megyesi et al, 1975, 1976). The elevations of the insulin-like activity were quantitated in bioassays and in insulin receptor assays and were sufficient to account for the patient's hypoglycemia. Elevated levels of insulin-like growth factor activity (IGF-II) were detected in radioreceptor assays by some investigators but not by others (Daughaday et al, 1981; Widmer et al, 1982; Froesch et al, 1982; Merimee, 1986). Technical differences in the way the samples were assayed may explain the discrepancy (Gorden et al, 1981, 1982). The failure of all groups to detect elevated concentrations of IGF-like activity may be explained by recent evidence indicating that the IGF-II-like material produced by some neoplasms is more labile than normal IGF-II, probably owing to reduced concentrations of the IGF carrier proteins (Daughaday et al, 1981;

TABLE 10–19   Laboratory Findings in Hypoglycemia Associated with Extrapancreatic Neoplasms

Insulin radioimmunoassay	Low
IGF-I radioimmunoassay	Low
IGF-II radioimmunoassay	Normal
Receptor assay for IGF-II-like material	Normal or Increased

Problems: 1. Binding proteins for the IGFs may interfere with the assays
2. IGFs may be rapidly degraded unless samples are collected in the presence of trypsin inhibitor.
3. The results of radioreceptor assays are variable in different research laboratories.

Merimee, 1986). Production of large amounts of IGF-II mRNA by one hemangiopericytoma that caused hypoglycemia strengthens the evidence that a substance closely related to the IGFs is produced by some extrapancreatic neoplasms (Roth et al, 1987).

Concentrations of the IGFs, determined in specific immunoassays for the insulin-like growth factors, are low (IGF-I) or normal (IGF-II) (see Table 10–19) (Zapf et al, 1981).

OTHER CAUSES OF HYPOGLYCEMIA

Hypoglycemia may develop in a variety of other conditions, including adrenal insufficiency (Wajchenberg et al, 1964; Kahn, 1978a), myxedema (Royce, 1971), glucagon deficiency (Bleicher et al, 1970), advanced liver disease, cirrhosis with septicemia (Nouel et al, 1981), renal disease (Rutsky et al, 1978), and malnutrition (Elias and Gwin, 1982; Santiago et al, 1982). In each of these conditions the insulin concentrations are appropriately suppressed during hypoglycemia. Specific tests of adrenal, thyroid, and pituitary function and measurement of glucagon and liver function tests establish the diagnosis. The finding of a plasma alanine concentration less than 0.1 mM is consistent with hypoglycemia due to inanition.

Alcohol-Induced Hypoglycemia

Alcohol has several effects on metabolism that can lead to hypoglycemia, particularly if glycogen stores are reduced by prior fasting. Infusion of alcohol can induce hypoglycemia in normal volunteers who have fasted from 36 to 72 hours (Eisenstein, 1982). Insulin levels are appropriately suppressed, and glucagon levels are high.

Drug-Induced Hypoglycemia

Hypoglycemia secondary to pharmacologic agents can occur as an unexpected reaction to normal doses of a prescribed drug (idiosyncratic reaction), by accidental exposure to a combination of factors predisposing to hypoglycemia, and following intentional drug overdosage (Seltzer, 1972). Many cases of accidental drug-induced hypoglycemia occur in children who are more susceptible to these effects or in adults receiving one or more drugs known to cause hypoglycemia at a time when other predisposing factors such as fasting, alcohol ingestion, or exercise are present. In the elderly and in patients with underlying hepatic or renal disease, the clearance of some drugs may be prolonged, and toxic levels may accumulate. Many drug interactions are possible, and the physician must always be alert to this possibility, especially when oral hypoglycemic agents are prescribed.

In nearly half of the cases of drug-induced hypoglycemia reported by Seltzer a sulfonylurea was involved, either alone or in combination with another medication (see Table 10–5). Usually a long-acting prepa-

ration that has biologically active metabolites is at fault, and the patients are often elderly, have underlying renal disease, have ingested alcohol, or have fasted. Profound hypoglycemia may occur in neonates whose mothers have taken sulfonylureas during the third trimester of pregnancy.

Quinine, when used for the treatment of falciparum malaria, may stimulate insulin secretion, leading to profound hypoglycemia with elevated insulin to glucose ratios. Pregnant women and patients with severe malaria appear to be particularly at risk (White et al, 1983). Pentamidine isethionate, which is being used increasingly in the treatment of *Pneumocystis carinii* pneumonia, may lead to hypoglycemia (Sharpe, 1983; Ganda, 1984). The quinidine-like cardiac antiarrhythmic disopyramide may also produce hypoglycemia, perhaps through a mechanism similar to that of quinine (Stapleton and Gillman; 1983). Finally, a first-dose interaction between the nonsteroidal inflammatory agent azapropazone with tolbutamide was recently reported (Waller and Waller, 1984).

Spurious hypoglycemia due to glucose consumption in vitro in blood samples, especially with high white blood counts, may occasionally be misleading. Appropriate handling of blood samples will avoid this artifact. Patients who have been chronically infused with dextrose may develop transient hypoglycemia if the infusion is rapidly discontinued. Particularly susceptible are patients who have received hyperalimentation and in whom endogenous substrates for gluconeogenesis may be limited because of illness and malnutrition.

BIBLIOGRAPHY

Anderson JH Jr., Blackwood WG, Goldman J, et al. Diabetes and hypoglycemia due to insulin antibodies. Am J Med 1978; 64:868.

Anderson JW, Herman RH. Classification of reactive hypoglycemia. Am J Clin Nutr 1969; 22:646.

Anderson JW, Herman RH. Effects of carbohydrate restriction on glucose tolerance of normal men and reactive hypoglycemia patients. Am J Clin Nutr 1975; 28:748.

Anthony D, Dippe S, Hoefeldt FD, et al. Personality disorder in reactive hypoglycemia: a quantitative study. Diabetes 1973; 22:664.

Arky RA, Arons DL. Hypoglycemia in diabetes mellitus. Med Clin North Am 1971; 55:919.

Becker HD, Arnold R, Borger HW, et al. Effect of selective proximal vagotomy on serum concentration of GIP, insulin and gastrin in duodenal ulcer patients. Gastroenterology 1978; 74:1007.

Blackshear PJ, Rotner IIE, Krisuciunas KAM, et al. Reactive hypoglycemia and insulin autoantibodies in drug-induced lupus erythematosus. Ann Intern Med 1983; 99:182.

Bleicher SG, Levy LF, Zarowitz H, et al. Glucagon deficiency hypoglycemia: A new syndrome. Clin Res 1970; 18:355.

Bloom SR, Royston CMS, Thomson JPS. Enteroglucagon release in the dumping syndrome. Lancet 1972; 2:789.

Breuer RI, Moses H III, Hagen TC, et al. Gastric operations and glucose homeostasis. Gastroenterology 1972; 62:1109.

Buss RW, Kansal PC, Roddam RF, et al. Mixed meal tolerance test and reactive hypoglycemia. Horm Metab Res 1982; 14:2871.

Cahill GF Jr, Soeldner JS. A non-editorial on non-hypoglycemia. N Engl J Med 1974; 291:905.

Chalew SA, McLaughlin JV, Mersey JH, et al. The use of the plasma epinephrine response in the diagnosis of idiopathic postprandial syndrome. JAMA 1984; 251:612.

Charles MA, Hoefeldt F, Shackleford A, et al. Comparison of oral glucose tolerance tests and mixed meals in patients with apparent idiopathic postabsorptive hypoglycemia. Absence of hypoglycemia with meals. Diabetes 1981; 30:465.

Cohen RM, Given BD, Licinio J, et al. Proinsulin radioimmunoassays in the evaluation of insulinomas and familial hyperproinsulinemia. Metabolism 1986; 35:1137.

Cohen RM, Camus F. Update on insulinomas or the case of the missing (pro) insulinoma. Diabetes Care 1988; 11:506.

Cole RA, Benedict W, Margolis S, et al. Blood glucose monitoring in symptomatic hypoglycemia. Diabetes 1976; 25:984.

Conn JW. Interpretation of the glucose tolerance test. The necessity of a standard preparatory diet. Am J Med Sci 1940; 199:555.

Conn JW, Seltzer HS. Spontaneous hypoglycemia. Am J Med 1955; 19:460.

Creutzfeldt W, Ebert R, Arnold R, et al. Serum gastric inhibitory polypeptide response in patients with duodenal ulcer. Gastroenterology 1977; 72:814.

Daughaday WH, Trivedi B, Kapadia M. Measurement of insulin-like growth factor II by a specific radioreceptor assay in serum of normal individuals, patients with abnormal growth hormone secretion and patients with tumor-associated hypoglycemia. J Clin Endocrinol Metab 1981; 53:289.

Diaz JL, Wilkin T. Differences in epitope restriction of autoantibodies to native human insulin (IAA) and antibodies to heterologous insulin (IA). Diabetes 1987; 36:66.

Dons R, Hodge J, Ginsberg B, et al. Anomalous glucose and insulin responses to fasting in insulinoma patients: caveats for diagnosis. Presented at the 7th International Congress for Endocrinology, Quebec City, 1984 (abs. #612).

Eastman RC, Rittmaster R, Kahn CR. Hypoglycemia. In: Kohler PO, ed. Basic clinical endocrinology. New York: John Wiley and Sons, 1986.

Eisenstein AB. Nutritional and metabolic effects of alcohol. J Am Diet Assoc 1982; 81:247.

Elias AN, Gwin UP. Glucose-resistant hypoglycemia in inanition. Arch Intern Med 1982; 142:743.

Ensick JW, Williams RH. Disorders causing hypoglycemia. In: Williams RH, ed. Textbook on endocrinology. Philadelphia: WB Saunders, 1974:627.

Fajans SS, Floyd JC. Fasting hypoglycemia in adults. N Engl J Med 1976; 294:766.

Fajans SS, Knopf RF, Floyd JC Jr, et al. The experimental induction in man of sensitivity to leucine hypoglycemia. J Clin Invest 1963; 42:216.

Fajans SS, Schneider JM, Schteingart DE, et al. The diagnostic value of sodium to tolbutamide in hypoglycemic states. J Clin Endocrinol 1961; 21:371.

Felig P, Cherif A, Minagawa A. Hypoglycemia during prolonged exercise in normal men. N Engl J Med 1982; 306:895.

Flier JS, Car RS, Muggeo M, et al. The evolving clinical course of patients with insulin receptor antibodies: spontaneous remission or receptor proliferation with hypoglycemia. J Clin Enocrinol Metab 1978; 47:985.

Freinkel N, Metzgher BE. Oral glucose tolerance and hypoglycemias in the fed state. N Engl J Med 1969; 280:820.

Froesch ER, Zapf J, Widmer V. Hypoglycemia associated with non-islet cell tumor and insulin-like growth factors [letter]. N Engl J Med 1982; 306:1178.

Ganda OP. Pentamidine and hypoglycemia [letter]. Ann Intern Med 1984; 100:464.

Gastineau CF. Is reactive hypoglycemia a clinical entity? Mayo Clinic Proc 1983; 58:545.

Gorden P, Kahn CR, Roth J, et al. Hypoglycemia associated with non-islet cell tumor and insulin-like growth factors. N Engl J Med 1982; 306:1179.

Gorden P, Hendricks CM, Kahn CR, et al. Hypoglycemia associated with non–islet cell tumor and insulin-like growth factors. N Engl J Med 1981; 305:1452.

Gorden P, Roth J, Freychet P, et al. The circulating proinsulin-like components. Diabetes 1972; 21:673.

Groen J, Kamminga CE, Willebrands AF, et al. Evidence for the presence of insulin in blood serum. A method for an approximate determination of the insulin content of blood. J Clin Invest 1952; 31:97.

Grunberger G, Weiner JL, Silverman R, et al. Factitious hypoglycemia due to surreptitious administration of insulin. Ann Intern Med 1988; 8:252.

Gutman RA, Lazarus NR, Penhos JC, et al. Circulating proinsulin-like material in patients with functioning insulinomas. N Engl J Med 1971; 284:1003.

Hadji-Georgopoulos A, Schmidt MI, Margolis S, et al. Elevated hypoglycemic index and late hyperinsulinism in symptomatic postprandial hypoglycemia. J Clin Endocrinol Metab 1981; 50:371.

Hirata Y. Methimazole and insulin autoimmune syndrome with hypoglycemia [letter]. Lancet 1983; 2:1037.

Hirata Y, Tominaga J, Jun-ichi I, et al. Spontaneous hypoglycemia with insulin autoimmunity in Graves' disease. Ann Intern Med 1974; 81:214.

Hoefeldt FD. Reactive hypoglycemia. Metabolism 1975; 24:1193.

Hoefeldt FD, Dippe S, Forsham PH. Diagnosis and classification of reactive hypoglycemia based on hormonal changes in response to oral and intravenous glucose administration. Am J Clin Nutr 1972; 25:1193.

Hoefeldt FD, Lufkin E, Hagler L, et al. Are abnormalities in insulin secretion responsible for reactive hypoglycemia? Diabetes 1974; 23:589.

Hogan MJ, Service FJ, Sharbrough FW, et al. Oral glucose tolerance test compared with a mixed meal in the diagnosis of reactive hypoglycemia. A caveat on stimulation. Mayo Clinic Proc 1983; 58:491.

Horwitz DL, Kuzuya H, Rubenstein AH. Circulating serum C-peptide. A brief review of diagnostic implications. N Engl J Med 1976; 295:207

Johnson DD, Dorr KE, Swenson WM, et al. Reactive hypoglycemia. JAMA 1980; 243:1151.

Jung Y, Khurana RC, Corredor DG, et al. Reactive hypoglycemia in women. Diabetes 1971; 20:428.

Kahn CR. Hypoglycemia. In: Melmon KL, Morrelli HF, eds. Clinical pharmacology. Basic principles in therapeutics. New York: Macmillan, 1978a:536.

Kahn CR. The riddle of tumor hypoglycemia revisited. Clin Endocrinol Metab 1980; 9:335.

Kahn CR, Baird KL, Jarrett DB, et al. Direct demonstration that receptor cross linking or aggregation is important in insulin action. Proc Natl Acad Sci USA 1978b; 75:4209.

Kahn CR, Flier JS, Bar RS, et al. The syndromes of insulin resistance and acanthosis nigricans: insulin-receptor disorders in man. N Engl J Med 1976; 294:739.

Kahn CR, Goldfine ID, Neville DM, et al. Alterations in insulin binding induced by changes in vivo in the levels of glucocorticoids and growth hormone. Endocrinology 1978c; 103:1054.

Kahn CR, Rosen SW, Weintraub BD, et al. Eutopic production of chorionic gonadotropin and its subunits by islet-cell tumors: A specific marker for malignancy. N Engl J Med 1977; 297:565.

Kaplan E, Rubenstein AH, Evans R, et al. Further studies of calcium infusion in the diagnosis of insulinoma. Presented at the Endocrine Society 61st Annual Meeting, Anaheim, C. 1979:170.

Khurana RC, Klayton R, Jung Y, et al. Insulin and glucose patterns in control subjects and in proved insulinoma. Am J Med Sci 1971; 262:115.

Kreisberg RA, Pennington LF. Tumor hypoglycemia: a heterogeneous disorder. Metabolism 1970; 19:445.

Landsberg L, Young JB. The role of the sympathetic nervous system and catecholamines in the regulation of energy metabolism. Am J Clin Nutr 1983; 38:1018.

Lawrence AM, Hagin TC. Propanolol-associated hypoglycemia [letter]. N Engl J Med 1983; 309:1327.

Lev-Ran A, Anderson RW. The diagnosis of hypoglycemia. Diabetes 1981; 30:996.

Luyckx AS, Lefebvre PJ. Plasma insulin in reactive hypoglycemia. Diabetes 1971; 20:435.

May JM, Williams RH. The effect of endogenous gastric inhibitory polypeptide on glucose-induced insulin secretion in mild diabetes. Diabetes 1978; 27:849.

Megyesi K, Kahn CR, Roth J, et al. Circulating NSILA-s in man: Preliminary studies of stimuli in vivo and of binding to plasma components. J Clin Endocrinol Metab 1975; 41:475.

Megyesi K, Roth J, Kahn CR, et al. Radioreceptor assay for NSILA-s

Application to the study of serum NSILA in non–islet cell tumor hypoglycemias. International Symposium on Growth Hormone and Related Peptides. Amsterdam, Excerpta Medica, 1976:127.

Merimee TJ. Insulin-like growth factors in patients with nonislet cell tumors and hypoglycemia. Metabolism 1986; 35:360.

Merimee TJ, Tyson JE. Stabilization of plasma glucose during fasting. Normal variations in two separate studies. N Engl J Med 1974; 291:1275.

National Diabetes Data Group. Classification and diagnosis of diabetes mellitus and other categories of glucose tolerance. Diabetes 1979; 28:1039.

Nouel O, Bernuan J, Rueff B, et al. Hypoglycemia: a common complication of septicemia in cirrhosis. Arch Intern Med 1981; 141:1477.

Permutt MA, Delmaz J, Stenson W. Effects of carbohydrate restriction on the hypoglycemic phase of the glucose tolerance test. J Clin Endocrinol Metab 1976; 43:1088.

Permutt MZ, Kelly J, Bernstein R, et al. Alimentary hypoglycemia in the absence of gastrointestinal surgery. N Engl J Med 1973; 288:1206.

Popp DA, Tse TF, et al. Oral propranolol and metoprolol both impair glucose recovery from insulin-induced hypoglycemia in insulin-dependent diabetes mellitus. Diabetes Care 1984; 7:243–247.

Ross SA, Dupre J. Hypersecretion of gastric inhibitory polypeptide following oral glucose in diabetes mellitus. Diabetes 1977; 26:525.

Roth J, Lowe W, Tang Fui S, et al. Messenger RNA for IGF-II is increased in a hemangiopericytoma associated with hypoglycemia. Presented at the Endocrine Society 69th Annual Meeting, Indianapolis, 1987 (abs. #664).

Rowe JW, Young JB, Minaker KL. Effect of insulin and glucose infusions on sympathetic nervous system activity in normal man. Diabetes 1981; 30:219.

Royce PC. Severely impaired consciousness in myxedema—a review. Am J Med Sci 1971; 261:46.

Rutsky EA, McDaniel HG, Thorpe DC, et al. Spontaneous hypoglycemia in chronic renal failure. Arch Intern Med 1978; 138:1364.

Santiago JV, Pereira MB, Alvioli LA. Fasting hypoglycemia in adults. Arch Intern Med 1982; 142:465.

Scarlett JA, Mako ME, Rubenstein AH, et al. Factitious hypoglycemia. Diagnosis by measurement of serum C-peptide immunoreactivity and insulin binding antibodies. N Engl J Med 1977; 297:1029.

Schein PS, DeLellis RA, Kahn CR, et al. Islet cell tumors: current concepts and management. Ann Intern Med 1973; 79:239.

Seltzer HS. Drug-induced hypoglycemia. A review based on 473 cases. Diabetes 1972; 21:955.

Seltzer HS, Fajans SS, Conn JW. Spontaneous hypoglycemia as an early manifestation of diabetes mellitus. Diabetes 1956; 5:437.

Service FJ, Horwitz DL, Rubenstein AH, et al. C-peptide suppression test for insulinoma. J Lab Clin Med 1977; 90:180.

Service FT. Hypoglycemic disorders. Boston: GK Hall, 1983.

Sharpe SM. Pentamidine and hypoglycemia. Ann Intern Med 1983; 99:128.

Shultz KT, Neelon FA, Nilsen LB, et al. Mechanism of postgastrectomy hypoglycemia. Arch Intern Med 1971; 128:240.

Sisk CW, Burnham CE, Stewart J, et al. Comparison of the 50 and 100 g oral glucose tolerance test. Diabetes 1970; 19:852.

Stapleton JT, Gillman MW. Hypoglycemic coma due to disopyramide toxicity. South Med J 1983; 76:1453.

Statement on hypoglycemia. Diabetes 1973; 22:137.

Stuart CA, Prince MJ, Peters EJ, et al. Insulin receptor proliferation: a mechanism for tumor associated hypoglycemia. J Clin Endocrinol Metab 1986; 63:879.

Sussman KE, Stimmler L, Birenboim H. Plasma insulin levels during reactive hypoglycemia. Diabetes 1966; 15:1.

Taylor SI, Grunberger G, Marcus-Samuels B, et al. Hypoglycemia associated with antibodies to the insulin receptors. N Engl J Med 1982; 307:1422.

Turner RC, Heding LG. Plasma proinsulin, C-peptide and insulin in diagnostic suppression tests for insulinomas. Diabetologia 1977; 13:571.

Turner RC, Oakley NW, Nabarro JDN. Control of basal insulin secretion with special reference to the diagnosis of insulinomas. Br Med J 1971; 2:132.

Veverbrants E, Olsen W, Arky RA. Role of gastrointestinal factors in reactive hypoglycemia. Metabolism 1969; 18:6.

Wajchenberg BL, Pereira VG, Pupo AA, et al. On the mechanism of insulin hypersensitivity in adrenocortical insufficiency. Diabetes 1964; 13:169.

Waller DG, Waller D. Hypoglycemia due to azapropazone-tolbutamide interaction. Br J Rheumatol 1984; 23:24.

Walsh JH. Gastrointestinal peptide hormones. In: Sleisinger MH, Fordtran JS, eds. Gastrointestinal disease. Philadelphia: WB Saunders, 1978:133.

Welle S, Lilavivanthana U, Campbell RG. Increased plasma norepinephrine concentrations and metabolic rates following glucose ingestion in man. Metabolism 1980; 29:806.

White NJ, Warrell DA, Chantkavrich P, et al. Severe hypoglycemia and hyperinsulinemia in falciparum malaria. N Engl J Med 1983; 309:61.

Widmer V, Zapf J, Froesch ER. Is extrapancreatic tumor hypoglycemia associated with elevated levels of insulin-like growth factor II? J Clin Endocrinol Metab 1982; 55:833.

Wilkin TJ, Nicholson S. Autoantibodies against human insulin. Br Med J 1984; 288:349.

Wilkin T, Nicholson S, Casey C. A micro enzyme-linked immunosorbent assay for insulin antibodies in serum. J Immunol Methods 1985; 76:185.

Wolfsdorf JI, Sadeghi-Nejad A, Senior B. Ketonuria does not exclude hyperinsulinemic hypoglycemia. Am J Dis Child 1984; 138:168.

Yager J, Young RT. Non-hypoglycemia is an epidemic condition. N Engl J Med 1974; 291:907.

Yalow RS, Berson SA. Dynamics of insulin secretion in hypoglycemia. Diabetes 1965; 14:341.

Zaloga GP, Chernow B. Postprandial hypoglycemia after nissen fundoplication for reflux esophagitis. Gastroenterology 1983; 84:840.

Zapf J, Walter H, Froesch ER. Radioimmunological determination of insulin-like growth factors I and II in hormonal subjects and in patients with growth disorders extrapancreatic tumor hypoglycemia. J Clin Invest 1981; 68:1321.

Zieve L, Jones DG, Aziz MA. Functional hypoglycemia and peptic ulcer. Postgrad Med 1964; 40:159.

11

Aldosterone Disorders

David H.P. Streeten, M.B., D.Phil., F.R.C.P.
Gunnar H. Anderson Jr., M.D.

L ike other mineralocorticoids, aldosterone has predominant actions on the excretion of sodium and potassium. In general, aldosterone promotes the uptake of potassium and the extrusion of sodium from most cells. By these actions on the secreting cells, aldosterone increases the potassium and decreases the sodium concentration in urine, feces, saliva, sweat, and probably other secretions and excretions.

These actions play important physiologic roles in conserving sodium and in maintaining plasma and extracellular fluid volumes in the face of diminished sodium intake or excessive sodium losses in urine, sweat, stools, and gastrointestinal and other secretions. When aldosterone production is excessive as a primary disorder, the end results include depletion of cellular and extracellular potassium content because of chronic potassium losses in the urine, excessive retention of sodium, replacement of intracellular potassium by sodium, and hypervolemic hypertension. Interpretation of the procedures used to diagnose the syndromes resulting from primary excess or deficiency of aldosterone production requires an understanding of the physiologic and pathologic mechanisms leading to aldosterone secretion by the adrenal cortex.

CONTROL OF ALDOSTERONE PRODUCTION

Aldosterone production is controlled by (1) variations in *renin release* by the renal juxtaglomerular apparatus mainly in response to changes in extracellular fluid volume and renal blood flow; variations in plasma renin concentration lead to appropriate changes in plasma angiotensin I and II concentrations with direct effects of the latter on secretion of aldosterone by the zona glomerulosa; (2) variations in *adrenocorticotropic hormone (ACTH) release*, which have transient effects on aldosterone secretion; (3) fluctuations in *serum potassium* concentration, which directly influence aldosterone production and release; and (4) possible effects on other influences such as beta-lipotropin (Matsuoka and Mulrow, 1980), beta-endorphin (Güllner and Gill, 1983; Kem et al, 1985), and dopamine (Edwards et al, 1975; Carey et al, 1979).

It is important to appreciate that normality of the secretion rate, plasma level, and urinary excretion of aldosterone cannot be determined without reference to the prevailing state of sodium and potassium repletion or depletion, the presence of stress, and the posture of the subject. Random measurements of aldosterone concentration in the plasma or excretion in the urine are difficult to interpret and often valueless in the absence of such information.

Although aldosterone is the only mineralocorticoid secreted in physiologically effective amounts by normal human subjects, disorders of adrenal steroidogenesis, such as that resulting from 11-beta-hydroxylase deficiency, may result in excessive release of 11-desoxycorticosterone (DOC), another potent mineralocorticoid with physiologic effects similar to those of aldosterone. Primary hyperaldosteronism must be differentiated from the effects of DOC excess as well as from mineralocorticoid effects such as might result from endogenous or exogenous hypercortisolism, excessive ACTH activity from the pituitary or ectopic sources or injection, and pseudohyperaldosteronism resulting from Liddle's syndrome (Liddle et al, 1963), a large intake of licorice (Wilson and Goetz, 1964), or fludrocortisone by mouth or DOC by injection.

As is the case with other syndromes resulting from excess of a hormone, primary hyperaldosteronism may be recognized by five groups of measurements:

1. Demonstration of excessive secretion rate, excretion rate, or plasma concentration of the hormone, in this case aldosterone
2. The finding of excessive metabolic actions of aldosterone on serum, sweat, salivary and fecal electrolyte concentrations, mucosal electrical potential, plasma renin activity (PRA) or concentration, and blood pressure
3. Evidence of resistance to suppression of production of aldosterone by intravenous saline loading, sodium retention induced by other mineralocorticoids, reduction of plasma angiotensin II concentrations, e.g., by converting enzyme inhibitors
4. Observations of subnormal or abnormal aldosterone responses to the stimulatory actions of infused an-

201

giotensin II, corticotropin (ACTH), or orthostasis alone or together with sodium depletion

5. Physical evidence, obtained by radiographs, computed tomographic (CT) scans, magnetic resonance imaging (MRI), scintiscanning, phlebography, and other techniques, of a single adenoma or bilateral hyperplasia or other lesions of the adrenal gland(s).

The diagnosis of disordered aldosterone secretion involves three steps that are necessary for appropriate therapy:

1. Screening tests involving clinical studies and relatively simple laboratory procedures
2. Definitive laboratory measurements conclusively establishing the presence of excessive or subnormal production, excretion, or plasma concentration of aldosterone
3. Investigations demonstrating, as far as possible, the cause or mechanisms of the disorder

The known types of aldosterone disorders are listed in Tables 11–1 and 11–2. Aldosterone hypersecretion generally leads to evidence of excessive action of the steroid (Conn, 1955) except in pseudohypoaldosteronism, which has clinical manifestations of hypoaldosteronism resulting from tissue resistance to the action of the excessive circulating levels of aldosterone. On the other hand, subnormal aldosterone secretion usually gives rise to clinical and biochemical evidence of aldosterone defi-

ciency except when hypoaldosteronism is associated with excessive action of another endogenous or exogenous mineralocorticoid.

Although the Glasgow group has mustered evidence that led it to conclude that hyperaldosteronism of bilateral origin (idiopathic adrenal hyperplasia [IAH]) is essentially no different from low-renin hypertension (Davies et al, 1979; Padfield et al, 1981; McAreavey et al, 1983), the invariable occurrence of hyperaldosteronism in patients with IAH and its absence in patients with low-renin hypertension continue to provide strong evidence that the two are separable disorders, albeit both still idiopathic.

SCREENING TESTS FOR ALDOSTERONE DISORDERS

Clinical Measurements.   Hypertension, occasionally severe or malignant (Kaplan, 1963; Brown et al, 1964; del Greco et al, 1966; Clarke et al, 1979), is almost always present, with few exceptions (Snow et al, 1976; Zipser and Speckart, 1978), in patients with primary hyperaldosteronism and in patients under the chronic influence of excessive amounts of other mineralocorticoids. Orthostatic hypotension is found, if carefully looked for (Streeten, 1987), in almost all patients with hypoaldosteronism (Wilson and Goetz, 1964; Streeten, 1987; Thomas, 1984; Kokko, 1985; Schambelan et al, 1972; Findling et al, 1987).

TABLE 11–1   Causes of Hyperaldosteronism

I. Primary
  A. Aldosterone-producing adenoma (APA)
  B. Bilateral adrenal (glomerulosa) hyperplasia, idiopathic (IAH)
  C. ''Indeterminate hyperaldosteronism''
  D. Dexamethasone-suppressible hyperaldosteronism
  E. Adrenocortical carcinoma
II. Secondary to
  A. Excessive renin release
    1. With hypervolemia and hypertension
      a) Renal ischemic lesions: renal arterial stenosis, infarction, necrotizing arteriolitis, intrinsic renal diseases, perirenal constriction, cholesterol embolization
      b) Renin-producing tumors: hemangiopericytoma, nephroblastoma
      c) Aortic coarctation
      d) Bartter's syndrome
    2. Caused by negative sodium balance and hypovolemia: normotensive or hypotensive
      a) Natriuretic drugs
      b) Sodium deprivation
      c) Watery diarrheas, gastrointestinal or biliary fistulas
      d) Excessive sweating
      e) Sodium-losing nephropathy
      f) Blood loss
      g) Hypoproteinemia
    3. Most types of generalized edema
  B. Excessive renin substrate: estrogen excess
  C. ACTH excess: usually transient

TABLE 11–2   Causes of Hypoaldosteronism

I. Primary: Caused by intrinsic adrenal disorders
    A. Associated with hypocortisolism and orthostatic hypotension
        1. Structural abnormalities
           a) Autoimmune adrenal insufficiency
           b) Adrenal destruction or ablation by tuberculosis (Addison's disease), metastatic tumors, bilateral adrenalectomy
           c) Aplasia or hypoplasia, congenital
           d) Adrenal hemorrhage
        2. Enzymatic disorders—Congenital adrenal hyperplasia with C21-hydroxylase deficiency
    B. Associated with mineralocorticoid excess and hypertension
        1. Congenital adrenal hyperplasia with C11-beta-hydroxylase or 17-alpha-hydroxylase deficiency
        2. DOC-producing tumors
        3. Licorice ingestion
    C. Hypoaldosteronism with normal or excessive cortisol and DOC production plus orthostatic hypotension
        1. Congenital enzymatic disorders
           a) Corticosterone methyl oxidase Type I deficiency
           b) Corticosterone methyl oxidase Type II deficiency
        2. Critical illness
        3. Drug: heparin, spironolactone
        4. Hemochromatosis of adrenal

II. Secondary to
        1. ACTH deficiency
           a) Hypopituitarism (sometimes),
           b) Administration of glucocorticoids (long-term) or steroidogenesis inhibitors (e.g., metyrapone, aminoglutethimide)
        2. Renin-angiotensin deficiencies
           a) Hyporeninemic disorders: diabetes mellitus; congenital; renal amyloid; idiopathic; autonomic insufficiency; indomethacin therapy
           b) Angiotensin converting enzyme inhibition: e.g., from captopril, enalapril, or idiopathic

III. Pseudohypoaldosteronism

Serum Electrolyte Concentrations.   Primary hyperaldosteronism is commonly but not invariably associated with hypokalemia that may disappear on a low-sodium diet (Conn et al, 1966; Creditor and Loschky, 1968; Streeten et al, 1979; Bravo et al, 1983). Metabolic alkalosis is also common, and mild hypernatremia may be present. Hypoaldosteronism is frequently associated with hyperkalemia and less frequently with metabolic acidosis and hyponatremia (Wilson and Goetz, 1964; Streeten, 1987; Thomas, 1984; Kokko, 1985; Schambelan et al, 1972; Findling et al, 1987).

Measurements of Plasma Aldosterone Concentrations.   These measurements are useful. Plasma aldosterone concentrations in normal subjects on a high sodium intake (above 100 mmol per day), after lying down for 1 hour, are usually below 10 and almost always below 15 ng per deciliter (Table 11–3A). In individuals whose "regular diet" has been high in sodium or augmented by sodium chloride tablets, 2 g three times a day, for 3 days, plasma aldosterone concentrations above 15 or 20 ng per deciliter while the patient is in the recumbent posture are suggestive of hyperaldosteronism, either primary or secondary (see Table 11–1). The use of plasma aldosterone concentrations as a screening test for hypoaldosteronism has not been standardized.

Urinary Aldosterone Excretion.   Urinary aldosterone excretion may be measured as the acid-labile metabolite, aldosterone-18-glucuronide, or as tetrahydroaldosterone. On a high-sodium diet, the acid-labile metabolite excretion is below 17 to 20 μg per day (Bravo et al, 1983; Laragh et al, 1966; Streeten et al, 1969; Crane and Harris, 1976) and TH aldosterone excretion is about four

TABLE 11–3A   Plasma Aldosterone Concentration

Method

    Blood drawn for plasma aldosterone concentration by RIA after unrestricted (not low) sodium intake for 3 days and after recumbency for at least 1 hr.

Normal

    Plasma aldosterone should be below 15 ng/dl (usually below 10 ng/dl)

Uses

    Diagnosis of hyperaldosteronism

Problems

    Does not differentiate primary from secondary hyperaldosteronism. Intake of Na may be inadequate: check Na in 24-hr urine collected the previous day.

to five times as high in normal subjects (Gomez-Sanchez and Holland, 1981). Excretion of the acid-labile metabolite usually exceeds normal limits in patients with primary hyperaldosteronism (Streeten et al, 1979), but there are many exceptions, particularly in older individuals (Streeten et al, 1979; Bravo et al, 1983; Laragh et al, 1966; Streeten et al, 1969; Crane and Harris, 1976; Gomez-Sanchez and Holland, 1981; Hegstad et al, 1983). The measurement should not be performed unless the 24-hour urine test is complete and the patient has adhered to a high-sodium diet or received sodium chloride supplements (2 g three times a day) for at least 3 days (Table 11–3B).

DEFINITIVE TESTS FOR ALDOSTERONE DISORDERS

Suppressive Tests

Suppressive tests are used for the diagnosis of primary hyperaldosteronism and comprise measurements of the plasma concentration, urinary excretion, or blood secretion rate of aldosterone under conditions of increased total body sodium resulting from sodium loading and/or mineralocorticoid (deoxycorticosterone acetate [DOCA] or fludrocortisone) administration (Table 11–3A).

Intravenous Saline Infusion. Two liters of 0.9 percent sodium chloride solution given over 3.5 to 4 hours and measurement of plasma aldosterone concentration at the conclusion of the infusion, after recumbency for at least the last hour of the infusion, were first used by Kem and associates (1971). Plasma aldosterone concentration fails to fall below 5 (Kem et al, 1971), 8.5 (Streeten et al, 1979), or 10 ng per deciliter (Holland et al, 1984) in most but not all patients with primary hyperaldosteronism (Streeten et al, 1979) and also in many pa-

tients with secondary hyperaldosteronism, such as patients with angiotensinogenic hypertension (Streeten et al, 1979) (Table 11–3C). Our studies on 820 hypertensive patients have shown that this test of primary hyperaldosteronism has a sensitivity of 77 percent and a specificity of 97 percent. It is, of course, very important to avoid causing congestive heart failure, inducing angina, or dangerously aggravating the hypertension by careful observation and appropriate blood pressure monitoring in these patients. These side effects have been rapidly overcome when they have occurred (in less than 1 percent of our patients) by prompt cessation of the infusion and by intravenous injection of furosemide, 40 mg.

DOC Suppression Test. The DOC suppression test comprises measurement of urinary aldosterone excretion on the third day of administration of a high-sodium diet (more than 100 mmol daily) and DOCA, 10 mg intramuscularly every 12 hours (Streeten et al, 1979; Biglieri et al, 1967; Slaton et al, 1969; Biglieri et al, 1972; Biglieri, 1976). Urinary aldosterone excretion fails to fall into the normal range below 17 μg per day on the third day of DOCA administration (Biglieri et al, 1967). In fact, DOCA administration suppressed urinary aldosterone below 12 μg per day in patients with other types of hypertension (Biglieri et al, 1967) or below 8 μg per day in our studies (Streeten et al, 1979). This has been a reliable test of primary hyperaldosteronism except in "indeterminate hyperaldosteronism" (Biglieri et al, 1972), a variant of primary hyperaldosteronism associated with excessive aldosterone production that is suppressible with DOCA (Biglieri et al, 1972; Biglieri, 1976). The test can be simplified by measuring plasma aldosterone (rather than urinary aldosterone) that exceeds 8.5 ng per deciliter between 0800 and 0900 hours after recumbency for 1 hour on the morning after the last dose of DOCA in patients with primary hyperaldosteronism (Streeten et al, 1979). The remote possibility of precipitating or severely aggravating congestive heart failure by this test must be considered (Table 11–3D).

TABLE 11–3B   Urinary Aldosterone Excretion

Method

   After high sodium intake (increased, if necessary, by NaCl tablets, 2 g t.i.d) for 3 days, collect 24-hr urine in refrigerator for aldosterone output, measured as acid-labile metabolite or as tetrahydroaldosterone.

Normal

   Acid-labile metabolite (aldosterone-18-glucuronide): < 17–20 μg/day, tetrahydroaldosterone: below about 70 μg/day.

Uses

   Diagnosis of pathologic hyperaldosteronism

Problems

   Urine collection may be incomplete and patient may not have adhered to high sodium intake (check 24-hr urinary Na output). Does not differentiate primary from secondary hyperaldosteronism. Normal output of aldosterone is lower in older subjects.

TABLE 11–3C   Intravenous Saline Infusion Test

Method

   Plasma aldosterone concentration is measured by RIA after a 2-L 0.9% saline infusion given intravenously over 3–4 hr in recumbency

Normal

   Plasma aldosterone concentration falls below 8.5–10 ng/dl.

Uses

   Diagnosis of all types of hyperaldosteronism

Problems

   Does not differentiate primary from secondary hyperaldosteronism, and has poor sensitivity. Test contraindicated in presence of congestive heart failure and other edematous states.

TABLE 11–3D Deoxycorticosterone (DOC) and Fludrocortisone Suppression Tests

Method

24-hr urinary excretion of aldosterone is measured by RIA on the day before and the third day of administration of deoxycorticosterone acetate (DOCA, 10 mg IM) or fludrocortisone (0.2 mg PO) every 12 hr for 3 days. Alternatively plasma aldosterone concentration can be measured by RIA after recumbency for at least 1 hr before the first dose and 12 hr after the last dose of the drug. Dietary salt intake should exceed 100 mEq daily.

Normal

Urinary aldosterone should fall below 8 μg/day and plasma aldosterone concentration below 8.5 ng/dl after DOCA or fludrocortisone.

Uses

To diagnose primary hyperaldosteronism by failure of aldosterone excretion or plasma aldosterone concentration to fall normally.

Problems

It may be difficult to obtain accurate 24-hr urine collections. The test does not differentiate between APA and IAH.

TABLE 11–3E Aldosterone Measurement on a High Sodium Diet

Method

When the patient has been taking a high sodium diet (100–200 mEq/day) without diuretics for at least 4–7 days, 24-hr urinary aldosterone excretion or plasma aldosterone after quiet recumbency for 1 hr, is measured by RIA.

Normal

Urinary aldosterone excretion is below 17–20 μg/day and recumbent plasma aldosterone below 15 ng/dl (usually below 8.5 ng/dl).

Uses

Screening test for primary hyperaldosteronism.

Problems

Low sensitivity; affected by age

Fludrocortisone Suppression Test. This test, introduced like the DOC suppression test by Biglieri and co-workers (1970), has also been reliable (Padfield et al, 1975; Lund and Nielsen, 1980) and can be used for outpatients provided they can be relied on to take 0.2 mg of Florinef by mouth every 12 hours and to ingest a high-sodium diet (at least 100 mmol daily) for 3 days. Criteria for the diagnosis of primary hyperaldosteronism are the same as those for the DOC suppression test: urinary aldosterone excretion on the third day greater than 8 μg per day (Streeten et al, 1979) or 18 to 20 μg per day (Padfield et al, 1975) or plasma aldosterone concentration above 8.5 ng per deciliter on the fourth day, between 0800 and 0900 hours, after recumbency for at least 1 hour (Streeten et al, 1979). The test results are not useful in differentiating patients with aldosterone-producing adenoma (APA) from those with IAH (Padfield et al, 1975).

Aldosterone Measurements on a High-Sodium Diet. In patients with primary hyperaldosteronism, sodium intake that is known to exceed 100 or (preferably) 200 mmol per day fails to suppress the excretion of acid-labile aldosterone into the normal range (below 17 to 20 μg per day) in 43 percent (Lund and Nielsen, 1980), 53 percent (Streeten et al, 1979), and 85 percent (Slaton et al, 1969) of patients (Table 11–3E). This is clearly not a sensitive test, though its sensitivity might be increased by relating aldosterone excretion to the age of the patient (Crane and Harris, 1976; Hegstad et al, 1983).

Captopril Test. The plasma aldosterone concentration is dependent on the plasma angiotensin II concentration in normal subjects and in patients with secon-

dary hyperaldosteronism but is elevated in spite of low plasma angiotensin II levels in primary hyperaldosteronism. Lyons and colleagues (1983) have exploited this difference by measuring the plasma aldosterone and PRA levels before and 2 hours after the administration of captopril, 25 mg by mouth in the seated posture. In nine normotensive controls, PRA rose (2.7 $\pm$ 0.7 to 14.2 $\pm$ 3.9 ng per milliliter per hour) and plasma aldosterone concentration fell (13.7 $\pm$ 5.0 to 2.1 $\pm$ 0.7 ng per deciliter). Results were similar in patients with essential hypertension, in nine out of 10 of whom plasma aldosterone concentration fell below 15 ng per deciliter after administration of captopril. Captopril had no significant effect on PRA or plasma aldosterone concentration in 12 patients with primary hyperaldosteronism. After the captopril was given, plasma aldosterone concentration remained above 15 ng per deciliter in all seven patients with APAs and in four of the five patients with IAH. The aldosterone to PRA ratio fell below 50 in the controls but was above 50 in all patients with APA and in four of the five patients with IAH (Table 11–3F).

Dexamethasone Suppression Test. Because, in patients with primary hyperaldosteronism, aldosterone secretion is largely under ACTH control and correlates closely with cortisol secretion (Kem et al, 1973), it is not surprising that dexamethasone administration reduces plasma concentrations and urinary excretion of aldosterone (Slaton et al, 1969; Kem et al, 1973; Ganguly et al, 1977; Wenting et al, 1978), albeit transiently, in these patients (Ganguly et al, 1977; Wenting et al, 1978). However, plasma aldosterone concentration and urinary aldosterone excretion are not suppressed into the normal range, except in a rare form of inherited, dexamethasone-suppressible hyperaldosteronism described by Sutherland and associates (1966), further studied by Salti and co-workers (1969), and confirmed by others (New et al, 1973; Gill and Bartter, 1981; Connell et al, 1986). In this variant of primary hyperaldosteronism, small doses of dex-

TABLE 11-3F   Captopril Test

Method

Plasma aldosterone and PRA levels before and 2 hr after the administration of captopril 25 mg by mouth in the seated posture.

Normal

A rise in the PRA and a fall in plasma aldosterone in normals. Plasma aldosterone concentration remains above 15 ng/dl in patients with APA and IAH. Aldosterone:PRA ratio falls in normals to less than 50, but remains above 50 with APA and IAH.

Uses

Differentiating APA and IAH from normals.

Pitfalls

Does not separate IAH from APA and may not separate IAH from patient with low renin essential hypertension. Needs confirmation by other workers.

---

amethasone (1 to 2 mg per day) have reduced plasma aldosterone concentration and urinary aldosterone excretion persistently into the normal range while correcting the associated metabolic derangements (hypokalemia, metabolic alkalosis, hypertension). It should be appreciated that if doses of dexamethasone higher than approximately 0.5 to 0.75 mg per day are required to inhibit hyperaldosteronism in these patients, the continued use of such therapy would be likely to convert the disorder from hyperaldosteronism to iatrogenic Cushing's syndrome, with questionable benefit to the patient (Table 11–3G).

TABLE 11-3G   Dexamethasone Suppression Test

Method

24-hr urinary aldosterone excretion is measured by RIA, before and on the 2nd or 3rd day of dexamethasone administration (0.5 mg PO q6h) on a 100–200 mEq sodium diet.

Normal

Aldosterone excretion is <20 μg/day before and during dexamethasone administration.

Uses

To diagnose dexamethasone-suppressible hyperaldosteronism in which aldosterone excretion falls from elevated to normal levels during dexamethasone administration.

Problems

Incorrectly collected 24-hr urines lead to erroneous conclusions. Even if true, the test should be repeated at approximately physiologic glucocorticoid dosage (e.g., 0.25 mg dexamethasone b.i.d.) to determine therapeutic usefulness of the result.

Stimulatory Tests

Stimulatory tests have been used mainly for the diagnosis of hypoaldosteronism (Kokko, 1985; Vagnucci, 1969; Sunderlin et al, 1981) but are also of value in the diagnosis of primary hyperaldosteronism (Streeten et al, 1979; Streeten and Anderson, 1982).

Sodium Deprivation.   On a daily sodium intake of 10 mmol per day, urinary excretion of acid-labile aldosterone increases to between 18 and 70 μg per day (Streeten et al, 1969) in normal subjects but increases subnormally in patients with hypoaldosteronism. At 0900 to 1000 hours, after the patient has been standing for 1 to 2 hours on the morning after the 3 days of restricted sodium intake, plasma aldosterone concentration fails to rise above 15 ng per deciliter in hypoaldosteronism. If PRA is measured at the same time, hypoaldosteronism can be recognized as being of the hyporeninemic type (if PRA fails to rise above 1.7 ng per milliliter per hour) or due to a primary defect in aldosterone secretion by the zona glomerulosa (if PRA rises normally, or excessively to above 8.5 ng per milliliter per hour) (Table 11–3H).

Furosemide Administration and Orthostasis.   These provide a useful stimulus for aldosterone secretory activity that is practicable in some outpatient settings. Furosemide, 40 mg, is injected intravenously, and the patient is told to lie down to promote diuresis for 1 hour, followed by standing and leisurely ambulation for 1 to 2 hours. Afterward, blood is drawn for meaurements of plasma aldosterone concentration and PRA (Streeten et al, 1975; Streeten and Anderson, 1979). In normal subjects, PRA rises to 1.7 to 8.5 ng per milliliter per hour (Streeten et al, 1975) and plasma aldosterone concentration increases to 13 to 50 ng per deciliter. In patients with hypoaldosteronism, plasma aldosterone concentration fails to rise normally, whereas PRA rises normally or excessively in primary dysfunction of the zona glomerulosa but rises subnormally (to less than 1.7 ng per milliliter

TABLE 11-3H   Sodium Deprivation Test for Hypoaldosteronism

Method

24-hr urinary aldosterone excretion is measured by RIA after 3–4 days on a diet containing 10 mmol sodium/day.

Normal

Acid-labile aldosterone excretion is 20–70 μg/day

Uses

To diagnose hypoaldosteronism, in which urinary aldosterone is <20 μg/day on low Na diet.

Problems

Adherence to a 10 mmol Na diet is difficult to verify, and 24 hour urines may be inaccurately collected.

per hour) in hyporeninemic hypoaldosteronism (Table 11–3I).

Somewhat to our surprise, we have found that in patients with primary hyperaldosteronism, plasma aldosterone concentration rises normally or excessively—to greater than 40 ng per deciliter (Streeten and Anderson, 1982) in 70 percent of patients—despite the characteristic, subnormal, or immeasurable rise in PRA in response to the stimuli of natriuresis and orthostasis. Thus, the plasma aldosterone concentration to PRA ratio (expressing plasma aldosterone concentration in nanograms per deciliter and PRA in nanograms per milliliter per hour), which was 26.5 ± 6.2 in essential hypertensive patients (n = 126), was 196.3 ± 61.9 (SEM) in 21 patients with primary hyperaldosteronism. This apparently anomalous response might result from the effects of a mild increase in plasma ACTH concentration—to which patients with primary hyperaldosteronism are exquisitely sensitive (see later)—brought about by the "stress" of standing for 2 hours after furosemide-induced volume depletion (Streeten and Anderson, 1982). Since patients with APA are insensitive to angiotensin II, it is difficult to explain in any other way this striking discordance between the subnormal rise in PRA and the excessive increase in plasma aldosterone concentration that they manifest in response to furosemide and the upright posture.

Orthostasis Without Antecedent Natriuresis.
Orthostasis without antecedent natriuresis will raise PRA and plasma aldosterone concentration in healthy individuals. However, the normal responses to this stimulus have not been sufficiently well defined to make this a definitive test for hypoaldosteronism unless plasma aldosterone concentration is extremely low, say less than 3 ng per deciliter after standing for 1 hour. The orthostatic stimulus has been of greater use in the diagnosis

of primary hyperaldosteronism. Whereas standing from 0800 to 1200 hours consistently stimulates a rise in plasma aldosterone concentration in normal subjects, patients with essential hypertension, and individuals with IAH, it is associated with no change or a fall in plasma aldosterone concentration in most patients with APA (Ganguly et al, 1973a, 1973b), in 78 percent (Ganguly, 1973b), 100 percent (Schambelan et al, 1976), 78 percent (Lund and Nielsen, 1980), 76 percent (Biglieri et al 1974), and 67 percent (Streeten et al, 1979) in reported series.

ACTH Infusion.   The normal plasma aldosterone response to ACTH infusion, e.g., cosyntropin (Cortrosyn), 0.25 mg in 5 percent dextrose solution over 4 to 8 hours, is measurable but slight in the absence of antecedent sodium depletion. When the ACTH infusion is administered after sodium depletion such as induced by adherence to a 10-mmol sodium diet for 3 days, or 3 hours after furosemide, 40 mg given intravenously, the rise in plasma aldosterone concentration is considerably magnified (Kem et al, 1975). Failure of plasma aldosterone concentration to rise above 10 to 15 ng per deciliter in response to ACTH infusion after sodium depletion by the described procedures occurs in hypoaldosteronism. Although the aldosterone response to ACTH has not been used for the diagnosis of primary hyperaldosteronism, this response to ACTH infusions is excessive in patients with primary aldosteronism associated either with an adrenal adenoma or with hyperplasia (Slaton et al, 1969; Kem et al, 1978; Sanita et al, 1979; Guthrie, 1981) (Table 11–3J).

Aldosterone Response to Angiotensin II Infusion.
Angiotensin II infusions at 3, 6, and 9 ng per kilogram per minute, each for 20 minutes, increase plasma al-

---

TABLE 11–3I   Furosemide Administration and Orthostasis

Method

> Furosemide, 40 mg, is injected intravenously followed by recumbency for 1 hr and standing (preferably) or sitting for 1 hr. Plasma renin activity and plasma aldosterone concentration are measured by RIA at the end of the standing period.

Normal

> Plasma aldosterone rises to 13–50 ng/dl.

Uses

> In primary hyperaldosteronism, plasma aldosterone rises above 25 ng/dl and PAC/PRA above 40, usually above 100. Plasma aldosterone fails to rise above 12 ng/dl, and PRA remains below 1.7 ng/ml/hr in hyporeninemic hypoaldosteronism while PRA rises above 8.5 ng/ml/hr in primary failure of zona glomerulosa function.

TABLE 11–3J   ACTH Infusion Test for Hypoaldosteronism

Method

> Antecedent sodium depletion is induced by a 10 mmol sodium diet for 3 days or an IV injection of furosemide, 40 mg, 2 hr before ACTH infusion (cosyntropin 0.25 mg in 5% dextrose solution) over 8 hr. Plasma aldosterone is measured before and after 4 and 8 hr of the ACTH infusion. Patient stands for the 2nd hr after furosemide and PRA is measured.

Normal

> Plasma aldosterone rises above 15 ng/dl.

Uses

> Plasma aldosterone fails to rise above 15 ng/dl and PRA is low in hyporeninemic hypoaldosteronism while PRA is elevated in zona glomerulosa failure.

Problems

> Standing after furosemide often causes orthostatic hypotension which may result in syncope.

dosterone concentration in normal subjects (see Table 11–4). It is evident that, like the ACTH test, this stimulatory procedure is considerably more effective when used after sodium depletion, which increases the sensitivity of the zona glomerulosa to angiotensin II (Oelkers et al, 1974). Patients with hypoaldosteronism show a subnormal rise in plasma aldosterone concentration in response to all three rates of angiotensin II infusion, and the abnormality is particularly evident when the infusion is given after restriction of sodium intake to 10 mmol per day for 3 days.

Angiotensin II infusions have not been systematically utilized to distinguish patients with APA from those with bilateral adrenocortical (zona glomerulosa) hyperplasia (Table 11–3K). However, there is little doubt that patients with APA show subnormal, negligible, or only occasionally normal increases in plasma aldosterone concentration in response to angiotensin II infusions (Sanita et al, 1979; Anderson and Streeten, 1986), whereas many patients with IAH respond excessively to this stimulus, as Wisgerhof and colleagues have reported (1978, 1981). Angiotensin II is no longer generally available for clinical use in the United States.

Measurements of the Physiologic Effects of Aldosterone

PRA. The well-documented role of the renin-angiotensin system as the major mechanism controlling aldosterone production can be utilized effectively in the diagnosis of aldosterone disorders.

In primary hyperaldosteronism, the sodium retention and hypervolemia resulting from the excessive action of aldosterone cause severe suppression of renin release (Conn et al, 1964; Gross et al, 1965; Ferriss et al, 1978). This phenomenon is best exploited by measuring PRA after applying standardized stimuli to its release. After adherence to a 10-mmol sodium diet for 3 days and while the patient is standing for 2 hours, or after furosemide, 40 mg, is given intravenously and while the patient is standing for 1 or 2 hours, PRA rises in normal subjects to 1.7 to 8.5 ng per milliliter per hour. In most patients with primary hyperaldosteronism, stimulated PRA is subnormal—in 95 percent of patients in our series (Streeten et al, 1979). PRA measurements in the recumbent posture after an unrestricted or a low-sodium diet have been of little value, however, since only 50 percent of patients with primary hyperaldosteronism had subnormal PRA levels in the series of 80 patients reported by Bravo and associates (1983). The ranges of normal PRA measurements listed here are for assays performed at physiologic blood pH (Goodfriend, 1973; Haber et al, 1969). Normal ranges are higher when the assay is performed after acidification of the plasma to pH 5.4 (Menard and Catt, 1972) (Table 11–3L).

In hypoaldosteronism, PRA measurements are useful in indicating whether subnormal aldosterone production results from an intrinsic zona glomerulosa defect, when PRA will be normal or elevated, or from a defect in renin release resulting from a renal disorder, autonomic insufficiency, diabetes mellitus, or other causes (Schambelan et al, 1972; Hudson et al, 1957; Arora et al, 1977; Perez et al, 1977; Phelps et al, 1980; Monnens et al, 1983; Landier et al, 1984).

Rectal Mucosal Electrical Potential. This potential is maintained within the normal range partly by the action of aldosterone on sodium-potassium exchange. Colonic potential difference was elevated in primary

---

TABLE 11–3K Angiotensin II Infusion Test

Method

Angiotensin II is infused in recumbency at 3, 6, and 9 ng/kg/min, each for 20 min, with measurements of plasma aldosterone before and after each infusion rate.

Normal

Plasma aldosterone rises above 17 ng/dl in normal subjects

Uses

In hypoaldosteronism, plasma aldosterone fails to rise above 17 ng/dl; in hyperaldosteronism with APA, plasma aldosterone is raised slightly or not at all above baseline levels by angiotensin II, and in hyperaldosteronism with IAH, plasma aldosterone rises excessively during angiotensin II infusion.

Problems

Angiotensin II is no longer marketed as a pharmaceutical. Sensitivity and specificity of angiotensin II responses have not been defined

---

TABLE 11–3L Plasma Renin Activity (PRA)

Method

PRA is measured by RIA after stimulation with sodium depletion (e.g., furosemide, 40 mg IV) and standing for 1 hr.

Normal

1.7–8.5 ng/mL/hr (higher values if PRA is measured at pH 5.4)

Uses

Stimulated PRA is subnormal in primary hyperaldosteronism, and in hyporeninemic hypoaldosteronism; it is elevated in hypoaldosteronism due to primary adrenal failure.

Problems

In the absence of primary disorders of aldosterone production, PRA is frequently subnormal (in low renin hypertension, some types of renal insufficiency, during beta-blocker therapy) and is often elevated (in CHF, cirrhosis with ascites, nephrotic syndrome, high-renin hypertension).

hyperaldosteronism (Edmonds and Godfrey, 1970), and the difference between the rectal and oral mucosal poten tial has been found to be consistently increased in hyperaldosteronism (Skrabal et al, 1978) (Table 11–3M).

Other Adrenal Steroid Measurements

Cortisol. Hypoaldosteronism may be a manifestation of complete adrenal insufficiency or Addison's disease. Hypopituitarism with ACTH deficiency may reduce the aldosterone response to sodium depletion. For these reasons, it is important to document in patients with suspected hypoaldosteronism the presence of normal cortisol production by measurements of urinary 17-hydroxycorticosteroids or of plasma cortisol before and after stimulation by ACTH and, preferably, also by metyrapone and/or an insulin tolerance test (Streeten et al, 1984).

Hypercortisolism is not associated with hyperaldosteronism except in some patients with adrenocortical carcinoma in whom there is characteristically excessive production of many different steroids, which may include aldosterone (Arteaga et al, 1984).

18-Hydroxycorticosterone (18–OHB). Measurements of plasma 18–OHB, urinary 18–OHB, or the predominant urinary metabolite of this steroid, 18–hydroxy compound A, are of use in both hyperaldosteronism and hypoaldosteronism. In primary hyperaldosteronism, plasma 18–OHB is present in excessive concentrations. Plasma 18–OHB concentrations at 0800 hours virtually always exceed 100 ng per deciliter in patients with APA but are less obviously elevated, almost always below 100 ng per deciliter, in patients with IAH (Biglieri et al, 1979; Biglieri and Schambelan, 1979; Kem et al, 1985b).

The concomitant presence of high concentrations of 18–OHB and low concentrations of aldosterone in the plasma provides the best means of diagnosing hypoaldosteronism due to a defect in corticosterone methyl oxidase Type II (Kokko, 1985; Ulick et al, 1964; Ulick, 1976; Lee et al, 1986; Veldhuis et al, 1980, 1983; Veldhuis and Melby, 1981). If both 18–OHB and aldosterone concentrations in the plasma are subnormal, but the plasma concentration of corticosterone is elevated, hypoaldosteronism is likely to be the result of a defect in corticosterone methyl oxidase Type I (Visser and Cost, 1964; Degenhart et al, 1966). Since both disorders are best treated with fludrocortisone, this differentiation is not essential for effective therapy in these patients (Table 11–3N).

DOC and Corticosterone. Pellnitz and co-workers (1978) have shown that serum concentrations of DOC, corticosterone, and cortisol are lower in patients with IAH than in patients with APA studied on a regular diet during dexamethasone administration (2 mg twice a day). Multiplication of the three steroid concentrations in each subject improved the differentiation of the two types of primary hyperaldosteronism.

Adrenal Vein Steroid Measurements. In patients with APA, plasma aldosterone concentrations in the adrenal vein draining the adenoma are elevated (usually above 200 ng per deciliter), whereas plasma aldosterone levels in the adrenal vein draining the contralateral gland (in which aldosterone production is usually negligible because of suppressed circulating angiotensin II levels) are no higher than in the inferior vena cava below the level of the adrenals. In IAH, plasma concentrations of al-

---

TABLE 11–3M   Rectal Mucosal Electrical Potential

Method

  Rectal mucosal potential or the difference between rectal and oral mucosal potentials is measured with special equipment (Adrenosonde, 80) on normal Na intake.

Normal

  Rectal potential difference (RPD) = 40.0 ± (S.D.) 7.3 mV

  Rectal-oral potential difference (R–OPD) = 11.5 ± 8.7 mV

Uses

  In primary hyperaldosteronism RPD = 68.3 ± 13.9, R–OPD = 46.1 ± 15.1 mV

  In adrenal insufficiency RPD = 23.0 ± 10.4, R–OPD = –10.6 ± 8.6 mV

Problems

  Confirmatory studies are needed.

TABLE 11–3N   Plasma 18-Hydroxycorticosterone (18–OHB) Levels

Method

  Plasma 18–OHB is measured by RIA with concomitant measurement of plasma aldosterone.

Normal

  Plasma 18–OHB: 23.3 ± (SEM) 12.2 ng/dl (range varies in different laboratories)

  Plasma 18–OHB/aldosterone ratio: 2.58 ± (SEM) 0.15

Uses

  On a high sodium diet in patients with primary hyperaldosteronism, plasma 18–OHB is elevated above 100 ng/dl in APA, and less elevated, seldom above 100 ng/dl, in IAH. With hypoaldosteronism, low plasma aldosterone and raised plasma 18–OHB levels indicate corticosterone methyl oxidase type II defect, while low plasma 18–OHB and aldosterone together with high plasma corticosterone levels indicate a defect in corticosterone methyl oxidase type I.

Problems

  Measurements of 18–OHB are available only in very few laboratories

dosterone in the adrenal veins on both sides are elevated considerably above inferior vena caval levels (Table 11–3O).

It is always important to measure the concentration of an independent hormone (usually cortisol or epinephrine) in all venous samples to facilitate interpretation of the adrenal vein aldosterone concentrations. If one sample, thought to have been obtained from an adrenal vein, was actually derived partly from the inferior vena cava or from some other venous source, the level of plasma cortisol or epinephrine (Levinson et al, 1982) in that sample will not be elevated, as it should be, above the concentration in the inferior vena cava. False conclusions from the determined plasma aldosterone concentrations may thus be avoided. When it has been possible to obtain blood from adrenal veins on both sides, this procedure has been very effective in demonstrating and localizing APA (Melby et al, 1967; Weinberger et al, 1979; Streeten et al, 1979; Vaughan et al, 1981).

Studies of Adrenal Morphology

Because the treatment of the two main types of primary hyperaldosteronism differs radically (surgical excision for APA, spironolactone for IAH), physical methods of determining adrenal morphology are of great value. Frequently these procedures will show the presence of a simple adenoma (APA) or bilateral hyperplasia or apparently normal-sized glands, thus facilitating therapeutic decisions.

Computed Tomography.   CT scans will reveal the presence of most adrenal adenomas unless they are smaller in diameter than 3 to 5 mm. An excrescence or

TABLE 11–3O   Adrenal Vein Steroid Measurements

Method

Blood is sampled under fluoroscopic control, from both adrenal veins and from the inferior vena cava below the level of the adrenals, for measurements of plasma aldosterone and either cortisol or epinephrine concentrations.

Normal

If both adrenal veins are successfully catheterized, plasma aldosterone, cortisol and epinephrine concentrations should be approximately equal in both adrenal veins and almost always (under the "stress" of the catheterization) higher than in the inferior vena cava. Absolute normal ranges of adrenal vein steroid levels depend upon the "stress" of the procedure.

Uses

To determine the unilaterality of excessive aldosterone secretion characteristic of APA.

Problems

If the blood sampled from an adrenal vein is diluted with blood from the inferior vena cava or a renal or hepatic vein, this fact will be reflected in a lower cortisol or epinephrine concentration than in blood from the contralateral vein. These findings are essential for the interpretation of the plasma aldosterone concentrations measured in the blood purported to have come from the adrenal veins.

excessive plumpness or fullness between the observed λ-shaped adrenal suggests a small adenoma, whereas tumors as large as 1 to 1.5 cm in diameter are more conclusively recognizable (Fig. 11–1A and B) (White et al, 1980; Linde et al, 1979; Abrams et al, 1982).

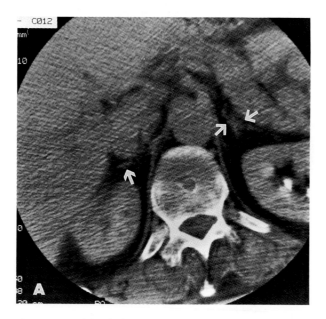
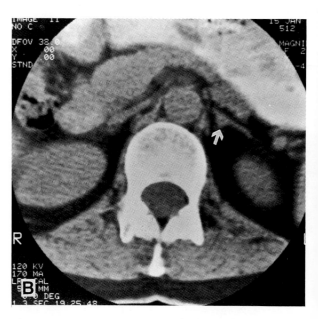

Figure 11–1   Abdominal CT scans with arrows pointing to both adrenals of a normal subject (A) and to the left adrenal of a patient with a small, rounded excrescence typical of an APA (B).

Magnetic Resonance Imaging. At present, MRI is thought to be less useful than CT scanning, which provides better resolution.

131I-19-Iodocholesterol Scintigraphy. This radionuclide is concentrated by the adrenal cortex. In the presence of an APA, concentration of the isotope is evident by gamma camera imaging in the tumor alone (Conn et al, 1971, 1972; Hogan et al, 1976; Gross et al, 1983), particularly if cholesterol uptake by both zonae fasciculatae is inhibited by antecedent dexamethasone administration (Conn et al, 1976).

Adrenal Phlebography. The characteristic venous pattern encircling an adrenocortical adenoma has provided an effective means of identifying and localizing adrenal adenomas in many patients (Conn et al, 1969). The two main reasons why this procedure has fallen largely into disuse are, first, that the adrenal veins are often difficult to find and to inject and, second, that adrenal infarction has resulted from this procedure (Fellerman et al, 1970), with potentially serious consequences.

Ultrasound Examination. Ultrasound is sometimes useful in detecting large adrenal tumors (Kehlet et al, 1976) but cannot be relied on to show the presence of more than a modest percentage of small aldosteronomas.

SECONDARY HYPERALDOSTERONISM

Secondary hyperaldosteronism is an appropriate response of the zona glomerulosa to excessive stimulation by the normal mechanisms—usually excessive renin release and angiotensin formation. As such, it should be recognized as a pathogenetic component of many disorders summarized in Table 11–1 and as the mechanism

of renal sodium retention and potassium excretion. Secondary hyperaldosteronism can be recognized clinically by the presence of its causes and by its characteristic manifestations: edema, hypertension, and/or hypokalemia and potassium depletion. Recognition of the role of secondary hyperaldosteronism facilitates understanding of the mechanisms of many states of disordered fluid and electrolyte homeostasis and may be useful in choosing appropriate therapy. There is seldom a need to document the presence of secondary hyperaldosteronism. When this is needed, however, measurements of PRA and plasma aldosterone concentration under standardized conditions of sodium intake and posture will demonstrate the presence of secondary hyperaldosteronism (Fig. 11–2).

SENSITIVITY AND SPECIFICITY OF TEST PROCEDURES

Because hypoaldosteronism is relatively rare, the sensitivity and specificity of the various tests used to diagnose this disorder have not been determined.

There are larger numbers of patients with primary hyperaldosteronism, and we have been able to estimate the sensitivity and specificity of individual and combined procedures used in making this diagnosis. The following diagnostic procedures have been performed on 820 consecutive patients with hypertension of unknown types:

1. Serum sodium and potassium concentrations in the untreated state
2. PRA and plasma aldosterone concentration 3 hours after furosemide, 40 mg intravenously, and after 2 hours in the upright posture

Figure 11–2 Pathogenesis of primary and secondary forms of hyper- and hypoaldosteronism.

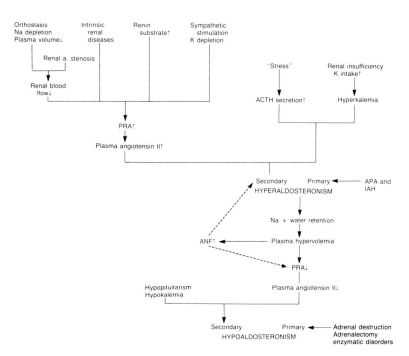

3. Plasma aldosterone concentration after intravenous infusion of 0.9 percent sodium chloride solution, 2 L over 3.5 to 4 hours

Table 11–5 lists the sensitivities and specificities of each diagnostic procedure, as well as of selected combinations of the procedures. The final diagnoses on which these calculations of sensitivity and specificity were based were established by confirmatory evidence of subnormal aldosterone suppressibility in response to DOCA, 10 mg intramuscularly every 12 hours for 3 days, or fludrocortisone, 0.2 mg by mouth every 12 hours for 3 days, as described previously, and by the surgical removal of an adrenocortical adenoma in the nine (of 22) patients who were diagnosed as having APA and operated on.

It is evident from Table 11–5 that unsatisfactory levels of sensitivity or specificity were derived from any one of the procedures used. Thus, for instance, hypokalemia (serum potassium less than 3.5 mmol per liter) was present in only 53 percent of the patients with hyperaldosteronism, suppressed PRA was present not only in the patients with primary hyperaldosteronism but also in another 28 percent of the 820 hypertensive patients who had low renin hypertension, and the saline infusion failed to suppress plasma aldosterone concentration in only 88 percent of the patients with primary hyperaldosteronism. However, it also failed to do so in 20 percent of patients with secondary hyperaldosteronism resulting from high-renin, angiotensinogenic hypertension (i.e., 3 percent of the 820 patients). When the results of two tests were combined, the sensitivity was reduced (as expected), but the specificity of the diagnostic results improved and usually exceeded 94 percent. The most effective and most generally useful test combinations were:

1. Stimulated PRA less than 1.7 ng per milliliter per hour and serum potassium less than 3.5 mmol per liter
2. Stimulated PRA less than 1.7 ng per milliliter per hour and stimulated plasma aldosterone concentration greater than 26.5 ng per deciliter
3. Stimulated PRA less than 1.7 ng per milliliter per hour and suppressed plasma aldosterone concentration greater than 8.5 ng per deciliter.
4. Serum potassium less than 3.5 mmol per liter and suppressed plasma aldosterone concentration greater than 8.5 ng per deciliter.

Lyons and associates (1983) reported a captopril test for primary hyperaldosteronism that had a sensitivity of 92 percent and specificity of 90 percent, in the relatively small number of patients studied.

RECOMMENDED DIAGNOSTIC PROCEDURES

There is clearly room for differences of opinion about the most useful diagnostic procedures for hypoaldosteronism and hyperaldosteronism since no comparative studies of the many available tests have been reported. The procedures selected will depend on their availability in the parts of the world where they are to be performed.

Our suggestions are as follows:

Primary Hyperaldosteronism

The following screening procedures are recommended:

1. Hypokalemia in the untreated state on a high sodium intake
2. Recumbent plasma aldosterone concentration greater than 8.5 ng per deciliter after a 2-L sodium chloride infusion

The following definitive procedures can be used:

1. PRA less than 1.7 ng per milliliter per hour and plasma aldosterone greater than 26.5 ng per deciliter after furosemide and standing, with or without spontaneous hypokalemia
2. PRA less than 1.7 ng per milliliter per hour after furosemide and standing plus plasma aldosterone greater than 8.5 ng per deciliter after a 2-L 0.9 percent sodium chloride infusion; with or without spontaneous hypokalemia
3. Captopril test with or without spontaneous hypokalemia

These tests should be confirmed by the fludrocortisone suppression test and, if positive, should be followed by CT scan of the adrenals and adrenal vein catheterization for aldosterone and cortisol measurements or plasma 18–OHB determinations (if available).

TABLE 11–4   Plasma Aldosterone Responses (mean ± SEM) to Angiotensin II Infusion in 16 Normal Subjects

Sodium intake	0	Angiotensin II infusion rates (ng/kg/min)		
		3	6	9
High-sodium diet (100–200 mmol/day)	6.0 ± 0.7	12.7 ± 1.2	17.1 ± 1.5	23.0 ± 1.9
Low-sodium diet (10 mmol/day)	18.8 ± 3.7	33.3 ± 4.2	48.2 ± 6.1	57.1 ± 6.5

TABLE 11-5   Reliability of Single and Multiple Diagnostic Procedures for Primary Hyperaldosteronism[*]

Procedure(s)	Sensitivity	Specificity
Serum potassium < 3.5 mmol/L	53	93
PRA (stim.) < 1.7 ng/ml/hr	82	69
PAC (stim.) > 26.5 ng/dl	72	54
PAC (supp.) > 8.5 ng/dl	88	94
Serum potassium < 3.5 mmol/L and PRA < 1.7 ng/ml/hr	46	97
Serum potassium < 3.5 mmol/L and stim. PAC > 26.5 ng/dl	59	97
Serum potassium < 3.5 mmol/L and supp. PAC > 8.5 ng/dl	56	98
PRA < 1.7 ng/ml/hr and supp. PAC > 8.5 ng/dl	73	99
PRA < 1.7 ng/ml/hr and stim. PAC > 26.5 ng/dl	61	94
PAC/PRA (stim.) > 40	63	87

PRA = plasma renin activity; PAC = plasma aldosterone concentration; stim. = stimulated by furosemide and orthostasis; supp. = suppressed by sodium chloride infusion.
[*] Results were obtained in hypertensive patients untreated for at least 1 week.

Hypoaldosteronism

Screening procedures reveal unexplained hyperkalemia and/or hyponatremia and/or orthostatic hypotension.

Definitive procedures show plasma aldosterone concentration less than 10 to 15 ng per deciliter both (1) after administration of furosemide, 40 mg intravenously, and standing, and (2) at 4 and 8 hours after the beginning of an 8-hour infusion of cosyntropin (Cortrosyn), 0.25 mg in 5 percent dextrose solution. If these results reveal hypoaldosteronism, plasma 18-OHB and corticosterone concentrations will usually reveal the presence of a corticosterone methyl oxidase Type I or II defect, though this is not necessary for therapeutic purposes.

BIBLIOGRAPHY

Abrams HL, Siegelman SS, Adams DF, et al. Computed tomography versus ultrasound of the adrenal glands: A prospective study. Radiology 1982; 143:121.

Anderson GH Jr, Streeten DHP. 1982 Unpublished observations.

Arora KK, Pfeifer MA, Walter C, et al. Hyperkalemia due to selective hypoaldosteronism. South Med J 1977; 70:634.

Arteaga E, Biglieri EG, Kater CE, et al. Aldosterone-producing adrenocortical carcinoma. Preoperative recognition and course in three cases. Ann Intern Med 1984; 101:316.

Biglieri EG. A perspective on aldosterone abnormalities. Clin Endocrinol 1976; 5:399.

Biglieri EG, Schambelan M. The significance of elevated levels of plasma 18-hydroxycorticosterone in patients with primary aldosteronism. J Clin Endocrinol Metab 1979; 49:87.

Biglieri EG, Schambelan M, Brust N, et al. Plasma aldosterone concentration. Further characterization of aldosterone producing adenomas. Circ Res 1974; 34(Suppl 1):183.

Biglieri EG, Schambelan M, Hirai J, et al. The significance of elevated levels of plasma 18-hydroxycorticosterone in patients with primary aldosteronism. J Clin Endocrinol Metab 1979; 49:87.

Biglieri EG, Slaton PE, Kronfield SJ, et al. Diagnosis of an aldosterone-producing adenoma in primary aldosteronism. An evaluative maneuver. JAMA 1967; 201:510.

Biglieri EG, Stockigt JR, Schambelan M. Adrenal mineralocorticoids causing hypertension. Am J Med 1972; 52:623.

Biglieri EG, Stockigt JR, Schambelan M. A preliminary evaluation for primary aldosteronism. Arch Intern Med 1970; 126:1004.

Bravo EL, Tarazi RC, Dustan HP, et al. The changing clinical spectrum of primary aldosteronism. Am J Med 1983; 74:641.

Brown JJ, Davies DL, Lever AF, et al. Plasma renin in a case of Conn's syndrome with fibrinoid lesions: Use of spironolactone in treatment. Br Med J 1964; 2:1636.

Carey RM, Thorner MO, Ortt EM. Effects of metoclopramide and bromocriptine on the renin-angiotensin-aldosterone system in man. Dopaminergic control of aldosterone. J Clin Invest 1979; 63:727.

Clarke D, Wilkinson R, Johnston IDA, et al. Severe hypertension in primary aldosteronism and good response to surgery. Lancet 1979; 1:482.

Conn JW. Presidential address. Part I. Painting background. Part II. Primary aldosteronism, a new clinical syndrome. J Lab Clin Med 1955; 45:3.

Conn JW, Beierwaltes WH, Lieberman LM, et al. Primary aldosteronism: Preoperative tumor visualization by scintillation scanning. J Clin Endocrinol Metab 1971; 33:713.

Conn JW, Cohen EL, Herwig KR. The dexamethasone-modified adrenal scintiscan in hyporeninemic aldosteronism (tumor versus hyperplasia). A comparison with adrenal venography and adrenal venous aldosterone. J Lab Clin Med 1976; 88:841.

Conn JW, Cohen EL, Rovner DR. Suppression of plasma renin activity in primary aldosteronism. JAMA 1964; 190:213.

Conn JW, Morita R, Cohen El, et al. Photoscanning of tumors in primary aldosteronism: Possible distinction from "idiopathic" aldosteronism. Hypertension 1972. Berlin: Springer-Verlag, 1972:299.

Conn JW, Rovner DR, Cohen EL, et al. Normokalemic primary aldosteronism. Its masquerade as "essential" hypertension. JAMA 1966; 195:21.

Conn JW, Rovner DR, Cohen EL, et al. Preoperative diagnosis of primary aldosteronism. Arch Intern Med 1969; 123:113.

Connell JMC, Kenyon CJ, Corrie JET, et al. Dexamethasone-suppressible hyperaldosteronism. Adrenal transition cell hyperplasia? Hypertension 1986; 8:669.

Crane MG, Harris JJ. Effect of aging on renin activity and aldosterone excretion. J Lab Clin Med 1976; 87:947.

Creditor MC, Loschky UK. Incidence of suppressed renin activity and of normokalemic primary aldosteronism in hypertensive Negro patients. Circulation 1968; 37:1027.

Davies DL, Beevers DG, Brown JJ, et al. Aldosterone and its stimuli in normal and hypertensive man: Are essential hypertension and primary hyperaldosteronism without tumour the same condition? J Endocrinol 1979; 81:79P.

Degenhart HJ, Frankena L, Visser HKA, et al. Further investigation of a new hereditary defect in the biosynthesis of aldosterone: Evidence for a defect in the 18-hydroxylation of corticosterone. Acta Physiol Pharmacol Neerl 1966; 14:88.

del Greco F, Dolkart R, Skom J, et al. Association of accelerated (malignant) hypertension in a patient with primary aldosteronism. J Clin Endocrinol 1966; 26:808.

Edmonds CJ, Godfrey RC. Measurement of electrical potentials of the human rectum and pelvic colon in normal and aldosterone-treated patients. Gut 1970; 11:330.

Edwards CRW, Miall PA, Hanker JP, et al. Inhibition of the plasma-aldosterone response to frusemide by bromocriptine. Lancet 1975; 2:903.

Fellerman H, Dalakos TG, Streeten DHP. Remission of Cushing's syndrome after unilateral adrenal phlebography. Apparent destruction of adrenal adenoma. Ann Intern Med 1970; 73:585.

Ferriss JB, Beevers DG, Brown JJ, et al. Clinical, biochemical and pathological features of low-renin ("primary") hyperaldosteronism. Am Heart J 1978; 95:375.

Findling JW, Adams AH, Raff H. Selective hypoaldosteronism due to an endogenous impairment in angiotensin II production. N Engl J Med 1987; 316:1632.

Ganguly A, Chavarri M, Luetscher JA, et al. Transient fall and subsequent return of high aldosterone secretion by adrenal adenoma during continued dexamethasone administration. J Clin Endocrinol Metab 1977; 44:775.

Ganguly A, Dowdy AJ, Luetscher JA, et al. Anomalous postural response of plasma aldosterone concentration in patients with aldosterone-producing adrenal adenoma. J Clin Endocrinol Metab 1973a; 36:401.

Ganguly A, Melada GA, Luetscher JA, et al. Control of plasma aldosterone in primary aldosteronism: Distinction between adenoma and hyperplasia. J Clin Endocrinol Metab 1973b; 37:765.

Gill JR Jr, Bartter FC. Overproduction of sodium-retaining steroids by the zona glomerulosa is adrenocorticotropin-dependent and mediates hypertension in dexamethasone-suppressible aldosteronism. J Clin Endocrinol Metabl 1981; 53:331.

Gomez-Sanchez CE, Holland OB. Urinary tetrahydroaldosterone and aldosterone-18-glucuronide excretion in white and black normal subjects and hypertensive patients. J Clin Endocrinol Metab 1981; 52:214.

Goodfriend TL. Radioimmunoassay of angiotensins and renin activity. In: Berson SA, Yalow R, eds. Methods of investigation and diagnostic endocrinology. Amsterdam and London: North Holland Co., 1973:1158.

Gross F, Brunner H, Ziegler M. Renin-angiotensin system, aldosterone, and sodium balance. Recent Progr Horm Res 1965; 21:119.

Gross MD, Shapiro B, Grekin RJ, et al. The relationship of adrenal gland iodomethylnorcholesterol uptake to zona glomerulosa function in primary aldosteronism. J Clin Endocrinol Metab 1983; 57:477.

Güllner H-G, Gill JR Jr. Beta endorphin selectively stimulates aldosterone secretion in hypophysectomized, nephrectomized dogs. J Clin Invest 1983; 71:124.

Guthrie GP. Multiple plasma steroid responses to graded ACTH infusions in patients with primary aldosteronism. J Lab Clin Med 1981; 98:364.

Haber E, Koerner T, Page LB, et al. Application of radioimmunoassay for angiotensin I to the physiological measurements of plasma renin activity in normal human subjects. J Clin Endocrinol Metab 1969; 29:1349.

Hegstad R, Brown RD, Jiang N-S, et al. Aging and aldosterone. Am J Med 1983; 74:442.

Hogan MJ, McRae J, Schambelan M, et al. Localization of aldosterone-producing adenomas with ^{131}I-19-iodocholesterol. N Engl J Med 1976; 294:410.

Holland OB, Brown H, Kuhnert LV, et al. Further evaluation of saline infusion for the diagnosis of primary aldosteronism. Hypertension 1984; 6:717.

Hudson JB, Chobanian AV, Relman AS. Hypoaldosteronism. A clinical study of a patient with isolated adrenal mineralocorticoid deficiency resulting in hyperkalemia and Stokes-Adams attacks. N Engl J Med 1957; 257:529.

Kaplan NM. Primary aldosteronism with malignant hypertension. N Engl J Med 1963; 269:1282.

Kehlet H, Blichert-Toft M, Hancke S, et al. Comparative study of ultrasound, ^{131}I-19-iodocholesterol scintigraphy, and aortography in localizing adrenal lesions. Br Med J 1976; 2:665.

Kem DC, Feldman M, Starkweather G, et al. Effect of human β-endorphin on plasma aldosterone concentrations in normal human subjects. J Clin Endocrinol Metab 1985a; 60:440.

Kem DC, Gomez-Sanchez C, Kramer NJ, et al. Plasma aldosterone and renin activity response to ACTH infusion in dexamethasone-suppressed normal and sodium-depleted man. J Clin Endocrinol Metab 1975; 40:116.

Kem DC, Tang K, Hanson CS, et al. The prediction of anatomical morphology of primary aldosteronism using serum 18-hydroxycorticosterone levels. J Clin Endocrinol Metab 1985b; 60:67.

Kem DC, Weinberger MH, Gomez-Sanchez C, et al. Circadian rhythm of plasma aldosterone concentration in patients with primary aldosteronism. J Clin Invest 1973; 52:2272.

Kem DC, Weinberger MH, Higgins JR, et al. Plasma aldosterone response to ACTH in primary aldosteronism and in patients with low renin hypertension. J Clin Endocrinol Metab 1978; 46:552.

Kem DC, Weinberger MH, Mayes DM, et al. Saline suppression of plasma aldosterone in hypertension. Arch Intern Med 1971; 128:380.

Kokko JP. Primary acquired hypoaldosteronism. Kidney Int 1985; 27:690.

Landier F, Guyene TT, Boutignon H, et al. Hyperreninemic hypoaldosteronism in infancy: A familial disease. J Clin Endocrinol Metab 1984; 58:143.

Laragh JH, Sealey JE, Summers SC. Patterns of adrenal secretion and urinary excretion of aldosterone and plasma renin activity in normal and hypertensive subjects. Circ Res 1966; 18(Suppl 1):158.

Lee PDK, Patterson BD, Hintz RL, et al. Biochemical diagnosis and management of corticosterone methyl oxidase type II deficiency. J Clin Endocrinol Metab 1986; 62:225.

Levinson PD, Zadik Z, Hamilton BPM, et al. Adrenal vein epinephrine levels: A useful aid in venous sampling for primary aldosteronism. Ann Intern Med 1982; 97:690.

Liddle GW, Bledsoe T, Coppage WS Jr. A familial renal disorder simulating primary aldosteronism but with negligible aldosterone secretion. Trans Assoc Am Physicians 1963; 76:199.

Linde R, Conlam C, Battino R, et al. Localization of aldosterone-producing adenoma by computed tomography. J Clin Endocrinol Metab 1979; 49:642.

Lund JO, Nielsen MD. Fludrocortisone suppression test in normal subjects with essential hypertension and in patients with various forms of aldosteronism. Acta Endocrinol (Copenh) 1980; 93:100.

Lyons DF, Kem DC, Brown RD, et al. Single dose captopril as a diagnostic test for primary aldosteronism. J Clin Endocrinol Metab 1983; 57: 892.

Matsuoka H, Mulrow PJ. β-Lipotropin: A new aldosterone-stimulating factor. Science 1980; 209:307.

McAreavey D, Murray GD, Lever AF, et al. Similarity of idiopathic aldosteronism and essential hypertension. A statistical comparison. Hypertension 1983; 5:116.

Melby JC, Spark RF, Dale SL, et al. Diagnosis and localization of aldosterone-producing adenomas by adrenal vein catheterization. N Engl J Med 1967; 277:1050.

Menard J, Catt KJ. Measurement of renin activity, concentration and substrate in rat plasma by radioimmunoassay of angiotensin I. Endocrinology 1972; 90:422.

Monnens L, Fischer T, Bos B, et al. Hyperreninemic hypoaldosteronism in infancy. Nephron 1983; 35:140.

New MI, Siegal EJ, Peterson RE. Dexamethasone-suppressible hyperaldosteronism. J Clin Endocrinol Metab 1973; 37:93.

Oelkers W, Brown JJ, Fraser R, et al. Sensitization of the adrenal cortex to angiotensin II in sodium-deplete man. Circ Res 1974; 34:69.

Padfield PL, Allison MEM, Brown JJ, et al. Response of plasma aldosterone to fludrocortisone in primary hyperaldosteronism and other forms of hypertension. Clin Endocrinol 1975; 4:493.

Padfield PL, Brown JJ, Davies D, et al. The myth of idiopathic hyperaldosteronism. Lancet 1981; 2:83.

Pellnitz W, Schöneshöfer M, Oelkers W. Differentiation between subtypes of primary hyperaldosteronism by multiple steroid measurement after dexamethasone administration. Klin Wochenschr 1978; 56:855.

Perez GO, Lespier LE, Oster JR, et al. Effect of alterations of sodium intake in patients with hyporeninemic hypoaldosteronism. Nephron 1977; 18:259.

Phelps KR, Lieberman RL, Oh MS, et al. Pathophysiology of the syndrome of hyporeninemic hypoaldosteronism. Metabolism 1980; 29:186.

Salti IS, Stiefel M, Ruse JL, et al. Non-tumorous primary aldosteronism: I. Type relieved by glucocorticoid (glucocorticoid-remediable aldosteronism). Can Med Assoc J 1969; 101:1.

Sanita T, Okuno T, Eguchi T, et al. Responses of aldosterone-producing adenomas to ACTH and angiotensins. Acta Endocrinol (Copenh) 1979; 92:702.

Schambelan M, Brust NL, Chang BCF, et al. Circadian rhythm and effect of posture on plasma aldosterone concentration in primary aldosteronism. J Clin Endocrinol 1976; 43:115.

Schambelan M, Stockigt JR, Biglieri EG. Isolated hypoaldosteronism in adults. A renin-deficiency syndrome. N Engl J Med 1972; 287:573.

Skrabal F, Aubock J, Edwards CRW, et al. Subtraction potential difference: In-vivo assay for mineralocorticoid activity. Lancet 1978; 1:298.

Slaton PE Jr, Schambelan M, Biglieri EG. Stimulation and suppression of aldosterone secretion in patients with an aldosterone-producing adenoma. J Clin Endocrinol 1969; 29:239.

Snow MH, Nichol P, Wilkinson R, et al. Normotensive primary aldosteronism. Br Med J 1976; 1:1125.

Streeten DHP. Orthostatic disorders of the circulation. New York: Plenum, 1987:111.

Streeten DHP, Anderson GH Jr. Outpatient experience with saralasin. Kidney Int 1979; 15:S44.

Streeten DHP, Anderson GH Jr. Simplified screening procedures for primary aldosteronism. Studies on the mechanism of the hyperresponsiveness to furosemide and standing. Clin Exp Hypertens [A] 1982; 4:1663.

Streeten DHP, Anderson GH Jr, Dalakos TG, et al. Normal and abnormal function of the hypothalamic-pituitary-adrenocortical system in man. Endocr Rev 1984: 5:371.

Streeten DHP, Anderson GH Jr, Freiberg JM, et al. Use of an angiotensin II antagonist (saralasin) in the recognition of "angiotensinogenic" hypertension. N Engl J Med 1975; 292:657.

Streeten DHP, Schletter FE, Clift GV, et al. Studies of the renin-angiotensin-aldosterone system in patients with hypertension and in normal subjects. Am J Med 1969; 46:844.

Streeten DHP, Tomycz N, Anderson GH Jr. Reliability of screening methods for the diagnosis of primary aldosteronism. Am J Med 1979; 67:403.

Sunderlin FS, Anderson GH Jr, Streeten DHP, et al. The renin-angiotensin-aldosterone system in diabetic patients with hyperkalemia. Diabetes 1981; 30:335.

Sutherland DJA, Ruse JL, Laidlaw JC. Hypertension, increased aldosterone secretion and low plasma renin activity relieved by dexamethasone. Can Med Assoc J 1966; 95:1109.

Thomas JP. Aldosterone deficiency in a patient with idiopathic haemochromatosis. Clin Endocrinol 1984; 21:271.

Ulick S. Diagnosis and nomenclature of the disorders of the terminal portion of the aldosterone biosynthetic pathway. J Clin Endocrinol Metab 1976; 43:92.

Ulick S, Gautier E, Vetter KK, et al. An aldosterone biosynthetic defect in a salt-losing disorder. J Clin Endocrinol Metab 1964; 24:669.

Vagnucci A. Selective aldosterone deficiency. J Clin Endocrinol Metab 1969; 29:279.

Vaughan NJA, Jowett TP, Slater JDH, et al. The diagnosis of primary hyperaldosteronism. Lancet 1981; 1:120.

Veldhuis JD, Kulin HE, Santen RJ, et al. Inborn error in the terminal step of aldosterone biosynthesis. Corticosterone methyl oxidase type II deficiency in a North American pedigree. N Engl J Med 1980; 303:117.

Veldhuis JD, Kulin HE, Wilson TE, et al. Detection of isolated aldosterone deficiency in the neonate. J Pediat 1983; 102:83.

Veldhuis JD, Melby JC. Isolated aldosterone deficiency in man: Acquired and inborn errors in the biosynthesis or action of aldosterone. Endocr Rev 1981; 2:495.

Visser HKA, Cost WS. A new hereditary defect in the biosynthesis of aldosterone: Urinary C_{21}-corticosteroid pattern in three related patients with a salt-losing syndrome, suggesting an 18-oxidation defect. Acta Endocrinol 1964; 47:589.

Weinberger MH, Grim CE, Hollifield JW. Primary aldosteronism: Diagnosis, localization and treatment. Ann Intern Med 1979; 90:386.

Wenting GJ, Man in 't Veld AJ, Derkx FH, et al. ACTH-dependent aldosterone excess due to adrenocortical adenoma: A variant of primary aldosteronism. J Clin Endocrinol Metab 1978; 46:326.

White EA, Schambelan M, Rost CR, et al. Use of computed tomography in diagnosing the cause of primary aldosteronism. N Engl J Med 1980; 303:1503.

Wilson ID, Goetz FC. Selective hypoaldosteronism after prolonged heparin administration. Am J Med 1964; 36:635.

Wisgerhof M, Brown RD, Hogan MJ, et al. The plasma aldosterone response to angiotensin II infusion in aldosterone-producing adenoma and idiopathic hyperaldosteronism. J Clin Endocrinol Metab 1981; 52:195.

Wisgerhof M, Carpenter PC, Brown RD. Increased adrenal sensitivity to angiotensin II in idiopathic hyperaldosteronism. J Clin Endocrinol Metab 1978; 47:938.

Zipser RD, Speckart PF. "Normotensive" primary aldosteronism. Ann Intern Med 1978; 88:655.

12   Adrenal Medullary Function

Emmanuel L. Bravo, M.D.

The definitive diagnosis of pheochromocytoma rests primarily on the measurement of norepinephrine, epinephrine, or their urinary metabolites, usually the metanephrines and vanillylmandelic acid (VMA). A logical approach to the laboratory assessment of patients suspected of having adrenal medullary hyperfunction is based on a thorough understanding of the biochemistry and physiology of the sympathoadrenomedullary system, the biochemistry of pheochromocytoma, and finally, an awareness of the limitations and pitfalls of some methods of analyzing catecholamines and their metabolites in biologic fluids.

BIOCHEMISTRY OF CATECHOLAMINES

The catecholamines are the products of the amino acid tyrosine. The initial step in the sequence is the hydroxylation of tyrosine to dihydroxyphenylalanine (L-dopa) by the action of the enzyme tyrosine hydroxylase and then to dopamine by the enzyme dopa decarboxylase. Dopamine is then actively transported into intracellular vesicles, where it is converted to norepinephrine by dopamine-beta-hydroxylase (DBH). Most of the norepinephrine is stored as a nondiffusible complex. In the adrenal medullary chromaffin cell, norepinephrine is converted further to epinephrine by the enzyme phenylethanolamine-n-methyltransferase (PNMT), which is found almost exclusively in the adrenal medulla.

In a normal adrenal medulla, the concentration of epinephrine is about four times that of norepinephrine, and the same ratio is found in the adrenal venous effluent. However, in plasma, norepinephrine is about eight to ten times that of epinephrine. Norepinephrine in plasma is derived almost exclusively (about 98 percent) from axon terminals of sympathetic postganglionic neurons; the remaining 2 percent derive from adrenal medullary secretion. On the other hand, all of the circulating epinephrine originates from the adrenal medulla. Centrally synthesized catecholamines do not contribute to the plasma pool of catecholamines.

The catecholamines are metabolized principally by two enzymes (Fig. 12–1): monoamine oxidase (MAO), which is found principally within adrenergic neurons, and

catechol-O-methyltransferase (COMT), which is localized for the most part in nonneural tissues. The action of COMT results in the formation of the metanephrines; further oxidation of the amines by MAO leads to the formation of VMA. With the use of radioactively labeled norepinephrine, it is estimated that of the circulating norepinephrine, 5 percent appears in urine as the free form and 8 percent is conjugated; 20 percent appears as free and conjugated normetanephrines; 23 percent as free and conjugated 3, 4-dihydroxyphenylethyleneglycol; and 30 percent as VMA (Maas and Landis, 1971). The free forms, metanephrine, and VMA are commonly assayed to assess adrenomedullary activity.

PLASMA CATECHOLAMINES

Two assay methods for determination of plasma norepinephrine and epinephrine levels are commercially available. The isotope derivative (or radioenzymatic) assay utilizes enzymatic conversion of catecholamines to tritium-labeled O-methyl derivatives to metanephrine and normetanephrine by COMT, followed by extensive purification of the derivatives by thin-layer chromatography (Peuler and Johnson, 1977). This assay is sensitive to 5.0 pg per 50 μl of plasma for either catecholamine; it is highly reproducible, but technically demanding. A second method employs high-pressure liquid chromatography (HPLC) to separate catecholamines in a plasma extract, with measurement by electrochemical detection (Goldstein et al, 1981). Results from this assay correlate well with those of the radioenzymatic assay. Although less sensitive, it is acceptable for clinical applications.

Reported normal supine values for plasma norepinephrine and epinephrine for the radioenzymatic (COMT) method average 227 ± 119 (SD) pg per milliliter and for HPLC, 353 ± 94 (SD) pg per milliliter. In our normal population studies, supine resting plasma norepinephrine concentrations, measured by the radioenzymatic method, average 218 ± 92 (SD) pg per milliliter, and plasma epinephrine concentrations average 42 ± 18 (SD) pg per milliliter (Table 12–1). No sex differences or age relationships were found in this group of 38 men and 22 women (age range, 22 to 72 years).

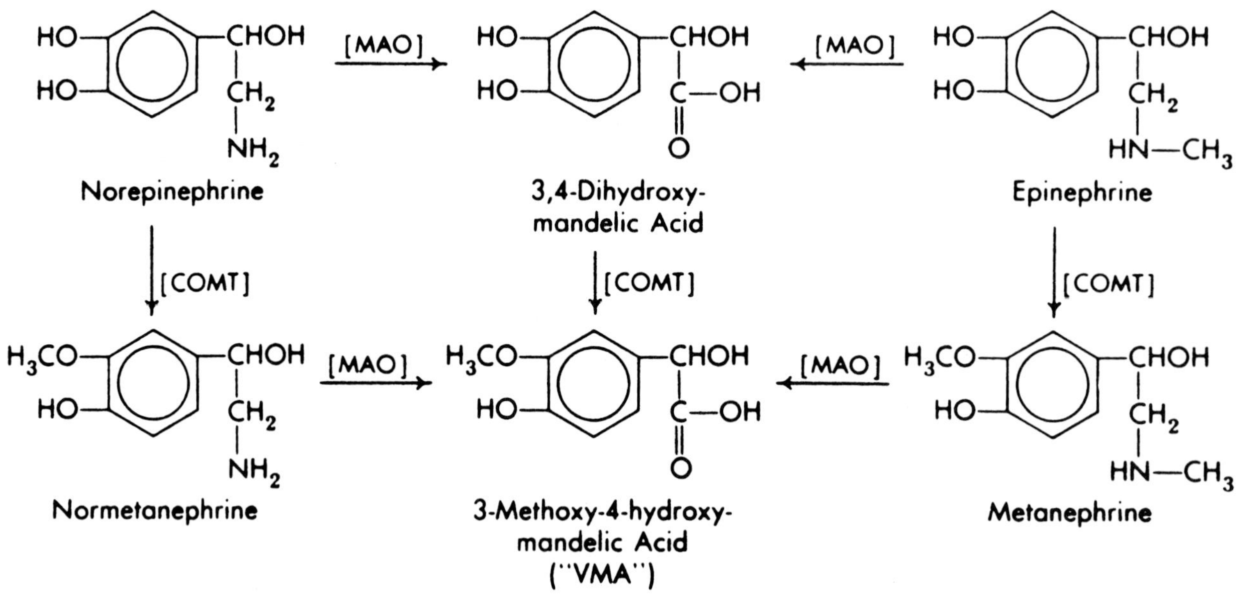

Figure 12-1   Metabolism of norepinephrine and epinephrine. COMT = catechol-O-methyltransferase; MAO= monoamine oxidase. (Modified from Mayer SE. In: Goodman LS, Gilman AG, eds. The pharmacological basis of therapeutics. 6th ed. New York: McGraw-Hill, 1980; with permission.)

Twofold to threefold increases in plasma norepinephrine levels occur in the upright position, whereas the plasma epinephrine level remains unchanged. Threefold to fourfold increments in plasma norepinephrine and 50-fold increments in plasma epinephrine occur during insulin-induced hypoglycemia (Cryer, 1980).

Certain precautions are worth emphasizing. Because of the lability of plasma catecholamines, rigidly controlled environmental conditions must be ensured during patient sampling and subsequent storage of samples. Basal levels are preferably drawn by means of an indwelling 21-gauge butterfly needle and kept patent with heparinized saline solution, following an overnight fast and 20 minutes of supine rest. Blood samples should be collected with either heparin or ethylenediaminetetraacetic acid (EDTA), kept in ice, spun in a refrigerated centrifuge at 4 °C within 1 hour, and then stored at −70 °C until processing. No coffee, tea, or smoking should be allowed for at least 3 hours prior to testing.

Careful consideration should be given to some clinical disorders that may elevate plasma catecholamines. These include marked volume depletion and the presence of other concomitant diseases such as angina pectoris, chronic obstructive pulmonary disease, chronic congestive heart failure, chronic renal failure, transient ischemic attacks, depression, hypothyroidism, and ketoacidosis. Spuriously low values could result from errors in blood sampling and in the handling and subsequent storage of samples.

A variety of drugs can alter the levels of circulating catecholamines (Table 12–2). Drugs that inhibit central sympathetic outflow (i.e., clonidine, methyldopa, guanabenz, bromocriptine, haloperidol) decrease plasma catecholamines in normal and hypertensive subjects but have little effect on the excessive catecholamine secretion by pheochromocytoma. Drugs that tend to increase plasma catecholamines do so only slightly, and levels of plasma catecholamines do not approach those usually encountered in pheochromocytoma. However, two drug-related conditions can produce levels of plasma catecholamines (greater than 2,000 pg per milliliter) that approach those of patients with pheochromocytoma: during sudden clonidine withdrawal and during vasodilator therapy with either hydralazine or minoxidil.

URINARY CATECHOLAMINES AND METABOLITES

Two major metabolites of the catecholamines, the metanephrines and VMA, are commonly assayed to assess sympathoadrenomedullary activity. These tests are relatively easy to perform and are usually readily available. In most circumstances a diagnosis can be confirmed or excluded on the basis of properly collected 24-hour urine samples. However, problems with urine collections and spurious results from drug or dietary interference aside, reliance on urinary determinations alone as indexes of catecholamine production can be misleading. The amounts and types of metabolites excreted in urine depend on the excretory function of the kidneys (Baines et al, 1979) and on the activities of synthesizing and degradative enzymes within the tumor (Jarrott and Louis, 1977). These relationships are discussed in later sections. Table 12–3 shows the effects of various drugs on simultaneously measured urinary free catecholamines, VMA, and metanephrine.

TABLE 12-1   Plasma Catecholamines

Uses

Diagnosis of pheochromocytoma

Method

Radioenzymatic and HPLC
Samples drawn in basal state using indwelling 21-gauge needle
with heparinized saline
Overnight fast and 20 minutes so supine rest samples collected
with heparin or EDTA, iced, spun in a refrigerated centrifuge at
4° C within one hour and stored at -70° C until processing.
No caffeinated beverages or smoking 3 hours before test.

Normal Values

Norepinephrine 218 ± 92 (SD) pg/ml radioenzymatic
Epinephrine   42 ± 18 (SD) pg/ml radioenzymatic

Interpretation

Values ≥ 2,000 pg/ml are usually associated with
pheochromocytoma. Values between 1,000 and 2,000 pg/ml are
equivocal and require a suppression test. Values ≤ 1,000 pg/ml
require a stimulation test (glucagon) if warranted by the
clinical setting.

Pitfalls

Disorders which elevate plasma catecholamines
Volume depletion, COPD, angina, CHF, chronic renal failure,
TIAs, depression, hypothyroidism, and ketoacidosis
Low Values
Errors in sampling, handling, and storage of samples
Drugs which alter levels (see Table 12-2).

NOTE: Clonidine withdrawal and vasodilator therapy with
hydralazine or minoxidil may elevate levels into the
pheochromocytoma range.

Reprinted with permission from *Endocrinology and Metabolism Continuing Education,* March 1984, Volume 2, No. 9, page 2, Table 1. Copyright
American Association for Clinical Chemistry, Inc.

CATECHOLAMINE PRODUCTION IN PHEOCHROMOCYTOMA

In pheochromocytoma, the activities of the enzymes involved in catecholamine synthesis (tyrosine hydroxylase, aromatic amino acid decarboxylase, and DBH) are markedly enhanced, whereas the activities of the enzymes involved in catecholamine catabolism (MAO and COMT) are reduced (Jarrott and Louis, 1977). Thus, excess amounts of newly synthesized norepinephrine that cannot be stored in the filled catecholamine storage vesicles may not be degraded and could diffuse from the pheochromocytoma into the circulation. This could result in large amounts of circulating norepinephrine with relatively small increases in urinary catecholamine metabolites.

Crout and Sjoerdsma (1964) have also demonstrated that the size of the tumor might be an important determinant of the relative amounts of catecholamine excretory products. They reported that small tumors weighing less than 50 g have rapid turnover rates with small catecholamine content. These tumors release mainly unmetabolized catecholamines into the circulation, resulting in low concentrations of metabolites relative to free catecholamines in the urine. On the other hand, large tumors weighing more than 50 g have slow turnover rates with large catecholamine content. These tumors release mainly metabolized catecholamines into the circulation, resulting in high concentrations of metabolites relative to free catecholamines in the urine.

These observations have important clinical implications. Because they release free unmetabolized catecholamines into the circulation, small tumors may tend to produce more symptoms and are best diagnosed by the measurement of plasma catecholamines. On the other hand, patients who have large tumors that metabolize most of the secreted catecholamines tend to have fewer

TABLE 12-2   Drugs that Spuriously Alter Urinary Excretion of Catecholamines and their Metabolites

Catecholamine/Metabolite	Increase	Decrease
Free catecholamines (<100 µg/24 hours)	Methyldopa L-dopa Prochlorperazine (Compazine) Amphetamine Clonidine withdrawal	Clonidine
VMA (<6.8 mg/24 hours)	Chlorpromazine Nalidixic acid Glycerol guaiacolate Methocarbamol (Robaxin) Clonidine withdrawal	MAO inhibitors Radiographic contrast material Clonidine
Metanephrines (<1.3 mg/24 hours)	MAO inhibitors Clonidine withdrawal Labetalol	Clonidine Clofibrate Nalidixic acid Radiographic contrast material

From Bravo EL. Plasma catecholamines: Their measurement and clinical utility. Lab Med, September 1986; with permission.

TABLE 12-3   Effect of Drugs on Plasma Norepinephrine Levels

Increase	Decrease	Uncertain*
Slight to moderate increase:	Clonidine (Catapres)	Propranolol (Inderal)
Phenoxybenzamine (Dibenzyline)	Methyldopa (Aldomet)	Nadolol (Corgard)
Phentolamine (Regitine)	Guanabenz (Wytensin)	Metoprolol (Lopressor)
Prazosin (Minipress)	Guanethidine (Ismelin)	Atenolol (Tenormin)
Tricyclic antidepressants	Reserpine (Serpasil)	Timolol (Blocadren)
Metoclopramide (Reglan)	Bromocriptine (Parlodel)	
Labetalol (Normodyne)	Haloperidol (Haldol)	
Amphetamines	Chlorpromazine (Thorazine)	
Ephedrine	Alpha-methyltyrosine (Demser)	
Methylxanthines	Cimetidine (Tagamet)	
Nifedipine (Procardia)	Thyroxine	
Thyrotropin-releasing hormone (protirelin)		
Naloxone		
Marked increase:		
Minoxidil (Loniten)		
Hydralazine (Apresoline)		
Acute clonidine withdrawal (Catapres)		

* Reported as either increased or unchanged.
From Bravo EL. The syndrome of primary aldosteronism and pheochromocytoma. In: Schrier RW, Gottschalk CW, eds. Diseases of the kidney. Vol II. 4th ed. Boston: Little, Brown, 1988; with permission.

symptoms, relatively lower circulating free catecholamines, but high urinary catecholamine metabolites.

PLASMA CATECHOLAMINES AND URINARY CATECHOLAMINE METABOLITES IN PHEOCHROMOCYTOMA

Figures 12–2 and 12–3 depict plasma catecholamine levels in a group of patients with documented pheochromocytoma. Their values are compared with those of subjects with essential hypertension. It is clear that the majority of patients with pheochromocytoma have markedly elevated plasma catecholamine levels that exceed those seen in other conditions. Three patients had plasma norepinephrine values that fell within the upper 95 percent confidence limits for values obtained in patients with essential hypertension (i.e., 811 pg per milliliter). None had values that fell within the range for sex- and age-matched normotensive subjects (i.e., 402 pg per milliliter). It is evident that the plasma epinephrine concentration has little value in predicting the location of a tumor. Although some patients with adrenal pheochromocytomas have plasma epinephrine values within normal range, some patients with extra-adrenal tumors have values that are distinctly above the normal range (see Fig. 12–3).

It is useful to record the blood pressure during plasma sampling for catecholamine measurements. Normal plasma catecholamine values obtained when the patient is normotensive and asymptomatic do not exclude the presence of a pheochromocytoma. *However, normal plasma catecholamine values in a hypertensive and symptomatic patient make the diagnosis of pheochromocytoma highly unlikely.*

Figure 12–4 shows the results of comparing simul-

taneously measured plasma catecholamines and urinary metanephrine and VMA in patients who had surgically confirmed pheochromocytoma (Bravo and Gifford, 1984). With the use of measurements in patients with essential hypertension as reference values, it can be shown that 25 of the 43 patients had false-negative results for uri-

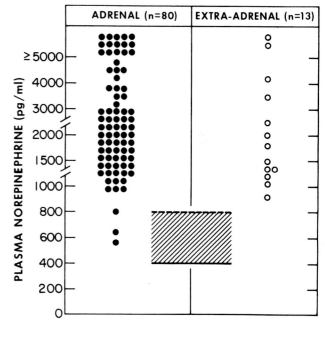

PLASMA EPINEPHRINE IN PHEOCHROMOCYTOMA

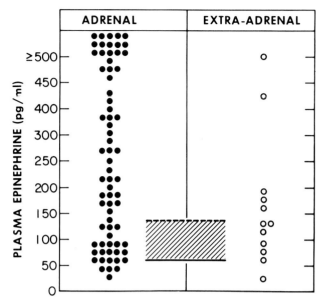

Figure 12-3 Plasma epinephrine values in pheochromocytoma. The cross-hatched area represents the mean (59 pg per milliliter) and the 95 percent upper confidence limits (135 pg per milliliter) of values obtained from 104 essential hypertensives.

degradation of catecholamines in pheochromocytomas (see earlier). Further, they suggest that of the urinary catecholamine metabolites, urinary metanephrine provides a more reliable clue to the presence of pheochromocytoma than does urinary VMA and that plasma catecholamine measurements are at least as reliable as the measurement of urinary metanephrine in predicting the presence of pheochromocytoma.

SENSITIVITY AND SPECIFICITY OF VARIOUS BIOCHEMICAL TESTS

The sensitivity and specificity of the various biochemical tests are as follows (Table 12–4): Measurement of plasma catecholamines appears to have the highest sensitivity and specificity, and the measurement of urinary VMA the lowest. However, all three tests provide excellent specificity when values are elevated.

The availability of tests in any given center will necessarily determine investigation in an individual patient, and debate over the relative merits of various tests will continue. However, it seems likely that if reliably carried out, any test will serve as well as another provided the investigator is aware of the limitations and pitfalls of some methods of analysis. However, because the metabolism of catecholamines in patients with pheochromocytoma may be modified by either a lack or an excess of metabolizing enzymes, both plasma catecholamines and catecholamine metabolites in urine (preferably metanephrine) should be measured in equivocal cases.

PHARMACOLOGIC TESTS FOR PHEOCHROMOCYTOMA

In most cases the demonstration of increased levels of plasma or urinary catecholamines and their metabolites should suffice to confirm the diagnosis of pheo-

nary VMA. On the other hand, only nine had false-negative results for urinary metanephrine. In one patient all three biochemical measurements were within the range of values in patients with essential hypertension. In another patient an elevated level of urinary metanephrine was the only biochemical abnormality, and in three patients the only abnormal result was an elevated level of plasma catecholamines. These findings are in accord with the demonstration of variable metabolism and

Figure 12-4 Comparison of simultaneously measured indexes of catecholamine production in 43 patients with surgically confirmed pheochromocytoma. The horizontal broken lines represent the 95 percent upper confidence limits of values for urinary vanillylmandelic acid (VMA) (i.e., 11 mg per 24 hours) and urinary metanephrines (MN) (i.e., 1.8 mg per 24 hours) in 30 subjects with essential hypertension. NE + E denotes norepinephrine plus epinephrine. Solid symbols denote false-negative tests. (From Bravo EL, Gifford RW. Pheochromocytoma: Diagnosis, localization and management. N Engl J Med 1984; 311:1298; reprinted with permission of *The New England Journal of Medicine*.)

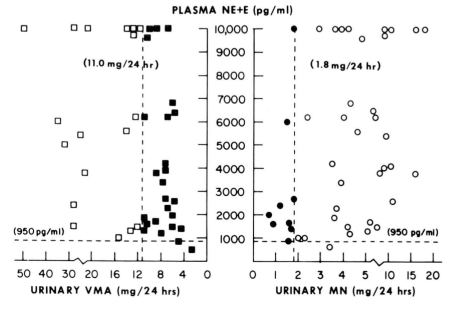

TABLE 12–4   Sensitivity and Specificity of Various Biochemical Tests

Biochemical Test	Standard*	Sensitivity (% range)†	Specificity (% range)
Plasma NE + E	>950 pg/ml	88–100	93–101
Urinary NMN + MN	>1.8 mg/24 hours	67– 91	83–103
Urinary VMA	>11.0 mg/24 hours	28– 56	98–102

NE + E = norepinephrine plus epinephrine; NMN + MN = normetanephrine plus metanephrine; VMA = vanillylmandelic acid.
* Upper 95% confidence limits obtained from essential hypertension subjects under basal conditions.
† Values are expressed as % ± 2 SE.
From Bravo EL. Pheochromocytoma: Current concepts in diagnosis, localization, and management. Primary Care 1983; 10:82; with permission.

chromocytoma (Table 12–5). However, when the biochemical tests are equivocal and the diagnosis is still open to question, a pharmacologic approach has been used. A provocative test is usually employed when the clinical findings are highly suggestive of pheochromocytoma but the blood pressure is normal or only slightly increased (160/100 mm Hg or lower) and catecholamine production is nearly normal. In patients with moderate increases in plasma catecholamines (between 1,000 and 2,000 pg per milliliter) with or without hypertension, a suppression test is employed.

The glucagon stimulation test (Lawrence, 1967) is widely used as a provocative agent because it has fewer side effects (Table 12–6). Glucagon is given as an intravenous bolus dose of 1.0 to 2.0 mg after determination of the patient's pressor response to a cold pressor test. A positive glucagon test requires a clear increase (at least threefold or over 2,000 pg per milliliter in plasma catecholamines, 1 to 3 minutes after drug administration. A simultaneous increase in blood pressure of at least 20/15 mm Hg above the pressor response to a cold pressor test is desirable but not essential.

TABLE 12–5   Urinary Catecholamines and Metabolites

Uses

   For the diagnosis of pheochromocytoma

Method

   HPLC: 24-hour urines collected in plastic bottles with acid preservatives; refrigerated during collection.

Normal values

Free norepinephrine	≤100 µg/24 hr
Free epinephrine	≤25 µg/24 hr
Metanephrines	≤300 µg/24 hr
Normetanephrines	≤620 µg/24 hr
MN & NMN	≤820 µg/24 hr
VMA	≤6.0 µg/24 hr

Pitfalls

   Drugs interfering with the tests are found in Table 12–2.
   Tumors that lack the enzyme MAO produce normal amounts of VMA.
   Tumors that lack the enzyme COMT produce normal amounts of both metanephrines and VMA.

The clonidine suppression test (Bravo et al, 1981) uses the ability of clonidine, a centrally acting alpha-adrenergic agonist, to suppress the release of neurogenically mediated catecholamine release (Table 12–7). The test is based on the principle that normal increases in plasma catecholamines are mediated through activation of the sympathetic nervous system, whereas in patients with pheochromocytoma, the increases result from diffusion of excess catecholamines from the tumor into the circulation, bypassing normal storage and release mechanisms. Therefore, clonidine should not be expected to suppress the release of catecholamines in patients with pheochromocytoma.

Figure 12–5 shows the results of the clonidine suppression test in patients with proven pheochromocytoma. The results were compared with those into sex-matched and age-matched subjects with essential hypertension. Of the 40 patients, 27 had adrenal pheochromocytoma and 13 had extra-adrenal pheochromocytoma. After clonidine had been administered, plasma catecholamine values fell below 500 pg per milliliter in all but one hypertensive patient. All but one patient with pheochromocytoma had plasma catecholamine values above 500 pg per milliliter. *Based on this experience, a normal clonidine suppression test should consist of a fall in the basal values of plasma norepinephrine plus epinephrine to a level below 500 pg per milliliter at 2 or 3 hours after the oral administration of 0.3 mg of clonidine.* It is important to record blood pressure and heart rate responses and any effects related to the central nervous system, as these signs and symptoms reflect completeness of the gastrointestinal absorption of clonidine.

A potential hazard during the performance of the test is hypotension. Experience with the test over the years indicates that in the untreated patient, symptomatic hypotension is not a problem. All reported cases of severe hypotension requiring treatment have occurred in patients who were receiving antihypertensive medications or had other conditions that would tend to augment the effects of any antihypertensive agent (Burris and D'Angelo, 1982; Given et al, 1983). In particular, marked volume depletion should be avoided, and any beta-adrenergic blocking agent should be discontinued about 48 hours before the test is performed. Since clonidine has a potent vagotonic effect, concomitant beta-adrenergic

TABLE 12-6   Glucagon Stimulation Test

Uses

Diagnosis of pheochromocytoma

Clinical Indications

In any patient with signs and symptoms suggestive of pheochromocytoma but normal or near-normal plasma catecholamines and diastolic blood pressure ≤ 100 mm Hg

Clinically asymptomatic patients with any of the following:
  • history of familial pheochromocytoma
  • an endocrine abnormality that is associated with MEA syndromes (e.g., hyperparathyroidism, medullary carcinoma of the thyroid)
  • clinical syndromes associated with pheochromocytoma (i.e., von Hippel Lindau syndrome, von Recklinghausen's neurofibromatosis)
  • significant pressor response to anesthetic agents or paradoxical hypertension with use of reserpine or guanethidine

Preparation

Fast for 10 hours overnight
Discontinue all drugs that act on the sympathetic nervous system at least 48 hours prior to testing. Procardia 10 mg, sublingual, may be administered 30 minutes prior to testing if elevation of blood pressure is a serious concern.
Have ready for IV injection 10 mg Regitine in 10 ml of 0.9 percent sodium chloride solution
Commence study after 30 min supine rest and insertion of a 19- to 21-gauge scalp vein needle into the forearm vein, which is kept patent with 0.9 percent sodium chloride solution containing two units of heparin per ml.

Test Performance

Determine arterial blood pressure and heart rate three times at 1-minute intervals.
Draw 5 ml blood for plasma catecholamines
Give 2.0 mg glucagon (in 10 ml 0.9 percent sodium chloride solution) intravenously over 60 sec
Measure blood pressure every 30 sec
Draw blood for plasma catecholamines at 1 and 2 min after glucagon injection

Interpretation

A positive response consists of at least a 3-fold rise and ≥ 2,000 pg/ml in plasma catecholamines 1 to 2 min after glucagon injection. A simultaneous increase in arterial blood pressure by 25/15 mm Hg is desirable, but not essential.

Pitfalls

Leakage of glucagon into the subcutaneous tissue or failure to properly sample blood at designated times makes interpretation of the test difficult.

blockade could lead to marked bradycardia, with further decreases in stroke volume and cardiac output resulting in severe hypotension.

Certain pitfalls must be avoided when the clonidine suppression test is performed. Beta-adrenergic blockers can prevent the plasma catecholamine–lowering effect of clonidine in a patient without pheochromocytoma because of the ability of such agents to interfere with hepatic clearance of catecholamines (Esler et al, 1981). Only assays that measure free catecholamines should be used. Assays that measure conjugated catecholamines give false-positive results (Aron et al, 1983) because conjugated catecholamines have long half-lives that are influenced by even mild degrees of renal functional impairment.

Pentolinium, 2.5 mg given intravenously, has been used by Brown and co-workers (1981) to detect small pheochromocytomas in patients. They found that the plasma epinephrine concentration, which was invariably increased in these patients, was not suppressed by pentolinium administration. However, this drug, which can produce acute urinary retention in susceptible persons, is not available in the United States.

LOCALIZATION OF PHEOCHROMOCYTOMA

Once the diagnosis has been confirmed, anatomic localization is mandatory because of the variable location of these tumors. Ninety-seven percent are found in the abdominal region. Less likely sites are the thorax (2 to 3 percent) and the neck (1 percent). The majority are found in the adrenal glands. Multiple tumors may

TABLE 12–7 Clonidine Suppression Test

Clinical Indications

Patient requiring a provocative test where further increases in blood pressure would be hazardous
To rule out the diagnosis of pheochromocytoma in the hypertensive patients with borderline increases in plasma and/or urinary catecholamines and symptoms suggestive of pheochromocytoma
Unexplained increases in plasma and/or urinary catecholamine levels
Adrenal mass but with questionable clinical manifestations and borderline increases in plasma and/or urinary catecholamine levels

Preparation

Discontinue all drugs that act on the sympathetic nervous system at least 48 hours prior to testing
Fast for 10 hours overnight
Bring patient into a quiet, warm, well-lighted room
Insert 19- to 21-gauge scalp vein needle into a forearm vein and keep patent with 0.9 percent sodium chloride solution containing 2 U heparin per ml
Commence study after 30 min of supine rest and insertion of needle

Test Performance

Determine arterial blood pressure and heart rate three times at 1-min intervals
Draw 5 ml of blood for plasma catecholamines
Give clonidine (Catapres) orally (0.3 mg) with 250 ml of water
Determine arterial blood pressure and heart rate at 30-min intervals for 3 hours
Sample blood (5.0 ml) for plasma catecholamines at 2 and 3 hours following oral clonidine

Blood Collection

Do not use a tourniquet
Draw blood samples into 10-ml plastic syringes and immediately transfer into heparin-treated tubes on ice
Separate in a refrigerated centrifuge at 4° C within 1 hour
Store plasma at -70° C until processing

Precautions

Sit patient up slowly after the test to prevent symptomatic orthostatic hypotension
Instruct patient not to drive a car for at least 8 hours after test

Interpretation

A normal response is a fall of plasma norepinephrine and epinephrine to ≤ 500 pg/ml and a fall of at least 40 percent from basal values

Pitfalls

Only techniques that measure *free* norepinephrine and epinephrine in plasma should be used
In tumors producing exclusively or predominantly epinephrine, plasma norepinephrine values will be reduced by clonidine
Beta-adrenergic blockers tend to increase the half-life of circulating catecholamines and may produce false-positive tests

arise in 10 percent of adults. Familial pheochromocytomas are frequently bilateral or arise from multiple sites. Pheochromocytomas occurring in children are commonly bilateral and more frequently lie outside the adrenals than in adults.

Current experience suggests that the use of computed tomographic (CT) scanning should all but eliminate the need for potentially hazardous arteriographic studies in the preoperative detection and localization of pheochromocytoma (Fig. 12–6). The procedure is noninvasive and nontoxic, appears to detect tumors larger than 1.0 cm accurately, and has a localizing precision of about 96 percent (Stewart et al, 1978). It is now suggested that CT scanning be selected as the initial localizing procedure. If the CT scan fails to demonstrate the presence of a tumor, selective arteriography can be performed. Selective caval sampling for catecholamine levels is reported to have a success rate of 97 percent (Allison et al, 1983), but the procedure is necessary only when an extra-adrenal tumor is suspected and when the presence of an adrenal tumor cannot be demonstrated satisfactorily by other techniques.

A recently developed technique for the localization of neoplastic chromaffin tissues uses ^{131}I-metaiodobenzylguanidine (MIBG), a radioactive compound selectively taken up by adrenergic cells (Sisson et al, 1981). Initial results suggest that it may be most useful in locating small multicentric sites and metastatic tumors or in proving that a mass demonstrated by other imaging techniques is an adrenergic tumor (Fig. 12–7). Scanning within ^{131}I-MIBG is reported to have an overall sensitivity of 77 percent, a specificity of 96 percent, and an accuracy of 86 percent (Swensen et al, 1985). Ultrasonography can be useful in determining whether a mass is solid or cystic.

EVALUATION OF THE PATIENT SUSPECTED OF HAVING PHEOCHROMOCYTOMA

Priority of evaluation is given to patients with the clinical characteristics described in Table 12–8. Concentrations of total plasma catecholamines are measured after the patient has rested in a supine position for at least 30 minutes. Values over 2,000 pg per milliliter are considered pathognomonic of pheochromocytoma. When

PHEOCHROMOCYTOMA

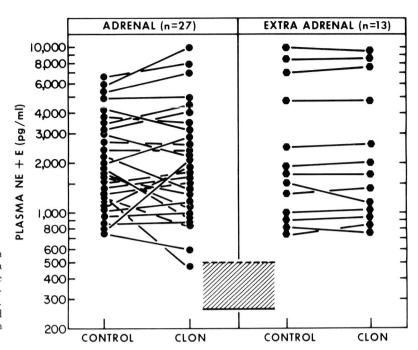

Figure 12–5 The clonidine suppression test in pheochromocytoma. The cross-hatched area represents the mean (218 pg per milliliter) and the 95 percent upper confidence limits (500 pg per milliliter) of values obtained from 47 normal subjects. Values shown represent the lowest values reached (at either 2 or 3 hours) after oral administration of 0.3 mg clonidine.

patients have values between 1,000 and 2,000 pg per milliliter, a clonidine suppression test is performed. An abdominal CT scan is then performed in patients with clinical and biochemical features suggestive of pheochromocytoma (Fig. 12–8).

A small percentage (about 9 percent) of patients may have moderate elevations in plasma catecholamine levels—that is, less than 1,000 pg per milliliter. Therefore, whenever the clinical presentation is suggestive of pheochromocytoma and plasma catecholamine levels are only slightly or moderately increased, further evaluation should be performed. Repeat testing, including the measurement of urinary catecholamine metabolites, should be done for confirmation. Such cases will require either a provocative test or a suppression test for a more definitive diagnosis. However, a provocative test should not be performed when the arterial blood pressure is 160/100 mm Hg or higher or when the patient has concomitant problems that might make sudden increases in blood pressure risky. In such cases, the clonidine suppression test should be employed.

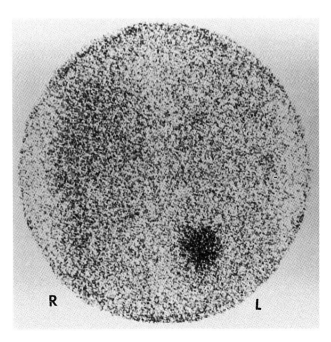

Figure 12–6 Localization of pheochromocytoma by abdominal CT scan. (k=kidney; v=inferior vena cava; a=aorta; p=pheochromocytoma.)

Figure 12–7 Localization of pheochromocytoma employing ^{131}I-MIBG. Uptake of ^{131}I-MIBG by the same tumor shown in Figure 12–6, 72 hours after radiosotope injection.

SIMPLIFIED APPROACH TO PHEOCHROMOCYTOMA

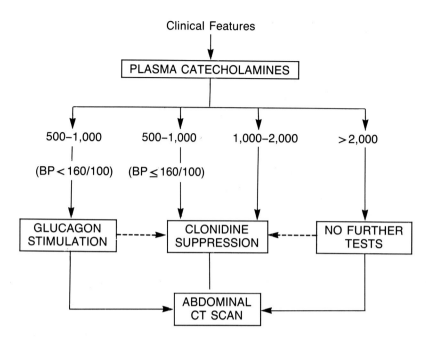

Figure 12-8 An algorithm recommended in the evaluation of patients suspected of having pheochromocytoma. (Modified from Bravo EL. The syndrome of primary aldosteronism and pheochromocytoma. In: Schrier RW, Gottschalk CW, eds. Diseases of the kidney. Vol II. 4th ed. Boston: Little, Brown, 1988; with permission.)

TABLE 12-8   Clinical Characteristics Warranting Priority of Evaluation for Pheochromocytoma

Accelerated or malignant hypertension

Refractoriness to medical antihypertensive therapy

Paroxysmal symptoms and hypertensive crises precipitated by mental stresses or during induction of general anesthesia or use of desipramine

Paradoxical hypertension with use of reserpine or guanethidine (both drugs have in common the property of acutely releasing stored catecholamines)

Presence of mucocutaneous familial disorders
  von Recklinghausen's neurofibromatosis
  Mucocutaneous neuromata with bilateral adrenal tumors, medullary carcinoma of thyroid, and ganglioneuromata of the visceral plexuses (multiple endocrine neoplasia type IIb)

Other related disorders
  von Hippel–Lindau disease (angiomata of the retina with cystic hemangioblastoma of the cerebellum)
  Sipple's syndrome (bilateral adrenal tumors, medullary carcinoma of the thyroid, and hyperparathyroidism, multiple endocrine neoplasia type IIa)
  Ectopic adrenocorticotropic hormone syndrome

BIBLIOGRAPHY

Allison DJ, Brown MJ, Jones DH, et al. Role of venous sampling in locating a pheochromocytoma. Br Med J 1983; 286:1122.

Aron DC, Bravo EL, Kapcala LP. Erroneous plasma norepinephrine levels in radioimmunoassay. Ann Intern Med 1983; 98:1023.

Baines AD, Craan AA, Chan W, et al. Tubular secretion and metabolism of dopamine, norepinephrine, methoxytryamine and normetanephrine by the rat kidney. J Pharmacol Exp Ther 1979; 208:144.

Bravo EL, Gifford RW Jr. Pheochromocytoma: Diagnosis, localization and management. N Eng J Med 1984; 311:1298.

Bravo EL, Tarazi RC, Fouad FM, et al. Clonidine-suppression: A useful aid in the diagnosis of pheochromocytoma. N Engl J Med 1981; 305:623.

Brown MJ, Allison DJ, Jenner DA, et al. Increased sensitivity and accuracy of pheochromocytoma diagnosis achieved by use of plasma-adrenaline estimations and a pentolinum-suppression test. Lancet 1981; 1:174.

Burris JF, D'Angelo LJ. Complications of clonidine suppression test for pheochromocytoma. N Engl J Med 1982; 307:756.

Crout JR, Sjoerdsma A. Turnover and metabolism of catecholamine in patients with pheochromocytoma. J Clin Invest 1964; 43:94.

Cryer PE. Physiology and pathophysiology of the human sympathoadrenal neuroendocrine system. N Engl J Med 1980; 303:436.

Esler IM, Jackman G, Leonard P, et al. Effect of propranolol on noradrenaline kinetics in patients with essential hypertension. Br J Clin Pharmacol 1981; 12:375.

Given BD, Taylor T, Lily LS, et al. Symptomatic hypotension following clonidine suppression test for pheochromocytoma. Arch Intern Med 1983; 143:2195.

Goldstein DS, Fenerstein GI, Izzo JL Jr, et al. Validity and reliability of fluid chromatography with electrochemical detection for measuring plasma levels of norepinephrine and epinephrine in man. Life Sci 1981; 28:467.

Jarrott B, Louis WJ. Abnormalities in enzymes involved in catecholamine synthesis and catabolism in pheochromocytoma. Clin Sci 1977; 53:529.

Lawrence AM. Glucagon provocative test for pheochromocytoma. Ann Intern Med 1967; 66:1091.

Maas JW, Landis DH. The metabolism of circulating norepinephrine by human subjects. J Pharmacol Exp Ther 1971; 177:600.

Peuler JD, Johnson GA. Simultaneous single isotope radioenzymatic assay of plasma norepinephrine, epinephrine, and dopamines. Life Sci 1977; 21:625.

Sisson JC, Frager MS, Valk TW, et al. Scintigraphic localization of pheochromocytoma. N Engl J Med 1981; 305:12.

Stewart BH, Bravo EL, Haaga J, et al. Localization of pheochromocytoma by computed tomography. N Engl J Med 1978; 299:460.

Swensen SJ, Brown ML, Sheps SG, et al. Use of ^{131}I-MIBG scintigraphy in the evaluation of suspected pheochromocytoma. Mayo Clin Proc 1985; 60:299.

13

The Hypothalamic-Pituitary-Ovarian Axis

Daniel Spratt, M.D.
Jacquelyn Loughlin, M.D.

The reproductive system in women is regulated by a fascinating and complex set of hormonal interactions. Since reproduction is essential to the propagation of a species, it is not surprising that multiple levels of checks and balances have evolved. Nor is it surprising that abnormalities can and do occur in any component of the reproductive axis and its related hormones. Endocrine testing, understanding of reproductive hormone disorders, and treatments employing gonadotropins and gonadotropin-releasing hormone (Gn-RH, also called luteinizing hormone – releasing hormone) and its analogs have all rapidly advanced over the past several years. Effective application of this new information must be undertaken with continued appreciation of the basic operating principles of the reproductive axis.

Clinical assessment of disorders of the hypothalamic-pituitary-ovarian (HPO) axis relies heavily on laboratory measurements of serum hormone levels as well as on observation of end-organ hormonal effects. Such evaluation is usually undertaken for one of three reasons: (1) to assess causes of infertility, (2) to determine if menstrual irregularities reflect more serious underlying disorders or the onset of menopause, or (3) to evaluate premature or delayed sexual development. The principal goal of this evaluation is to locate the abnormality within the system so that appropriate therapy can be determined.

This chapter describes common endocrine testing of the female reproductive axis and related hormones and discusses the application and interpretation of those tests in clinical situations. Difficulties in interpreting laboratory tests often result from certain characteristics of this system, which may be beneficial to list at the onset of this discussion. In addition to cyclical variations, some hormones of this axis (particularly luteinizing hormone [LH] and progesterone) are often secreted in pulses so that concentrations in the blood may change from minute to minute. Furthermore, the effects of most hormones are related to the sum of the hormone secreted over time. Therefore, a determination of a blood concentration at a single point in time may not always reflect accurately the status of the system. Tests of end-organ hormone effect are often more useful. Second, changes in these hormones are so closely interrelated over the monthly cycle that each hormone cannot be considered in isolation. As with all hormones, a value in the "normal range" is not always normal for the individual under consideration and must be weighted with respect to the clinical situation and other hormones. As a final precaution, the roles of many tests of the HPO axis or of fertility remain controversial. Other tests such as the Gn-RH or clomiphene stimulations are now relegated chiefly to use in research settings. The status of these tests is specified later in this chapter. Ordering and interpretation of any endocrine testing should be tempered by each patient's history and physical findings.

OVERVIEW OF THE MENSTRUAL CYCLE

Reproductive function in women is characterized by the cycles of hormones described by Ross and colleagues (Fig. 13–1) that occur at approximately monthly intervals (hence, *menses*, the plural of the Greek word *mensis*, meaning "month"). Shortly after birth, the HPO axis is activated for several months and then is relatively quiescent until puberty. The gonads are activated at puberty by enhanced secretion of Gn-RH, the decapeptide hypothalamic hormone responsible for stimulating the anterior pituitary to release the gonadotropins, LH and follicle-stimulating hormone (FSH) (Fig. 13–2). At gonadarche, Gn-RH secretion rises, resulting in increased release of LH and FSH, which in turn stimulates follicular maturation in the ovary. In 2 to 3 years, regular ovulatory cycles are established that persist until the onset of menopause. The control mechanisms responsible for the enhancement of Gn-RH secretion are unclear. However, the burgeoning knowledge of the roles of endorphins and neurotransmitters (such as dopamine and the catecholamines) in regulation of Gn-RH may lead to a greater understanding of the mechanisms of puberty and menstrual disturbances.

The first detailed depiction of hormonal events in the menstrual cycle was derived from several sources. Ross and others' description of cyclical changes in LH, FSH, and ovarian steroids was obtained by sampling blood daily across the menstrual cycle. Other studies defined nega-

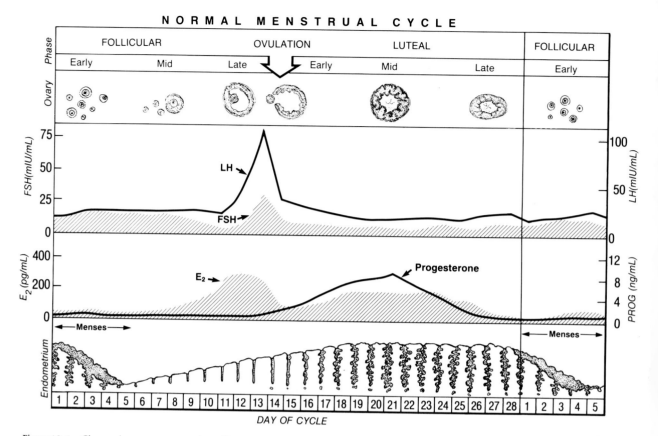

Figure 13-1 Changes in serum concentrations of LH, FSH, estradiol, and progesterone and in the endometrium that accompany follicular maturation, ovulation, and corpus luteum function across the menstrual cycle. Measurements of these hormones and their effects on the body temperature, the endometrium, the cervical mucus, and vaginal cytology are employed in the diagnosis of reproductive disorders. (Adapted from Ross GT. Disorders of the ovary and female reproductive tract. In: Wilson JD, Foster DW, eds. Williams textbook of endocrinology, 7th ed. Philadelphia: WB Saunders, 1985:224–225.)

tive and positive feedback control of gonadotropin secretion by the ovarian steroids. Morphologic and biochemical studies described the maturing follicle, the corpus luteum, and the progressive changes occurring in the endometrium.

Each menstrual cycle begins with recruitment and stimulation of a cohort of primordial follicles from which a dominant follicle is eventually selected during the follicular phase (see Fig. 13–1). The falling levels of progesterone, estrogen, and inhibin associated with the end of the previous cycle contribute to decreased negative feedback on Gn-RH and gonadotropin secretion. Thus, follicular recruitment begins near the initiation of menses under the influence of rising FSH levels. The enlarging follicles produce increasing amounts of estradiol, which at levels of less than 200 to 300 pg per milliliter have a negative feedback effect on LH and FSH secretion. The increasing estrogen secretion from an emerging dominant follicle contributes to atresia of the other follicles by suppressing FSH levels in the late follicular phase. Rising concentrations of estrogen also promote proliferation of the endometrium and changes in the vaginal epithelium, the cervical mucus, and the fallopian tubes that help maximize fertility.

Estradiol secretion from the mature follicle results in serum levels above 200 to 300 pg per milliliter, at which point the negative feedback on the hypothalamus and pituitary switches to positive feedback. The follicle is usually 17 to 25 mm in diameter at this time. The positive feedback results in an outpouring of Gn-RH and LH (the midcycle surge). Ovulation ensues within 20 hours. By that time, cervical mucus is in optimal condition for sperm transport.

Immediately following ovulation, the corpus luteum ("yellow body," named for its histologic appearance due to its abundance of steroid hormones) forms and begins secreting both estradiol and progesterone to initiate the luteal phase. During the late follicular phase, FSH induces the formation of LH receptors on granulosa cells. Following the midcycle surge, LH becomes the dominant gonadotropin stimulating the corpus luteum to produce estradiol and progesterone. Progesterone alters the cervical mucus so that it is less conducive to sperm transport. However, the most notable effects of progesterone are on the endometrium. Glands are stimulated, and the proliferative endometrium is converted to a secretory endometrium, creating an environment favorable for implantation and nurturing of a fertilized ovum. The many

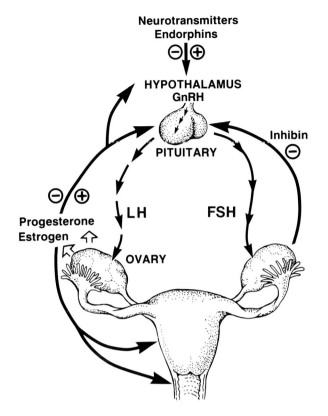

Figure 13-2 The hypothalamic-pituitary-ovarian axis. Pulsatile secretion of Gn-RH stimulates episodic release of LH and, less apparent, FSH from the anterior pituitary. The gonadotropins stimulate ovarian function. Ovarian steroids and inhibin in turn modulate hypothalamic-pituitary function.

HYPOTHALAMIC-PITUITARY PHYSIOLOGY AND CLINICAL TESTING

Physiology

The preceding picture of the menstrual cycle was supplemented by two important discoveries at the beginning of the 1970s that led to the explosion of knowledge in reproductive neuroendocrinology. The structure of Gn-RH was determined by Schally and Guillimen, and this permitted intensive research in hypothalamic-pituitary physiology. At the same time, Knobil and others found that Gn-RH is not secreted tonically but in pulses every 1 to 2 hours during the follicular phase. Pulsatile release of Gn-RH is absolutely required for normal function of the reproductive axis. It results in episodic secretion of LH and, to a lesser extent, FSH, which follows a distinctive set of changing patterns throughout the menstrual cycle (Fig. 13-3). However, this change in Gn-RH pulse patterns does not appear absolutely necessary for ovulation. A second major influence on gonadotropin secretion is the changing levels of gonadal steroids throughout the menstrual cycle. As mentioned, the negative feedback effect of low levels of estrogen suppresses FSH in the late follicular phase and promotes the emergence of a single dominant follicle. The positive feedback of high levels of estradiol at midcycle leads to the LH surge that causes ovulation. Modulation of Gn-RH secretion by endorphins and neurotransmitters also occurs. Recent information indicates that Gn-RH probably works in concert with an FSH-releasing hormone and a gonadotropin release–inhibiting hormone. Continued refinements in our knowledge of the hypothalamic-pituitary axis have permitted new understandings of and therapies for reproductive disorders.

proteins secreted by the endometrium are in the early stages of identification and evaluation. Hence, their function and disorders resulting from their improper secretion are not yet well understood.

If a fertilized ovum does not implant, the corpus luteum regresses 11 to 16 days following its formation. The resulting decline in estrogen and progesterone levels withdraws support of the vascular supply to the endometrium, resulting in necrosis of its inner margins, sloughing of the tissue, menses, and the initiation of a new cycle.

Multiple novel gonadal peptides that appear to play active roles in regulating the menstrual cycle are currently being evaluated and characterized. Foremost among these are the related hormones, inhibin and activin, which modulate FSH secretion and ovarian function. Müllerian inhibitory substance (MI) appears to have actions on ovum maturation in female fetuses in addition to its suppression of müllerian ducts in male fetuses. The roles of follistatin, growth factors, and other peptides are being defined and may play major roles in the diagnosis and treatment of HPO axis disorders in the near future. However, clinical knowledge of these peptides is not sufficiently advanced to be included in the following discussion.

Static Measurements of LH and FSH

Peripheral serum concentrations of Gn-RH are generally too low to be detected in available assays (Table 13-1). Therefore, serum levels of the gonadotropins are relied on to reflect Gn-RH secretion as well as pituitary gonadotrope function. Gonadotropin levels are influenced by hypothalamic and pituitary functional status as well as by levels of gonadal steroids. The best established diagnostic use of LH and FSH concentrations is to differentiate primary ovarian failure from other causes of amenorrhea. Gonadotropin levels can also be useful as collaborative evidence of polycystic ovarian syndrome (PCOS) or gonadotropin-secreting pituitary adenomas. Currently, serum LH and FSH concentrations are measured by radioimmunoassay (RIA) and usually expressed in milli-International units per milliliter or micrograms per milliliter. Principles for RIA are elegantly reviewed in earlier chapters of this text and elsewhere. Until recently, most LH-RIAs also detected human chorionic gonadotropin (hCG) owing to the similarity of structure

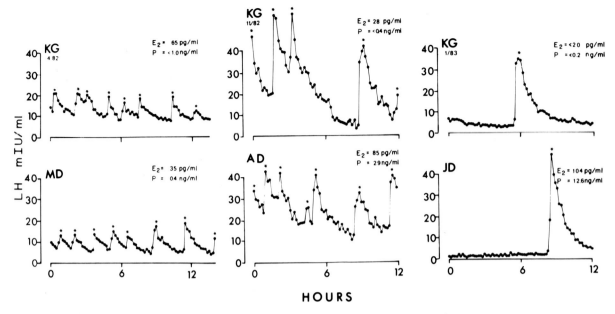

Figure 13-3 Pulsatile secretion of LH across the menstrual cycle. Typical patterns of LH secretion are shown for the follicular phase (*left*), just following the midcycle surge (*middle*), and the late luteal phase (*right*). Small, discrete pulses of LH occur about every 60 to 100 minutes during the follicular phase. During the midcycle surge, both the amplitude and frequency of LH pulses markedly increase. Slowing of LH pulses occurs throughout the luteal phase. The importance of this progression of pulse patterns is not completely understood. The upper panel depicts LH secretory patterns at different times in a woman with hypothalamic amenorrhea. The lower panel depicts LH secretory patterns determined by sampling LH at 10-minute intervals for 12 hours in three normal women. Note the similarity in secretory patterns. However, concurrent levels of ovarian steroids are inappropriate in the woman with amenorrhea. (From Crowley WF, Filicori M, Spratt DI, Santoro NF. The physiology of gonadotropin-releasing hormone (GnRH) secretion in men and women. Recent Prog Horm Res 1985; 41:473; with permission.)

of LH and hCG causing cross-reaction of hCG with LH antiserum used in RIAs. hCG is the dominant gonadotropin during pregnancy, is produced by the placenta and probably by the fetal kidney, and has actions similar to those of LH. Thus, with the older assay methods, LH may appear elevated in pregnancy or with hCG-producing tumors, when it is actually hCG that is elevated. This problem is largely avoided with the new monoclonal antibodies.

Normal ranges for serum concentrations of LH and FSH are derived from single samples from many women in different phases of the menstrual cycle. Reference laboratories do not use normative data obtained from pooled specimens (combining multiple samples in each patient). Therefore, although *pooling of blood samples* has been advocated to avoid peaks and valleys of hormone pulses, this technique is not generally used by endocrinologists and is not advisable in view of the nature of normative data currently available.

Enzyme-linked measurements of LH in the urine at midcycle are now available in kits designed for home use to detect the midcycle LH surge for prediction of ovulation (Table 13-2). Other new assay techniques for serum LH and FSH such as enzyme-linked immunoassays or chemoluminescent assays may soon replace RIA.

TABLE 13-1   Static Measurements of Serum LH and FSH

Methods:	1. RIA 2. Enzyme-linked or chemoluminescent assays (in near future)
Normal (for RIA):	Varies with the stage of the menstrual cycle (see Fig. 13-4)
Uses:	1. Differentiating primary ovarian failure from other causes of amenorrhea 2. Collaborative data for diagnosis of PCOS or gonadotropin-secreting pituitary adenomas
Pitfalls:	1. Cross-reactivity with hCG in pregnancy or hCG-producing tumors (older assays) 2. May be normal in early menopause or in hypothalamic or pituitary disorders

TABLE 13-2   Home Monitoring of Urine for Midcycle LH Surge

Method:	Enzyme-linked colorimetric assay of spot urine
Normal:	Test device (dipstick or paper) turns blue when LH surge occurs
Uses:	To predict or confirm ovulation in patients attempting pregnancy with (1) irregular cycles, (2) clomiphene therapy (with or without artificial insemination), and (3) ovulation induction with Gn-RH
Pitfalls:	Occasional false-negative results
Alternative methods for confirming ovulation: Basal body temperature charts or luteal phase progesterone levels	

Difficulties in Interpreting Serum Gonadotropin Concentrations

As mentioned, the greatest utility of serum gonadotropin determinations is in differentiating primary ovarian failure from other causes of amenorrhea. Several pitfalls occur in using LH and FSH determinations in other situations. The pulsatile and cyclical nature of gonadotropin secretion can make interpretation of single serum determinations difficult. Concurrent levels of gonadal steroid feedback must also be considered when interpreting LH and FSH determinations. Furthermore, LH and FSH levels can fluctuate in disorders of the HPO axis. Serum LH and FSH concentrations in the normal range at a single point in time do not always indicate normal pituitary and ovarian function. The following are examples of this difficulty in common clinical situations.

Menopause.   In menopause, LH and FSH are typically elevated, with an FSH predominance and low estradiol levels (Fig. 13–4). However, in the perimenopausal period, ovarian function can wax and wane, causing corresponding changes in LH and FSH levels. Even worse, these changes are not always simultaneous. Thus, as the ovary is failing, normal estrogen levels may be observed with normal or high FSH levels, or low estrogen levels can be observed with normal FSH. Endocrine testing can be confusing in early ovarian failure. However, as a rule, if an elevation of FSH is observed in a clinical situation consistent with menopause, permanent cessation of ovarian function is almost certain to follow within months

to 1 or 2 years. Gonadotropin-secreting pituitary adenomas provide a rare exception to this rule. They may be differentiated from menopause by normal or high estradiol levels in the presence of elevated FSH concentrations in women of premenopausal age.

Hypothalamic Amenorrhea.   Diagnosis of hypothalamic amenorrhea by gonadotropins is often not reliable. The use of this term should be clarified. First, the term has been applied both to secondary amenorrhea related to weight loss, exercise, and unknown causes and to primary amenorrhea caused by congenital deficiency of Gn-RH secretion. The latter condition is known as idiopathic hypogonadotropic hypogonadism (IHH), idiopathic gonadotropic deficiency (IGD), or, if anosmia or hyposmia is also present, Kallmann's syndrome. IHH is usually diagnosed by the total lack of spontaneous puberty, with gonadotropins in the low or low-normal range with minimal concentrations of estrogen (see Fig. 13–4), and must be differentiated from amenorrhea caused by tumors in the areas of the hypothalamus and pituitary.

Hypothalamic amenorrhea associated with strenuous exercise or weight loss is usually secondary in onset and often has no identifiable cause. Gonadotropin secretion patterns vary widely, and serum gonadotropin concentrations may be normal or low. LH pulses may be absent or may appear normal even with extensive serum sampling (see Fig. 13–3). Either the progression of the gonadotropin pulse patterns or the concurrent sex steroid levels may be inappropriate. Low gonadotropin levels increase the suspicion of destructive lesions but may also be present in hypothalamic amenorrhea of unknown cause. Thus, serum gonadotropin concentrations are not reliable for differentiating causes of amenorrhea.

Polycystic Ovarian Syndrome.   PCOS (previously termed Stein-Leventhal syndrome) is often reported to have a characteristic LH to FSH ratio of 2 to 1 or 3 to 1 with a low-normal FSH and high serum concentrations of LH. However, studies using frequent serum sampling demonstrate that LH to FSH ratios vary widely among patients with PCOS (Fig. 13–5). LH pulses may also have increased amplitude resulting in moment to moment variations in the LH to FSH ratio in the same patient. Consequently, these ratios cannot be used to rule out PCOS.

Dynamic Testing of Pituitary Function

Dynamic testing has little place in the diagnosis of HPO axis disorders and infertility. Clomiphene citrate historically has been used to assess the status of the hypothalamic-pituitary portion of the reproductive axis. The principle of this test is that clomiphene competitively blocks estrogen receptors, thus decreasing estrogen negative feedback to the hypothalamus and pituitary. The more the hypothalamus, gonadotropes, and ovaries are functioning, the greater will be the LH and FSH increase following administration of clomiphene. The test is per-

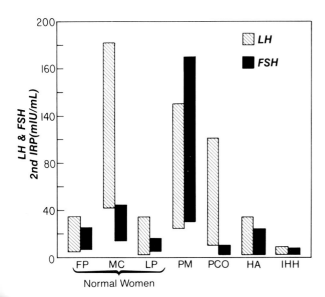

Figure 13–4 Serum concentrations of LH and FSH measured using the second IRP-hMG standard in normal women during the follicular phase (FP), midcycle (MC), and the luteal phase (LP) compared with those of postmenopausal woman (PM) and women with PCOS, hypothalamic amenorrhea (HA), and idiopathic hypogonadotropic hypogonadism (IHH).

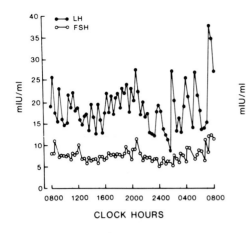
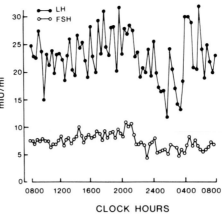

Figure 13–5 Patterns of LH and FSH secretion in two women with PCOS. Note the variation in the LH to FSH ratio both between patients and from moment to moment in the same patient. (From Yen SSC, Jaffe R, eds. Reproductive endocrinology. Philadelphia: WB Saunders, 1986; with permission.)

formed by administering 100 mg of clomiphene daily for 5 days to the amenorrheic patient with concurrent measurements of serum LH and FSH concentrations. This test is cumbersome and not recommended. Except in research settings, clomiphene should be used in women for ovulation induction therapy only. With the availability of Gn-RH, clomiphene testing largely gave way to the Gn-RH stimulation test.

In its turn, the Gn-RH stimulation test is no longer widely used clinically since it often fails to distinguish normal from abnormal gonadotrope function or pituitary from hypothalamic disease. It is performed by measuring baseline LH and FSH concentrations, then injecting 100 µg of Gn-RH intravenously or subcutaneously and determining LH and FSH levels again at approximately 15, 30, 45, and 60 minutes. Since pituitary gonadotropin secretion may appear normal in hypothalamic amenorrhea, it is not surprising that responses to Gn-RH are often normal in these disorders.

Finally, the estrogen provocation test has been used to assess the functional status of the hypothalamic-pituitary unit with respect to potential success of clomiphene for ovulation induction. Estradiol benzoate is administered as a single 1-mg intramuscular injection. Serum concentrations of estradiol, LH, and FSH are assayed daily during the ensuing 72 hours to monitor for evidence of positive feedback on the pituitary. Patients who do not respond with positive feedback reportedly are unlikely to undergo successful ovulation induction with clomiphene. This test is rarely used in the United States. An alternative to the estrogen provocation test is simple assessment of the estrogen secretory status by progesterone withdrawal (see later).

OVARIAN PHYSIOLOGY AND CLINICAL TESTING

Physiology

The ovary produces a mature ovum each month. As indicated, ovarian secretion of steroids is closely coordinated with ovulation in order both to regulate the menstrual cycle and to promote changes in the endometrium, cervical mucus, and fallopian tubes that are beneficial for fertilization and implantation.

The chief ovarian steroids are estradiol and progesterone. Estradiol was the first steroid hormone to be isolated in the 1930s and is named for its association with estrus in animals. The word *estrus* is derived from the Greek *oistros*, meaning "gadfly." The gadfly's behavior yielded a later meaning of *oistros*, "mad desire," whose association with animal behavior at midcycle is clear. Any association of estrogen with libido is much more subtle in humans. However, the preovulatory rise in estradiol levels has several effects on the vaginal epithelium, the cervical mucus, and the endometrium that permit assessment of the estrogen secretory status. Progesterone promotes gestation by its effects on the endometrium during the luteal phase. Morphologic assessment of these effects during the luteal phase is used to judge the adequacy of corpus luteum function.

The dominant follicle produced each cycle is selected from a cohort of primordial follicles whose maturation begins just prior to menses. The follicle is surrounded by the basal lamina (Fig. 13–6). Inside the basal lamina are the granulosa cells, which are closely associated with the ovum and secrete estradiol under the influence of FSH. Just outside the basal lamina are the theca cells, which are stimulated by LH and chiefly produce androgens. These androgens, androstenedione and testosterone, diffuse either into capillaries and the circulation or into granulosa cells. Aromatization into estrone and estradiol respectively occurs both peripherally and in the granulosa cells. Estradiol is the predominant estrogen secreted particularly at midcycle and in the luteal phase. Granulosa cells are sensitive to the amount of androgens that the thecal cells provide, and excess androgens in the microenvironment of the follicle suppress aromatization and can lead to follicular atresia and menstrual dysfunction.

During the first few days of the follicular phase, both ovaries produce equivalent amounts of sex hormones. As a dominant follicle begins to emerge in one ovary, greater amounts of estrogen are secreted by that ovary. The dominant follicle produces estrogen with increasing efficiency and begins synthesizing inhibin. In the late follicular phase, the rising levels of estrogen and inhibin suppress FSH secretion. The loss of FSH stimulation and other factors leads to atresia of the less efficient non-dominant follicles. The mature dominant follicle pro-,duces circulating estradiol levels (greater than 200 to 300 pg per milliliter) sufficient to cause positive feedback at the level of the hypothalamus and pituitary, leading to the LH surge and ovulation.

After the follicle ruptures, theca and granulosa cells intermingle and are transformed into the estradiol- and progesterone-secreting cells of the corpus luteum. These hormones change the proliferative endometrium into a secretory endometrium in preparation for implantation and nurturing of a fertilized ovum. As the luteal phase progresses, pulsatile secretion of progesterone becomes increasingly evident (Fig. 13–7). The timing of luteinization is critical, and premature luteinization has recently been described in association with suppression of ovulation.

Assessment of Estradiol Secretion

Estradiol secretion (Table 13–3) is generally assumed to be normal in a woman with regular menstrual cycles. Assessment of estrogen levels is usually done only in patients with amenorrhea or precocious sexual development, in postmenopausal women suspected of having inappropriate estrogen secretion, and during ovulation induction with human menopausal gonadotropins (hMG, or Pergonal) or Gn-RH. Estrogen evaluation can be accomplished by direct measurement of serum estradiol concentrations by RIA, by observing biologic effects of estrogen in the patient (cervical mucus, vaginal epithelium), or by progestin-induced withdrawal bleeding. A large proportion of circulating estradiol is protein bound (particularly by sex hormone–binding globulin), and most RIAs measure total (bound plus free) serum concentrations. In addition, extraction procedures improve the specificity of the assay. Most clinically available assays are unextracted and have detection limits of 20 to 25 pg per milliliter.

The disadvantage of direct measurements of serum estradiol is that these determinations represent only a single point in time. In addition, normal levels of estrogen vary between individuals and throughout the cycle. Thus, except for monitoring ovulation induction or diagnosing precocious puberty, serum estradiol levels are not often obtained. Rather, end-organ effects are used to assess the biologic activity of estradiol. This approach reflects the body's response to estrogen secretion integrated over time and can be accomplished in several ways.

Progestin-induced withdrawal bleeding (Table 13–4) takes advantage of the estrogen-stimulated proliferation of the endometrium. If significant amounts of estrogen are present, the endometrium will grow. Administration of a progestational agent will result in secretory changes

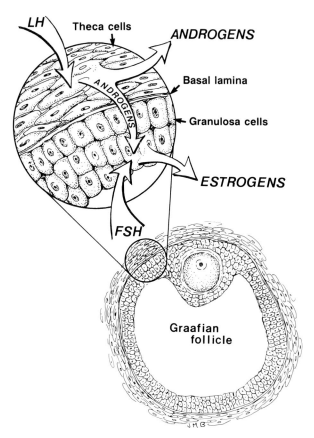

Figure 13–6   The maturing follicle with associated theca and granulosa cells. Theca cells under the influence of LH produce chiefly androgens. These androgens are converted to estrogens by the granulosa cells under the influence of FSH. Granulosa cells are also the chief source of inhibin and activin in women.

in the endometrium. Following progesterone withdrawal, the secretory endometrium will be shed. Thus, any uterine bleeding within 10 days of the withdrawal yields information regarding the level of endogenous HPO axis activity (reflected by the presence of estradiol-17β [E_2] stimulation of the endometrium) and the patency of the uterine cavity and the cervix.

Progestin withdrawal is accomplished by administering either medroxy-progesterone acetate (Provera), 10 mg daily for 5 to 10 days, or a single intramuscular injection of progesterone in oil (100 mg). Lack of withdrawal bleeding indicates either minimal activity of the HPO axis or an abnormal endometrium or cervical stenosis. If uterine synechiae (Asherman's syndrome) are suspected, conjugated estrogens (2.5 mg daily) should be given for 25 days, with concomitant progesterone the last 10 days, to assess endometrial withdrawal bleeding when both estrogen and progesterone are provided. Lack of withdrawal bleeding suggests Asherman's syndrome or cervical stenosis but may also be caused by hyperandrogenemia or noncompliance. The cervix should be sounded and, if patent, hysterosalpingography or hysteroscopy considered.

The progestin-induced withdrawal bleed is useful to assess estrogen status in several situations. Several

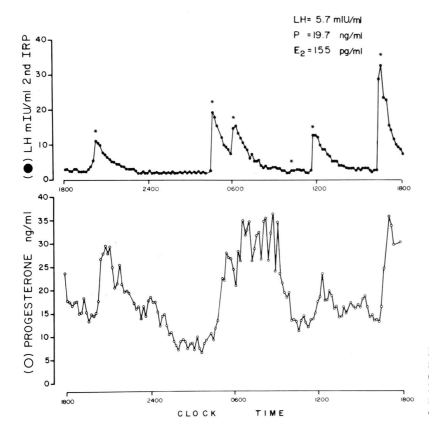

Figure 13-7 LH and progesterone pulses of a normal woman in the midluteal phase of the cycle. (From Crowley WF, Filicori M, Spratt DI, Santoro NF. The physiology of gonadotropin-releasing hormone (GnRH) secretion in men and women. Recent Prog Horm Res 1985; 41:473; with permission.)

groups have reported that infertile anovulatory patients who fail to respond to this test are unlikely to respond to ovulation induction with clomiphene. Some groups bypass clomiphene therapy in such patients and proceed to hMG (Pergonal), hCG, or Gn-RH therapy. However, most groups recommend initial therapy with clomiphene in patients whose pituitaries are otherwise intact. This test is also helpful in determining the presence of unopposed estrogen stimulation of the endometrium, which is accompanied by an increased risk of endometrial cancer. If no bleeding occurs and structural abnormalities have been excluded, the estrogen deficiency increases the risk of osteoporosis, and cyclical or continuous estrogen and progesterone supplementation may be considered. This latter issue is still undergoing evaluation.

TABLE 13-3   Evaluation of Estradiol Secretion

Methods:
1. Direct measurement of serum levels by RIA
2. Inspection of cervical mucus or vaginal epithelium
3. Progestin-induced withdrawal bleeding

Normal values for a typical unextracted RIA:

Early follicular phase:	30–100 pg/ml
Preovulatory:	200–400 pg/ml
Luteal phase:	50–150 pg/ml
Postmenopausal/prepubertal:	< 20 pg/ml
On oral contraceptives:	< 50 pg/ml

Uses:
1. Monitoring ovulation induction therapy (see text)
2. Screening for precocious puberty
3. Confirming estrogen secretory status in amenorrheic patients when results of other testing are equivocal

Pitfalls of RIA:
1. May not accurately reflect integrated estradiol secretion
2. May be normal in early menopause
3. Occasionally insufficiently sensitive as an index of suppression of estradiol secretion

TABLE 13-4   Progestin-Induced Withdrawal Bleeding

Methods:
1. Administration of either medroxyprogesterone acetate (Provera), 10 mg daily for 5 to 10 days, or a single intramuscular injection of progesterone in oil (100 mg)
2. If no bleeding from (1), then conjugated estrogens are administered, 2.5 mg daily for 21 days, with concurrent medroxyprogesterone, 10 mg for the last 10 days

Normal: Uterine bleeding within 10 days of the withdrawal

Uses:
1. Assessment of level of ovarian estrogen secretion in patients with amenorrhea
2. Evaluation of patency of outflow tract

Pitfalls:
1. May be abnormal with hyperandrogenemia or noncompliance
2. Estrogen plus Provera may occasionally require two cycles to be effective

TABLE 13-5   Inspection of Cervical Mucus

Method:	Specimen obtained from cervical os with suction, forceps, or spatula; air-dried on slide; and examined microscopically for ferning pattern
Normal:	See Figure 13-8
Uses:	Assessment of estrogen secretory status (usually in patients undergoing ovulation induction)
Pitfalls:	1. Not reliable with infections or damage of the cervix 2. Some variability of relation between estrogen levels and cervical mucus production between patients

Inspection of cervical mucus (Table 13–5) takes advantage of the principle that rising estrogen levels are accompanied by changes in cervical mucus. Through the second half of the follicular phase, secretion of cervical mucus increases tenfold. Protein, sodium chloride, and water content all increase dramatically. The mucus becomes clear and thick, resembling egg whites, and is increasingly elastic so that it can be drawn into threads (spinnbarkheit) usually 10 to 15 cm in length by the time of ovulation. Dried mucus crystallizes into increasingly profuse, frost-like patterns ("ferning"; Fig. 13–8). Permeability to sperm peaks by ovulation and rapidly declines afterward. These changes in the cervical mucus are accompanied by dilation of the cervical os to 3 to 4 mm at midcycle.

The advantage of inspecting cervical mucus is that it provides an immediate and inexpensive assessment of the estrogen status. Cervical mucus is most commonly inspected during monitoring of ovulation induction with clomiphene, hMG/hCG, or Gn-RH. Impending menarche in girls with primary amenorrhea may be signaled by ferning of the cervical mucus as well as development of secondary sexual characteristics. The first clue to inappropriate estrogen secretion by tumors in postmenopausal women may be an increased amount and ferning of cervical mucus. Inspection of cervical mucus can be useful in other situations as well.

Examination of vaginal cytology (Table 13–6) reflects the changes in the vaginal epithelium that occur in response to increasing levels of estrogen. The stratified squamous epithelium of the vagina consists of four nondiscrete layers: basal, parabasal, intermediate, and superficial. Estrogen promotes growth and maturation of the epithelial cells. Thus, the more estrogen present, the greater will be the percentage of superficial cells on the surface of the epithelium. The vaginal wall is characteristically moist and pink when it is well supplied with estrogen. This estrogen effect can be assessed by obtaining a smear of the surface epithelium from the lateral walls of the upper one-third of the vagina, with care taken to avoid the cervix. Specimens can be obtained with a cotton swab or wooden spatula. Immediate examination is done on a wet mount, and more detailed evaluation is performed on a specimen fixed and stained by the Papanicolaou method. Cells are counted according to their appearance (Fig. 13–9).

The most common cytologic rating scheme of vaginal epithelium is the maturation index (MI), which tallies the percentage of parabasal, intermediate, and superficial cells as a reflection of estrogen stimulation. The advantage of the MI is that it provides an immediate estimate of the state of estrogen production. The MI may also be a more sensitive indicator of estradiol levels than RIAs, with detection limits of 20 to 25 pg per milliliter. The disadvantages are twofold. First, preparation artifacts are easily produced by sampling the cervix, by

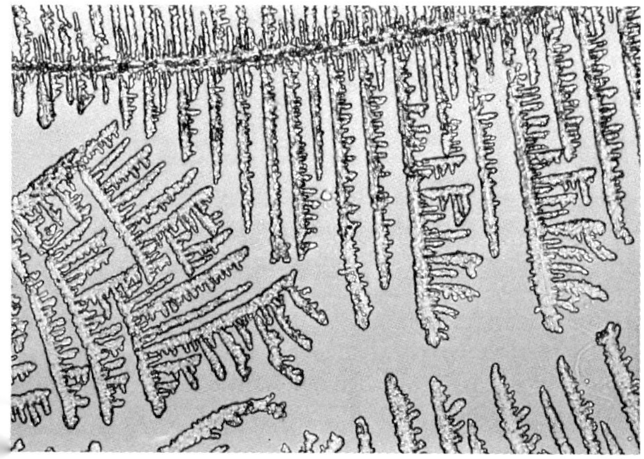

Figure 13-8   Cervical mucus examined under the microscope in a woman on the day before ovulation shows profuse ferning consistent with high E_2 levels.

TABLE 13-6   Maturation Index

Method:	A smear of the surface epithelium is obtained from the lateral walls of the upper one-third of the vagina, with care taken to avoid the cervix. Specimens can be obtained with a cotton swab or wooden spatula. Immediate examination can be done on a wet mount, and more detailed evaluation performed on a specimen fixed and stained by the Papanicolaou method. Cells are counted according to their appearance (Fig. 13–9).
Normal:	>30–50% superficial cells in cycling women
Uses:	Assessment of state of estrogen production during assessment of (1) HPO suppression, (2) suspected precocious puberty, and (3) efficacy of estrogen replacement when in doubt
Pitfalls:	1. Preparation artifacts are easily produced by sampling the cervix, by drying of the specimen, or by variations in fixation techniques 2. Differences in scoring may occur between observers

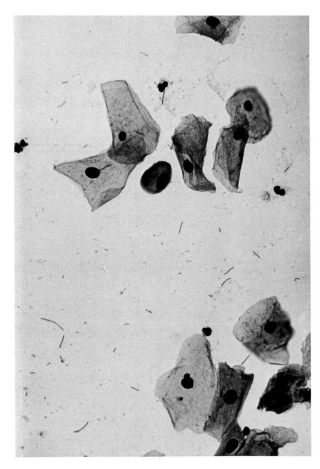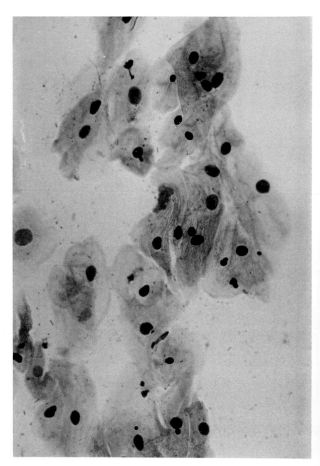

Figure 13-9 Vaginal epithelial smears in patients with (*left*) and without (*right*) estrogen deficiency. Note the larger number of cells with pyknotic nuclei and abundant cytoplasm (superficial cells) in the presence of estrogen. A parabasal cell is present on the left.

drying of the specimen, or by variations in fixation techniques. Second, the differences between basal and intermediate and between intermediate and superficial cells are sometimes subtle. Therefore, evaluation of poorly prepared specimens or by inexperienced observers may be misleading. In fact, the same specimen may often be evaluated differently by two observers. As a consequence, many laboratories entrust their vaginal cytology evaluation to one or two experienced technicians.

The MI is chiefly employed to confirm other clinical or laboratory assessments of estrogen production or replacement therapy when findings are equivocal. It is also commonly used to assess estrogen production when diagnosing precocious puberty in girls (less than 8 years old). However, vaginal smears are often unpleasant for these young patients. More recently, the MI has been used to assess the degree of HPO axis suppression during therapy with the Gn-RH agonist. Occasionally incomplete suppression will be detected by the MI but not by serum estradiol levels (particularly with imperfect compliance).

Bone densitometry is increasingly employed to assess the adverse effects of estrogen deficiency on bone. The accelerated loss of bone density following menopause is well documented. Since this issue has become increas-

ingly important and bone density measurements are often inappropriately ordered, techniques of bone density should be briefly discussed.

Four techniques are currently employed to measure bone density. They may measure cortical bone (the chief component of the axial skeleton, including the proximal femur) or trabecular bone (chief component of the vertebrae) or both. Estrogen deficiency may lead to either cortical or trabecular bone loss or both. Plain x-ray films are relatively insensitive to bone demineralization. Approximately 40 percent of bone loss occurs before it is detectable by conventional radiology. Single-energy photon absorptiometry is much more sensitive but measures only bone in the distal radius. These measurements do not correlate well with those in the hip or spine, where most serious fractures associated with estrogen deficiency occur. Consequently, dual-energy photon absorptiometry (DPA) was developed. This technique can measure both vertebral and hip bone densities and is currently the most common technique used in estrogen-deficient patients. However, certain caveats in clinical use must be observed. Estrogen deficiency is associated with an increased rate of bone loss in many but not all women. Once bone is lost, no effective therapies exist to restore mineralization.

Thus, the most effective screening for estrogen replacement therapy (which is preventive) would predict which women are going to lose significant bone mass or would quickly detect an accelerated rate of loss. No bone densitometry technique will determine which women will lose bone mass. The precision of current DPA techniques is not sufficient to assess an accelerated rate of loss over a short interval. Thus, DPA should not be used for widespread screening of perimenopausal or postmenopausal women to recommend estrogen therapy.

Computed tomography (CT) provides a more precise estimate of both cortical and trabecular bone density. However, it is relatively expensive and uses greater amounts of radiation. At present, CT bone densitometry must be carefully calibrated and may differ between institutions. Quantitative CT may use a single energy source (QCT-SE) or dual energy sources (QCT-DE). Dual energy techniques provide increased accuracy of measurements but also increase radiation exposure.

A promising new technique of bone density measurements is quantitative digital radiography, which uses x-rays of two energy peaks (QDR-DE). This approach is still being evaluated but appears to have similar accuracy to QCT-DE but with much less cost and radiation exposure.

All techniques of bone densitometry must still be considered to be in the developmental stages. Clinical applications are not yet firmly established. Therefore, bone density measurements should be carefully and conservatively applied.

Assessment of Progesterone Secretion

Progesterone, like estrogen, can be assessed either by direct measurements of serum concentrations by RIA or by observation of end-organ effects (Tables 13–7 to 13–9). RIA techniques are similar to those described for estradiol. An additional difficulty in interpreting progesterone determinations at a single point in time is the marked pulsation of progesterone secretion in the mid- to late luteal phase (see Fig. 13–7). At present, determinations of serum progesterone concentrations are used clinically almost exclusively to confirm ovulation. Levels greater than 3 to 5 ng per milliliter obtained 5 to 10 days prior to menses are consistent with ovulation and the formation of a corpus luteum. In the rare circumstance of luteinized unruptured follicle (LUF syndrome), progesterone levels will rise without ovulation. More recently, premature luteinization of the follicle has been described that suppresses normal ovulation. If this syndrome is suspected by unexplained regression of a normally developing follicle, progesterone determinations in the preovulatory period may be useful.

The utility of serum progesterone levels to screen for inadequate luteal phase is questionable. Indices of integrated progesterone secretion (serial basal body temperatures [BBT] or endometrial biopsies) are considered more accurate in the diagnosis of this disorder. One effect of progesterone is to mildly increase the body temperature. If body temperatures are measured before arising in the morning (BBT), ovulation is usually reflected by a rise in the BBT by 0.3° to 0.6 °F following ovulation. The length of the BBT rise usually reflects the life span of the corpus luteum. Thus BBTs may be used both to document ovulation and to screen for short luteal phases as a cause of infertility. Several limitations of BBT tracking exist. It is *not predictive* of ovulation. A slight decrease in the temperature may sometimes occur just prior to ovulation but is not a reliable observation. Second, a luteal rise in BBT can be lacking even when ovulation does occur. Finally, a BBT rise for 11 days or more does not confirm normal corpus luteum function.

The endometrial biopsy taken during the luteal phase takes advantage of the progesterone-induced change in endometrial morphology to assess corpus luteum function. The endometrium demonstrates progressive changes with characteristic histologic appearances each day of the luteal phase (Figs. 13–1 and 13–10). The biopsy is performed in cycles of normal length in patients with unexplained infertility. Biopsies are usually performed on day 26 of the 28-day cycle just prior to menses. Concomitant BBT tracking or urinary monitoring of the LH surge is useful to confirm the date of ovulation. If the biopsy has a morphologic appearance that is incon-

---

TABLE 13–7   Measurement of Serum Progesterone Concentrations

Method:	RIA
Normal:	1. > 5 ng/ml confirms ovulation
	2. Value demonstrating normal corpus luteum function is controversial
Uses:	Confirmation of ovulation
Pitfalls:	1. Borderline levels of 3 to 5 ng/ml are equivocal evidence of ovulation
	2. Pulsatile progesterone in the mid- to late luteal phase renders assessment of corpus luteum function difficult by single blood samples
Alternative methods:	1. Basal body temperature
	2. Home urine LH monitoring kits

TABLE 13-8   Basal Body Temperature

Method:	Oral temperatures are measured before arising each morning (BBT) with concomitant recording of the day of the cycle
Normal:	1. Ovulation is usually reflected by a rise in the BBT by 0.3° to 0.6° F 1 to 2 days after ovulation 2. Temperature rise of ≥ 11 days' duration
Uses:	1. Confirmation of ovulation 2. Evaluation of length of luteal phase
Pitfalls:	1. Ovulation occasionally is not followed by a discrete rise in BBTs 2. With LUF syndrome, BBT will rise despite the ovum's not being released 3. Short luteal phases occasionally in normal women
Alternative methods:	Luteal phase progesterone or home urine LH monitoring kits for confirmation of ovulation

sistent by 2 or more days with the day of the menstrual cycle, corpus luteum insufficiency is suspected. Several warnings must be issued in considering the endometrial biopsy. (1) The day of the menstrual cycle, of ovulation, and of onset of the subsequent period should be recorded for interpretation. (2) Inadequate luteal phases occasionally occur in normal women. Thus, two consecutive abnormal biopsies are usually required to establish a convincing diagnosis of inadequate luteal phase. With these criteria, the incidence of inadequate luteal phase is low (less than 5 percent). (3) Some studies have noted a degree of subjectivity in interpretation of endometrial biopsies, with significant differences in interpretations between experienced pathologists.

From an endocrine standpoint, endometrial biopsies are performed for two reasons: (1) to evaluate for inadequate luteal phase in the couple with unexplained infertility or recurrent spontaneous abortion after other more common mechanical and endocrine etiologies have been eliminated, and (2) to rule out endometrial abnormalities in patients with amenorrhea associated with unopposed estrogen stimulation or with hyperandrogenemia, or in postmenopausal patients beginning or undergoing estrogen replacement therapy. The frequency with which the latter should be undertaken is not well established. As a minimum, any patient who experiences irregular bleeding or spotting on estrogen replacement therapy should receive an endometrial biopsy. The efficacy of detecting and treating inadequate luteal phase in infertile couples is not well established.

Assessment of Androgen Secretion

Serum androgen levels in women are usually measured only in patients with hirsutism or virilization or with unexplained infertility. Androgens are secreted by both the ovary and the adrenal gland in women (Fig. 13–11). Dehydroepiandrosterone sulfate (DHEAS) and androstenedione are relatively weak androgens with precursors that include 17OH-progesterone (see Chapter 5). The synthetic pathways beginning with cholesterol are similar in the ovary and the adrenal cortex except that the ovary generates minimal amounts of DHEA and DHEAS (see Fig. 13–11). Thus, DHEAS is generally a good marker to differentiate adrenal androgen excess from ovarian androgen excess. It should be noted that because serum DHEAS levels decrease with age, normal values in postmenopausal women are lower than those in ovulating women. Recent reports indicate that measurements of serum concentrations of androstanediol glucuronide, the metabolite of DHT, may provide an index of peripheral androgen action and may therefore be a more useful clinical marker of hyperandrogenemia. Further experience with this test is required.

The greatest utility of serum androgen determina-

TABLE 13-9   Endometrial Biopsy

Method:	Obtain biopsy of the endometrium 1 to 2 days before expected menses (day 26 of a 28-day cycle), and compare morphology with standards
Normal:	Morphology within 2 days of standard from a normal menstrual cycle
Uses:	1. To evaluate for inadequate luteal phase in the couple with unexplained infertility or recurrent spontaneous abortion after other more common mechanical and endocrine etiologies have been eliminated 2. To rule out endometrial abnormalities in patients with amenorrhea associated with unopposed estrogen stimulation or with hyperandrogenemia, or in postmenopausal patients beginning or undergoing estrogen replacement therapy
Pitfalls:	1. "Inadequate" luteal phases occasionally occur in normal women; thus, two consecutive abnormal biopsies are required for diagnosis of inadequate luteal phase 2. Significant differences in interpretations may occur between experienced pathologists 3. Effective therapy for "inadequate" luteal phase not well established

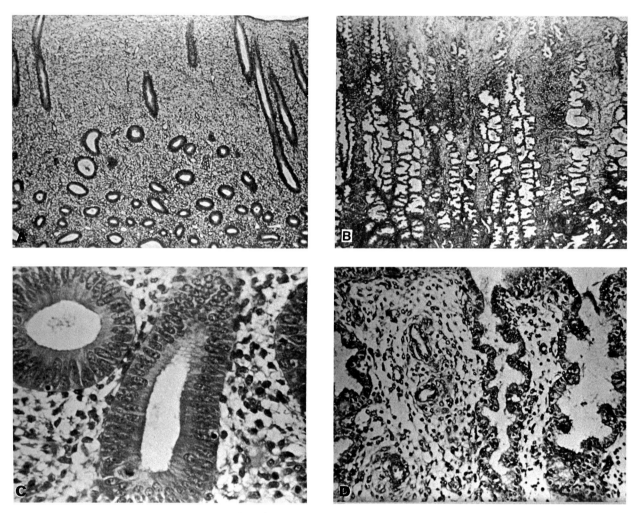

Figure 13-10 Endometrial biopsies (*A*) in the midproliferative phase of the menstrual cycle and (*B*) in the late secretory phase. Note the increased tortuosity of glands and increased secretory activity as the luteal phase advances. (Courtesy of Frank Vellios, M.D.)

tions in patients who have signs of increased production of androgens (hirsutism, acne developing after puberty, or virilization) is as a screen for androgen-producing tumors and as markers to assess the efficacy of therapy in these patients. DHEAS and testosterone and the usual androgen markers. DHEAS levels of greater than 7 μg per milliliter or total serum testosterone concentrations of greater than 200 ng per deciliter are usually considered worrisome, and further exploration for a tumor is indicated. If the clinical evidence of androgen excess seems excessive for the DHEAS or total testosterone determinations, further evaluation should also be undertaken. Free testosterone levels may be elevated in the presence of normal total testosterone concentrations secondary to reduced sex hormone–binding globulin concentrations associated with obesity and other causes (Table 13–10). Serum levels of androstenedione or urinary 17-ketosteroids may rarely be elevated despite normal DHEAS and testosterone levels and should be determined if clinically indicated.

Levels of 17OH-progesterone are used exclusively in

the diagnosis of congenital adrenal hyperplasia (21-hydroxylase deficiency). In patients with a family history of hirsutism, congenital adrenal hyperplasia of late onset should be considered (see Chapter 5). DHEAS may be

TABLE 13-10   Sex Hormone–Binding Globulin

Method: If abnormalities in sex hormone–binding globulin (SHBG) are suspected, free (unbound) hormone levels are usually measured to circumvent the problem. Direct measurement is rarely justified clinically but is performed by RIA.

Situations in which SHBG levels are altered:

High SHBG	Low SHBG
Elevated estrogens	Elevated androgens
Oral contraceptives	Hypothyroidism
Pregnancy	Progestin administration (except medroxyprogesterone)
Hyperthyroidism	Acromegaly
	Cushing's syndrome
	Obesity

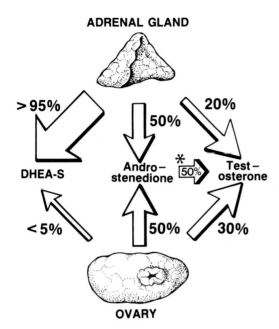

ADRENAL GLAND

OVARY

Figure 13–11   Relative contributions of the adrenal gland and the ovary to circulating levels of androgens. (*Fifty percent of circulating testosterone is derived from peripheral conversion of androstenedione.)

axis are Cushing's syndrome, adrenal insufficiency, and poorly controlled diabetes. Screening for these serious diseases should be conducted if clinically indicated.

Nonendocrine Testing of the Reproductive Axis

Several techniques are used to assess the structural and genetic aspects of the reproductive system in the female. Karyotypes and buccal smears are used to assess patients with suspected genetic disorders. The karyotype is the more precise of the two techniques and is usually applied only in patients with primary amenorrhea. Turner's syndrome (gonadal dysgenesis) is the only common genetic disorder associated with reproductive dysfunction. Hysterosalpingograms are useful for assessing patency of the fallopian tubes as well as uterine structural abnormalities. Hysteroscopy is used to confirm uterine synechiae and other uterine abnormalities. Diagnostic laparoscopy is most commonly performed to identify endometriosis and tubal, ovarian, and adnexal abnormalities. Evaluation for structural abnormalities of the reproductive system should take precedence when no ovulatory or hormonal disorder is suggested by the history or physical examination and when the history reveals possible causes of structural abnormalities such as pelvic procedures or infections. A laparoscopy or hys-

normal in these patients, and stimulated serum concentrations of 17OH-progesterone are required for diagnosis of this disorder.

With the advent of reliable RIAs for serum DHEAS, 17OH-progesterone, androstenedione, and testosterone, urinary measurements of androgens (the 17-ketosteroids) are now rarely used in endocrinology. Urinary 17-ketosteroid measurements are often subject to cross-reacting substances. In rare cases, androgen-secreting tumors have been found in obviously virilized patients in whom 17-ketosteroids have been elevated (usually greater than 50 mg per 24 hours) despite normal serum DHEAS, androstenedione, and testosterone. Twenty-four-hour urine collections are now usually reserved for the occasional patient in whom an androgen-secreting tumor is suspected (because of virilization) but serum androgen levels are unexpectedly normal or minimally elevated.

OTHER HORMONES THAT AFFECT THE HPO AXIS

Many hormones appear to modulate the activity of the reproductive axis. The most common disturbances of these hormones that cause reproductive abnormalities are hyperprolactinemia, hypothyroidism, and hyperthyroidism (Table 13–11). The incidence of these disorders is relatively high, and their presentation can be subtle, as described in other chapters. Therefore, screening for these endocrinopathies should be routinely undertaken during evaluations of reproductive disorders. Less common hormonal imbalances known to affect the HPO

TABLE 13–11   Causes of Amenorrhea

I.	Hypothalamic/pituitary
	A. ''Hypothalamic amenorrhea''
	1. Exercise induced
	2. Weight loss related
	3. Etiology not defined (? stress)
	B. PCOS*
	C. Congenital Gn-RH deficiency (IHH or Kallmann's syndrome)
	D. Tumors/infiltrative lesions
	E. Trauma/infections
	F. Surgery/radiotherapy
	G. Drugs/chronic diseases
	H. Sheehan's syndrome
	I. ? Obesity
II.	Ovarian
	A. Ovarian failure
	1. Senescence
	2. Autoimmune
	3. Chemotherapy/surgical removal
	B. Resistant ovary syndrome
III.	Uterine
	A. Pregnancy
	B. Uterine synechiae (Asherman's syndrome)
	C. Cervical stenosis
IV.	Other endocrinopathies
	A. Hyperprolactinemia
	B. Hyperandrogenemia
	C. Hyperthyroidism or hypothyroidism
	D. Cushing's syndrome
	E. Poorly controlled diabetes

* Etiology controversial

terosalpingogram should be performed prior to initiating gonadotropin or Gn-RH therapy for ovulation induction even when there is no history to suggest a structural abnormality. Use of these tests is further discussed in subsequent sections.

SYNOPSIS OF ENDOCRINE TESTING IN DIAGNOSIS OF COMMON REPRODUCTIVE DISORDERS

Ovarian Failure

When menopause or premature ovarian failure is suspected clinically, gonadotropin determinations are the most reliable diagnostic test. In women with obvious menopause (older than 45 years of age, cessation of periods, and symptoms of estrogen deficiency), clinical evidence may not require laboratory confirmation. With loss of negative feedback from ovarian steroids and inhibin, FSH demonstrates the greater rise and is the most valuable laboratory test for the diagnosis of menopause. As mentioned, ovarian steroid levels may wax and wane in the perimenopausal period, and a normal estradiol level in the presence of elevated gonadotropins by no means rules out menopause. However, in the younger woman in whom ovarian failure is being considered, gonadotropin-producing pituitary adenomas must also be considered. These tumors have been reported to constitute 2 to 5 percent of all pituitary tumors and may secrete FSH alone, both FSH and LH, or, very rarely, LH alone. A disproportionately low LH level and/or lack of signs or symptoms of estrogen deficiency justify a CT or nuclear magnetic resonance scan to rule out such a tumor in the young woman with an elevated serum concentration of FSH and menstrual irregularities. Anti-ovarian antibodies are frequently present in women with premature ovarian failure. However, determination of antibody titers does not significantly contribute to diagnosis or treatment of most of these patients.

Amenorrhea

The central focus of the endocrine evaluation of amenorrhea is differentiating identifiable abnormalities (see Table 13-11) from hypothalamic amenorrhea. Hypothalamic amenorrhea is a diagnosis of exclusion. Thus, a reasonable evaluation of all other possible etiologies must precede this diagnosis. The assessment of primary amenorrhea differs from that of secondary amenorrhea in the greater consideration of chromosomal, congenital, or developmental abnormalities. Karyotypes are not usually obtained in secondary amenorrhea if more than one period has occurred. Karyotypes are more definitive than buccal smears in patients suspected of having genetic syndromes.

Relevant data from the history and physical examination guide the laboratory work-up. Laboratory testing is intended to differentiate between hypothalamic-

pituitary, ovarian, uterine, and other hormone disorders. Table 13-12 lists a common scheme for evaluation of amenorrhea. Gonadotropin, prolactin, beta-hCG (for pregnancy), and thyroid function determinations are obtained initially since disorders of these hormones are not always clinically apparent. When pregnancy has been excluded, a progestin-induced withdrawal bleeding test is administered as previously described. The gonadotropin levels differentiate primary ovarian failure from other causes of amenorrhea. An increased LH to FSH ratio suggests PCOS. Gonadotropin levels are not reliable for differentiating PCOS from other causes of amenorrhea. The progestin withdrawal test estimates the degree of endogenous estrogen secretion and indicates uterine patency.

Tumors in the area of the hypothalamus and pituitary rarely present as isolated amenorrhea, but suspicion increases with minimal activity of the HPO axis. Similarly, hyperandrogenemia usually is signaled by hirsutism or virilization. However, if no other causes of the amenorrhea are apparent, hypothalamic-pituitary imaging and determination of androgen levels are recommended. If no diagnosis has been made after these procedures and a careful review of the history and physical examination reveals no other clues, the patient is considered to have hypothalamic amenorrhea. Clues suggesting other endocrine diseases should be pursued, as described in the other chapters of this book.

Oligomenorrhea and Polycystic Ovarian Syndrome

Oligomenorrhea should be evaluated similarly to amenorrhea except that progestin withdrawal as a test of estrogen status is unnecessary and hypothalamic-pituitary imaging is not undertaken unless hyperprolactinemia or

---

TABLE 13-12   Evaluation of Amenorrhea

1. History and physical examination
2. Initial laboratory tests (if no cause is apparent from history and physical examination):
   a. Prolactin
   b. LH and FSH
   c. Thyroxine and thyroid-stimulating hormone
   d. Pregnancy test
3. Secondary laboratory testing:

a. Prolactin >50 to 100 ng/ml	Pituitary imaging
b. LH and FSH low	Hypothalamic and pituitary imaging
c. LH and FSH high	Consider ovarian failure versus gonadotropin-secreting tumor
d. Thyroid tests abnormal	Treat thyroid disease
e. Initial testing normal	Progestin withdrawal testing; testosterone and DHEAS levels

other indications of hypothalamic-pituitary disease are present. Prolactin and thyroid function should be determined initially. LH and FSH levels provide little information except to suggest the possibility of PCOS.

PCOS refers to a heterogeneous group of disorders characterized by menstrual irregularities and hyperandrogenemia that usually appear about the time of puberty. Obesity or an increased LH to FSH ratio may or may not be present. The ovaries are classically described as enlarged and containing multiple subcapsular cysts, but they may have an entirely normal appearance. Some patients have clear increases in LH to FSH ratios with menstrual irregularities in the absence of clinical or laboratory evidence of hyperandrogenemia. Currently, the term *polycystic ovarian syndrome* covers a wide spectrum of disorders without clear agreement on the boundaries of this diagnosis. As these disorders are better understood, more precise classifications and terminology will undoubtedly evolve. Although serum levels of LH and FSH may be helpful, serum androgen levels (testosterone and DHEAS) in conjunction with historical and physical findings are the most useful endocrine tests for the diagnosis of PCOS.

Hirsutism

The criteria for abnormal distribution of terminal hair (Tables 13-13 and 13-14) in women are reviewed elsewhere. Initial evaluation of serum androgen levels is intended to screen for adrenal or ovarian androgen-secreting tumors and to provide a marker to assist in monitoring subsequent therapies. As described earlier, this is usually done by determination of serum concentrations of DHEAS and testosterone. Some authors also advocate the use of stimulated 17OH-progesterone levels in the initial screening of hirsutism, although the yield without a suggestive family history is low and the test is expensive. Various strategies of testosterone sampling have been advocated since testosterone elevations may be intermittent. Some authors recommend multiple determinations if initial values are normal. Free (unbound) testosterone concentrations are more sensitive indicators of testosterone elevations, particularly in obese patients. However, testosterone elevations secondary to tumors are almost always apparent with total testosterone determinations.

We suggest single determinations of DHEAS and testosterone (free testosterone in obese women) to screen for worrisome causes of hirsutism. Levels suggestive of tumors (DHEAS greater than 7 μg per milliliter, testosterone greater than 200 ng per deciliter) should be confirmed. If both DHEAS and testosterone are normal, more detailed studies using catheterization and selective sampling of adrenal and ovarian veins have demonstrated that in the great majority of patients ovarian androgen production is increased. Thus, for practical purposes, patients with mild to moderate hirsutism and normal DHEAS and testosterone levels can be considered to have increased production of ovarian androgens and may be

TABLE 13-13   Causes of Hirsutism

I. Androgen dependent
   A. Ovary
      1. PCOS
      2. Hyperthecosis
      3. Androgen-secreting tumors
   B. Adrenal
      1. Congenital adrenal hyperplasia
      2. Cushing's syndrome
      3. Idiopathic
      4. Tumors
   C. Iatrogenic
      1. Danazol
      2. 19-Nor progestins
      3. Anabolic steroids
II. Androgen independent

treated accordingly. Urinary steroid measurements are no longer commonly used. Elevations of DHEAS above 7 μg per milliliter require further evaluation with dexamethasone suppression (1 mg daily for 14 days to suppress the DHEAS into the normal range) and an adrenal CT scan. Testosterone levels consistently exceeding 200 ng per deciliter require pelvic ultrasonography and a CT scan of the adrenals to rule out the rare testosterone-secreting adrenal adenomas. Laparotomy with ovarian biopsy may be necessary to exclude small ovarian tumors in patients with normal radiographic findings and persistent testosterone elevations in the "tumor" range. Additional workup should be guided by the degree of the patient's hirsutism or virilization in relation to the patient's ethnic

TABLE 13-14   Evaluation of Hirsutism

1. History and physical examination
2. Initial laboratory tests:*
   a. DHEAS: Premenopausal normal values, 0.4 to 4.3 μg/ml
      Postmenopausal normal values, 0.1 to 1.9 μg/ml
   b. Total or free testosterone: Normal value <80 ng/dl
   c. Stimulated 17OH-progesterone (if congenital adrenal hyperplasia suspected)
   d. Androstanediol glucuronide (clinical value not yet established)
3. Secondary laboratory testing:
   a. If total testosterone persistently >200 ng/dl:
      Sonography of ovaries
      CT of adrenals
      Consider ovarian biopsy
   b. If DHEAS >7 μg/ml:
      CT of adrenals
      Trial of dexamethasone for suppression
   c. If testosterone and DHEAS are unexpectedly low for clinical presentation:
      Androstenedione
      24-hour urine collection for 17OH and ketosteroids

* Normal ranges vary.

background. A virilized patient requires a detailed evaluation of all serum androgens and urinary 17-ketosteroids if initial screening does not lead to a diagnosis.

Infertility With Regular Menstrual Cycles and Without Hirsutism

Most endocrine causes of infertility are manifested by menstrual irregularities. Hyperprolactinemia can be an exception to this rule. Thus, prolactin determinations should be obtained at the initiation of infertility evaluations. Current claims of luteal phase rises in prolactin or normal prolactin levels being causally related to infertility are not yet well established. In the woman with regular cycles, further endocrine evaluation should await semen analysis of the partner, postcoital testing, and evaluation of structural abnormalities of the fallopian tubes and uterus. If these evaluations are normal, a luteal phase endometrial biopsy may be undertaken for consideration of inadequate luteal phase. Criteria for diagnosis of inadequate luteal phase are described earlier in this chapter. Laparoscopy is indicated to exclude endometriosis or subtle tuboperitoneal factors if these tests are completed and normal.

More recently described disorders such as LUF syndrome and premature luteinization of the follicle seem to occur rarely but must also be considered. The latter may be diagnosed by abnormal elevations of progesterone in the preovulatory period. The role of other fertility tests such as sperm antibodies and hamster egg penetration is still being evaluated and is reviewed elsewhere.

Monitoring of Ovulation

Prediction of ovulation is important for timing of intercourse and artificial insemination in women attempting to become pregnant. As mentioned, BBT tracking cannot be used prospectively to predict ovulation. The simplest means of prediction is cervical mucus changes or the previously mentioned kits that detect increases in urinary LH levels during the midcycle surge just prior to ovulation. These home monitoring kits are particularly useful in women with irregular periods, as well as those undergoing clomiphene or Gn-RH therapy.

Monitoring hMG therapy is more complex. Since a midcycle LH surge and ovulation do not usually occur with hMG therapy, an injection of hCG must be administered when the follicle is mature in order to mimic the LH surge. The appropriate timing of the hCG injection is determined by serum estradiol levels in conjunction with serial ultrasound evaluations of the follicles. The diameter of the mature follicle and accompanying serum levels of estradiol may vary greatly between patients. Follicular diameters of 16 to 25 mm and serum estradiol levels of 500 to 1,100 pg per milliliter are most common when the follicle is ripe for ovulation during hMG therapy. This estradiol level contrasts with midcycle peak levels of 200 to 400 pg per milliliter during normal spontaneous cycles. Abundant, clear cervical mucus with profuse ferning and a dilated cervical os help verify preovulatory levels of estrogen.

If hCG is to be used in conjunction with clomiphene, some means of determining when the follicle is mature is critical, since premature administration of hCG will be ineffective. Cervical mucus changes are a good screening observation, but these may be compromised by clomiphene. The status of the follicle should be confirmed by at least an ultrasound examination and possibly an estradiol determination prior to administration of hCG.

BIBLIOGRAPHY

Physiology and General References

Clarke IJ, Cummins JT. Pulsatility of reproductive hormones: Physiologic basis and clinical implications. Clin Endocrinol Metab 1987; 1:1.

Crowley WF, Filicori M, Spratt DI, Santoro NF. The physiology of gonadotropin-releasing hormone (GnRH) secretion in men and women. Recent Prog Horm Res 1985; 41:473.

Donahoe PK, Cate RL, MacLaughlin DT, et al. Mullerian inhibiting substances: Gene structure and mechanism of action of a fetal regressor. Recent Prog Horm Res 1987; 43:431.

Filicori M, Santoro N, Merriam GR, Crowley WF. Characterization of the physiological pattern of episodic gonadotropin secretion throughout the human menstrual cycle. J Clin Endocrinol Metab 1986; 62:1136.

Frisch RE. Fatness and fertility. Sci Am 1988; 258:88.

Jansen RPS. Endocrine response in the fallopian tube. Endocr Rev 1984; 5:525.

Knobil E. The neuroendocrine control of the menstrual cycle. Recent Prog Horm Res 1980; 36:53.

Knobil E, Neill JD. The physiology of reproduction. New York: Raven Press, 1988.

Lenton EA, Sulaiman R, Sobowale O, et al. The human menstrual cycle: Plasma concentrations of prolactin, LH, FSH, oestradiol and progesterone in conceiving and non-conceiving women. J Reprod Fertil 1982; 65:131.

McLachlan RI, Robertson DM, deKretser D, Burger HG. Inhibin—a non-steroidal regulator of pituitary follicle stimulating hormone. Clin Endocrinol Metab 1987; 1:89.

Ross GT, Cargille CM, Lipsett MB, et al. Pituitary and gonadal hormones in women during spontaneous and induced ovulatory cycles. Recent Progr Horm Res 1970; 26:1.

Sherman BM, Korenman SG. Hormonal characteristics of the human menstrual cycle throughout reproductive life. J Clin Invest 1975; 55:699.

Soules MR, Clifton DK, Steiner RA, et al. The corpus luteum: Determinants of progesterone secretion in the normal menstrual cycle. Obstet Gynecol 1988; 71:659.

Vale W, Rivier C, Hsueh A, et al. Chemical and biological characterization of the inhibin family of protein hormones. Recent Prog Horm Res 1988; 44:1.

Yen SSC, Jaffe RB, eds. Reproductive endocrinology: Physiology, pathophysiology and clinical management. Philadelphia: WB Saunders, 1986.

Ying SY. Inhibins, activins, and follistatins: Gonadal proteins modulating the secretion of follicle-stimulating hormone. Endocr Rev 1988; 9:267.

Pituitary Gonadotropins

Bullen BA, Skrinar GS, Bertins IZ, et al. Induction of menstrual disorders by strenuous exercise in untrained women. N Engl J Med 1985; 312:1349.

Elkind-Hirsch K, Goldzieher JW, Gibbons WE, et al. Evaluation of the ovustick urinary luteinizing hormone kit in normal and stimulated menstrual cycles. Obstet Gynecol 1986; 67:450.

Henley K, Vaitukaitus JL. Exercise-induced menstrual dysfunction. Ann Rev Med 1988; 39:443.

Knee GR, Feinman MA, Strauss JF, et al. Detection of the ovulatory luteinizing hormone (LH) surge with a semiquantitative urinary LH assay. Fertil Steril 1985; 44:707.

Rebar R, Judd HL, Yen SSC, et al. Characterization of the inappropriate gonadotropin secretion in polycystic ovary syndrome. J Clin Invest 1976; 57:1320.

Sheehan HL, Davis JC. Pituitary necrosis. Br Med Bull 1968; 24:59.

Schlaff WD. Dynamic testing in reproductive endocrinology. Fertil Steril 1986; 45:589.

Snyder PJ, Sterling FH. Hypersecretion of LH and FSH by a pituitary adenoma. J Clin Endocrinol Metab 1976; 42:544.

Yen SSC, Tsai CC, Naftolin F, et al. Pulsatile patterns of gonadotropin release in subjects with and without ovarian function. J Clin Endocrinol Metab 1972; 34:671.

Yen SSC, Rebar R, VandenBerg G, et al. Pituitary gonadotropin responsiveness to synthetic LRF in subjects with normal and abnormal hypothalamic-pituitary-gonadal axis. J Reprod Fertil 1973; 20:137.

Ovaries, Endometrium, and Cervix

Abdulla V, Diver MJ, Hipkin LJ, et al. Plasma progesterone levels as an indicator of ovulation. Br J Obstet Gynaecol 1983; 90:543.

Aiman J, Smentek C. Premature ovarian failure. Obstet Gynecol 1985; 66:9.

Bryce RL, Shuter B, Sinosich MJ, et al. The value of ultrasound, gonadotropin, and estradiol measurements for precise ovulation prediction. Fertil Steril 1982; 37:42.

Check JH, Chase JS, Adelson HG, et al. New approaches to the diagnosis and therapy of the luteinized unruptured follicle syndrome. Int J Fertil 1986; 30:29.

Downs KA, Gibson M. Basal body temperature graph and the luteal phase defect. Fertil Steril 1983; 40:466.

Genant HK, Cann CE, Ettinger B, Gordan GS. Quantitative computed tomography of vertebral spongiosa: A sensitive method for detecting early bone loss after oophorectomy. Ann Intern Med 1982; 97:699.

Israel R, Mishell DR, Stone SC, et al. Single luteal phase serum progesterone assay as an indicator of ovulation. Am J Obstet Gynecol 1972; 112:1043.

Keenan JA, Herbert CM, Bush JR, Wentz AC. Diagnosis and management of out-of-phase endometrial biopsies among patients receiving clomiphene citrate for ovulation induction. Fertil Steril 1989; 51:964.

Kerin JF, Kirby C, Morris D, et al. Incidence of the luteinized unruptured follicle phenomenon in cycling women. Fertil Steril 1983; 40:620.

Kletzky OA, Davajan V, Nakamura RM, et al. Clinical categorization of patients with secondary amenorrhea using progesterone-induced uterine bleeding and measurement of serum gonadotropin levels. Am J Obstet Gynecol 1975; 121:695.

Leader A, Wiseman D, Taylor PF. The prediction of ovulation: A comparison of the basal body temperature graph, cervical mucus score, and real-time pelvic ultrasonography. Fertil Steril 1985; 43:395.

Lenton EA, Weston GA, Cooke ID. Problems in using basal body temperature recordings in an infertility clinic. Br Med J 1977; 1:803.

Lenton EA, Landgren BM, Sexton L. Normal variation in the length of the luteal phase of the menstrual cycle: Identification of the short luteal phase. Br J Obstet Gynecol 1984; 91:685.

Magyar DM, Boyers SP, Marshall JR, et al. Regular menstrual cycles and premenstrual molimina as indicators of ovulation. Obstet Gynecol 1979; 53:411.

McNeely MJ, Soules MR. The diagnosis of luteal phase deficiency: A critical review. Fertil Steril 1988; 50:1.

Midgley AR Jr, Niswender GD, Gay VL, et al. Use of antibodies for characterization of gonadotropins and steroids. Recent Prog Horm Res 1971; 27:235.

Moghissi KS. Cyclic changes of cervical mucus in normal and progestin-treated women. Fertil Steril 1966; 17:63.

Noyes RW, Hertig AT, Rock J. Dating the endometrial biopsy. Fertil Steril 1950; 1:3.

Noyes RW, Haman JO. Accuracy of endometrial dating. Fertil Steril 1953; 4:504.

Papanicolaou GN. General survey of vaginal smear and its use in research and diagnosis. Am J Obstet Gynecol 1946; 52:1023.

Quagliarello J, Arny M. Inaccuracy of basal body temperature charts in predicting urinary luteinizing hormone surges. Fertil Steril 1986; 45:334.

Rebar RW, Erickson GF, Yen SSC. "Idiopathic premature ovarian failure": Clinical and endocrine characteristics. Fertil Steril 1982; 37:35.

Rosenfeld DL, Chudow S, Bronson RA. Diagnosis of luteal phase inadequacy. Obstet Gynecol 1980; 56:193.

Wathen NC, Perry L, Lilford RJ, et al. Interpretation of single progesterone measurement in diagnosis of anovulation and defective luteal phase: Observations on analysis of the normal range. Br Med J 1984; 288:7.

Wentz AC. Endometrial biopsy in the evaluation of infertility. Fertil Steril 1980; 33:121.

Wied GL. Suggested standard for karyopyknosis: Use in hormonal reading of vaginal smears. Fertil Steril 1955; 6:61.

Yamashita T, Okamato S, Thomas A, et al. Predicting pregnancy outcome after in vitro fertilization and embryo transfer using estradiol, progesterone, and human chorionic gonadotropin B-subunit. Fertil Steril 1989; 51:304.

Androgens, Hirsutism, and Polycystic Ovary

Abraham GE. Ovarian and adrenal contributions to androgens during the menstrual cycle. J Clin Endocrinol Metab 1974; 39:340.

Anderson DC. Sex hormone-binding globulin. Clin Endocrinol (Oxf) 1974; 3:69.

Bardin CW, Lipsett MB. Testosterone and androstenedione blood production rates in normal women and women with idiopathic hirsutism or polycystic ovaries. J Clin Invest 1967; 46:891.

DeVane GW, Czekala NM, Judd HL, Yen SSC. Circulating gonadotropins, estrogens, and androgens in polycystic ovarian disease. J Obstet Gynecol 1973; 121:496.

Hoffman DI, Klove K, Lobo RA. The prevalence and significance of elevated dehydroepiandrosterone sulfate levels in anovulatory women. Fertil Steril 1984; 42:76.

Judd HL, Scully RE, Herbst AL, et al. Familial hyperthecosis: Comparison of endocrinologic and histologic findings with polycystic ovarian disease. Am J Obstet Gynecol 1973; 117:976.

Kirshner A, Jacobs J. Combined ovarian and adrenal vein catheterization to determine the site(s) of androgen overproduction in hirsutism. J Clin Endocrinol Metab 1971; 33:199.

Korenman SG, Kirschner MA, Lipsett MB. Testosterone production in normal and virilized women and in women with the Stein-Leventhal syndrome or idiopathic hirsutism. J Clin Endocrinol Metab 1965; 25:798.

Korth-Schutz S, Levine LS, New MI, Chow DM. Dehydroepiandrosterone sulfate (CDS) levels, a rapid test for abnormal adrenal androgen secretion. J Clin Endocrinol Metab 1976; 42:1005.

New MI, Dupont B, Pang S, et al. An update of congenital adrenal hyperplasia. Recent Prog Horm Res 1981; 37:105.

Rittmaster R, Loriaux DL. Hirsutism. Ann Intern Med 1987; 106:96.

Wajchenberg BL, Marcondes JA, Mathor MB, et al. Free testosterone levels during the menstrual cycle in obese versus normal women. Fertil Steril 1989; 51:535.

White PC, New MI, Dupont B. Congenital adrenal hyperplasia (1). N Engl J Med 1987; 316:1519.

White PC, New MI, Dupont B. Congenital adrenal hyperplasia (2). N Engl J Med 1987; 316:1580.

Yen SSC. The polycystic ovary syndrome. Clin Endocrinol (Oxf) 1980; 12:177.

Related Testing

Ayvaliotis B, Bronson R, Rosenfeld D, et al. Conception rates in couples where autoimmunity to sperm is detected. Fertil Steril 1985; 43:739.

Ben David M, Schenker JG. Transient hyperprolactinemia: A correctable cause of idiopathic female infertility. J Clin Endocrinol Metab 1983; 57:442.

Badawy SZA, Shaykh ME, Shulman S, et al. Circulating sperm antibodies: Indications for testing in infertile couples. Int J Fertil 1984; 29.159.

Boccuzzi G, Angeli A, Bisbocci D, et al. Effect of synthetic luteinizing hormone releasing hormone (LH-RH) on the release of gonadotropins in Cushing's disease. J Clin Endocrinol Metab 1975; 40:892.

Bronson R, Cooper G, Rosenfeld D. Sperm antibodies: Their role in infertility. Fertil Steril 1984; 42:171.

Damewood MD, Zacur HA, Hoffman GJ, et al. Circulating antiovarian antibodies in premature ovarian failure. Obstet Gynecol 1986; 68:850.

Del Pozo E, Wyss H, Tolis G, et al. Prolactin and deficient luteal function. Obstet Gynecol 1979; 53:282.

Rogers J. Menstruation and systemic disease: Thyroid disorders. N Engl J Med 1958; 259:721.

Vazquez AM, Kenny FM. Ovarian failure and anti-ovarian antibodies in association with hypoparathyroidism, moniliasis, and Addison's and Hashimoto's diseases. Obstet Gynecol 1973; 41:414.

14 Disorders of Male Reproductive Function

Howard R. Nankin, M.D.

Tu Lin, M.D.

Richard V. Clark, M.D., Ph.D.

During the past two decades there has been a major increase in our understanding of male reproductive physiology, made possible by a variety of disciplines, both basic and clinical. In this chapter, the approach to clinical and laboratory investigation of male gonadal disorders is reviewed.

NORMAL PHYSIOLOGY OF THE HYPOTHALAMIC-PITUITARY-TESTICULAR AXIS

Structure and Anatomy of Testes

The normal adult testis measures about 3 by 5 cm, has a volume of 15 to 25 ml, and has a rubbery, firm consistency. It consists of two major components: seminiferous tubules and the interstitial compartment. The major secretory product of Leydig's cells in the small (10 percent) interstitial compartment is testosterone, which serves as a circulating hormone and as a prohormone for dihydrotestosterone (DHT) and estradiol. Seminiferous tubules are composed of germ cells and Sertoli's cells (Fig. 14-1). These tubules comprise 90 percent of testis volume. Generally, there is a good correlation between normal testes size and normal function and sperm counts.

Luteinizing Hormone and Follicle-Stimulating Hormone

Testicular function is primarily under the control of luteinizing hormone (LH) and follicle-stimulating hormone (FSH) secreted by the anterior pituitary gland. FSH, LH, thyroid-stimulating hormone (TSH), and human chorionic gonadotropin (hCG) are structurally similar, each composed of two glycopeptide chains (alpha and beta). The alpha chains of these hormones have a common sequence of 96 amino acids. The beta chain is u ique to each and confers receptor-binding specificity. FSH-beta and LH-beta contain 115 amino acids; hCG-beta contains 147 amino acids. Two complex carbohydrate side chains are attached to the alpha subunits. The beta chain of hCG has five complex carbohydrate side chains; FSH-beta and LH-beta each have two. A terminal sialic acid is present on the carbohydrate chains of hCG-beta and FSH-beta. Sialic acid decreases the metabolic clearance of these hormones. Consequently, FSH and hCG have longer plasma half-lives than LH. The two chains (subunits) are synthesized separately and assembled and glycosylated prior to secretion from the pituitary. At normal rates of secretion, there is an excess of alpha-chain synthesis, and free alpha subunit can be detected in the serum by radioimmunoassay. Elevated alpha subunits are without known effect on gonadal function (Table 14-1). Under conditions of hypersecretion, a small amount of free beta chain can also appear in the serum. Both FSH and LH are synthesized in common gonadotropic cells, which make up 5 to 9 percent of the pituitary cell population.

Gonadotropin-Releasing Hormone

LH, and to a lesser extent FSH, is secreted into the peripheral circulation in a pulsatile fashion (Fig. 14-2). The secretion of gonadotropins is regulated by the episodic stimulation of the pituitary gland by luteinizing hormone (gonadotropin)–releasing hormone (LH-RH or Gn-RH). Gn-RH is a decapeptide that is synthesized by hypothalamic neurons and secreted episodically into the hypothalamo-hypophyseal portal system, where it is carried into the anterior pituitary gland. Gn-RH binds to specific high-affinity receptors on the plasma membrane of pituitary gonadotropes and stimulates the release of both LH and FSH. The effects of Gn-RH on gonadotropin release are calcium dependent, mediated by increased phospholipid turnover (hydrolysis of phosphatidylinositol, 4,5-bisphosphate), formation of diacylglycerol and inositol trisphosphate, and activation of calcium- and phospholipid-dependent protein kinase (protein kinase C). Studies by Knobil (1980) in nonhuman primates

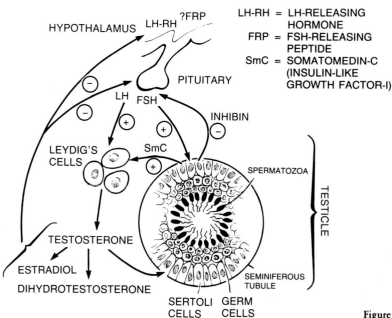

LH-RH = LH-RELEASING
HORMONE
FRP = FSH-RELEASING
PEPTIDE
SmC = SOMATOMEDIN-C
(INSULIN-LIKE
GROWTH FACTOR-I)

Figure 14-1 The hypothalamic-pituitary axis in the male.

demonstrated that a pulsatile, as opposed to a continuous, pattern of Gn-RH stimulation of the pituitary was essential for induction and maintenance of normal gonadotropin release. It has been documented that low-dosage, pulsatile Gn-RH can induce normal testicular development and function in patients with endogenous Gn-RH deficiency. Administration of high continuous doses of Gn-RH or superactive Gn-RH analogues can severely suppress gonadotropin release and testicular function and has been used as a method of medical castration in patients with prostatic cancer, as treatment for boys with precocious puberty, and also as a male contraceptive (the last use has not been as effective as the former two).

Hypothalamic Gn-RH synthesis and release are regulated by neurons, stimulatory and inhibitory neurotransmitters (e.g., catecholamine, serotonin, and amino acids), and neuropeptides (opioid peptides such as beta-endorphin, met-enkephalin, dynorphin, and other neuropeptides such as substance P, neuropeptide Y, and vasoactive intestinal peptide). Gn-RH provides a link between the central nervous system and the pituitary gland. Since secretion is controlled by neural mechanisms and these are, of necessity, dependent on cyclic rather than

continuous transmission, LH pulsatility is a strict reflection of Gn-RH pulsatility (see Fig. 14–2). However, the pulsatility may not be necessary for gonadal function. The gonads of both sexes may respond to supraphysiologic treatment with exogenous gonadotropins with very long half-lives (e.g., hCG).

Feedback (Testosterone, Estradiol, and Inhibin)

Testosterone and estradiol independently control LH secretion at two separate anatomic sites, the hypothalamus and pituitary. Testosterone can be converted to estradiol by the enzyme aromatase. However, the inhibitory effect of testosterone on LH release persisted even in the presence of aromatase inhibitor. Furthermore, nonaromatizable androgen, such as DHT, inhibits LH release without a concomitant increase in estradiol concentration. Androgens and estrogens produce differential effects on the frequency of pulsatile LH secretion as well as on its amplitude. The effect of testosterone is mediated mainly through the hypothalamus by decreased Gn-RH pulse frequency. Whether testosterone has an effect at the pituitary gland remains unclear. In contrast to testosterone, the early effect of estrogen on LH release is decreased pulse amplitude mediated by a direct pituitary action. Estrogen also has a major effect on the hypothalamus by inhibiting Gn-RH release. Aromatase has been localized in the hypothalamus. Progesterone and 17OH-progesterone exert feedback inhibition also.

Mottram and Cramer (1923) observed severe morphologic changes in the anterior pituitary gland of a male rat whose testicular germinal elements had been damaged by radiation. This observation led to the suggestion that the pituitary gland is in some way regulated by a testicular factor other than steroid hormones. McCullagh

TABLE 14-1   Conditions in Which Alpha Subunits are Elevated

Ovulatory surge
Menopause
Primary gonadal failure
Primary hypothyroidism
Renal failure
Pituitary tumors
Gn-RH stimulation
Thyrotropin-releasing hormone
stimulation

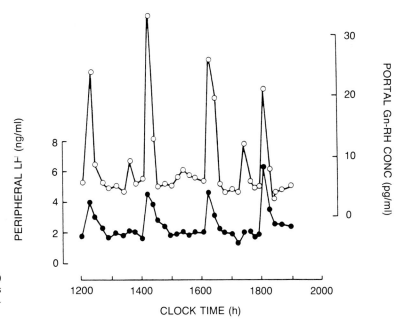

Figure 14-2   Concentrations of Gn-RH (*open circles*) in pituitary portal plasma and peripheral LH levels (*closed circles*) of sheep. (Adapted from Clarke IJ, Cummings JT. Endocrinology 1982; 111:1737.)

(1932) coined the name *inhibin* for this hypothetical testicular substance. Inhibin is currently defined as a peptide factor that selectively inhibits the release of pituitary FSH without affecting circulating levels of other pituitary hormones. There is strong indirect evidence for the existence of inhibin in humans based on various physiologic and pathologic states in which FSH secretion varies inversely with the adequacy of gametogenesis. Inhibin has been purified from bovine and porcine ovarian follicular fluid as heterodimers with a molecular weight of 32,000. Two forms of inhibin, designated inhibin A and B, have been identified that consist of a common alpha subunit (MW 18,000) and one of two distinct but highly homologous beta chains (MW 14,700 and MW 14,000). These are extremely potent and specific inhibitors of FSH

in pituitary primary culture bioassay, having a median effective dose of approximately 1 ng per milliliter. The sequences of the precursors of porcine, bovine, and human inhibin alpha subunits and beta subunits have been deduced from complementary DNA sequences. The sequence of inhibin is partially homologous to transforming growth factor–beta (TGF-beta) and müllerian inhibiting factor. Inhibin has been shown to inhibit the release of basal FSH, but not LH in vivo and in vitro. A recent surprising discovery was that homodimers of the smaller beta subunit of inhibin isolated from porcine follicular fluid stimulated FSH release from pituitary cells in vitro, in contrast to inhibin, which inhibits FSH release. This has been named activin or FSH-releasing peptide (FRP) (Fig. 14–3).

Figure 14-3   Schematic representation of structures of inhibin and activin. (Adapted from Ying S-Y. Inhibins, activins and follistatins: Gonadal proteins modulating the secretion of follicle-stimulating hormone. Endocr Rev 1988; 9:267.)

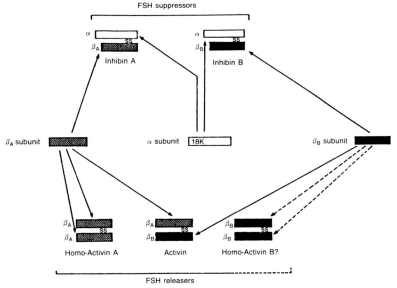

Regulation of Testes

Leydig's cells are scattered in the interstitial compartment of the testis and constitute about 2 percent of total testicular volume. Steroidogenesis in these cells is regulated mainly by LH. LH binds to specific, high-affinity membrane receptors on Leydig's cells and stimulates androgen biosynthesis via a cyclic adenosine monophosphate (cAMP)–dependent pathway, causing increased cholesterol transport into the mitochondria and increased cytochrome P450 side-chain cleavage enzyme, which enhances the conversion of cholesterol to pregnenolone, the rate-limiting step of testosterone formation. High intraluminal testosterone concentration is maintained in the seminiferous tubule by the binding of testosterone to androgen-binding protein (ABP), which is important for normal spermatogenesis. ABP is produced by Sertoli's cells under the influence of FSH and testosterone.

Many other factors besides LH have been reported to modulate Leydig's cell function. When FSH is administered to men with isolated gonadotropin deficiency during long-term hCG treatment, testosterone levels were further increased. FSH can induce LH receptors. The effect of FSH probably is mediated indirectly by products secreted by Sertoli's cells since Leydig's cells do not have specific receptors of FSH. Prolactin can also induce LH receptors but has no significant effect on LH-stimulated androgen response. In men with hyperprolactinemia, plasma testosterone is often reduced, probably owing to inhibition of Gn-RH release. The role of growth hormone (GH) on Leydig's cell function has been partially elucidated. In children with growth hormone deficiency, puberty is often delayed. Treatment with GH causes normal growth and sexual maturation at the same time. GH enhances hCG-stimulated testosterone secretion in GH-deficient subjects. The effect of GH on Leydig's cells is

mediated by somatomedin-C, a polypeptide produced mainly in the liver (also called insulin-like growth factor-I). Somatomedin-C can enhance Leydig's cell steroidogenesis, and Leydig's cells contain specific, high-affinity receptors for somatomedin-C. There are morphine-like substances in the testis that appear to be involved in Leydig's cell function (Fig. 14–4).

FSH binds to specific receptors on the plasma membrane of Sertoli's cells and probably spermatogonia of the seminiferous tubules. FSH binding to the membrane receptor results in increased cAMP formation, activation of cAMP-dependent protein kinase, and protein phosphorylation. FSH increases formation of a variety of proteins that are important in spermatogenesis (ABP and transferrin) and feedback control of FSH release (inhibin) and modulation of Leydig's cell function (Fig. 14–5).

The hormonal milieu necessary for the initiation and maintenance of spermatogenesis in man is not clear. Spermatogenesis requires FSH for its initiation. Spermatogenesis is not initiated in prepubertal hypogonadotropic hypogonadism and not maintained in men who acquire gonadotropin deficiency as adults (e.g., hypopituitarism as a result of hypophysectomy or pituitary tumor). A series of recent studies by Matsumoto and Bremner (1987) suggest that normal serum levels of FSH are not required for qualitatively normal spermatogenesis in humans. However, to achieve quantitatively normal levels of sperm production, FSH replacement was required. There also seem to be differences in the necessity for FSH in the initiation and maintenance of sperm production. Once sperm production is initiated with hCG and FSH in hypogonadotropic hypogonadal men, it can often be maintained by treatment with hCG alone. High intratesticular testosterone levels (50 to 100× serum) are normally present and are of major importance in spermatogenesis. Testosterone pellets implanted in testes of hypopituitary animals can maintain local spermatogenesis.

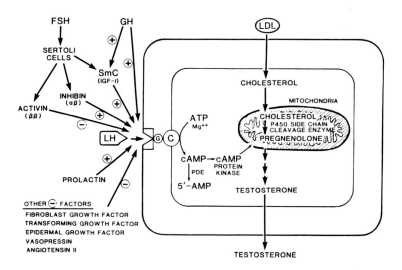

Figure 14–4 Hormones and factors modifying Leydig's cell steroidogenesis. Leydig's cells have specific binding sites (receptors) for somatomedin-C (SmC), also called insulin-like growth factor-I (IGF-I); prolactin; fibroblast growth factor; transforming growth factor-beta; epidermal growth factor; vasopressin; and angiotensin II. Many steps of the steroidogenic pathway are affected by these substances.

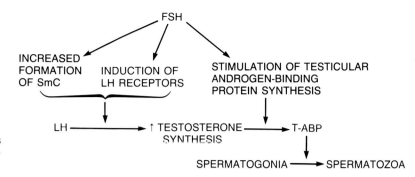

Figure 14-5 Follicle-stimulating hormone actions directly affect Sertoli's cells and indirectly modulate Leydig's cells.

Testosterone, Bioavailable Testosterone

The major androgen secreted by the testes is testosterone—approximately 7,000 μg daily. Most of the circulating testosterone is bound to protein (55 percent bound to testosterone-estrogen–binding globulin (TeBG) or sex hormone–binding globulin (SHBG), with 42 percent bound to albumin), and only about 2 to 3 percent of testosterone is free. Recent studies suggest that about 50 percent of albumin-bound testosterone is also bioactive. Non-TeBG-bound testosterone concentrations, determined after differential ammonium sulfate precipitation, correlated with availability of testosterone entry into brain and other tissues. Androgen effects in tissues are usually mediated by androgen receptors (Fig. 14–6). The original two-step model of steroid hormone action, binding to cytoplasmic receptors followed by translocation to the nucleus, has been revised in the light of recent evidence that estrogen receptors are predominantly concentrated in the cell nucleus at all times. Both the traditional cytosolic and nuclear forms of the receptor normally reside in the nuclear compartment, and the more loosely associated unoccupied receptors escape into the cytosol during fractionation of intracellular components. The cytosolic receptor is probably the result of a preparation artifact. The activated receptor may acquire increased affinity for regulatory elements within the nucleus rather than undergo physical translocation from cytosol to nucleus. Testosterone itself may be biologically active, or in some organs 5-alpha-reductase must produce DHT from the precursor androgen. Androgen receptors bind both testosterone and DHT. The affinity of androgen receptor for DHT is seven fold higher than for testosterone. However, testosterone is an effective androgen. It is responsible for virilization of the wolffian duct during embryogenesis, may mediate spermatogenesis in men, and mediates postnatal partial virilization in men with 5-alpha-reductase deficiency. These men virilize, but prostate growth, beard growth, and male pattern balding do not occur. Absence of androgen receptors impairs the response of target tissues to androgen. As a consequence, the masculinization of internal (development of wolffian duct derivatives) and external (derived from the genital tubercule, groove, and swelling) sex characteristics is impaired, resulting in testicular feminization or androgen resistance syndrome (Table 14–2).

ONTOGENITY OF THE HYPOTHALAMIC-PITUITARY-TESTICULAR AXIS

Overview

Within the first few weeks after birth, circulating levels of placental-derived chorionic gonadotropin rapidly fall and endogenous pituitary gonadotropin levels rise. Testosterone levels increase for the first few months of neonatal life and can reach substantial levels of about 350 ng per deciliter. After 6 months or so, both gonadotropins and testosterone levels decline, and all reach the prepubertal nadir and remain there until the onset of

Figure 14-6 Androgens have several mechanisms of action.

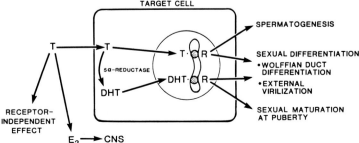

TABLE 14-2   Androgen Resistance Syndromes

	External Phenotype	Internal Phenotype	Karyotype	Inheritance	Serum Testosterone
5-alpha-reductase deficiency	Female genitalia at birth; variable virilization at expected time of puberty	Testes, epididymides, vasa deferententia present	46, XY	Autosomal recessive	Normal
Complete testicular feminization	Female external genitalia with a blind-ending vagina, female habitus and breast development, paucity of axillary and pubic hair	Testes present, absent wolffian and müllerian derivatives	46, XY	X-linked recessive	Normal or high male plasma levels
Incomplete testicular feminization	Female habitus and breast development, normal axillary and pubic hair, clitoromegaly, and partial fusion of the labioscrotal folds	Testes present, underdeveloped wolffian duct derivatives	46, XY	X-linked recessive	Normal or high
Reifenstein syndrome	Male with perineoscrotal hypospadias, normal axillary and pubic hair	Testes and wolffian duct structure present, varying in the degree of male development	46, XY	X-linked recessive	Normal or high
Infertile male syndrome		Testes with oligospermia or azoospermia	46, XY	Probably X-linked	Normal

+ = frequency

puberty. In normal boys, puberty characteristically begins between 10 and 15 years of age and takes about 3 to 3½ years to complete. At that time men have the secondary sex characteristics resulting from exposure to testosterone and within 1 year of onset of ejaculation should have normal levels of sperm in their semen. Peak sexual function occurs in men from 20 to 40 years of age. Starting at age 45 to 50 years, circulating gonadotropin levels progressively rise. Elevations in FSH are usually more pronounced than rises in LH. Serum testosterone levels remain relatively constant until far-advanced old age, although many studies suggest lower limits to the normal ranges with old age and beyond. However, beginning in middle age and thereafter, there is general agreement that testosterone available to the tissues begins to undergo reductions (free testosterone and non-TeBG-T, also called non-SHBG-T). There are sex-hormone-independent changes in libido and potency as men reach middle age and old age; however, men should

remain potent unless certain clinical disorders arise. In men 65 years of age and older, the Leydig cells no longer respond to exogenous LH-like stimulation (hCG). There appear to be age-related changes in steroidogenic capacity. What evidence is available suggests that if an aged man can ejaculate, he is probably capable of fertility, although epidemiologic data suggest that with advancing age it is more difficult for man to impregnate his partner than it is for a young man.

Puberty

An as yet unidentified mechanism initiates the hypothalamus to release Gn-RH in episodic pulses. This results in the episodic release of LH and FSH from the gonadotropes of the pituitary. The pulses begin shortly before puberty but are of small magnitude. With the onset of puberty, the variation between lower awake and higher sleep-related LH levels in serum is substantial. In

TABLE 14–2   Androgen Resistance Syndromes (Continued)

Serum Estradiol	LH	FSH	Pathogenesis		
Normal	Normal or slightly increased	Normal	Inability to form dihydrotesterone		
			ANDROGEN RECEPTOR DEFECTS		
			Absent	Qualitatively Abnormal	Decreased Amount
Higher than in normal men	Elevated	Normal	+ + +	+	+
Higher than in normal men	Elevated	Normal		+ +	+
Higher than in normal men	Elevated	Normal		+	+ +
Higher than in normal men	Elevated (usually)	Normal		+ +	+ +

addition, there are large increments of circulating testosterone in sleeping pubertal boys. These sleep-related differences persist throughout puberty and disappear when adulthood is reached. Daytime pubertal levels of gonadotropins and testosterone gradually rise to reach adult levels by the end of puberty. By definition, the prepubertal penis is less than 2 cm wide and the prepubertal testis is less than 2 cm in longest diameter. The earliest sign of puberty is testicular enlargement, which is followed by the changes consistent with increasing testosterone levels.

ROUTINE TESTING

Hormone Levels

Laboratory analyses of circulating gonadotropins and testosterone have become available throughout the world. In general, the enhanced accuracy of making a diagnosis based on multiple determinations must be weighed against the cost per determination. LH is released in normal men in pulses that occur about every 2 hours, and since the peak-to-nadir difference can be substantial (average 50 percent), it is more precise to draw three specimens 20 minutes apart or on consecutive days than it is to rely on one sample. There is no diurnal variation for gonadotropins in adults; they can be drawn anytime throughout the day. FSH has a much longer half-life, and the differences caused by pulsatile release are much smaller. One or two blood samples should suffice to give a representative value. Legal and illegal narcotics, street drugs, and alcohol reduce Gn-RH, resulting ultimately in reduced testosterone from lowered levels of LH and FSH. Estrogens, androgens, and digitalis can reduce the gonadotropins.

Assay Techniques

Since the mid-1960s, radioimmunoassay (RIA) has been used to determine circulating and urinary concentrations of both gonadotropins. The technology has progressively improved, resulting in increased specificity and sensitivity. Differentiating low normal from subnormal adult circulating concentrations and normal from subnormal prepubertal circulating concentrations has been difficult because of the limited low-range assay sensitivity. A little-used but capable discriminator involves 6- to 24-hour urine collections. Kulin and Santner (1977) have shown the advantages of urinary collections analyzed by RIA techniques when blood levels cannot differentiate the reproductive status. New technology for RIA involves monoclonal antibodies and the use of two antibodies to the hormone in question. Other techniques involve antibodies with enzymatic labels or labels that can be made to fluoresce. The clinician should become familiar with the expertise of a capable laboratory for the best patient outcomes (Table 14–3).

The in vitro LH bioassay is based on the short-term (usually 3-hour) dose-related testosterone response of testicular interstitial cells to gonadotropin in vitro. Testosterone production by dispersed rat or mouse interstitial cells to unknown samples is compared with the responses evoked by standard hormones. The assay termed as rat interstitial cell testosterone (RICT) and described by Dufau and colleagues in the 1970s. LH bioassay has been applied to the measurement of pituitary and serum LH and LH-like gonadotropin from humans. The RICT assay is five to ten times more sensitive than RIA for measurement of circulating LH.

The plasma levels of bioactive LH in men and postmenopausal women have been generally higher than those measured by RIA, although the two values are frequently closer to unity. There is an increase in the bioactive to immunoreactive (B:I) ratio at the midcycle surge of LH. Hypogonadism has been caused by anomalous LH, which is immunologically active but devoid of biologic activity. Serious illness can reduce the B:I ratios (Table 14–4).

Serum Testosterone Levels

Although sporadic pulsatile elevations may occur, serum testosterone has a diurnal rhythm with highest values occurring between 6 and 9 AM. There is progressive decline throughout the day, and lowest levels occur late at night and in the early hours of the new day. The difference from peak to nadir values can be between 20 and 50 percent. Thus, testosterone values should be obtained in the early morning for most accurate results, particularly in young men and even in older men. There is some controversy about whether the diurnal rhythm persists in men 65 years of age and older; however, studies agree that there is a diurnal rhythm but that it might not be as great as that seen in younger men.

In normal young men, about 55 percent of circulating testosterone is tightly bound to SHBG (TeBG), about 42 percent is bound to albumin, and the remaining fraction is free. For many years it was thought that free testosterone exerted the physiologic action of testosterone (Table 14–5). More recently, it has been demonstrated that a large proportion of albumin-bound testosterone (about 50 percent) is available to tissues, and the best estimates of biologically active testosterone include that contributed by free testosterone and albumin-bound

TABLE 14–3 Hypogonadism

Hypogonadotropic (Decreased LH and FSH Levels)	Hypergonadotropic (Increased LH and FSH Levels)
Pituitary disorders	
Prolactinoma	Chromosomal abnormalities
Acromegaly	Klinefelter's syndrome—e.g., 47XXY, 46XY/47XXY, 48 XXXY
Nonfunctioning tumors	Streak gonads— XY karyotype
Craniopharyngioma	Noonan's syndrome (male Turner's syndrome)
Histiocytosis X	Congenital adrenal hyperplasia—defective androgen synthesis
Empty sella syndrome	Orchitis, mumps
Autoimmune hypophysitis	Surgical castration
Infarction	Myotonic dystrophy
Trauma (including breech delivery)	Drug induced—nitrogen mustard, cyclophosphamide, chlorambucil, procarbazine
Postsurgery/radiation	Irradiation
Gn-RH and/or gonadotropin deficiency	Renal failure
Gn-RH deficiency (isolated or combined)	Cirrhosis of liver
Isolated LH deficiency (rare)	Spinal cord injury
Isolated FSH deficiency (rare)	Celiac disease
Kallmann's syndrome	Sickle cell disease
Prader-Willi syndrome	Others
Other disorders and states	Rudimentary testes syndrome
Hemochromatosis	Vanishing testes syndrome
Male anorexia nervosa and depression	Lead, cadmium exposure
Sarcoidosis	Endocrine autoimmune syndrome
Extensive burns	Bioinactive LH
Severe illness	
Street drugs, narcotics, ethanol	

TABLE 14-4   Bioactive LH

Method	Patient's serum stripped of most endogenous steroids using charcoal, incubated in vitro with mouse or rat interstitial cells for about 3 hours; changes in incubation medium testosterone compared to LH standards
Normal Values	Bioactive to immunoactive ratio about 3 to 5
Uses	Useful in evaluating patients suspected of having bio-inactive LH; assay is 5 to 10 times as sensitive as LH RIA
Problems	Tedious; other peptides/factors in serum may influence Leydig cell responses; largely a research tool.

testosterone. There are several ways to estimate the amount of androgen available to tissues. This can be done reasonably well by methods that determine the non-SHGT-T, analyzing circulating levels of SHBG and calculating the various components, or calculating an index in which serum testosterone is divided by SHBG or some estimate of SHBG binding. SHBG binds (with decreasing affinity) DHT, testosterone, and estradiol. It is produced in the liver and increases in hyperthyroid states, as men age, and with exposure to estrogens. Circulating levels, on the other hand, are reduced by testosterone (Table 14-6). Men have "normal" levels of estradiol, estrone, progesterone, and 17OH-progesterone. Some of these steroids have diurnal rhythms (Table 14-7).

Gn-RH Stimulation

Stimulation of the pituitary gland itself can be accomplished using synthetic Gn-RH. The decapeptide is identical to endogenously occurring Gn-RH, is commercially available, and can be given by intravenous or sub-cutaneous injection: 100 μg is the standard test dose. In normal prepubertal youngsters, the gonadotropin elevations are small, and FSH increases more than LH. In adults there should be a two- to five-fold rise of LH and a smaller, but discernible rise of FSH. In individuals who have a Gn-RH deficiency, the pituitary may not respond to the initial injection. If such individuals are given daily injections of this material over 1 week and then tested, a response is usually seen (Table 14-8). Mortimer and colleagues (1973) have reported a comprehensive study of Gn-RH for diagnostic testing. They found that in 31 patients with hypogonadism due to nonfuctioning pituitary tumors (chromophobe adenomas), 11 had normal LH responses, 19 were impaired, and only one had an absent LH response. Patients with isolated gonadotropin deficiency, presumably due to hypothalamic disease, had impaired or absent responses in 11 of 15 cases. More than half of the patients with craniopharyngiomas who had hypothalamic or stalk lesions had impaired to absent responses to Gn-RH. Therefore, long-standing hypothalamic disease probably causes a loss of pituitary gland

TABLE 14-5   Serum Free Testosterone Analysis

Method	Several methods are used: 1) determine total testosterone and SHBG and calculate free; 2) the gold standard is using dialysis; 3) ultrafilterable testosterone correlates well with dialysis; and 4) using analog tracers of testosterone which do not bind to plasma protein and performing RIA.
Normal Values	50–210 pg/ml (Nichols Institute, using dialysis); 203 ± 26 pg/ml (SD), range 159 to 250 pg/ml in normal young men, 178 ± 38 pg/ml, range 146 to 238 pg/ml in 65- to 85-year-old men, in our lab using ultrafiltration (Nankin and Calkins, 1986).
Uses	A better reflection of tissue available testosterone than is total; it may be replaced by non-SHBG-T (see text)
Problems	Assays using analog tracers need further standardization; in our hands data did not directly compare with ultrafiltration results; dialysis assay is tedious; non-SHBG-T appears to correlate better with bio-available testosterone and is technically easier to do than dialysis; calculating free hormone after SHBG determination requires several assumptions to ger results

TABLE 14-6 SHBG (TeBG)·

Assay Method

Radioreceptor assay—Using tritiated DHT as ligand, reflecting the affinity of the specific androgen-binding site on SHBG

Direct radioimmunoassay—Reflecting total mass of the protein

Increased SHBG levels in

Thyrotoxicosis
Chronic liver disease
Primary testicular failure
Estrogen administration
Congenital hyper-SHBG-emia

Decreased SHBG levels in

Obesity
Hypothyroidism
Androgen administration
Congenital hypo-SHBG-emia

* Elevated in men with testicular dysfunction, resulting in a reduction of the free testosterone level.

responses to Gn-RH. There have been excellent studies reporting that Gn-RH-deficient individuals can be treated every 2 hours with pulses of Gn-RH and over several months will undergo pubertal maturation, and fertility can be accomplished.

Clomiphene Citrate Testing

Clomiphene citrate, a weak estrogen that functions as an antiestrogen in adults, has been shown to block feedback, probably at the hypothalamic level, and stimulates both LH and FSH levels. This also results in an increase in testosterone. In prepubertal individuals and boys up until late puberty, the weak estrogen actions predominate. In adults, the usual dosage is 50 mg given every 8 hours for 1 week. LH, FSH, and testosterone levels should double on the last day and the day after the medication is discontinued when compared to baseline mean levels of each hormone from at least two separate samples. Clomiphene tests the integrity of the whole feedback system; Gn-RH tests the pituitary.

hCG Testing

With present concerns about the acquired immunodeficiency syndrome (AIDS) and Jakob-Creutzfeldt disease, the use of biologic materials of human origin (pituitary or urine) cannot be guaranteed free of transmissible disease. Therefore, the hCG testing is described for historical completeness until data are available ensuring the safety of this material (Table 14-9).

Although LH of human pituitary origin has been used to stimulate testosterone production, commercially produced hCG has been available for several decades and has been used as a direct stimulator of Leydig's cells for many years. This LH-like material has a long half-life

TABLE 14-7 Circulating Hormone Levels in Men

Hormone	Normal Range*	Diurnal Rhythm
LH	5–20 mIU/ml†	Sleep elevations in puberty
FSH	2–20 mIU/ml	None apparent
Testosterone	420–1,100 ng/dl†	Early morning (6–9 AM) peak in adults (there are reports of afternoon peaks in late fall/early winter in some men); sleep-related rises in puberty
Estradiol	10–50 pg/ml	No
Estrone	15–65 pg/ml	? (may vary with adrenal function)
Progesterone	<25 ng/dl	No
17OH-progesterone	50–250 ng/dl	Yes, AM values greater
Dihydrotestosterone	25–75 ng/dl	? (probably present)
TeBG (SHBG)	0.2–1.4 µg DHT-bound/dl	?; may change with activity
Non-SHBG-T	150–350 ng/dl†	No clinical data, but probably mirrors testosterone rhythm
Free testosterone	50–210 pg/ml†	No clinical data, but probably mirrors testosterone rhythm
Dehydroepiandrosterone	180–1,250 ng/dl†	Yes, AM values greater
Androstendione	50–250 ng/dl	Yes, AM values greater

* Varies from laboratory to laboratory; normal adult ranges given.
† Age variations; young adult male range given.

TABLE 14–8   Gn-RH (Gonadorelin, Factrel) Stimulation Test

Method

Fasting overnight, bed rest preferred but can
be done fasting and ambulatory.
Two baseline venous blood samples.
Gn-RH 100 μg IV over 30 seconds.
Obtain venous blood samples at 15, 30, 45,
and 60 minutes after Gn-RH administration.

Limitations

The test may not differentiate hypothalamic from
pituitary disorders.
Small responses to Gn-RH prior to puberty.

Interpretation

There is no general agreement about whether results
are best interpreted with respect to peak response,
area under the response curve, absolute change in
gonadotropin level, or percent change. An LH rise of
10 to 20 mIU/ml is usually considered normal, while
FSH responses are of smaller magnitude.

and is well tolerated. After a single adminstration of 3,000 units of hCG, serum testosterone levels are obtained daily for 5 days. Serum testosterone levels should rise above 200 ng per deciliter after 72 hours in any normal prepubertal individual. Failure to demonstrate a rise suggests that either Leydig's cells have not been exposed to LH or that they are incapable of responding. When LH deficiency is suspected, the injections can be maintained for 6 to 8 weeks, using 3,000 units twice a week by intramuscular injection. Serum testosterone levels may be obtained at weekly intervals. In our experience, doing this with youngsters who had Gn-RH deficiency, the testosterone levels began to rise by about the sixth week. In healthy adult males ranging from 20 to 40 years of age, a single injection of about 3,000 units of hCG causes a two- to threefold rise of testosterone at 48 to 72 hours with a mean value of 1,350 ng per deciliter.

TABLE 14–9   hCG Stimulation Test*

Method

3000 units IM
Serum testosterone levels are obtained daily for
5 days beginning on day 0, before injection given.

Limitations

This test is insensitive to differentiate normal
function from mild testicular failure.
Absent response—Anorchia in "cryptorchid"
with nonpalpable testes; primary testicular failure
Normal prepubertal response: testosterone
increases to 200 ng/dl or more. Young normal
men demonstrate 2 to 2.5-fold rises. Men 65 years
and older respond poorly.

* Material of human origin, see text.
Adapted from Saez JM, Forest MG. Kinetics of human chorionic gonadotropin-induced steroidogenic response of the human testis. I. Plasma testosterone: Implications for human chorionic gonadotropin stimulation test. J Clin Endocrinol Metab 1979; 49:278; and Forest MG, Lecoq A, Saez JM. J Clin Endocrinol Metab 1979; 49:132.

CLINICAL INDICATIONS FOR TESTING

The discussion does not deal with most neonatal and congenital disorders.

Precocious Puberty

Precocious puberty by definition is sexual maturation in a boy before age 10 years. The majority of such individuals have significant abnormalities, with less than half finally diagnosed as idiopathic (Fig. 14–7). The defect could be a Gn-RH-producing tumor of the hypothalamus or a variety of posterior hypothalamic tumors that may be associated with central nervous system disorders. Such tumors should increase LH and FSH, and testicular enlargement and evidence of virilization should occur. When central-type precocious puberty is suspected, a full neurologic evaluation, including computed tomography (CT) and magnetic resonance imaging (MRI) studies, should be performed to rule out disorders such as astrocytomas, hypothalamic harmartomas, neuroblastomas, and optic gliomas. hCG can be produced by several malignancies, including hepatoblastomas and choriocarcinomas (of the testis, mediastinum, or the brain). hCG has LH-like activities and primarily stimulates Leydig's cells to produce testosterone. The beta subunit of chorionic gonadotropin (beta-hCG) levels can be determined in blood and urinary pregnancy tests (which require very high hCG levels for positive results), and more sensitive quantitative excretion of hCG can be determined in the urine. Adrenal tumors or Leydig's cell tumors could produce androgens that result in early sexual maturation. Gonadotropin levels should be low with either. Hypothyroidism has been associated with early maturation by increased gonadotropin levels. Adrenal enzyme defects, including 21-hydroxylase deficiency, can result in early puberty. The evaluation should include a thorough physical examination and measurement of gonadotropin and testosterone levels (Table 14–10). If any enzyme defect is suspected, urine can be collected for 17-ketosteroids, and blood can be collected for dehydroepiandrosterone sulfate (DHEAS). Albright's syndrome (McCune-Albright) is characterized by café au lait spots and bone lesions and occurs more commonly in females. It can occur with precocious puberty, bone cysts causing fractures and a variety of central nervous system problems, and other endocrine disorders. The bone problems usually ameliorate when growth is complete. The pathophysiology for the precocious puberty in this disorder has not been elucidated.

Delayed Puberty

Delayed puberty is a common complaint. The prognosis for males with delayed puberty is much better than it is for those with precocious development. The diagnosis is considered in a prepubertal 15-year-old and in

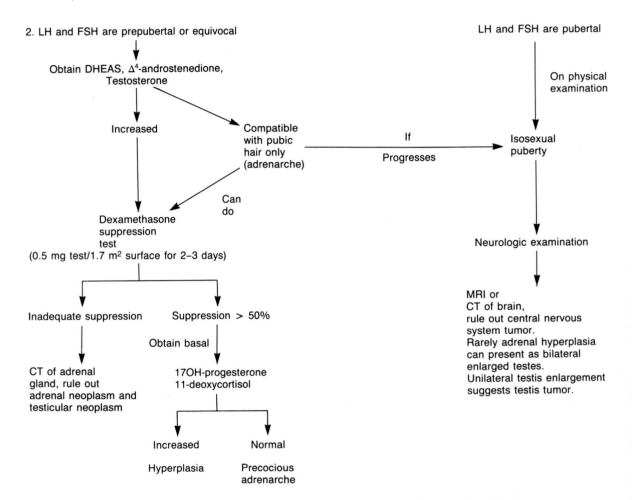

Evaluation of Precocious Puberty
(Exclude factitious and iatrogenic)

Serum LH and FSH × 3

1. If LH is markedly elevated, obtain beta subunit of hCG (blood and urine).

Rule out: gonadotropin-producing neoplasm
hepatoblastoma
pineal or testicular or mediastinal teratoma

2. LH and FSH are prepubertal or equivocal

Obtain DHEAS, Δ^4-androstenedione, Testosterone

Increased

Compatible with pubic hair only (adrenarche)

If Progresses

LH and FSH are pubertal

On physical examination

Isosexual puberty

Can do

Dexamethasone suppression test
(0.5 mg test/1.7 m² surface for 2–3 days)

Neurologic examination

Inadequate suppression

Suppression > 50%

Obtain basal

CT of adrenal gland, rule out adrenal neoplasm and testicular neoplasm

17OH-progesterone
11-deoxycortisol

MRI or CT of brain, rule out central nervous system tumor. Rarely adrenal hyperplasia can present as bilateral enlarged testes. Unilateral testis enlargement suggests testis tumor.

Increased   Normal

Hyperplasia   Precocious adrenarche

Figure 14–7   Evaluation of precocious puberty, excluding factitious and iatrogenic causes. (Modified from Odell WD. The physiology of puberty: Disorders of the pubertal process. In: DeGroot LJ, Cahill GF, Martin L, et al, eds. Endocrinology. Vol 3. New York: Grune & Stratton, 1979:1376.)

boys with incomplete pubertal development 36 months after starting puberty or at age 18 years. The evaluation should include a complete history and physical examination and careful determination of testicular and penile sizes. If the gonadotropin levels are elevated, primary testicular failure is suspected, including Klinefelter's syndrome. The association of anosmia or hyposmia with small testicles and low gonadotropin and androgen levels suggests Kallmann's syndrome—abnormal development of the olfactory bulbs and the hypothalamus with congenital absence of Gn-RH. There may be a variety of other abnormalities. Isolated Gn-RH deficiency also

occurs, but high-resolution CT or MRI should be performed to exclude a hypothalamic or pituitary lesion. Specific disorders are described subsequently; however, most individuals who begin puberty late will go on to normal sexual maturation (Table 14–11).

Hypogonadism

In young adult males who have gone through normal puberty, subsequent hypogonadism is unusual. Testicular torsion is a painful event, beginning usually on one side with a high probability of occurring on the con tralateral side. Mumps orchitis occurs in postpubertal males. Orchitis of one testis may have as a late consequence bilateral Leydig's cell and seminiferous tubule failure, occurring 20 or 30 years later.

Anytime an individual is being evaluated for hypogonadism, gonadotropin and testosterone levels should be requested. Low testosterone with high gonadotropin levels suggest primary testicular failure. Therefore, testicular disorders can be divided into two major categories: those with low-normal or low gonadotropin levels and those associated with elevated gonadotropin levels (Table 14–12). Current RIAs of gonadotropin in serum are not sensitive enough to differentiate low from low-normal values. Testicular dysfunction associated with low or low-normal gonadotropin levels is usually due to either hypothalamic or pituitary disorders. In patients with suspected pituitary or hypothalamic disorders, the function of other pituitary hormones should be evaluated (Table 14–13). Serum LH, FSH, and testosterone levels of hypogonadotropic, hypogonadal men are indistinguishable from those of prepubertal boys. Since gonadotropin responsiveness to clomiphene does not appear normally until midpuberty and gonadotropin response to Gn-RH adminstration may be similar in both hypogonadal patients and normal boys, neither of these tests may be of value in youngsters and youths. The presence of nocturnal LH release in early pubertal boys may help to establish that puberty has been initiated. The prolactin response to thyrotropin-releasing hormone (TRH) or chlorpromazine may be used to differentiate isolated gonadotropin deficiency from delayed puberty. The release of prolactin in normal pubertal boys is normal, whereas among hypogonadotropic individuals, it is often impaired.

HYPOGONADOTROPIC HYPOGONADISM

Prader-Willi Syndrome

Prader-Willi syndrome is an association of Gn-RH deficiency, obesity, hypotonia, various degrees of mental retardation, very small testes, and failure of maturation. The disorder can be sporadic, or several family members can be affected. It is associated with a partial deletion of the long arm of chromosome 15.

Kallmann's Syndrome

Kallmann's syndrome is associated with deficiency of smell and delayed sexual maturation. It is inherited as an autosomal dominant disorder with incomplete penetrance or as an autosomal recessive disorder. It may also be associated with other anomalies, such as mental retardation, color blindness, syndactyly, strabismus, spina bifida occulta, nerve deafness, cerebellar ataxia, ichthyosis, harelip, cleft palate, and unilateral cryptorchidism.

TABLE 14–10   Causes of Precocious Puberty

Central nervous system tumors
  Neurofibroma
  Hamartoma
  Pinealoma
  Astrocytoma
  Fibrous dysplasia
  Ganglioneuroma
  Ependymoma
Steroid-producing neoplasms
  Adrenal adenoma
  Adrenal carcinoma
  Gonadal neoplasms
Gonadotropin-producing neoplasms
  Teratoma
    Gonadal
    Pineal
    Mediastinal
  Hepatoblastoma
Exogenous hormones (iatrogenic)
  Steroids
  Gonadotropins
  Drugs
Familial
ACTH-producing neoplasm
Hypothyroidism, primary
Cushing's disease
Congenital adrenal hyperplasia
  21-Hydroxylase deficiency
  11-Hydroxylase deficiency
Idiopathic isosexual precocious puberty
Polyostotic fibrous dysplasia (Albright's syndrome or McCune-Albright's syndrome)

This disorder is mainly due to a hypothalamic defect, secondary to defective development of the rhinencephalon and the production site of Gn-RH in the hypothalamus. The rhinencephalon defects have been demonstrated by MRI in these patients. Low circulating gonadotropin levels usually rise in response to administration of Gn-RH. Serum testosterone levels are often less than 50 ng per deciliter. Testes are soft and are much smaller than 2 cm in diameter. Normal pubertal development and spermatogenesis can be achieved by pulsatile administration of Gn-RH in some of these men. There have been case reports of occasional male patients responding to chronic treatment with clomiphene.

Isolated LH Deficiency

In patients with isolated LH deficiency, testicular size may be small or normal, but some active spermatogenesis is present on biopsy and sperm may be present in the ejaculate, although the semen volume is low. These men are undermasculinized, are eunuchoid in appearance, and have gynecomastia. Although serum FSH is normal, serum levels of LH and testosterone are low. This is called

TABLE 14-11   Evaluation of Delayed Puberty

Initial session

 History and physical examination
 Childhood and growth pattern
 Testicular size, penile size, sexual hair assessment

 Radiology: Bone age and skull radiograph (sella turcica)

 Blood: Thyroxine RIA, THBR (T_3), TSH
          DHEAS
          Testosterone
          LH and FSH, possibly prolactin

 Urine: LH and FSH

 Olfactory threshold (sense of smell)

First follow-up (3–5 months from initial review) if no progress in maturation

 Radiology: CT scan or MRI of brain and pituitary gland

 Blood: Prolactin
          Multiple samples for LH and FSH
          GH provocative tests
          Gn-RH stimulation test
          hCG stimulation test

 Urine: LH and FSH

 Visual field examination

Second follow-up (6–10 months from initial review) if no progress in maturation

 Blood: LH and FSH
          Repeat Gn-RH stimulation test

 Urine: LH and FSH

 Others: Testicular biopsy if LH and/or FSH increased
          Trial with sex steroid
          Chromosome analysis

Modified from Santen R, Kulin H. Evaluation of delayed puberty and hypogonadism. In: Santen RJ, Swerdloff RS, eds. Male reproductive dysfunction. New York: Marcel Dekker, 1987:145.

the fertile eunuch syndrome. LH or hCG treatment should help normalize these men.

Hemochromatosis

Hypogonadism occurs in 19 to 75 percent of men with hereditary hemochromatosis. Gonadal insufficiency is due to iron-induced damage of either testicular Leydig's cells or pituitary gonadotropes and the hypothalamus. In a 1984 report by Kelly and associates of 41 men with hereditary hemochromatosis, five had hypogonadism. One man had primary hypogonadism, and four had secondary hypogonadism. Improvement of gonadal function was seen in two of the five hypogonadal men after chronic phlebotomy. This suggests that some of the damage by iron deposition is reversible.

Hyperprolactinemia

Hypogonadism is common among men with prolactin-producing pituitary adenomas. Circulating testosterone, LH, and FSH levels are usually reduced. The defect is due to effects of elevated prolactin level on pulsatile hypothalamic Gn-RH release. The frequency of spontaneous LH secretory episodes was reduced in hyperprolactinemic men, and this can be restored by bromocriptine.

Anorexia Nervosa

Anorexia nervosa is very uncommon in men. Plasma LH, FSH, and testosterone levels are low but increase after weight is regained.

Burn Patients

Patients with burn injuries frequently complain of impotence and decreased libido. Serum total and free testosterone levels are low. LH levels are also decreased. This abnormality develops within 24 to 48 hours after burn injury and persists for the duration of in-hospital recovery. The patients with the most severe burns tend

TABLE 14–12   Usual Gonadotropin and Sex Hormone Relationships with Illness and Conditions

	Testosterone	Estradiol	FSH	LH	Prolactin
Renal failure	↓	N or ↓	N or ↑	↑	N or ↑
Cirrhosis	↓	↑	N	N or ↓	N or ↑
Hemochromatosis	↓	—	↓	↓	↓
Sickle cell anemia	↓	—	↑	↑	—
Leprosy	↓	↓	↑	↑	—
Myotonia dystrophica	↓	—	↑	↑	—
Paraplegia	N or ↓	N or ↑	N	—	—
Hyperthyroidism	↑	↑	↑	↑	—
Hypothyroidism	↓	—	—	—	↑
Diabetes	N	—	N or ↓	N or ↓	—
Cushing's syndrome	↓	—	↓	↓	—
Protein-calorie malnutrition	↓	↓	↓	↓	↓
Obesity	↓	↑	N	N	—
Strenuous exercise	N or ↑	—	N	N	—
Critical illness	↓	—	↓	↓	—

— = uncertain; N = normal.
Modified from Morley JE, Melmed S. Gonadal dysfunction in systemic disorders. Metabolism 1979; 28:1051.

to have the lowest testosterone levels. The mechanism responsible for the decreased testosterone levels remains unclear. It is probably due to multiple factors, such as stress and increased cortisol, epinephrine, and interleukin-1 levels. It is also possible that opiate analgesics contribute to decrease LH and testosterone levels.

Critical Illness

The effects of systemic illnesses on the pituitary-thyroid axis have been extensively investigated. In contrast, alterations in gonadal function in men have been investigated only recently. Patients with acute brain injury resulting in coma, myocardial infarction, and elective surgery uniformly develop transient hypogonadotropic hypogonadism. Serum total and free testosterone levels decreased within 24 hours of the illness. LH levels

are also low, but the response to Gn-RH stimulation is unaltered. This suggests that critical illness has associated hypothalamic dysfunction.

Cushing's Syndrome

Gonadal and sexual disturbances are common in Cushing's syndrome. Males have loss of libido, impotence, oligospermia, and histologic changes in the testes. Testosterone levels are low. Basal LH and FSH levels are decreased, and the response to Gn-RH is impaired. These data suggest that these males have hypogonadotropic hypogonadism. Glucocorticoids have a direct inhibitory effect on the function of Leydig's cells. Exogenous adrenocorticotropic hormone (ACTH) is known to decrease plasma testosterone with no change in plasma LH levels.

TABLE 14–13   Combined Pituitary Testing Protocol*

Plasma/Serum Hormone Assayed	Time after Infusion (Minutes)						
	0	10	15	30	45	60	90
IR-ACTH	X	X			X	X	
IR-Cortisol	X				X	X	
IR-FSH	X				X	X	
IR-LH	X		X	X			
IR-TSH	X		X	X			
IR-prolactin	X	X	X				
IR-GH	X				X	X	X

* Combined schedule for assaying plasma hormone levels during combined anterior pituitary function test (ovine corticotropin-releasing hormone, 1 µg/kg; Gn-RH 100 µg; human GH-releasing hormone, 1 µg/kg; and TRH, 200 µg). IR = immunoreactive.
Modified from Sheldon WR, DeBold CR, Evans WS, et al. Rapid sequential intravenous administration of four hypothalamic releasing hormones as a combined anterior pituitary function test in normal subjects. J Clin Endocrinol Metab 1985; 60:623.

HYPERGONADOTROPIC HYPOGONADISM

Klinefelter's Syndrome

Klinefelter's syndrome is a well-recognized form of hypogonadism related to aberrations of the sex chromosomes. The incidence of chromatin-positive Klinefelter's syndrome includes 0.1 to 0.21 percent of all phenotypic boys and 20 percent of azoospermic adults. Adults with Klinefelter's syndrome usually have small, firm testes less than 2.5 cm in diameter. Azoospermia is the rule, and testicular biopsy reveals tubular hyalinization, which increases with age. The presence of bilateral gynecomastia is variable, being reported in 20 to 80 percent of these subjects. Other common features of Klinefelter's syndrome reflect the lack of androgen effects, including sparse body hair, poor muscular development and strength, a eunuchoidal body habitus, and excessive height. The increased length of the lower segment, from pubis to sole, is present before puberty and is not due solely to delayed epiphyseal closure. Arm span is also increased. Serum testosterone levels are low or low-normal, and LH and FSH levels are markedly elevated. Severely affected males are easily recognized; however, many men with Klinefelter's syndrome have subtle forms of the disease that manifest as diagnostic challenges. Chromosomal analyses of the peripheral blood of patients with Klinefelter's syndrome commonly reveal a 47,XXY karyotype, although various forms of mosaicism occur in about 20 percent of these men.

Mumps Orchitis

In postpubertal males, mumps (parotitis) often results in orchitis—very painful, swollen testicular enlargement. The orchitis is usually unilateral but may be bilateral. The afflicted testis often atrophies, but testosterone levels commonly remain normal with unilateral diseases. However, there may be late (20 years and more) failure of the apparently spared testis.

Spinal Cord Injury

Patients with spinal cord injury usually have normal libido, but the ability to have erections and ejaculations depends on the level of neurologic deficits. Mean serum testosterone levels are usually normal or slightly reduced. Serum LH and FSH levels are usually elevated, suggesting primary testicular failure. Impaired scrotal cooling may contribute to testis failure.

Myotonic Dystrophy

Myotonic dystrophy is inherited as an autosomal dominant disorder. It is associated with myotonia, progressive muscular weakness, cataracts, and frontal balding. Decreased libido and impotence are common. Serum testosterone levels are often low, and LH and FSH levels are increased.

Celiac Disease

Moderate impairment of libido and potency occurs in about 25 percent with severe celiac disease. Sperm motility is reduced in 75 percent of subjects. Serum total and free testosterone levels are elevated, and serum DHT levels are often low. LH and FSH levels are also frequently elevated. Sperm density may be increased in some patients with celiac disease with the institution of a gluten-free diet.

Sickle Cell Disease

In patients with sickle cell anemia there is impairment of skeletal and sexual maturation in early adolescence. Hypogonadism and testicular atrophy occur in 30 percent of afflicted individuals. Serum testosterone, androstenedione, and DHT levels are low, whereas LH and FSH levels are elevated, suggesting primary testis failure. The disorder can be associated with zinc deficiency, so zinc supplements may help these men.

Chronic Renal Failure

Spermatogenesis in patients with renal failure undergoing hemodialysis is impaired. Serum LH and FSH levels are usually elevated, and plasma testosterone levels are low. The initial response of LH and FSH to Gn-RH stimulation is normal. Therefore, pituitary function in patients with uremia remains intact. The elevated LH levels may be due to decreased metabolic clearance rate. Elevated prolactin levels, zinc deficiency, and LH unresponsiveness have been reported in the patients.

OTHER HYPOGONADAL DISORDERS

Obesity

Obese men who are otherwise healthy are often found to have low serum testosterone levels. However, most men have normal testicular size, libido, potency, and normal spermatogenesis. The lower total testosterone levels are usually offset by a higher percentage of dialyzable free fractions, often resulting in normal free testosterone concentrations. The responses of LH and FSH to Gn-RH and clomiphene are also normal. Some men with morbid obesity (over 250 percent of ideal body weight) do have subnormal serum free testosterone levels and inappropriately low LH and FSH levels in the blood. Serum estrone and estradiol are elevated in obese men. The abnormal serum estrogen and androgen levels are reversible with weight loss. Prominent breasts are usually a combination of fat and glandular tissue.

Total fasting rapidly alters hypothalamic-pituitary-gonadal function in men. Moderately obese men undergoing a 10-day therapeutic fast have blunted serum FSH responses to Gn-RH, decreased serum FSH and testosterone, and increased urinary excretion of LH and FSH, all of which are probably due to increased clearance of renal gonadotropin secondary to ketosis.

Diabetes Mellitus

Impotence is common among diabetic patients. Previous studies on the effects of diabetes on pituitary-gonadal function have been conflicting. Plasma testosterone levels have been found to be normal or low in impotent patients. Most recently, in a group of diabetic patients with organic impotence, urinary LH levels were found to be elevated and plasma free testosterone levels were reduced. Impotence in these men responded to androgen therapy.

Strenuous Physical Exercise

Strenuous physical exercise alters the integrity of various neuroendocrine systems. Female ballet dancers and athletes frequently develop hypothalamic amenorrhea and altered release of Gn-RH. In a group of male marathon runners who were running 125 to 200 km per week, the mean frequency of spontaneous LH pulses was diminished as compared with that in healthy controls. The amplitude of the pulses were also low in the runners, and the response of LH to Gn-RH was decreased. Since each pulse of LH is a direct consequence of a burst of secretion of hypothalamic Gn-RH, the diminished frequency of LH pulses observed may reflect a failure of the pulse generator of the hypothalamic Gn-RH. Plasma testosterone levels were similar in the two groups and increased equally in response to hCG administration. During short-term intense physical exercise, the plasma gonadotropin levels in the athletes remained stable, but significant elevations of plasma cortisol, prolactin, and testosterone occurred. Therefore, decreased Gn-RH release may be due to the prolonged, repetitive elevations of gonadal steroids that are elicited by their daily exercise. Clinically, none reported any sexual problems or had signs of hypogonadism on physical examination, and all had normal plasma testosterone levels. These hormone relationships were different from those of female athletes, who frequently developed amenorrhea and had low levels of estrogens. Overtrained male athletes develop apathy, a heavy-legged feeling, and impaired racing time. The plasma cortisol, ACTH, GH, and prolactin responses to insulin hypoglycemia are impaired; however, LH, TSH, and prolactin responses to Gn-RH and TRH are normal.

Biologically Inactive with Elevated Immunologically Active LH

A male patient who had normal primary sex characteristics failed to enter puberty spontaneously. The plasma total testosterone level was low, and the plasma LH level by RIA was elevated. The excretion rate of bioassayable urine gonadotropin was increased in the rat ovarian weight assay and the mouse uterine weight assay. Bioassay using rat interstitial cells was not performed. These findings suggested primary gonadal failure. The patient, however, responded to exogenous LH and hCG with higher plasma testosterone levels and developed secondary sex characteristics. In response to Gn-RH, plasma LH levels by RIA rose markedly, but plasma FSH and testosterone levels remained unaltered. These findings suggest that this syndrome is attributable to the presence of an abnormal LH, which is biologically inactive in the affected patients but biologically active in rodents.

Chronic Alcoholic Liver Disease

Alcoholic liver disease may lead to impotence, infertility, and feminization in men. Gynecomastia is found in about 40 percent and testicular atrophy in 60 percent of these patients. Prostatic size is reduced, and a decreased incidence of benign prostatic hypertrophy is seen. Alcohol has a direct toxic effect on the gonads, causing impaired spermatogenesis and decreased testosterone formation. In patients with no signs of hypogonadism, pulsatility of LH is preserved and mean concentrations of the hormone are increased. This is similar to primary testicular failure. In the patients with overt gonadal failure, the pulsatility and release of LH are also impaired, consistent with hypothalamic defects.

GYNECOMASTIA

Gynecomastia is a common disorder. Histologic evidence of gynecomastia was present in 40 percent of 447 men examined at autopsy. Clinically evident gynecomastia was present in about 30 percent of outpatient adult subjects. It may present as a discrete, palpable, subareolar plate or a more diffuse mass that may resemble surrounding fat. Growth and development of breasts are under the control of both stimulatory (estrogens) and inhibitory (androgens) hormones. Estrogen stimulates the cellular growth and proliferation of parenchymal epithelium to form ductal and stromal elements. These appear as discs of breast tissue. In later stages, these are replaced by fibrosis and hyalinization, with regression of epithelial proliferation (fibroglandular). Testosterone mainly exerts inhibitory effects on breast development. In men, the circulating ratio of testosterone to estradiol is 200:1, and the production ratio is 100:1. Most gynecomastia can be attributed to ratio changes of androgen to estrogen, i.e., either excess of circulating estrogen or androgen deficiency. Absent or defective androgen receptors, as found in patients with testicular feminization syndrome or related disorders, may also contribute to enlarged breasts. Drugs can cause breast growth also by a variety of mechanisms. Elevated prolactin by itself usually does not cause gynecomastia or galactorrhea in men—estrogen must form breast tissue first; then prolactin may stimulate growth and cause lactation.

Neonatal gynecomastia is thought to be related to gestational estrogens and should disappear after a few weeks. Pubertal gynecomastia occurs 1 to 2 years after the onset of sexual maturation in 50 to 80 percent of males. It varies from a small, unilateral disk to bilateral prominent breasts, usually more apparent in obese boys. The ratio of testosterone to estradiol is decreased in puberty. There have been studies showing a relative increase in free estradiol in maturing boys with breast tissue. This breast tissue usually resolves spontaneously in 1 to 2 years. In a small percentage of these boys, there is persistent gynecomastia. Cosmetic removal of this breast tissue by a skilled surgeon usually has a good psychological impact on any youngster teased or concerned about the breast tissue. This surgery should be made available to any youngster who has good reason to ask for it. As men reach late middle age and beyond, gynecomastia again occurs. This is also thought to be related to alterations in circulating steroid hormone concentrations. However, since the appearance of breast tissue may be an indication of serious underlying disease or drugs, physiologic causes are diagnoses of exclusion.

A variety of disorders and drugs can cause enlarged breasts; therefore an evaluation should include a detailed drug history and consideration of systemic hepatic, renal, cardiac, pulmonary, and thyroid disorders and underlying malignancy. Physical examination should include careful assessment of testes and prostate. A small prostate suggests a long-standing androgen deficiency. The work-up is outlined in Table 14–14.

Gynecomastia can occur in both primary and secondary testicular failure. Serum testosterone levels are low or low-normal, and estradiol levels are usually normal or slightly elevated, resulting in increased estrogen to testosterone ratios. A variety of tumors can cause gynecomastia by producing hCG. These tumors include both testicular and nontesticular tumors, such as carcinoma of the lung and gastrointestinal tract. Many medications have been reported to be associated with gynecomastia. Spironolactone and cimetidine cause gynecomastia by competitive displacement of DHT binding to androgen receptors. Spironolactone also inhibits androgen biosynthesis. Digitalis preparations may also cause gynecomastia. They probably cause enlarged breasts through a "refeeding" mechanism in debilitated men with congestive heart failure. Abnormal estrogen production should result in relative suppression of the gonadotropins and testosterone. Reduced responsiveness of target tissue is usually associated with normal or increased LH, FSH, and testosterone. Causes of gynecomastia are outlined in Table 14–15.

Useful screening tests for gynecomastia include measurement of serum beta-hCG subunit to rule out malignancy, chest radiograph and determination of serum estradiol and testosterone levels. Thyroid function tests and serum prolactin, LH, FSH, and DHEAS levels should be obtained if clinically indicated.

SEXUAL DYSFUNCTION

This section addresses men who have had an alteration in their ability to have sexual relations. Sexual activity is a pleasurable event even when not associated with procreation. It serves deeply felt personal needs, contributes to the stability of pair bonding, and contributes to the permanence of families and, in turn, societies. Although subject to wide variation in men, sexual activity gradually reduces from about three episodes per week at age 30 to approximately one episode every other week at age 70 and declines further thereafter. Most men remain sexually active into their sixties. In healthy elderly men, sexual activity was correlated with the characteristic frequency in youth. Several studies have demonstrat-

---

TABLE 14–14   Work-up for Gynecomastia

History
    Age of onset
    Duration, tenderness, progression
    Changes in libido
    Drug (legal and illicit) and alcohol history
    Constitutional symptoms

Physical examination
    Presence of a eunuchoid habitus
    Palmar erythema or spider angiomata
    Visual fields
    Goiter, lidlag, exophthalmos, onycholysis
    Breast size or tenderness
    Galactorrhea
    Hepatomegaly
    Testicular size and consistency, tumor
    Secondary sexual development
    Prostate

Laboratory tests
    Liver and renal function tests
    Serum beta-hCG, LH, and FSH
    Serum testosterone and estradiol levels
    Free or bioavailable testosterone and estradiol
    Serum prolactin level
    Thyroid function tests (triiodothyronine resin
        uptake, thyroxine assay, TSH)

Radiographic
    Chest radiographs
    CT of pituitary gland
    CT of adrenal glands
    Mammogram (if unilateral breast development
        and in the appropriate setting and/or cancer
        suspected)

TABLE 14-15   Causes of Gynecomastia

Physiologic
  Newborns
  Puberty
  Aging
  Refeeding

Pathologic
  Testosterone deficiency
    Congenital
      Congenital anorchia
      Klinefelter's syndrome
      Androgen resistance
        Complete (testicular feminization syndrome)
        Partial (Reifenstein, Lubs, Rosewater, and Dreyfus syndromes)
      Defects in androgen synthesis
    Testicular failure
      Viral orchitis; trauma; castration; granulomatous disease; varicocele
  Increased estrogen production
    Increased testicular estrogen secretion
      HCG-producing tumor; testicular tumor; bronchogenic
        carcinoma; gastrointestinal tumors; ectopic choriocarcinomas
    True hermaphroditism
    Estrogen-producing adrenal tumor
  Increased peripheral conversion
    Adrenal disease; liver disease (alcohol); starvation; thyrotoxicosis
  Increase in peripheral aromatose activity
    Heredity; Obesity
  Increased prolactin level
    Pituitary tumors (prolactinoma)
    Drugs that deplete catecholamine or catecholamine antagonists—
      sulpiride; phenothiazine; methyldopa; reserpine; tricyclic
      antidepressant; metoclopramide

Drugs
  Initiating or terminating exogenous androgens
  Estrogen and estrogen-like substances (estradiol, diethylstilbestrol,
    digitalis)
  Estrogen precursors—testosterone enanthate, testosterone propionate
  Drugs that enhance endogenous estrogen formation—hCG,
    clomiphene
  Drugs that inhibit testosterone synthesis and/or action, such as
    ketoconazole; alkylating agents; spironolactone; cimetidine;
    aminoglutethimide
  Others:
    Busulfan; ethionamide; isoniazid; D-penicillamine; diazepam;
    marijuana; heroin

Idiopathic

ed a decline in sexual performance and also interest with age, although a small percentage of older persons may actually increase their sexual activity. General health is the most important variable, and the health of the surviving spouse is the next most important aspect in determining the frequency and enjoyment of sexual activity. There are age-related alterations in sexual response, even in healthy men who remain sexually active. With age, there appears to be a longer duration of foreplay needed to obtain a full erection, a longer plateau phase, slower and less forceful orgasms, less forceful ejaculatory contractions, a diminished skin flush, less nipple erection and testis enlargement, more rapid detumescence, and a longer refractory interval before another erection can be achieved. In older men, orgasm is usually experienced as a shorter, one-stage experience, without the initial phase of "ejaculatory inevitability" that occurs in younger individuals. Some of these changes may be related to alterations of the fibroelastosis of the trabeculae in the corpora, combined with progressive sclerosis of both small arteries and veins. Although basal levels of testosterone may not decline significantly with aging, the portion of circulating testosterone that is available to tissues does decline with aging. This may also contribute to age-related alterations in sexual functioning. For several years it has been known that normal men experience firm erections related to rapid eye movement (REM) sleep. The frequency of erections is about twice as great in young adult men as it is in aged men. There are numerous studies in animals showing reduced sexual function in aging males, even if serum testosterone is maintained. Taken together, these data suggest that there is some organic basis for altered sexual performance with age and that this change is not entirely due to social, psychological, or general health status.

Sexual Physiology in the Male

There are four basic components of male sexuality: libido, erection, emission and orgasm, and ejaculation. Libido, the urge to have sex, depends greatly on the mental state, and it can be reduced by sedation, preoccupation with other activities, and the fear of failure. Testosterone appears to enhance normal male libido, and it is not clear whether this involves a minimum level or if there is a direct relationship to a physiologic range. An erection is a neurovascular reflex phenomenon that depends on reflex stimuli and a wide variety of psychogenic factors. Impulses from the cerebral cortex and limbic system are directed to the sympathetic ganglia and then to the sacral parasympathetic center. Cortical impulses can also act to suppress sexual arousal. Sexual dysfunction has been associated with certain types of cerebrovascular accidents, lesions, and temporal lobe epilepsy. Sometimes, epilepsy is not clinically apparent and is found on a screening electroencephalogram (EEG). Treatment of seizures may improve sexual performance. The local reflex loop has tactile sensory impulses carried by way of the pudendal nerves to an autonomic center in the spinal cord. The efferent impulses are transmitted by the sacral (S_2 to S_4) parasympathetic nerve plexus (nervi erigentes), and the nerve fibers form two separate nerves, one on each side of the penis. These course underneath the prostate gland on each side and then, after proceeding along the shaft of the penis, enter into the corporal tissues. The penile erectile tissues consist of two corpora cavernosa and a single corpus spongiosum. Smooth muscles appear to limit the entry of arterial blood into the corpora during the flaccid state, and these muscles can be relaxed by both sympathetic and parasympathetic fibers. A vasodilating substance, probably vasoactive intestinal polypeptide, appears to be involved in erections. There is also reduced venous outflow from the tumescent corpora. Erection is achieved when 20 to 50 ml of blood distends the corpora. The firmness of erection is due primarily to the two corpora cavernosa that are enclosed in a firm fibrous cover (tunica albuginea). Orgasm and emission occur simultaneously. Orgasm is a pleasurable sensation, and emission is the discharge of secretions from Cowper's glands, vasa deferentia, prostate, epididymides, and the seminal vesicles into the bulbar urethra. These two occurrences are probably related to a sympathetic reflex relayed from the lumbar sympathetic chain and the superior hypogastric plexus. Ejaculation directly follows as the bulbocavernous and ischiocavernous muscles contract rhythmically to discharge the seminal fluid. Ejaculation is thought to require both sympathetic and parasympathetic innervation, and this is followed by detumescence.

Types of Sexual Dysfunction

Sexual dysfunction is often a subjective assessment by the patient and by the partner. Dysfunction can take the form of reduced libido, impotence, failure to maintain an erection, premature ejaculation, failure of ejaculation, or a combination of these. In evaluating a patient, the physician must consider the overall health, use of medications or street drugs, stresses, home life, and the partner. Not every patient referred for sexual dysfunction should proceed with a work-up and treatment. The feelings of the partner should be assessed. A man with far-advanced malignancy, severe lung disease, incapacitating angina, or other advanced illnesses should be given reassurance and support, and he and his partner should be informed that there are other ways to manifest their affection for each other. They can still engage in caressing and manual stimulation and need not have vaginal sex. It is often reassuring to the couple that this is the best way to proceed. In a stable relationship the survival of the spouse is paramount, and in most couples, particularly those with long-standing marriages, failure to have vaginal sex does not have any deleterious effect on the relationship. By generally accepted definition, a man should be able to achieve an erection firm enough for vaginal penetration at least 75 percent of the time. It should be realized, however, that there are men who are happy if they can penetrate 50 percent of the time and men who are unhappy if they fail even once or twice. It is common for men to experience transient episodes of reduced libido or impotence; these are often associated with periods of stress, fatigue, depression, ill health, or marital problems. If the sexual dysfunction lasts for more than 2 months, medical evaluation can be undertaken.

Premature ejaculation is the too-rapid occurrence of orgasm and ejaculation. Although no precise definition is available, a man should be able to gain vaginal penetration and have the penis inserted into the vagina for longer than a few thrusts and for longer than 2 minutes before ejaculating. If this is a regular problem and no clinical abnormalities are noted on physical examination, the patient can be referred to a competent sex therapist for treatment. Failure of ejaculation can be due to three possibilities: (1) medications that may be interfering with ejaculation (particularly those that interfere with normal neurologic function); (2) nerve damage; and (3) psychological problems. If possible, the medications can be altered or discontinued. If the disorder is due to neuropathy, which may be very difficult to prove clinically, there may be no treatment. If the disorder is psychogenic, sex education and sex therapy should be of value. It is important to remember that the same factors that contribute to libido also contribute to potency. By far the most common dysfunction is erectile impotence.

TABLE 14-16   Sexual Function

Dysfunction (2 months or more)	Normal
Reduced/absent libido	Normal libido
Impotence (most common = 80%)	Vaginal penetration 75% of attempts
Premature ejaculation (<2 min)	Ejaculation 2 minutes or longer after penetration
Failure of ejaculation (when potent)	Able to ejaculate 85% + (when potent)

In some patients, in whom there is a concurrent reduction of libido and potency, an individual may not perceive a problem. Older men commonly report that longer intervals of sexual continence are acceptable. This may be related to some of the changes that occur with aging (Table 14–16).

Impotence

By definition, a man should be able to achieve a reasonably firm erection, have vaginal penetration, begin thrusting, and maintain an erection for a reasonable interval in more than three-fourths of attempts (and he should then have orgasm and ejaculation more than 85 percent of the time). Impotence is uncommon in men under the age of 45 years and progressively increases thereafter to become the most common form of sexual dysfunction (80 percent). The true incidence is difficult to ascertain. Assuming a man does not have a debilitating illness, the etiology of impotence can be divided into five likely causes: (1) psychological; (2) hormonal; (3) vascular (both reduced arterial perfusion and corporal incompetence); (4) drugs (legal and illegal); and (5) peripheral neuropathy and central nervous system disease (Table 14–17). Particularly as men get older and have medical problems, there can be multiple causes contributing to the sexual dysfunction. Sleep apnea is associated with hypogonadism and impotence.

Psychogenic Impotence

Depending on the referral population studied and the interests of the investigators, psychogenic impotence has been reported to be the primary etiology in 35 to 90 percent of impotent men. In general, psychogenic impotence occurs in younger individuals, tends to have an abrupt onset (rather than a slowly progressive onset as in organic impotence), may be selective with one partner but not with another partner, and may be associated with good nocturnal erections and the ability to masturbate with a firm erection. These individuals generally have a reduced libido. Psychogenic impotence is often associated with stressful situations such as family discord and states such as depression. When their spouses urge men to seek medical treatment, this may be perceived as an emotionally threatening act. Acute or chronic physical disabilities may alter sexual responsiveness—for example, because of concern for a possible heart attack—and may also lead to abstinence.

Hormonal Impotence

When serum testosterone levels are used, the incidence of hypogonadism varies between 13 and 35 percent of patients referred. The hypogonadism appears to be about equally divided between primary and secondary forms. Several groups throughout the world have reported impotent men with low serum testosterone levels, with normal or low-normal prolactin and gonadotropin values, and with no other demonstrable abnormality of the pituitary or hypothalamus. The pathophysiology behind the secondary forms remains unknown. A variety of animal studies have demonstrated that hormone replacement restored potency in castrated males. Testosterone increases male sexual activity; and libido, genital sensations, and pleasure may all be increased by androgens. Reduced male hormone can have a deleterious effect on sexual function in aging men. In a double-blind crossover study of six profoundly hypogonadal men, intramuscular testosterone enanthate increased spontaneous erections, increased coitus frequency, and improved the quality of orgasm. Our own data on 10 mildly hypogonadal (serum testosterone level less than 420 ng per deciliter) impotent men, using a double-blind crossover approach, demonstrated that intramuscular testosterone cypionate improved libido in all

TABLE 14-17   Causes of Impotence

1. Psychogenic (primary or contributory)
2. Hormonal
3. Vascular
   Arterial insufficiency
   Corporal incompetence
4. Medications/alcohol/street drugs
5. Neurogenic
   Peripheral neuropathy
   Spinal cord
   Central nervous system
6. Multiple causes (1 to 5)
7. Concurrent severe medical illness

individuals and restored potency in seven patients. It has been noted that some men lose sexual interest with serum testosterone levels close to average (approximately 500 ng per deciliter), and many hypogonadal men (with levels less than 200 ng per deciliter) have greatly improved potency when testosterone levels are raised to 600 to 700 ng per deciliter on replacement. Reports have demonstrated an improvement in sexual functioning with testosterone replacement even in young men. A few case reports indicate that castrated men can achieve erections without replacement therapy. In general, the ability of these men to achieve erections is largely short term after castration: it is much more difficult to achieve an erection and to maintain it, and these men do not have semen. Castrated men tend to lose their potency.

Elevated serum prolactin levels are associated with reduced libido and potency, independent of endogenous gonadotropin and testosterone levels. The threshold level to cause dysfunction is not certain, but levels up to twice the upper limit of normal may not cause significant dysfunction. If prolactin is elevated, and this cannot be corrected by medication adjustments, the etiology should be investigated. Uremia can be associated with zinc deficiency, Leydig cell insensitivity to LH, and hyperprolactinemia. Treatment of these men with exogenous testosterone does not restore potency. If a dopamine agonist (for example, bromocriptine) can normalize prolactin and testosterone, then sexual function is most commonly restored. If testosterone levels do not normalize during dopamine agonist therapy, the addition of testosterone should restore potency. Hyperprolactinemia of pituitary origin and uremia often respond to bromocriptine. The lowest dose of this medication that normalizes prolactin should be utilized. Blood levels of prolactin can be followed, and patients should be given a 3-month trial before proceeding to other forms of treatment. At present it is not clear what should be done if men must remain on drugs that elevate prolactin, other than to rule out other causes.

A wide variety of systemic disorders can be associated with gonadal dysfunction. These disorders include cirrhosis of the liver, obesity, malnutrition, kidney failure, diabetes mellitus, Cushing's syndrome, hypothyroidism and hyperthyroidism, myotonic dystrophy, hemochromatosis, sarcoidosis, and sickle cell disease. Whenever possible, the underlying disorder should be treated. Each patient or couple needs an individualized assessment regarding the possible benefits to be achieved with evaluation and treatment for sexual dysfunction.

Vascular Impotence

The firmness of erection appears to be related to the arterial pressure of the vessels supplying the corpora, primarily the profunda arteries that supply the corpora cavernosa. Reduced perfusion pressure, from any etiology, could contribute to impotence. Apparently, the reduced perfusion must be bilateral to cause impotence,

as there appear to be connections between both corpora cavernosa. Occlusive vascular disease was diagnosed as the basis for anywhere from 25 to 67 percent of patients in different reported studies. Other vascular etiologies include Peyronie's disease, in which there can be significant fibrosis of the corpora, complications of priapism, vascular surgical bypass in which the internal iliac arteries (which eventually perfuse the profunda arteries) are bypassed or occluded, and renal transplant surgery in which the internal iliac artery is used as the vascular supply for the kidney. Another mechanism for vasculogenic impotence is the pelvic steal syndrome, which is characterized by reasonably normal penile blood pressure at rest, but with vigorous pelvic thrusting there is siphoning of blood into the ileofemoral circulation, which dilates with the increased activity of the thigh and pelvic muscles. Corporal incompetence simply means that there is leakage of corporal blood so that an adequate pressure level cannot be maintained in the corpora. This can be due to such things as venous incompetence (the equivalent of varicose veins) or a fistula between the corpora cavernosa and the corpus spongiosum. The exact percentage of patients who have these two forms of impotence is unclear. We do diagnose the pelvic steal syndrome after appropriate testing in a reasonable number of our patients. Corporal incompetence is probably less common, but if it is diagnosed and surgically treated, about three out of four patients have the return of normal potency (see later).

Drug-Related Impotence

Legal and illegal drugs and alcohol can alter the normal functioning of the reproductive system by interfering with the hypothalamic-pituitary mechanism, by causing feedback inhibition of this system, by antagonizing the actions of androgens, and by interfering with normal neuromuscular function. Narcotic-type medications and alcohol stimulate endorphin release and reduce endogenous gonadotropin release from the pituitary, reducing circulating levels of testosterone. They may have other actions that also interfere with sexual functioning. Virtually all psychotropic drugs, most medications used to treat hypertension, most depressants, estrogens, spironolactone, antineoplastic drugs, nonspecific beta-blockers, and in higher doses the cardiac-specific beta-blockers, alpha-blockers, and anticholinergic drugs can reduce sexual function. Some of the new calcium-channel blockers have been associated with impotence as well as some of the currently used antiarrhythmic agents. The long-term use of digoxin has been associated with reduced testosterone and LH levels, increased estradiol level, and reduced sexual function. Currently, we believe that furosemide, hydralazine, the angiotensin-converting enzyme inhibitors, and perhaps low-dose prazosin are the medications to use in hypertensive patients to restore or maintain potency. Antihistamines have been associated with impotence, probably by causing sedation. Some medications cannot be switched or deleted. How this is managed depends on the illness (Table 14–18).

Neurologic Impotence

Neurologic impotence can manifest itself as part of a diffuse process of peripheral neuropathy, or it may be an isolated process. The causes include alcoholism, diabetes mellitus, multiple sclerosis, tumors involving the spinal cord, and other causes of peripheral neuropathy such as heavy-metal poisoning. There is a high incidence of neurologic impotence after certain surgical procedures, including resections of the lower colon and rectum, surgery on aortic aneurysms, and suprapubic and perineal prostatectomies, and it is estimated that this occurs after about 15 percent of transurethral prostatectomies. Walsh and colleagues have described nerve- and potency-sparing prostate resection techniques, and other groups have reported retained potency after colon and aortic surgery. Trauma may also result in nerve damage. The overall incidence for neuropathy is estimated at between 7 and 41 percent. Impotence has also been linked with central nervous system disease, including temporal lobe epilepsy and temporal lobe lesions that result in limbic disturbances.

Work-up of Impotence

At the time of the initial assessment, a decision should be made regarding the appropriateness of a work-up for impotence (Table 14–19) with the potential for the various forms of treatment to be utilized. The partner should be seen to assess the impact of sexual dysfunction on the couple. The partner can sometimes offer useful information about the possibility of nocturnal erections or morning erections that the patient either does not know about or does not admit to. The spouse may not be interested in sexual activity, and in those couples it is best for them to resolve their differences before

TABLE 14–18 Drugs Associated with Sexual Dysfunction

Legal or illicit narcotics, alcohol
Psychotropic medications
Thiazide-type diuretics (use furosemide)
Calcium-channel blockers, arrhythmia medications
Beta-blockers, alpha-blockers
Estrogens, spironolactone, cimetidine, digitalis
Antihistamines, anticholinergics, antispasmodics and muscle relaxers (for back pain)
Most antihypertensive medications (use angiotensin-converting enzyme inhibitors, hydralazine, low-dose prazosin)
Metoclopramide and any other dopamine antagonist (prolactin elevator)
Try to relate onset of impotence with drugs, delete or switch a possible causal drug whenever possible (some diseases preclude switching)

TABLE 14–19 Work-up for Impotence

Appropriateness for man and partner
Exclude alcoholic and illicit drug abusers
Exclude obese (>20–30%) men (encourage weight reduction)
Optimize poorly controlled men with diabetes mellitus or renal failure
Complete history and physical examination
Psychologic tests and/or assessment (see Table 14–20)
Penile blood pressure; rest and after exercise
Fasting 7–9 AM serum for testosterone (free or bioavailable preferred), LH and prolactin (more than one sample), other studies as indicated
Bulbocavernous reflex and bulvocavernous reflex latency time
Penile injections (papaverine ± phentolamine) (is erection possible?)
Sleep studies for tumescence evaluation

proceeding further. Any medical or gynecologic problems with the partner should be addressed.

We do not evaluate men on illicit drugs and active alcohol abusers. Men with overt metabolic problems should be appropriately treated and stabilized. Other medical disorders should be addressed. Men who are more than 20 to 30 percent over ideal weight should reduce their weight before initiating a work-up. Some hormone levels may be influenced by massive and morbid obesity. Some medical conditions are improved by weight reduction, and perhaps medications can be reduced or discontinued. The patient should undergo a complete medical history and physical examination. The onset of impotence, its progression, and prior episodes should be reviewed. Attention is paid to peripheral vascular diseases, neurologic status, relationship to the sex partner, current medical diagnoses and medications, and as part of the physical examination, the habitus, muscular pattern, breasts, sexual hair distribution, testicular and scrotal contents, prostate, and penis should be carefully assessed. A bulbocavernous reflex should be performed. To do this test, the physician places rubber gloves on both hands and performs a usual rectal examination. With the examining finger still in the rectum, a small amount of lubricant is placed on the thumb and index and middle fingers of the other hand, and the glans is pressed and allowed to pop out of those three fingers. This is done repetitively, and it should be followed by contractions of the perineal muscles. If these do not occur, there is a possibility of a neurologic disorder. In men with known or overt psychiatric problems, a psychiatric or psychological consultation should be obtained.

We routinely perform a Minnesota Multiphasic Personality Inventory (MMPI) on every patient. This test is interpreted by a clinical psychologist and helps in evaluating patients. Other tests have been used also (Table 14–20). Men with previously unrecognized significant psychopathology are referred for psychiatric consultation.

The MMPI may give clues to men with possible psychological impotence, but men may be perfectly normal on this test and still have psychogenic impotence.

Using a small digital blood pressure cuff and a Doppler sound detection probe, we attempt to find the systolic blood pressure in both profunda (cavernosal) arteries. The patient lies on his back, and the penis gently stretched and tilted to one side, and then the other side is evaluated. The systolic pressure is compared with the pressure in the brachial artery. In normal individuals the penile pressure should be 0.8 or greater when compared with the arm blood pressure. In patients with ratios between 0.6 and 0.8, vascular inflow is compromised, but the patients may be able to achieve reasonably firm erections. When the ratios decline to or are below 0.6, vascular impotence seems likely. We suspect that low systemic blood pressure may also result in impotence, but data to substantiate this are not available. Abnormal penile blood pressure should be confirmed at a later date. After the basal blood pressure is taken, we have the supine patient bend his legs at the hips and at the knees and then lift the buttocks off the examining table up and down repetitively for a total of 2 minutes. The penile blood pressure is again compared with the forearm blood pressure. If the ratios fall by 0.15 or more, or if the ratios approach 0.6, the patient is thought to have the pelvic steal syndrome. Arteriograms can confirm arterial diseases. A dynamic infusion cavernosogram can assess corporal incompetence.

Laboratory evaluation should include measurement of serum testosterone or an estimate of bioavailable testosterone (either free testosterone or non-SHBG-T), serum LH, and serum prolactin. The patients should arrive before breakfast in the fasting state, between 7 and 9 AM. Despite the added expense of having the specimens drawn more than once, at least two specimens should be drawn on separate days for each man. Any other appropriate laboratory studies could be performed such as thyroid functions, standard biochemical profile, blood count, urinalysis, and measurement of FSH if the testes appear small. Elevation of serum prolactin levels suggests specific disorders for exclusion before other treatment is done. Increased LH suggests testis failure. Low levels of circulating testosterone could result from altered function of the hypothalamus, pituitary, or testes.

Although only a small percentage of patients referred for impotence evaluation are found to have significant elevations of prolactin, such patients do exist and prolactin levels should be determined. Since there are sleep-related rises of prolactin, the samples should be drawn after the patients have been awake and about for 1 hour or more. With prolactin elevations up to twice the upper limit of normal, there does not seem to be interference with sexual function. With greater elevations, there can be a causal relationship between prolactin and sexual dysfunction; however, the exact threshold is not known.

For the bulbocavernous reflex latency time (a more precise version of the bulbocavernous reflex), short pulses of electrical stimulation of varying strength are used to stimulate the penis, and recording needles sensing responses are placed in the perineal muscles. The magnitude of stimulation required to generate a response is evaluated, and the time for a response to occur is also assessed, using equipment that averages the responses. There is a normal range for a response (between 30 and 44 ms). This study tests some of the nerves involved in sexual function but does not directly test the nerves involved with erection. An abnormal test helps to confirm a diagnosis of peripheral neuropathy, but we have followed a few patients in whom the test response was abnormally delayed who could achieve an erection after other therapeutic maneuvers.

Direct injections of a mixture of papaverine (30 mg per milliliter) and phentolamine (0.5 mg per milliliter) into the corpora cavernosa are used both as a diagnostic test and as treatment (see later). This combination of medications commonly causes firm erections in impotent men. Those individuals failing to respond are thought to have either corporal incompetence or severe vascular insufficiency. An initial test dose of 0.1 ml is injected into one corpus cavernosum, and the patients are instructed how to self-inject it. They are asked to remain in the office in case hyperresponsiveness occurs. After about 15 minutes, if there is no significant erectile response, the men are asked to attempt sexual activity within the next 15 to 30 minutes. If they achieve a firm erection with this dose, no further injections are indicated as part of the evaluation. If they do not achieve a firm erection, they self-inject 0.2 ml into the other corpus cavernosum that night or during the next few days. The injected

TABLE 14–20 Assessment of Sexual Dysfunction

Test	Items	Administration Time (Minutes)
Sexual interaction inventory	102	30 (LoPiccolo and Steger 1974)
Marital adjustment test	15	5 (Locke and Wallace 1959)
Sex anxiety inventory	38	15 (Janda and O'Grady 1980)
Sexual behavior and attitudes scale	10	5 (Sotile and Kilmann 1978)
Minnesota Multiphasic Personality Inventory	566	40 (Hathaway and McKinley 1984)

This table offers an example of an assessment battery that was used in a major outcome study that investigated the effects of different sex therapy treatments on erectile dysfunction (Kilmann et al 1987). Such a battery, coupled with the results of an in-depth interview, can identify aspects of the patient and/or relationship that require intervention. If administered before and after therapy, such a battery can offer valuable information about treatment effects.

material appears to cross to the other corpus. If a satisfactory erection is achieved with sexual activity, this phase of the evaluation is completed. If the erection is inadequate, the dose is increased by 0.2 ml, and the patients are to inject themselves once a week with the increasing dose (0.2 ml per week) until they achieve a firm erection or until they reach a total dose of 1.0 ml. If they fail to achieve a firm erection, either corporal incompetence or severe vascular insufficiency is diagnosed. If they do achieve a firm erection, those two problems can be largely excluded (but they may still have vascular impotence).

Response to the injections takes about 15 to 45 minutes. The patients can take the injection and then begin usual foreplay. After ejaculation, the penis should undergo detumescence within 15 to 20 minutes. If an erection lasts for 3 hours, the patients seek medical aid, and if the erection is still firm at 4 hours, medical treatment is begun. Several techniques are utilized to cause detumescence. If detumescence occurs within 6 hours, no clotting or significant problems should result. Treatment of prolonged erection can begin at 4 hours, with evacuation of 25 ml of blood from one corpus. If the erection recurs, then at 15-minute intervals, 10 ml of a saline solution with added epinephrine is put into the other corpus, and 25 ml of blood is removed. This is repeated at 15-minute intervals, altering the corpora, until detumesence occurs. The saline solution is 1,000 ml of normal saline with 1 ml of 1:1,000 aqueous epinephrine added. In our experience using penile injections on more than 40 men, only one man had a firm erection lasting more than 4 hours. He was one of our earlier patients and received as an initial dose 0.4 ml of the combined medications. Complete detumescence was achieved using the preceding approach without any residual problems. We then switched to an initial dose of 0.1 ml on each new patient, and no more prolonged tumescence occurred. One man developed transient orthostatic hypotension on that dose (0.1 ml), and not further injections were used.

Sleep studies are performed to document whether or not firm erections occur. It is known that during REM sleep, men achieve erections. About 80 percent of men with psychological impotence will have firm nocturnal erections. On the other hand, 20 percent of men who have primarily psychogenic impotence may not experience significant nocturnal erections. Thus, the documentation of firm erections is helpful. More recently, sleep apnea has been associated with hypogonadism and impotence. Such men typically have a history of loud snoring with irregular breathing at night. A third potential benefit of a complete sleep study would be an EEG to exclude the possibility of previously unrecognized epileptic disorders that may also be associated with hypogonadism and impotence. Candidates for penile prosthesis should be evaluated in a sleep laboratory to confirm the need for surgical intervention.

Sometimes, the history obtained from the patient or from his partner documents the presence of firm nocturnal erections. With this history in an impotent patient, strong consideration should be given to sex education and sex therapy. If this history is not clear, outpatient or inpatient studies can be done with the Snap-Gauge (DACOMED). This disposable band costs about $20 and is applied to the penis with a Velcro binding. Three plastic strips of increasing tensile strength bridge a gap opposite the Velcro bands. These usually tear with a "pop" if they are ruptured. The pop often awakens the patient, and they appreciate the fact that they have a firm erection. Normal tumescence should rupture at least two bands and commonly ruptures all three. There are problems using this apparatus: (1) Patients can take it on and off, and they sometimes tear the bands doing this; (2) the apparatus can fall off; (3) the glue holding the edges of the plastic strips to the bands sometimes gives away and the strips fall off rather than tear. We have tried several maneuvers to utilize these gauges more effectively. We apply the Snap-Gauge, tape the loose end to the band, and make pen marks where the tape joins the gauge. A thin vertical strip of tape is applied to the penis, extending about 1 inch above and below the Snap-Gauge. We prefer removing the unit the next morning. If this is not possible, the tape covering the tip of the Snap-Gauge with the pen marks is not applied. The patients are instructed to observe the bridging strips on arising in the morning and to remove the Snap-Gauge without tearing anything. The unit is delivered or mailed for confirmation.

Another method of monitoring nocturnal tumescence involves portable strain-gauge electronic units, with either direct printout of results or a memory chip. These can be used at home or in the hospital. After suitable calibration, a correct-size strain gauge (or two) is placed on the penis by a technician. Although most manufacturers suggest placing one at the base and one at the distal portion of the penis, using one strain gauge in about the middle of the penis will suffice. The strain gauges cost about $25 each and after sterilization can often be reused. The patients are instructed how to turn on the machine and plug in the strain gauge. These units show tumescence changes throughout the night and are less likely to be influenced by patient manipulation than the Snap-Gauge. If a man has no overt erections or erections that are less than 1.0 cm in maximum circumference, by definition, these are inadequate. If the nocturnal tumescence is greater than 1.0 cm, the erections may be partial or full. At this point, a Snap-Gauge could be used to assess the firmness of erection. In the past we have used artificial erections with the strain gauge in place. After a tourniquet is applied to the base of the penis, normal saline solution is injected into the corpora and the firmness is evaluated until firm erection is reached, or if the circumference change noted during sleep is reached and the erection is still partial, the study can be terminated. If a firm artificial erection could be produced with tumescence less than or the same as that achieved during sleep, the nocturnal erections were estimated as being firm. A more objective approach can be used (see later).

There are sophisticated approaches for evaluating for sleep apnea (see later), but it is feasible to screen patients overnight using a fingertip oximeter. If no significant desaturation occurs, it is unlikely that the patient is experiencing significant sleep apnea.

Complete sleep studies can be performed in patients who present diagnostic dilemmas. Fully equipped facilities can do polysomnography and nocturnal penile tumescence. This will include an EEG on at least the first night, and it can be set up to detect temporal lobe seizures. Monitoring will also include an electro-oculogram, an anterior tibial electromyogram, submental electromyogram, and nasal and oral air flow. Two mercury strain gauges can be applied to the penis and connected to the recording unit. Oxygen saturation can be evaluated using an ear or finger oximeter. Chest and abdominal expiratory effort can be monitored using pneumatic respiration transducers. Firmness of nocturnal erections can be quantitated using one of several measuring devices (such as the Chatillon Mechanical Dial Push/Pull Gauge, DPP 1kg, 1 kg by 10 g). In general, all studies are done the first night, and during the subsequent night or two, attention is focused on the presence or absence of tumescence. In most facilities, when the patient appears to achieve a maximum erection, the technician will awaken the patient, assess the firmness of erection, and take a photograph of the erection. There are small appliances that are left on the penis overnight to apparently directly quantitate the firmness of erection (Rigiscan, DACOMED). We have no experience using these, but there are potential advantages to such studies—cost, convenience, and less publicity. If a man gets a firm erection after one or two nights, no further studies are needed. In general, three nights without a firm erection are usually required to strongly suggest an organic cause for impotence, but even this does not exclude a psychogenic etiology.

Diagnostic and Therapeutic Trials for Impotence

Since impotence in an individual may have more than one contributing cause, the diagnostic work-up often lends itself to therapeutic trials. A patient may experience progressively improving sexual function as the trials continue. Those patients who have absolute causes of impotence (e.g., penile-brachial index 0.60 or lower, definite penile nerve damage) are not candidates for a therapeutic trial. For those men who may potentially benefit, medications may be switched or deleted. Narcotic medications and muscle relaxants should be discontinued if possible. Hypertension medications can be switched from those associated with impotence to those not usually linked to sexual dysfunction (there can be variations in response in an individual patient; what does not affect

one man may be deleterious to another). Control of diabetes mellitus should be optimized and weight reduction initiated for substantially obese men. Alcohol should be avoided or minimized, especially prior to sexual activity. Sometimes a vacation trip will result in enhanced sexual performance. This suggests a psychogenic component to impotence and the man (or couple) should be referred for sex education and therapy. In our experience virtually all couples who undergo this therapy are benefited, and in many potency is restored, especially when there are suggestions of a psychogenic component (see above). A 2-month trial of yohimbine may prove useful. In general, all of these trials should be for 2 to 3 months to assess their full impact.

If serum testosterone levels are below normal for the patient's age group (preferably estimates of free testosterone or non-SHBG-T), a trial of testosterone therapy is appropriate. Also, we have utilized this medication in middle-aged and older men who have average circulating testosterone values that are below the normal range for young men, but within the normal range for old men. For example, 420 ng per deciliter is our lower limit of normal for 20- to 40-year-old normal men, and 350 ng per deciliter is our lower limit of normal for men between the ages of 65 and 80 years. Therefore, an older man with testosterone levels between 350 and 420 ng per deciliter would also be offered a trial of injectable testosterone; many of these men experience improvement of libido and potency. Testosterone cypionate and enanthate appear to have similar actions. The injectable androgens have two advantages over oral preparations: (1) The levels can be measured in blood, and (2) there is no hepatotoxicity. We prefer giving 50 to 75 mg of depot testosterone intramuscularly at 1-week intervals to avoid the greater peaks and subsequent declines that larger, less frequent injections produce. A 3-month trial should be completed before accepting a failure to respond. The patients should be watched for side effects, including worsening sleep apnea, obstructive uropathy, and polycythemia. No man with a diagnosis of prostate cancer should be given testosterone.

If serum prolactin is elevated, and this cannot be normalized by medication adjustment, the etiology is investigated. Many drugs, including psychotropic medications, metoclopramide, and methyldopa, are associated with hyperprolactinemia. Impotence in a uremic man can be associated with zinc deficiency, insensitivity of Leydig's cells to luteinizing hormone, and hyperprolactinemia. Bromocriptine may normalize hyperprolactinemia of pituitary origin and that associated with uremia. A 3-month trial of dopamine agonist should be evaluated, and testosterone levels should also be determined. If the latter remains subnormal, testosterone may be needed as well. For a more detailed review of impotence therapy, particularly dealing with patients who fail to respond to the above trials, the reader is referred to the American Urological Association Update Series (1987).

MALE INFERTILITY

A couple is regarded as infertile if they have failed to achieve pregnancy after 1 year of unprotected intercourse. Approximately 15 percent of couples attempting pregnancy do not conceive in the first year, and about 5 to 10 percent are still barren at the end of 2 years. In practical terms, basic evaluation should begin after 1 year of infertility, whereas expensive and specialized procedures probably should be reserved until after 2 or more years. Either member of a couple can be the primary cause of infertility, as a male with azoospermia or a female with tubal obstruction. Usually, a combination of factors from both partners exists. Thus, a man with reduced sperm motility may not be able to impregnate a woman with mild endometriosis, though he might succeed with a woman who had no reproductive abnormality. This section outlines current techniques for evaluation of the infertile male. Although most infertile men have no identifiable cause of infertility, known factors must always be excluded (Table 14–21). Hypogonadism is usually associated with impaired sperm production (see the section on hypogonadism). In addition, the female partner must always be evaluated for a potential source of reproductive impairment.

At the initial evaluation, the male and his partner should be questioned regarding libido and erection, coital technique, and frequency and timing of intercourse. Although the phenomenon is uncommon, individuals lacking an understanding of simple reproductive physiology can reduce fertility by the practice of premature withdrawal, coitus associated with the time of menses rather than midcycle, or abstinence except for the perceived fertility period. Obviously, timing of intercourse close to the time of ovulation is essential. For most couples, this optimal time is about 11 to 13 days after the onset of menses. Basal body temperature records that rely on progesterone-induced temperature rise can be useful, but these records are often confusing to patients. Recently, home kits have become available to monitor the appearance of LH in a woman's urine. This indicates the preovulatory surge in LH and is predictive of ovulation in 12 to 36 hours.

As mentioned previously, a critical feature of the initial assessment is consideration of the female partner's reproductive potential. Though obvious menstrual irregularity can be ascertained by history, subtle dysfunction may require careful gynecologic evaluation. Frequently unrecognized female factors include cervical abnormality, tubal obstruction, shortened luteal phase, anovulation, and hyperprolactinemia. The evaluation of both partners often should proceed simultaneously. Frequently, correction of a female factor markedly improves fertility rates among couples in whom the problem initially had been assumed to be due to a male factor.

Male History

The medical history of the infertile male is directed toward identifying factors known to impair erectile or testicular function and excluding mild forms of systemic illness associated with reduced sperm production. Major risk factors are listed in Table 14–22. Failure of complete testicular descent or late descent can cause permanent germ cell injury. In utero exposure to diethylstilbestrol is associated with epididymal abnormalities which can cause obstructive azoospermia. Late or incomplete puberty can indicate hypogonadism especially when associated with partial or complete impotency. Failure to ejaculate (despite a normal erection and the sensation of orgasm) indicates retrograde ejaculation. Genital infections, especially chronic epididymitis and prostatitis, can markedly diminish sperm motility as well as fertility. Mumps orchitis (virtually always postpubertal) can cause progressive tubular sclerosis and irreversible damage to the seminiferous epithelium as well as to the Leydig cells. Personal habits can lead to testicular injury, especially heavy alcohol intake, bathing in hot baths, and frequent marijuana use. Occupational exposures to radiation and certain pesticides such as dibromochloropropane can be associated with reduced fertility. Treatment of cancer by radiation or chemotherapy can severely impair sperm production. Pelvic trauma or previous pelvic surgery such as prostatectomy can injure the gonads or the accessory organs and ducts and can also damage pelvic nerves,

TABLE 14–21 Causes of Male Infertility

Usually Irreversible	Potentially Reversible
Chromosomal abnormality	Vas or epididymal occlusion
Absent vas deferens	Retrograde ejaculation
Young's syndrome	Prostatitis, epididymitis
Nonmotile sperm	Gonadotropin deficiency
Mumps orchitis	Varicocele
Cryptorchidism	Drugs and/or toxins
Drugs and/or toxins	Heat or irradiation
Epididymal dysfunction	Sexual dysfunction
Androgen resistance	Immunologic
	Systemic illness

TABLE 14–22   Risk Factors for Male Infertility to Evaluate in History

Late or incomplete testicular descent
Abnormal pubertal development
Inadequate libido or potency
Retrograde ejaculation
Genital infections
Drugs including alcohol and marijuana
Toxins including pesticides and radiation
Heat including prolonged fever
Cancer therapy
Systemic illness

thereby causing erectile or ejaculatory dysfunction. A history of chronic sinopulmonary infections can indicate Young's syndrome.

Physical Examination

The infertile male usually has a normal physical examination; nevertheless, a thorough examination is important to detect any evidence of hypogonadism or potential causes of infertility. The degree of virilization can be an important index of hypogonadism. Usually, the normal male has full axillary and pubic hair with a male escutcheon, terminal hair on the face, upper chest, upper abdomen, and frequently over shoulders, male muscle pattern and mass, deep, "adult male" voice, and often temporal balding. The nipples and pectoral area should be palpated for any evidence of gynecomastia. The genitals should be examined carefully for phallic size (normally longer than 6 cm and more than 3 cm wide), location of the urethral opening and any hypospadias, testicular descent, and normal thinning of scrotal skin with rugal folds.

Testicular size and consistency are important indices of germ cell content. The testis grows from a neonatal size of 1 to 3 cc to an adult size of 20 to 30 cc. The normal adult seminiferous tubules are composed of several stages of development, with germ cells making up over 90 percent of the testicular volume and Leydig's cells contributing less than 1 percent. Adult testes that are soft in consistency or less than 20 cc in volume suggest hypogonadism and warrant a complete endocrinologic evaluation as described earlier. Testicular size is measured by volume with an orchidometer (see page 72) or as linear dimensions (short and long axes) using a ruler. Corresponding volumes and linear dimensions are shown in Table 14–23. Most examiners find the orchidometer easier to use and the measurements more reproducible. The testis, epididymis, and vas deferens should be palpated bilaterally for physical presence of any masses, nodules or tenderness. The presence of a varicocele can be assessed by palpation of the spermatic cord while the patient is standing and performing the Valsalva maneuver. The prostate should be palpated for size, consistency, tenderness, and evidence of masses or nodules. The examina-

tion should also exclude any evidence of systemic illness that might affect testicular function.

Semen Analysis

Semen analysis is the most readily available and most widely used diagnostic test in the evaluation of an infertile man. Semen analysis can provide valuable information about sperm number, motility, and morphology. However, results must be interpreted with caution as they are indirect measures of sperm function and do not correlate directly with fertilizing ability. Normal values are listed in Table 14–24 for sperm concentration (millions per milliliter), total sperm count, sperm morphology, sperm velocity, and semen volume.

Number and Motility

Sperm count and sperm velocity are the two most frequently abnormal semen characteristics in infertile males. Borderline values begin with sperm densities less than 20 million per milliliter or a total sperm count less than 60 million. Definite risk for infertility is found at sperm densities less than 10 million per milliliter or total count less than 20 million. Borderline values for percentage motile sperm are less than 60 percent, and poor values are less than 40 percent. Motility grade should be 3 or 4 for the majority of sperm. Possible causes of male infertility based on semen analysis are listed in Table 14–25.

While semen samples containing less than 5 to 10 million motile sperm are usually regarded as being of very low fertility potential, the low number of motile sperm is probably not the only cause of infertility. Studies on gonadotropin replacement in men with hypogonadotropic hypogonadism show that pregnancy can be achieved consistently even with counts less than 10 million total sperm when motility and morphology are normal. Such results suggest that multiple factors cause infertility in men with low sperm counts or reduced sperm motility.

Traditionally, semen analysis has been done with a hemocytometer to count the sperm and a covered drop of semen to estimate motility. Makler introduced a specialized chamber with a fixed depth (10 μm) in which both sperm count and motility estimation could be done. Although sperm counts from these devices can be very accurate, motility estimations are subjective and only utilize a scale of 0 (nonmotile) to +4 (rapid, forward progression). A few laboratories have utilized manual analysis of multiple exposure photography or videomicrography to develop more detailed assessments of sperm motility. Recently, automated systems using computer analysis of videomicrographic recordings have become available. These have greatly increased the reproducibility of velocity analysis and have provided much more subtle information on sperm motion. Velocity parameters that are especially useful include frequency distribution of linear

TABLE 14-23   Testicular Size

Volume (cc)	Dimensions (cm)	Adult Condition
2	2.0 × 1.2	Severe hypogonadism, such
4	2.5 × 1.5	as Klinefelter's syndrome
6	2.9 × 1.8	Moderate hypogonadism, such
10	3.4 × 2.1	as gonadotropin deficiency
15	4.1 × 2.5	or maturation arrest
20	4.3 × 2.8	Normal size, but may
25	4.7 × 3.1	include obstruction or
30	5.2 × 3.3	idiopathic oligospermia

velocity (μm per second), linear versus curvilinear velocity, and lateral head displacement about mean trajectory path. Presently, these devices are used primarily by research laboratories (because of the system expense and degree of expertise required for their regular use), though their speed and accuracy make them attractive to clinical laboratories.

Morphology

Sperm morphology is important to assess particularly as certain individuals may show unusually high percentages of abnormal forms, most often tapered heads or pin heads rather than normal oval forms. To assess morphology, semen is spread on a slide in a thin film, air dried, fixed in 95 percent ethyl alcohol (or a mixture of equal parts ethanol and ether), and stained. Staining is most frequently done by Papanicolaou or Giemsa methods, though other stains are also utilized. In addition to sperm, semen may contain significant numbers of other, nonflagellated cells (round cells)—which may include immature germ cells (spermatids, spermatocytes, spermatogonia)—and leukocytes such as lymphocytes and neutrophils. Distinction between immature germ cells and leukocytes is very useful as the former suggests disruption of the germinal epithelium with premature release of developing germ cells, while a predominance of leukocytes can indicate an infection or immune process. Considerable experience is necessary for proper classification of round cells. The Bryan-Leishman stain facilitates this, but it is a difficult procedure to perform. More recently, the use of monoclonal antibodies to specific cell types coupled with immunoperoxidase staining promises more facile identification of specific types of leukocytes.

Collection Techniques

Specimen collection techniques are an important factor in reliable semen analysis. Samples are collected by masturbation into a sterile container (as a urine col-

TABLE 14-24   Semen Analysis

Semen Characteristic	Category		
	Normal	Borderline	Poor
Total sperm/ejaculate	> 60 × 10⁶	40–59 × 10⁶	< 40 × 10⁶
Sperm density (per ml)	> 20 × 10⁶	10–19 × 10⁶	< 10 × 10⁶
Volume	> 2.0 ml	1.0–1.9 ml	< 1.0 ml
Motility	> 60%	40–59%	< 40%
Motility grade	> 3.0	2.5–2.9	< 2.5
Oval forms	> 60%	40–59%	< 40%

Method
  Hemocytometer
  Makler Chamber
  Coulter Counter
  Computed assisted videomicrography

Uses
  Screening male partners of infertile couples, follow-up evaluation of therapy

Problems
  Abstinence interval before collection should be 1–3 days.
  Specimen should be collected by masturbation into a sterile container, as a urine sample cup, and examined for motility within 1 hour.
    Individual variability may be high and require several samples for reasonable assessment of semen characteristics.

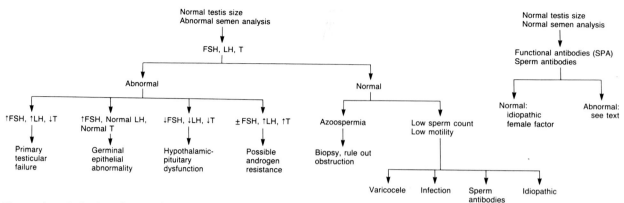

Figure 14-8   Evaluation of male infertility based on semen analysis and testicular size.

lection cup), and analyzed within 1 hour. Abstinence intervals of greater than 4 days can elevate total sperm count but depress sperm motility. Samples collected 24 to 72 hours after the last ejaculation seem to be most representative of mean semen characteristics. However, most men show a significant degree of variability in semen parameters from sample to sample. This can be especially significant in borderline samples, and several semen samples collected over 2 to 4 months may be necessary from such an individual to obtain a reasonable estimation of the semen characteristics. A manual on semen analysis developed by the World Health Organization is available from the American Fertility Society.

Azoospermia

Patients with azoospermia present a special situation. While this typically reflects a profound degree of damage to the seminiferous epithelium, usually associat-

ed with an elevated FSH, azoospermia may also indicate tubal obstruction, most commonly in the epididymis in which case FSH levels are usually normal. A fructose test should be done on the semen of azoospermic men to rule out the rare case of ejaculatory duct obstruction or agenesis of seminal vesicles (Table 14-26). Fructose comes primarily from the seminal vesicles and is analyzed by a colorimetric assay easily done by commercial laboratories. A testicular biopsy is warranted in persistent azoospermia to assess the seminiferous epithelium and rule out tubal obstruction. Silber and Rodriguez-Rigau have shown that more than 20 mature sperm per seminiferous tubule cross-section should be associated with the presence of sperm in the ejaculate, and azoospermia in these cases suggests ductal obstruction which is potentially correctable. Other than obstructive azoospermia, there are few conditions in which information from the biopsy will direct a therapeutic decision that may improve sperm production or fertility. The response of the seminiferous epithelium to a variety of injuries can be very similar, and the usual pathologic finding is one of maturation arrest or variable germ cell depletion.

Functional Tests of Sperm Fertility Potential

Direct assessment of fertility potential is done in animal husbandry by using aliquots of ejaculate from a particular animal for multiple inseminations. Fertility

TABLE 14-25   Etiology of Male Infertility Based on Semen Analysis

Azoospermia
  Seminiferous tubule sclerosis
  Germinal aplasia
  Maturation arrest
  Ductal obstruction
  Absent ejaculation

Nonmotile Sperm
  Kartagener's syndrome
  Metabolic defect
  Prolonged abstinence
  Idiopathic

Oligospermia
  Drug and/or toxin
  Varicocele
  Cryptorchidism
  Genital infection
  Systemic illness
  Idiopathic

Normal but Infertile
  Female abnormality
  Inadequate coital habits
  Immunologic
  Idiopathic

TABLE 14-26   Fructose Test

Method
  Fructose presence or concentration in semen
Normal
  Present in ejaculate, concentration 120–450 mg/dl
Uses
  Evaluation of azoospermia; absence of fructose suggests obstruction or lack of ejaculatory ducts or seminal vesicles
Problems
  Somewhat cumbersome assay, can be done by reference laboratory

rates between different males can be compared, and the most fertile selected for frequent breeding. Obviously this cannot be done with humans, and indirect measures of sperm fertilizing capacity have been developed. The zona-free hamster egg sperm penetration assay (SPA) is the most widely used test to estimate an individual's fertility potential (Table 14–27). The assay is complicated, requiring ovulation induction of the hamster, harvesting the oocytes, proper storage of the oocytes until they can be tested, removal of the cumulus from oocytes, incubating sperm and oocytes in a tissue culture chamber, and scoring which eggs, if any, have been penetrated based on presence of decondensed sperm nuclei within the ooplasm. Appearance of the sperm head within the egg presumes sperm capacitation followed by the acrosome reaction allowing fusion of the sperm head with the oocyte outer membrane. Proper handling of both sperm and oocytes is critical to the reproducibility of the assay. Most groups find a relatively good correlation between the SPA and subsequent fertility potential, especially with in vitro fertilization (IVF). However, several groups have questioned the predictability of outcome of IVF based on the heterologous SPA, and a negative SPA does not exclude attempts at IVF.

Although different laboratories must establish their own normal values, greater than 10 percent of the hamster ova should be penetrated by one or more sperm from fertile men. Lower penetration rates are associated with progressively poorer fertility. Recently, the split zona human oocyte has been advocated as a technique to study fertility potential using homologous oocytes. These are typically retrieved at oophorectomy or from cadavers. The split zona assay can allow comparisons between different semen samples, or different treatments of aliquots from the same ejaculate. Both procedures are difficult for routine laboratory use. However, the recent introduction of commercially available frozen hamster oocytes may facilitate clinical application at nonresearch laboratory centers.

Other sperm-function tests include evaluation of sperm–cervical mucus interaction and supravital staining. The postcoital test is a good in vivo method of evaluating cervical factors as causes of impaired sperm function. The test involves sampling of cervical mucus at different times for presence and number of motile sperm in the vaginal vault and cervical canal. Coitus is timed as closely to ovulation as feasible as the estrogen elevation at this time alters the cervical mucus to a condition receptive to spermatozoa. In addition, in vitro methods using the partners or animal cervical mucus are also available. Supravital staining of sperm is based on the uptake of stain by dead sperm due to loss of integrity of the plasma membrane. If there is a large number of nonmotile sperm, such a technique can differentiate live nonmotile sperm from dead sperm. The utility of this test is questionable as, currently, poor motility cannot be improved. However, a large fraction of nonmotile, live sperm suggests a flagellar defect.

Sperm Antibodies

Sperm antibodies can arise in either the male or female and can bind to the sperm surface, thus blocking molecules important in capacitation or egg binding. Sperm are sequestered cells that possess several cell surface antigens that are recognized as foreign and can incite an immune response and antibody formation in the male when exposed by vasectomy or trauma. Sperm antibodies have been clearly shown to develop in all species studied, including man after vasectomy. Sperm antigens can be found in the circulation bound to immune complexes, and sperm surface antibodies have been demonstrated to several sperm surface antigens. Following vasovasostomy, roughly 50 percent of men show antibodies binding to the sperm surface. Development of sperm antibodies also has been associated with testicular biopsy, cryptorchidism, varicocele, testicular cancer, and testicular inflammation (mumps orchitis).

Demonstration of sperm surface antibodies has been accomplished by three techniques using antihuman immunoglobulins bound to red blood cells, polyacrylamide beads, or fluorescent isotopes (Table 14–28). While the specificity of the probe depends on the anti-Ig antibody developed (most are polyclonal), the sensitivity depends on the particular probe. The most widely used probes now use either polyacrylamide beads (Immunobeads) or fluorescein. Tests are regarded as positive if more than 10 percent of sperm show binding. However, binding levels of 10 to 20 percent are considered borderline, while levels over 20 percent have a strong correlation with infertility.

The role of sperm antibodies in infertility is not clear. Studies in which sperm surface antibodies have been removed by specific proteases or by absorbent columns have shown recovery of heterologous ova penetration. This suggests that the surface antibodies are responsible for impaired sperm egg interaction. Other treatments have been very nonspecific (as with systemic glucocorticoids) and associated with severe side effects.

TABLE 14–27   Sperm Penetration Assay

Method
　Zona-free hamster oocytes

Normal
　Usually greater than 10% of oocytes penetrated

Uses
　Evaluation of male fertility potential

Problems
　Technically difficult assay that requires rigorous quality control with each assay using known donors as controls. There is significant interassay variation. Best performed at an experienced laboratory.

TABLE 14-28   Sperm Surface Antibodies

Method
   Mixed antiglobulin reaction
   Immunobeads
   Fluorescein labeled antibodies
Normal
   Less than 10% of sperm bind marker
Uses
   Screening for immunologic cause of male
   infertility. Tests can be performed on
   washed sperm (direct), or on sperm after
   exposure to spouse's serum or cervical
   mucus (indirect testing for female tract
   antibodies).
Problems
   Sensitivity and specificity vary with the
   method; immunofluorescence techniques
   are more sensitive, but more difficult to
   perform. Tests should be regarded more as
   qualitative than precisely quantitative due to
   variation and threshold nature of results.

Chromosomal Abnormalities

Certain chromosomal abnormalities are associated with impaired testicular function, sometimes dramatically. Klinefelter's syndrome (47,XXY) is the most common. The classic form—small testes, inadequate virilization, gynecomastia, and azoospermia—is relatively easy to recognize. However, patients can present with impaired sperm production and azoospermia, but with adequate androgen levels inducing normal virilization, libido, and potency. This is especially true of mosaic forms (46,XY/47,XXY). In mosaics, the testes are reduced in size, and serum gonadotropins are usually elevated though testosterone is typically normal. The spectrum can include patients with near normal parameters. Another disorder of sex chromosome number is XYY syndrome (47,XYY) in which there is an extra Y chromosome. Typically, these men have normal virilization and normal serum gonadotropins and testosterone, but show variable tubular abnormalities, from maturation arrest to tubular sclerosis, and have severe oligospermia or azoospermia. Autosomal chromosome abnormalities can be associated with testicular dysfunction, notably Down syndrome (trisomy 21), and balanced autosomal translocations. Interestingly, detailed chromosome analysis of oligospermic men or men whose wives have had frequent spontaneous abortions have shown a variety of subtle chromosomal abnormalities, indicating a role for genetic mechanisms in some cases of unexplained infertility. In general, a karyotype should be considered in men with reduced testicular size (less than 15 ml) and azoospermia.

Varicocele

Varicocele is clearly associated with infertility, and marked testicular atrophy can be found with large varicoceles. The general incidence of varicocele appears to be about 10 percent, and roughly one-half of men with varicoceles show reduced semen quality, either low sperm counts or reduced motility. Nevertheless, varicoceles are not uniformly associated with impaired fertility even in men with suboptimal semen characteristics. A recent report suggests that men with varicocele have evidence of a primary testicular defect having either elevated basal serum FSH or an exaggerated response of FSH and LH to GnRH stimulation whether they have normal or impaired semen characteristics or fertility.

Varicocele affects testicular function in a variety of ways, most likely by increased testicular temperature, altered blood flow, and possibly by venous reflux of metabolic wastes from the kidneys or of organ-specific compounds such as adrenal steroid or catecholamines. Varicocele occurs on the left side in about 90 percent of cases, probably related to the insertion of the left testicular vein into the left renal vein rather than the inferior vena cava, as on the right. The semen characteristics of infertile men with varicocele are not specific and show variable reductions in sperm count and motility and an increased percentage of tapered sperm and immature or amorphous forms.

In comparison to other therapies of oligospermia, surgical repair of varicocele may offer promising results. However, responses to treatment are not consistent. Published reports vary and indicate an improvement in semen quality ranging from 30 to 70 percent of patients and pregnancy in up to 25 percent of treated couples. Unfortunately, reported series differ on patient selection, on the degree of pre- and postvaricocelectomy evaluation, and on whether female factors were excluded. While there is no well-controlled study demonstrating statistically significant improvement in fertility after varicocele repair, studies comparing men electing either surgery or medical therapy indicate a positive response to surgery. Even more controversial is the issue of subclinical varicoceles identified only by Doppler stethoscope, radioisotopic scans, venography, or thermography. Whether these subclinical changes represent physiologically significant alterations in blood flow or temperature remains to be proven, as do benefits from their surgical repair.

Infections

Infections in the male reproductive tract can cause infertility. Clinically apparent infections of the testis, epididymis, or the prostate can lead to reduced sperm count or motility. Epididymitis is considered secondary to urethritis or cystitis, and the ipsilateral testis is usually involved. Causative organisms typically are *Neisseria gonorrhoeae* and *Chlamydia trachomatis* in sexually active men under 35 years of age and coliform bacteria in men over 35. A variety of other organisms have been associated with epididymitis, including *Mycobacterium tuberculosis, Ureaplasma urealyticum*, herpes simplex virus, and mumps virus. Mumps orchitis virtually always occurs in postpubertal males, in whom it occurs in about one-third of the cases of mumps parotitis; it can cause severe, irreversible tubular damage. Prostatitis can take several forms: acute or chronic, bacterial or nonbacterial, symptomatic or asymptomatic. The presence of excess leukocytes in the semen is suggestive or prostatitis (more than one leukocyte per 100 sperm). Physical examination often reveals a soft, tender, enlarged prostate gland. Culture is best obtained using a two or four-glass urine collection with prostatic massage. The most common infectious organism is *Escherichia coli*. Ureaplasma infections have been implicated in infertility, and treatment with doxycycline has been reported to improve sperm function or fertility, though a controlled study did not show an effect.

Conclusions

The infertile couple requires careful evaluation of both the male and female partner. While there are many treatable causes of male infertility, idiopathic infertility is the most common diagnosis. This remains a diagnosis of exclusion, and therapeutic options are poor. Medical treatment such as use of exogenous gonadotropins, aromatose inhibitors (testolactone), and anti-estrogens (clomiphene citrate) have not been shown efficacious in placebo-controlled trials. Therapies based on gamete manipulation such as intrauterine insemination with washed sperm or IVF using eggs with disrupted zonas are under active investigation with preliminary studies showing promising results.

BIBLIOGRAPHY

Aiman J, Griffin JE. The frequency of androgen receptor deficiency in infertile men. J Clin Endocrinol Metab 1982; 54:725.

Aitken RJ, Best FSM, Richardson DW, Djahanbakhch O, Templeton AA, Lees MM. An analysis of semen quality and sperm function in cases of oligozoospermia. Fertil Steril 1982; 38:705.

Amann RP. A critical review of methods for evaluation of spermatogenesis from seminal characteristics. J Androl 1981; 2:37-58.

American Urological Association Update Series. Treatment for organic impotence: Alternatives for the penile prosthesis. Parts I and II. Lessons 11 and 12, Vol VI. Padma-Nathan H, Payton T, Goldstein I. Houston: American Urological Association Office of Education, 1987.

Baker HWG, Burger HC, deKretser DM, Lording DW, McGowan P, Rennie GC. Factors affecting the variability of semen analysis results in infertile men. Int J Androl 1981; 4:609.

Bardin CW. Pituitary-testicular axis. In: Yen SSC, Jaffe RB, eds. Reproductive endocrinology. 2nd ed. Philadelphia: WB Saunders, 1986:177.

Barron JL, Noakes TD, Levy W, et al. Hypothalamic dysfunction in overtrained athletes. J Clin Endocrinol Metab 1985; 60:803.

Beard CM, Benson RC, Kelalis PP, Elveback L, Kurland LT. Incidence of mumps orchitis in Rochester, Minnesota, 1935 to 1974. Mayo Clin Proc 1977; 52:3.

Berger RE, Holmes KK. Infection and male infertility. In: Santen RJ, Swerdloff, RS eds. Male Reproductive Dysfunction. New York, Marcel Dekker, 1986:407.

Berger RE, Karp LE, Williamson RA, Koehler J, Moore DE, Holmes KK. The relationship of pyospermia and seminal fluid bacteriology to sperm function as reflected in the sperm penetration assay. Fertil Steril 1982; 37:557.

Blaivas JG, O'Donnell TF, Gottlieb P, Labib KB. Comprehensive laboratory evaluation of impotent men. J Urol 1980; 124:201.

Bronson RA, Cooper GW, Rosenfield D. Sperm antibodies: Their role in infertility. Fertil Steril 1984; 42:171.

Burger H, Rose N. Sexual impotence. Med J Aust 1979; 2:24.

Carlson HE. Gynecomastia. N Engl J Med 1980; 303:795.

Chandley AC, Edmond P, Gowans L, Fletcher J, Frackiewicz A, Newton M. Cytogenetics and infertility in man. I. Karyotype and semen analysis. Ann Hum Genet 1975; 39:231.

Clark RV, Sherins RJ. Treatment of men with idiopathic oligospermic infertility using the aromatase inhibitor, testolactone: Results of a double blinded, randomized placebo controlled trial with crossover. J Androl, in press.

Clark RV, Sherins RJ. Use of semen analysis in the evaluation of the infertile couple. In: Santen RJ, Swerdloff RS, eds. Male Reproductive Dysfunction. New York: Marcel Dekker, 1986: 253.

Clarke GN, Elliott PJ, Smalia C. Detection of sperm antibodies in semen using the immunobead test: A survey of 813 consecutive patients. Am J Reprod Immunol Microbiol 1985; 7:118.

Clifton DK, Bremner WJ. The effect of testicular X-irradiation on spermatogenesis in man. J Androl 1983, 4:387.

Cockett ATK, Urry RL, Dougherty KA. The varicocele and semen characteristics. J Urol 1979; 121:435.

Collins WE, McKendrup JBR, Silverman M, et al. Multidisciplinary survey of erectile impotence. Can Med Assoc J 1983; 128:1393.

Davidson JM, Chen JJ, Crapo L, et al. Hormonal changes and sexual function in aging men. J Clin Endocrinol Metab 1983; 57:71.

Deslypere JP, Vermeulen A. Leydig cell function in normal men: Effect of age, lifestyle, residence, diet, and activity. J Clin Endocrinol Metab 1984; 59:955.

Dubin L, Amelar RD. Varicocelectomy: 986 cases in a twelve-year study. Urology 1977; 10:446.

Dufau ML. Endocrine regulation and communicating functions of the Leydig cells. Ann Rev Physiol 1988; 50:483.

Dufau ML, Veldhuis JD. Pathophysiological relationships between the biological and immunological activities of luteinizing hormone. Baillieres Clin Endocrinol Metab 1987; 1:153.

Dunkel L, Perheentupa J, Sorva R. Single versus repeated dose human chorionic gonadotropin stimulation in the differential diagnosis of hypogonadotropic hypogonadism. J Clin Endocrinol Metab 1985; 60:333.

Eil C, Gamblin GT, Hodge JW, Clark RV, Sherins RJ. Whole cell and nuclear androgen uptake in skin fibroblasts from infertile men. J. Androl. 1985; 6:365.

Engle G, Burnham SJ, Carter MF. Penile blood pressure in the evaluation of erectile impotence. Fertil Steril 1978; 6:687.

Ertekin C, Reel F. Bulbocavernosus reflex in normal men and in patients with neurogenic bladder an/or impotence. J Neurol Sci 1976; 28:1.

Fariss BL, Fenner DK, Plymate SR, Brannen GE, Jacob WH, Thomason AM. Seminal characteristics in the presence of a varicocele as compared with those of expectant fathers and prevasectomy men. Fertil. Steril. 1981; 35:325.

Forest MG, David M, Lecoq A, et al. Kinetics of the hCG-induced steroidogenic response of the human testis. III. Studies in children of the plasma levels of testosterone and hCG: Rationale for testicular stimulation test. Pediatr Res 1980; 14:819.

Fraser HM, Baird DT. Clinical applications of LHRH analogues. Baillieres Clin Endocrinol Metab 1987; 1:43.

Freund M. Interrelationships among the characteristics of human semen and factors affecting semen-specimen quality. J Reprod Fertil 1962; 4:143.

Freund M. Standards for the rating of human sperm morphology. Int J Fertil 1966; 11:97.

Freund M, Carol B. Factors affecting hemocytometer counts of sperm concentrations in men. J Reprod Fertil 1964; 8:149.

Furlow W. Male sexual dysfunction. Urol Clin North Am 1981; 8:79.

Gordon DL, Herrigel JE, Moore DJ, Paulsen CA. Efficacy of Coulter counter in determining low sperm concentrations. Am J Clin Pathol 1967; 47:226.

Griffin JE, Wilson JD. Syndrome of androgen resistance. Hosp Pract 1987; 159.

Gump DW, Gibson M, Ashikaga T. Lack of association between genital mycoplasmas and infertility. N Engl J Med 1984; 310:937.

Gura V, Weizman A, Maoz B, et al. Hyperprolactinemia—a possible cause of sexual impotence in male patients undergoing chronic hemodialysis. Nephron 1980; 26:53.

Haas GG Jr, Cines DB, Schreiber AD. Immunologic infertility: Identification of patients with antisperm antibody. N Engl J Med 1980; 303:722.

Handelsman DJ, Conway AJ, Boylan LM, Turtle JR. Young's syndrome: Obstructive azoospermia and chronic sinopulmonary infections. N Engl J Med 1984; 310:3.

Hembree WC, Zeidenberg P, Nahas G. Marihuana effects of human gonadal function. In: Nahas G, Poton WDM, Idanpaan-Heittila J, eds. Marihuana: Chemistry, biochemistry, and cellular effects. New York, Springer Verlag, 1976: 521.

Hoffer LJ, Beitins IZ, Kyung H, Bistrian BR. Effects of severe dietary restriction on male reproductive hormones. J Clin Endocrinol Metab 1986; 62:288.

Karacan I. Evaluation of nocturnal penile tumescence and impotence. In: Guilleminault C, ed. Sleeping and waking disorders. Menlo Park, CA: Addison-Wesley, 1982:343.

Katz DF, Overstreet JW. Sperm motility assessment by videomicrography. Fertil Steril 1981; 35:188.

Kelly TM, Edwards CQ, Merkle AW, Kushner JP. Hypogonadism in hemochromatosis: Reversal with iron depletion. Ann Intern Med 1984; 101:629.

Kilmann PR, Auerbach R. Treatments of premature ejaculation and psychogenic impotence: A critical review of the literature. Arch Sex Behav 1979; 8:81.

Kilmann PR, Milan RJ, Boland JP, et al. Group treatment of secondary erectile dysfunction. J Sex Marital Ther 1987; 13:168.

Kinsey AC, Pomeroy WB, Martin CE. Sexual behavior in the human male. Philadelphia: WB Saunders, 1948.

Kirby RW, Kotchen TA, Rees ED. Hyperprolactinemia—a review of recent clinical advances. Arch Intern Med 1979; 129:1415.

Knobil E. The neuroendocrine control of the menstrual cycle. Recent Prog Horm Res 1980; 36:53.

Knuth UA, Honigl W, Bals-Pratsch M, Schleicher G, Nieschlag E. Treatment of severe oligospermia with human chorionic gonadotropin human menopausal gonadotropin: A placebo-controlled, double blind trial. J Clin Endocrinol Metab 1987; 65:1081.

Kulin HE, Santner SJ. Timed urinary gonadotropin measurements in normal infants, children, and adults, and in patients with disorders of sexual maturation. J Pediatr 1977; 90:760.

Labrie F, Dupont A, Belanger A. Treatment of prostate cancer with gonadotropin-releasing hormone agonists. Endocr Rev 1986; 7:67.

Lin T, Haskell J, Vinson N, et al. Characterization of insulin and insulin-like growth factor I receptors of purified Leydig cells and their role in steroidogenesis in primary culture: A comparative study. Endocrinology 1986; 119:1641.

Lipschultz LI, Caminos-Torres R, Greenspan C. Testicular function after unilateral orchiopexy. N Engl J Med 1976; 295:15.

Lubs HA. Testicular size in Klinefelter's syndrome in men over fifty—report of a case with XXY/XY mosaicism. N Engl J Med 1962; 267:326.

MacLeod J. Human seminal cytology as a sensitive indicator of the germinal epithelium. Int J Fertil 1964; 9:281

MacLeod J, Gold RZ. The male factor in fertility and infertility. II. Spermatozoon counts in 1000 men of known fertility and in 1000 cases of infertile marriage. J Urol 1951; 66:436.

Mahony MC, Alexander NJ, Swanson RJ. Evaluation of semen parameters by means of automated sperm motion analysis. Fertil Steril 1988; 49:876.

Makler A. The improved ten-micrometer chamber for rapid sperm count and motility evaluation. Fert Steril 1980; 33:337.

Mann A, Pardridge WM, Cefalu W, et al. Bioavailability of albumin-bound testosterone. J Clin Endocrinol Metab 1985; 61:705.

Marshall JC, Kelch R. Gonadotropin-releasing hormone: Role of pulsatile secretion in the regulation of reproduction. N Engl J Med 1986; 315:1459.

Matsumoto AM, Bremner WJ. Endocrinology of the hypothalamic-pituitary-testicular axis with particular reference to the hormonal control of spermatogenesis. Baillieres Clin Endocrinol Metab 1987; 1:71.

Mattson RH, Cramer JA. Epilepsy, sex hormones, and antiepileptic drugs. Epilepsia 1985; 26(Suppl 1):S40.

McCullagh GR. Dual endocrine activity of the testes. Science 1932; 76:19.

Milby TH, Whorton D. Epidemiological assessment of occupationally related, chemically induced sperm count suppression. J Occup Med 1980; 2:77.

Morley JE, Melmed S. Gonadal dysfunction in systemic disorders. Metabolism 1979; 28:1051.

Mortimer CH, Besser GM, McNeilly HS, et al. Luteinizing hormone-releasing hormone test in patients with hypothalamic-pituitary-gonadal dysfunction. Br Med J 1973; 4:73.

Mortimer D, Templeton AA, Linton EA, Coleman RA. Influence of abstinence and ejaculation-to-analysis delay on semen analysis parameters of suspected infertile men. Arch Androl 1982; 8:251.

Mottram JC, Cramer TV. On the general effects of exposure to radium on metabolism and tumor growth in the rat and the special effects on testis and pituitary. AMJ Exp Physiol 1923; 13:209.

Murono E, Nankin HR, Lin T, et al. The aging Leydig cell V. Diurnal rhythms in aged men. Acta Endocrinol 1982; 99:619.

Murono EP, Nankin HR, Lin T, et al. The aging Leydig cell VI. Response of testosterone precursors to gonadotropin in men. Acta Endocrinol 1982; 100:299.

Nagao RR, Plymate SR, Berger RE, Perrin EB, Paulsen CA. Comparison of gonadal function between fertile and infertile men with varicoceles. Fertil Steril 1986; 46:930.

Nankin HR. Hormone kinetics after intramuscular testosterone cypionate. Fertil Steril 1987; 47:1004.

Nankin HR, Calkins JH. Decreased bioavailable testosterone in aging normal and impotent men. J Clin Endocrinol Metab 1986; 63:1418.

Nankin HR, Harman SM. Gonadal function and sexual potency in the aging male. In: Exton-Smith AN, Weksler ME, eds. Practical geriatric medicine. London: Churchill Livingstone, 1985:308.

Nankin HR, Lin T, Osterman J. Chronic testosterone cypionate therapy in men with secondary impotence. Fertil Steril 1986; 46:300.

Nankin HR, Osterman J, Lin T, et al. A new alternative in evaluating and treating impotence in men: Direct injections of the corpora cavernosa. J SC Med Assoc 1987; 83:55.

Nankin HR, Pinto R, Fan D, et al. Daytime titers of testosterone, LH, estrone, estradiol, and testosterone-binding protein: Acute effects of LH and LH-releasing hormone in men. J Clin Endocrinol Metab 1975; 41:278.

Nankin HR, Yanaihara T, Troen P. Response of gonadotropins and testosterone to clomiphene stimulation in a pubertal boy. J Clin Endocrinol Metab 1971; 33:360.

Newton R, Schinfeld JS, Schiff I. The effect of varicocelectomy on sperm count, motility and conception rate. Fertil Steril 1980; 34:250.

Odell WD, Swerdloff RS. Abnormalities of gonadal function in men. Clin Endocrinol 1978; 8:149.

Oppermann D, Happ J, Mayr WR. Stimulation of spermatogenesis and biological paternity by intranasal (low dose) gonadotropin-releasing hormone (GnRH) in a male with Kallmann's syndrome: Intraindividual comparison of GnRH and gonadotropins for stimulation of spermatogenesis. J Clin Endocrinol Metab 1987; 65:1060.

Ory SJ. Clinical uses of luteinizing hormone-releasing hormone. Fertil Steril 1983; 39:577.

Partsch CJ, Hermanussen M, Sippell WG. Differentiation of male hypogonadotropic hypogonadism and constitutional delay of puberty by pulsatile adminstration of gonadotropin-releasing hormone. J Clin Endocrinol Metab 1985; 60:1196.

Pirke KM, Doerr P. Age-related changes in free plasma testosterone, dihydrotestosterone, and oestradiol. Acta Endocrinol (Copenh) 1975; 80:171.

Rechtschaffen A, Kales A, eds. A manual of standardized terminology, techniques and scoring system for sleep studies of human subjects. Los Angeles: Brain Information Service, 1977.

Rodriguez-Rigau LJ, Smith KD, Steinberger E. Varicocele and the morphology of spermatozoa. Fertil Steril 1981; 35:54.

Rogers BJ. The sperm penetration assay: Its usefulness reevaluated. Fertil Steril 1985; 43:821.

Rose LI, Underwood RH, Newmark SR, et al. Pathophysiology of spironolactone-induced gynecomastia. Ann Intern Med 1977; 87:398.

Santen RJ, deKretser DM, Paulsen CA, Vorhees J. Gonadotropins and testosterone in the XYY syndrome. Lancet 1970; 2:371.

Saypol DC. Varicocele. J Androl 1981; 2:61.

Schwartz D, Laplanche A, Jouannet P, David G. Within-subject variability of human semen in regard to sperm count, volume, total number of spermatozoa and length of abstinence. J Reprod Fertil 1979; 57:391.

Schilsky RL, Sherins RJ. Adverse effects of treatment: Gonadal dysfunction. In: DeVita VT Jr, Hellman S, Rosenberg SA eds: Cancer, principles and practice of oncology. Philadelphia, JB Lippincott, 1985: 2032.

Sheldon WR, DeBold CR, Evans WS, et al. Rapid sequential intravenous adminstration of four hypothalamic releasing hormones as a combined anterior pituitary function test in normal subjects. J Clin Endocrinol Metab 1985; 60:623.

Sherins RJ, Brightwell D, Steruthal PM. Longitudinal analysis of semen of fertile and infertile men. In: Troen P, Nankin HR, eds. The testis in normal and infertile men. New York: Raven Press, 1977: 473.

Shrom SH, Leif HE, Wein AJ. Clinical profile of experience with 130 consecutive cases of impotent men. Urology 1979; 13:511.

Siemons LJ, Mahler CH. Hypogonadotropic hypogonadism in hemochromatosis: Recovery of reproductive function after iron depletion. J Clin Endocrinol Metab 1987; 65:585.

Silber SJ, Rodriguez-Rigau LJ. Quantitative analysis of testicle biopsy: Determination of partial obstruction and prediction of sperm count after surgery for obstruction. Fertil Steril 1981; 36:480.

Skakkebaek NE, Zeuthen E, Nielsen J, Yde H. Abnormal spermatogenesis in XYY males: A report on four cases ascertained through a population study. Fertil Steril 1973; 24:390.

Slag MF, Morley JE, Elson MK, et al. Impotence in medical clinic outpatients. JAMA 1983; 249:1736.

Smith KD, Rodriguez-Rigau LJ, Steinberger E. Relation between indices of semen analysis and pregnancy rate in infertile couples. Fertil Steril 1977; 28:1314.

Sokol RZ, Steiner B, Bastillo M, Petersen G, Swerdloff RS. Controlled comparison of the efficacy of clomiphene citrate in male infertility. Fertil Steril 1988; 49:865.

Spark RF. Neuroendocrinology and impotence (editorial). Ann Intern Med 1983; 98:103.

Takihara H, Cosentino MJ, Sakatoka J, et al. Significance of testicular size measurement in andrology. II. Correlation of testicular size with testicular function. J Urol 1987; 137:416.

Thomas AJ Jr. Ejaculatory dysfunction. Fertil Steril 1983; 39:445.

Toth A, Lesser ML, Brooks C, Labriola D. Subsequent pregnancies among 161 couples treated for T-mycoplasma genital tract infection. N Engl J Med 1983; 308:505.

Tyler JPP, Crockett NG. Comparison of the morphology of vital and dead human spermatozoa. J Reprod Fertil 1982; 66:667.

VanThiel DH, Lester R, Sherins RJ. Hypogonadism in liver disease: evidence for a double defect. Gastroenterology 1974; 67:1188.

Vantman D, Koukoulis G, Dennison L, Zinaman M, Sherins RJ. Computer-assisted semen analysis: Evaluation of method and assessment determination. Fertil Steril 1988; 49:510.

Vermeulen A. Decline in sexual activity in aging men: Correlation with sex hormone levels and testicular changes. J Biosoc Sci [Suppl] 1979; 6:5.

Vogel AV, Peake GT, Radu RT. Pituitary-testicular axis dysfunction in burned men. J Clin Endocrinol Metab 1985; 60:658.

Wang C., Baker HWG, Burger HW, deKretser DM, Hudson B. Hormonal studies in Klinefelter's syndrome. Clin Endocrinol (Oxf) 1975; 4:399.

Wasserman MD, Pollak CT, Spielman AG, Weitzman ED. The differential diagnosis of impotence. JAMA 1980; 243:2038.

Weiss HD. The physiology of human penile erection. Ann Intern Med 1972; 76:793.

Whitehead ED, Leiter E. Genital abnormalities and abnormal semen analyses in male patients exposed to diethylstibestrol in utero. J Urol 1981; 125:47.

Wickings EJ, Freischem CW, Langer K, Nieschlag E. Heterologous ovum penetration test and seminal parameters in fertile and infertile men. J Androl 1983; 4:261.

Wolff H, Anderson DJ. Immunohistologic characterization and quantitation of leukocyte subpopulations in human semen. Fertil Steril 1988; 49:497.

Wilson JD, Aimen J, MacDonald PC. The pathogenesis of gynecomastia. Adv Intern Med 1980; 25:1.

Woolf PD, Hamill RW, McDonald JV, et al. Transient hypogonadotropic hypogonadism caused by critical illness. J Clin Endocrinol 1985; 60:444.

Wortsman J, Eagleton LE, Rosner W, Dufau ML. Mechanism for the hypotestosteronemia of the sleep apnea syndrome. Am J Med Sci 1987; 293:221.

Ying S-Y. Inhibins, activins and follistatins: Gonadal proteins modulating the secretion of follicle-stimulating hormone. Endocr Rev 1988; 9:267.

15

Ectopic Hormone Production by Tumors

Andrée de Bustros, M.D.
Stephen B. Baylin, M.D.

The purpose of this chapter is three-fold. First, it summarizes the current understanding of ectopic hormone production by tumors, emphasizing the relationships between events in the biosynthesis of these hormones and the status of cellular differentiation and malignant transformation. Second, it describes the well-defined clinical syndromes associated with hormone production by tumors and broadly outlines a practical diagnostic approach to these entities. Third, it gives a perspective for ongoing and future directions of research on the problem of "aberrant" production of hormones by cancer cells.

HISTORICAL PERSPECTIVE AND CHANGING CONCEPTS

In 1969, Liddle first used the term *ectopic hormone production* in conjunction with the elaboration by tumors of hormones that are usually not produced by the tissue of origin for a given neoplasm. Although this term remains useful in referring to the clinical manifestations of hormonal production by tumors ("ectopic" hormone syndromes), it has now become apparent that the types of normal cells capable of hormone production are far more widespread than originally thought. It is well established that polypeptide hormones are present in sites other than the specialized glandular tissues that contain the highest concentrations. For example, somatostatin, calcitonin, vasoactive intestinal polypeptide, as well as several other small peptide hormones have been detected in the brain, with the use of sensitive immunocytochemical techniques. Immunoreactive insulin, growth hormone (GH), human chorionic gonadotropin (hCG), adrenocorticotropic hormone (ACTH), and corticotropin-releasing factor (CRF) have been found in a variety of normal tissues. Whereas most of the preceding data has been derived using immunologic techniques, more sensitive and specific DNA-RNA hybridization assays are increasingly being used, and these also detect the presence of hormones in normal tissues. For example, messenger RNA (mRNA) for the ACTH precursor molecule, pro-opiomelanocortin (POMC), has been found in male rat testes and female rat ovaries and placenta.

It is fascinating that small polypeptide hormones classically considered only for their endocrine role in complex multicellular organisms have also been found in primitive organisms such as protozoa. In these cells, the identified peptides are presumed to act locally, and thus may play a role in the regulation of cell growth and differentiation. Such cellular self-regulation (autocrine secretion pattern), as well as control of adjacent cells by diffusion of regulatory substances through the extracellular space (paracrine secretion pattern), must also be at play in complex organisms. This may be true especially in early embryonic life, in which dramatic rates of growth are seen, long before the development of the complex circulatory and endocrine systems. Even in adult tissues, evidence is accumulating that hormones may play a role in the local regulation of cell growth and differentiation. For example, POMC mRNA is expressed in a stage-specific manner by spermatogenic cells, suggesting that it may act as an autocrine or paracrine factor important for testicular function.

One then must understand the presence of peptide hormones in tumor cells in the context of the preceding findings for normal cells. It is tempting to speculate that the malignant phenotype represents a state of aberrant cellular differentiation in which cellular events are accentuated that are normally most apparent in embryonic life or in the early differentiation steps of the adult cell system in which the tumor arises. The pattern of production of hormones by tumors could then be tightly linked to neoplastic transformation and to the degree of differentiation of the cells giving rise to tumors.

INCIDENCE OF ECTOPIC HORMONE SYNDROMES AND CRITERIA FOR DIAGNOSIS

The incidence of hormonal production by neoplasms is very difficult to assess. Not all hormones synthesized by tumors produce clinical symptoms, either because they are released in the blood in a biologically inactive form or because the secreted levels are not high enough to produce distant manifestations. For instance, the biologically inactive ACTH precursor, POMC, previously referred to as "Big" or "ProACTH," has been detected in the sera of many patients with lung cancer who do not suffer from Cushing's syndrome. One can then only guess how many hormones are produced and how often by tumors, since an endocrine evaluation is rarely done in patients with cancer who have no apparent endocrine abnormalities. A suggested list of criteria for the diagnosis of ectopic hormone production is presented in Table 15–1.

Radioimmunoassays, which still are the traditional means of measuring circulating hormones, are far from perfect in terms of sensitivity and specificity. The classic criteria for the demonstration of hormone synthesis by tumors, such as the presence of an arteriovenous gradient for a given hormone across the tumor, or the detection of immunoreactivity for such a hormone in tumor tissues, depend on these imperfect immunologic techniques. For example, parathyroid hormone (PTH) production by tumors in patients with cancer-related hypercalcemia has long remained a controversial issue, largely because of the technical limitations of the old PTH radioimmunoassays. The evolution of the techniques of molecular biology has provided a new perspective to the problem of hormone production by tumors. The advent of recombinant DNA techniques has allowed the characterization of most peptide hormone genes. Using cloned cDNA or genomic DNA fragments and highly sensitive and specific DNA-RNA hybridization assays, one can determine the level of a particular peptide hormone mRNA species in tumors. In the case of tumor-related hypercalcemia, this technique has now provided conclusive evidence that PTH is rarely if ever produced in nonparathyroid tumors (see discussion later). Furthermore, the potentially powerful technique of cytoplasmic in situ

hybridization can be used to study, in tumors, the distribution of a specific mRNA species at the cellular level, and thus it could help characterize the specific cell types involved in hormone production.

BIOLOGIC BASIS OF HORMONAL PRODUCTION BY TUMORS

Several theories have been proposed in an attempt to explain the production of hormones by tumors, and several classifications of hormone production by neoplasms have been put forward, based on the histology and embryogenesis of specific tumor types. The most frequently cited concept is that of the amine precursor uptake and decarboxylation (APUD) endocrine cell of origin and its relationship to cellular production of biologically active small polypeptide hormones. Initially, it appeared that this cell system originated solely in the embryologic neural crest. However, some APUD cells such as those found in the gastrointestinal tract appear to be of endodermal origin. Thus, the theory of a distinct class of cells derived from the neural crest and uniquely qualified to produce small polypeptide hormones seems inadequate to explain ectopic hormone production by tumors.

The level of production of hormones by a tumor and the form of the hormone are probably determined by the degree of endocrine differentiation of the neoplastic cells. An excellent example for this point is found among lung tumors. Tumors with neuroendocrine features, such as small cell lung carcinoma (SCLC), possess APUD characteristics and are most frequently responsible for producing endocrine syndromes secondary to excessive amounts of small polypeptide hormones. This is thought to result because SCLC arises from a separate cell of origin in the bronchial epithelium from the other major forms of lung cancer. However, there is firm evidence that other histologic types of lung neoplasms such as squamous cell carcinomas or adenocarcinomas can also have elevated levels of hormones such as ACTH and calcitonin, and even contain cell populations with APUD features. The various histologic types of lung tumors then may represent a spectrum of differentiation in a single cell system. In the laboratory, established lines of SCLC are observed to acquire, in late passages, a distinct non-SCLC phenotype and lose their APUD features. Also, in some patients, several histologic types of lung cancer can be found at different times during the evolution of the disease, and the various cell types may coexist in the same tumor tissue. APUD features, then, do not necessarily reflect tumor origin from an endocrine cell, but rather may arise as a consequence of a certain direction of differentiation, and the degree of endocrine differentiation may reflect the level of cell maturation along this pathway.

Production and release of a mature hormone with biologic activity require, in a cell, the presence of specific biochemical and structural features such as the process-

TABLE 15–1   Criteria for the Diagnosis of Ectopic Hormone Production

Presence of an endocrine syndrome in association with a tumor
Elevated serum or urine levels of the hormone involved
Presence of bioactive or immunoreactive hormone in the tumor tissue
Presence of an arteriovenous gradient for the hormone across the tumor
Presence of the hormone gene specific mRNA in the tumor itself or in cultured tumor cells

ing enzymes involved in the cleavage of inactive hormone precursors, neurosecretory granules in which mature hormones are stored, and intact secretory mechanisms. Thus, introduction of a proinsulin-SV40 recombinant vector into AT T-20 cells (an ACTH-secreting mouse pituitary cell line) results in a stably transformed cell line in which the cells are capable of proteolytic processing of proinsulin to insulin and of releasing insulin into the culture medium upon stimulation with secretagogues. By contrast, similarly transformed fibroblast L cells, which lack neuroendocrine differentiation features, secrete only proinsulin, and their secretion rate is unaffected by secretagogues.

Tumor cells with a significant degree of endocrine differentiation, such as SCLC cells, can produce and secrete mature hormones. Some tumor cells do not evolve the machinery needed for proteolytic processing of precursor hormones and thus only produce biologically inactive hormones. Tumor cells with an even lesser degree of APUD differentiation are, perhaps, only able to transcribe certain peptide hormone genes. In such tumors, the elaboration of hormones might be detectable only by a DNA-RNA hybridization assay. Finally, tumor cells completely devoid of APUD characteristics may not even transcribe polypeptide hormone genes.

Tumor evolution in the host is a dynamic process, and the ongoing movement of differentiation within a tumor may lead to the evolution of heterogeneous cell populations, with variable degrees of endocrine differentiation. For example, ACTH production and the ectopic Cushing's syndrome are seen to evolve only with the aggressive phase of certain tumors such as lung and prostatic carcinomas. The behavior of medullary thyroid carcinoma (MTC), a tumor of defined endocrine cell origin (C cell of the thyroid), also illustrates these points. Distinct stages of development have been defined for MTC (C cell hyperplasia, microscopic cancer, disseminated tumor), and intracellular concentrations of the hormone calcitonin decrease while those of the enzyme L-dopa decarboxylase (DDC), a key APUD marker, increase during tumor progression. Also, POMC-specific mRNA was detected in metastases but not in primary tumor in patients with MTC, implying that tumor progression may be accompanied by the emergence of a new cell population with distinct properties. Indeed, the fact that cell populations responsible for hormone production in tumors change during tumor progression may be the major limiting factor to the use of hormones as circulating markers for monitoring the clinical course of disease and the response to therapy.

The determination of coordinated regulation of gene expression in normal cells and the deviations that occur in tumor cells are poorly understood. Exciting work is ongoing in this area, however, and it is increasingly apparent that the tissue-specific expression of genes is due to the interaction of defined regulatory DNA regions within the gene and nuclear proteins. These proteins are usually present in tissues that highly express the gene and may be absent or present in lesser amounts in tissues that do not express the gene. For example, transcription of the GH gene is stimulated to a much greater extent by nuclear extracts from GH-expressing pituitary tumor cells than by extracts from nonexpressing HeLa cells. The degree of hormone gene expression by tumors then could be tightly linked to relationships between degree of endocrine cell differentiation and attendant levels of specific nuclear transcription factors. Also, abnormalities in regulation of given transcription factors relative to the degree of cell differentiation could produce some of the aberrant patterns of hormone production associated with neoplasms. Finally, single specific transcription factors could regulate synthesis of groups of hormones. This might explain why certain peptide hormones are produced more frequently than others in tumors, why these peptides are often simultaneously found in neoplasms, and why specific tumor types tend to be associated with specific hormones. For example, small polypeptide hormones such as ACTH, calcitonin, and somatostatin are usually produced by tumors exhibiting APUD characteristics such as SCLC, pancreatic islet cell tumors, and MTC. By contrast, placental hormones of larger molecular weight such as hCG tend to be produced by tumors lacking APUD characteristics such as large cell carcinomas of the lung.

Consistent with the aforementioned concept that regulation of hormone gene expression in tumors occurs at the transcriptional control level is the fact that, to date, no major structural differences have been defined in the coding regions of hormone genes expressed in normal versus tumor tissues. Hormone genes highly expressed in tumors exhibit DNA conformational characteristics similar to those found in normal cells that express the same genes. For example, the calcitonin gene is hypomethylated and in the "open" chromatin conformation typical of highly transcribed genes both in medullary thyroid carcinoma, which arises from the calcitonin-producing thyroid C cells, and in lung carcinomas, which express calcitonin ectopically.

In contrast to the DNA structural features, the transcriptional events for hormone genes expressed ectopically, including post-transcriptional processing steps, are often altered in tumors. As detailed in the individual ectopic hormone syndromes discussed later (Table 15–2), large unprocessed RNA transcripts and/or peptide precursors are a uniform feature of ectopic hormone production.

TUMOR–RELATED HYPERCALCEMIA

Biologic Aspects

Hypercalcemia is probably the most common endocrine manifestation of malignancy, occurring in 10 to 20 percent of all patients with cancer. In the general population, the frequency of malignancy as an etiologic factor for hypercalcemia is equal to that of primary hyperparathyroidism, whereas in hospitalized patients, malignancy is the most common cause of hypercalcemia.

TABLE 15-2   Ectopic Hormone Syndromes

Clinical Aspects	Hormones Involved
Hypercalcemia	PTH-like peptides, TGFs, OAF, 1,25-dihydroxyvitamin D, prostaglandins
Cushing's syndrome	POMC, CRF
SIADH	ADH
Acromegaly	GH, CRF
Hypoglycemia	IGF-II?
Precocious puberty or gynecomastia	hCG
Erythrocytosis	Erythropoietin
Osteomalacia	?
Hyperthyroidism	hCG
Hypertension	Renin
Watery diarrhea	Vasoactive intestinal polypeptide
Flushing	Pancreatic polypeptide
Gastric ulcers	Gastrin

Hypercalcemia in malignancy is associated with a well-defined group of tumors, in particular breast cancer; squamous cell carcinomas of the head, neck, and lung; renal carcinoma; and multiple myeloma. Other common types of cancers such as adenocarcinomas of the colon, stomach, and prostate and SCLC are rarely associated with hypercalcemia. Although many patients with tumor-related hypercalcemia have bone metastases that contribute to the elevation of the serum calcium, others have hypercalcemia in the absence of detectable bone lesions. There is, then, no unifying theory to explain all cases of tumor-related hypercalcemia. However, it has become clear that tumors can be placed into three overlapping groups according to the mechanism by which they cause hypercalcemia: (1) solid tumors, such as breast cancer, that produce hypercalcemia when associated with extensive bone metastases; (2) solid tumors, such as squamous carcinomas of the lung and renal carcinoma, that secrete circulating bone-resorbing substances; and (3) hematologic malignancies that release osteolytic factors locally in bone (Table 15-3).

In each of these groups, a key factor in the development of hypercalcemia due to malignancy is some form of increase in the rate of bone resorption. Usually the degree of osteolysis is high enough to overwhelm renal mechanisms for calcium excretion, the body's major defense mechanism against hypercalcemia. In some instances, such as in severe cases of multiple myeloma, decreased glomerular filtration rate may contribute to the severity of hypercalcemia.

Solid Tumors with Extensive Bone Involvement

The prototype of tumors in this group is breast cancer, which accounts for more than 25 percent of the total cases in this category. Most women with advanced breast cancer have bone metastases, and about a third of them develop hypercalcemia. The pathogenesis of hypercalcemia in such patients may appear straightforward, but in fact, little is known about precise mechanisms by which cancer cells in bone lead to increased bone resorption. In vitro studies have shown that breast cancer cells themselves have the capacity to resorb bone directly by producing collagenolytic and lysosomal enzymes. Also, several studies have implicated prostaglandins, which are released by breast cancer cells, as local mediators of bone resorption. Of clinical relevance is the fact that the administration of estrogens or antiestrogens to patients with advanced breast cancer may precipitate severe hypercalcemia. In vitro studies with the MCF-7 breast cancer cell line have shown that estrogen treatment induces a release of bone-resorbing activity that is accompanied by production of prostaglandin E and blocked by prostaglandin synthesis inhibitors such as indomethacin.

Solid Tumors with Humorally Mediated Hypercalcemia

Most of the recent advances in the understanding of tumor-related hypercalcemia have occurred in the group of solid tumors associated with hypercalcemia without skeletal involvement, such as squamous cell tumors of the head and neck, lung, cervix, and vulva. With such tumors, hypercalcemia is believed to be due to the secretion by the tumor cells of circulating substances that act on bone to activate osteoclasts and cause bone resorption. The possibility that tumors secrete such substances was recognized as early as 1941, when Fuller Albright, in discussing a patient with renal cell carcinoma and hypercalcemia, first suggested that tumors could cause hypercalcemia by secreting PTH. Subsequently,

TABLE 15-3   Mechanisms of Tumor-Related Hypercalcemia

Mechanism	Tumor Type	Mediator
Skeletal metastases	Breast cancer, SCLC, and adenocarcinoma of the lung	Direct tumor cell osteolysis Prostaglandins?
Production of circulating bone-resorbing factors	Squamous cell carcinomas of the head, neck, and lung; renal carcinoma	PTH-like peptides TGFs
Local production of osteolytic factors	Multiple myeloma, T-cell lymphoma	OAF 1,25-dihydroxyvitamin D

immunoreactive PTH was indeed identified in tumor extracts and/or sera of patients with hypercalcemia. Further studies, however, yielded conflicting data owing to (1) the heterogeneous populations of circulating PTH fragments; (2) the poor correlation between PTH levels measured by different assays; and (3) the assumption by some investigators that detectable PTH immunoreactivity in malignancies associated with hypercalcemia was definitive evidence for ectopic PTH secretion. Using cloned PTH DNA in a DNA-RNA hybridization assay, Simpson and colleagues failed to detect PTH mRNA in a series of human tumors, some derived from patients with hypercalcemia. This study provides convincing evidence for the lack of synthesis of PTH by these tumors. Since most cases of humoral hypercalcemia are now known not to be due to PTH, emphasis has shifted to other peptides that could be involved in the pathogenesis of hypercalcemia in solid tumors not associated with extensive bone metastases.

The factors currently receiving attention are as follows.

PTH-Like Substances. Studies by Stewart and associates revealed a distinct group of patients who had elevated nephrogenous cyclic adenosine monophosphate (cAMP) excretion but absent serum PTH immunoreactivity. Moreover, unlike patients with primary hyperparathyroidism, these patients had low plasma levels of 1,25-dihydroxyvitamin D and high fasting calcium excretion. These findings led to the suggestion that tumors produce factors that act like PTH in some, but not all, respects and that fail to react with PTH antisera.

Extracts of tumors from the aforementioned patients have been found to exhibit, in vitro, adenylate cyclase–stimulating activity owing to peptides that specifically bind to renal receptors. Such activity can be blocked by PTH antagonists but not by PTH antisera. Recently, the structure of a responsible peptide factor has been determined and partial homologies to the aminoterminal region of PTH have been identified. As in PTH, the 1-34 aminoterminal region of the peptide appears to be responsible for biologic activity. The factor also resembles PTH in its ability to interact with the PTH receptor, to stimulate adenyl cyclase production in the kidney, to promote phosphate excretion, and to enhance bone resorption in vitro and in vivo. The identification of this new PTH-like factor is a major step forward in the elucidation of tumor-related hypercalcemia. However, the actual demonstration that this factor circulates in the blood of patients with hypercalcemia awaits the availability of sufficient synthetic peptide to generate an antibody that can be used in a radioimmunoassay.

Transforming Growth Factors (TGFs). The other family of factors that has been implicated in humoral hypercalcemia of malignancy is the tumor-derived growth factors such as TGFs. TGFs are potent stimulators of cell growth and/or differentiation. TGF alpha interacts with the epidermal growth factor (EGF) receptor and causes many of the known biologic effects of EGF, including stimulation of osteoclast function. For example, extracts

of a transplantable rat Leydig's cell tumor, known to elicit hypercalcemia in the absence of bone metastases, have been shown to contain a bone-resorbing factor that co-purifies with TGF alpha. Human TGF alpha has also been shown to be a potent stimulator of bone resorption.

Hematologic Malignancies and Osteolytic Factors

The most important examples of hematologic malignancies associated with hypercalcemia are multiple myeloma and the recently recognized T-cell lymphoma. About 25 percent of patients with multiple myeloma develop hypercalcemia, usually in association with bone involvement. Early studies have suggested that cultured myeloma cells release an osteoclast-activating factor (OAF) that mediates the increased bone resorption. It has now become clear that OAF is not a discrete factor but rather comprises a family of proteins (lymphokines) secreted by normal or mitogen-activated lymphoid cells. In the syndrome of T-cell lymphoma, lymphokines produced by T cells transformed by the human T cell leukemia/lymphoma virus (HTLV-I) are thought to account for the very high incidence of hypercalcemia. Interleukin I, a monocyte product, has also been shown to stimulate osteolysis and may cause the hypercalcemia associated with some monocytic leukemias as well as some forms of lymphoma. There is also evidence that some solid tumors such as squamous cell carcinomas may produce colony-stimulating activity for leukocytes as well as osteoclastic bone activity. These tumors are associated with neutrophilia and hypercalcemia. Since bone-resorbing osteoclasts are believed to be derived from macrophages, it is tempting to speculate that factors that lead to stimulation of proliferation of macrophages could also stimulate osteoclastic bone resorption.

A role for vitamin D has also been suggested in the pathogenesis of hypercalcemia in hematologic malignancies. Breslau and co-workers (1984) found elevated plasma levels of 1,25-dihydroxyvitamin D in three patients with T-cell lymphoma. Subsequently, it was shown that normal human cord blood T-cell lymphocytes infected with the HTLV-I virus acquire the capacity to convert 25-hydroxyvitamin D to 1,25-dihydroxyvitamin D. Excessive production of this active vitamin D metabolite by lymphoma cells, with subsequent osteoclastic activation, must then be considered as a pathogenetic factor for hypercalcemia.

It is thus clear that hypercalcemia can result from activity of several pathways related to behavior of neoplastic cells. Although these pathways have been arbitrarily placed into three categories, as discussed previously, the distinction between them is not always easy to make clinically. Bone metastases may be difficult to demonstrate in any given patient, and more than one mechanism may be operative in any individual with a malignancy and hypercalcemia. Whatever mechanisms are responsible for hypercalcemia in a given patient, they are tied closely to the biology of the underlying tumor. The appreciation that lymphokines and other tumor-derived growth factors have bone-resorbing activity makes it likely that hypercalcemia is tightly linked to the neoplastic process and that osteolysis may actually play a role in the establishment and progression of some forms of cancer.

Diagnosis

The main differential diagnosis of hypercalcemia in a patient with cancer is primary hyperparathyroidism (Table 15-4). Primary hyperparathyroidism should be considered if the hypercalcemia is long-standing (more than 1 year) or if the patient has recurrent kidney stones or subperiosteal bone resorption. Measurement of circulating PTH levels can help in the diagnosis since the hormone is usually distinctly elevated in patients with primary hyperparathyroidism and suppressed in tumor-related hypercalcemia. Occasionally, however, as a result of technical problems with some PTH radioimmunoassays, PTH can be detectable and even somewhat elevated in tumor-related hypercalcemia. In such cases, effort should be made to rule out hyperparathyroidism by computed tomography (CT) or combined technetium and thallium scans of the neck and even selective venous catheterization. Removal of a parathyroid adenoma in a patient with cancer may significantly diminish the morbidity arising from hypercalcemia.

Once hyperparathyroidism has been ruled out, the approach to tumor-related hypercalcemia involves separating those patients with and without skeletal metastases. The presence of bone metastases can usually be ascertained with bone radiographs and scans, but occasionally, such lesions are difficult to document. The tumors in this group of patients are predominantly breast cancer, multiple myeloma, lymphomas, and usually SCLC and adenocarcinomas of the lung. In patients with these tumors, as well as hypercalcemia, and especially in those with breast cancer, the skeletal involvement is invariably extensive. In fact, the absence of defined bone metastases in a patient with breast cancer and hypercalcemia should raise the suspicion of coexistent primary hyperparathyroidism.

It is often more difficult to make the diagnosis of humoral hypercalcemia of malignancy, since existing diagnostic modalities cannot always rule out the presence of skeletal metastases. In fact, the only definitive diagnosis of this form of cancer-associated hypercalcemia must rely on the normalization of serum calcium after successful treatment of the associated tumor. Unfortunately, with present treatment modalities, the tumors in this group of patients, usually squamous cell tumors of the head, neck, and lung as well as renal carcinomas, are difficult to remove as the source of hypercalcemia. Measurement of PTH levels can help in diagnosis, because in the advanced states of cancers often associated with hypercalcemia, circulating PTH levels are usually not elevated. By contrast, urinary excretion of cAMP may be high owing to the effect of PTH-like substances on the kidney. Because, as discussed previously, many important bone-resorbing factors have been identified only recently, specific assays for their detection are still not available for clinical use. Measuring levels of 1,25-dihydroxyvitamin D may be useful since these levels tend to be low in the hormonally mediated hypercalcemia of malignancy and high in primary hyperparathyroidism. However, there is often overlap between the levels in these entities, and in some tumors, such as lymphomas, vitamin D is actually produced by the tumor and contributes to osteoclastic bone resorption.

THE ECTOPIC CUSHING'S SYNDROME

Biologic Aspects

The association of Cushing's syndrome with nonendocrine tumors was first recognized in 1928, when Brown described a patient with hypercortisolism and noted at autopsy the existence of an oat (small) cell carcinoma (SCLC) of the lung. The precise causal relationship between the two entities was not delineated. In 1961, corticotropic activity was measured in the plasma of two patients with cancer, using an adrenal weight maintenance assay. Shortly thereafter, an ACTH-like substance was identified in tumor tissues, thus tracing the origin of this hormonal material to a nonendocrine source. In his classic review in 1969, Liddle characterized further the syndrome of "ectopic" ACTH production and suggested that the "ectopic" ACTH molecule was similar to that of pituitary ACTH.

Tumors derived from APUD cells account for the vast majority of cases of ectopic Cushing's syndrome. SCLC is associated with more than 50 percent of reported cases. Pancreatic islet cell tumors, carcinoid tumors of the lung and thymus, medullary thyroid carcinomas, and pheochromocytomas are responsible, in comparable percentages, for the remaining 50 percent of cases.

The incidence of ectopic Cushing's syndrome is low, even in association with SCLC (3.2 to 4.8 percent of all patients with this neoplasm). By contrast, ACTH immunoreactivity is found in the majority of lung tumor extracts and in the plasma of many patients with lung cancer.

TABLE 15-4   Diagnostic Approach to Tumor-Related Hypercalcemia

Rule out primary hyperparathyroidism (history, PTH levels, neck scans, and selective venous catheterization if indicated).

Look for skeletal metastases by radiologic and nuclear medicine studies.

Look for evidence of PTH-like factors and other mediators of hypercalcemia: urine cAMP excretion, 1,25-dihydroxyvitamin D levels.

ACTH and POMC-Derived Peptides

The ACTH precursor molecule, or POMC, undergoes enzymatic cleavage with resultant production of ACTH and other POMC-derived peptides. In the anterior lobe of the pituitary, a first proteolytic step causes the release of an N terminal peptide, which includes ACTH as well as beta-lipotropic hormone (βLPH). Further cleavage results in the production of ACTH itself, γLPH, and beta-endorphin. In the intermediate lobe of the pituitary, further processing results in the production of melanocyte-stimulating hormones (MSHs).

Ectopic ACTH-producing tumors have been shown to produce βLPH, endorphin, and βMSH, suggesting that these peptides come from a common precursor as in the pituitary. This was confirmed when RNA extracted from a thymic carcinoid was found to direct the synthesis, in a cell-free translation system, of a protein with ACTH and beta-endorphin immunoreactivity, which was similar in size to the pituitary ACTH precursor molecule. Several studies, however, suggested that the post-transcriptional and post-translational processing of the POMC molecule was altered in nonpituitary tumors. In one study, the nonpituitary tumors, in comparison to pituitary cells, had exaggerated processing of the POMC molecule to γMSH and βMSH. Also, hybridization of a cDNA for bovine POMC to RNA extracted from carcinoid tumors revealed two species of POMC-specific mRNA. The predominant species was similar in size to pituitary POMC-specific mRNA (1,200 base pairs), and a minor, slightly larger species (approximately 1,400 base pairs) was also detected. These studies suggest that a similar POMC gene is expressed in both pituitary tissue and nonpituitary ACTH-producing tumors but that transcription and post-transcriptional steps may be somewhat different. The POMC mRNA species that is detected in low amounts exclusively in carcinoid tumors may represent an incompletely processed transcript of the POMC gene.

CRF

In 1971, Upton and Amatruda detected CRF-like activity, in addition to ACTH, in pancreatic and lung tumors of patients with the ectopic Cushing's syndrome. They proposed that the ectopic production of CRF may have stimulated production of ACTH. The biochemical and immunologic characterization of CRF was established several years later, when CRF was isolated from ovine hypothalami. The human CRF gene was subsequently cloned and characterized. Recently, several patients with ectopic CRF secretion has been reported, including one patient with prostatic carcinoma, one with an intrasellar gangliocytoma, and one with medullary thyroid carcinoma. The features of Cushing's syndrome associated with ectopic CRF production include hyperplasia of the ACTH-producing cells of the pituitary, a reflection of stimulation by CRF. This is in contrast to findings in patients with ectopic ACTH production in whom the pituitary gland ACTH secretion and growth of pituitary cells are suppressed. Cortisol production in the ectopic CRF syndrome, unlike in the ectopic ACTH syndrome, may be responsive to dexamethasone suppression and metyrapone stimulation. Thus, the dynamics of steroid secretion and synthesis in patients with tumor production of CRF may be indistinguishable from those of patients with pituitary-dependent Cushing's syndrome. There is, then, difficulty in making the diagnosis between these two entities.

Diagnosis

The recognition of the ectopic Cushing's syndrome is important because hypercortisolism can contribute significantly to the morbidity and mortality of patients with cancer. The most common type of tumor associated with the ectopic Cushing's syndrome, SCLC, progresses rapidly, and often, patients do not have time to develop the full phenotypic characteristics of Cushing's syndrome. Rather, the metabolic abnormalities associated with glucocorticoid excess (muscle weakness, mental disturbances, carbohydrate intolerance), mineralocorticoid excess (hypertension, edema, hypokalemic alkalosis), and androgen excess in women (hirsutism, menstrual irregularities) often dominate the clinical picture. In addition, the production of excessive amounts of melanotropic POMC products such as βLPH, γMSH, and βMSH may cause skin hyperpigmentation.

The diagnosis of ectopic Cushing's syndrome is, then, sometimes difficult to make, especially when the symptomatology is minimal. The stress alone on the patients with cancer who are undergoing traumatic hospital experiences may lead to elevations of plasma ACTH as well as to abnormal cortisol secretion dynamics. General guidelines for the differential diagnosis of the ectopic Cushing's syndrome are shown in Figure 15–1. Urinary free cortisol measurements are seldom affected by stress and hence should be used to document the presence of hypercortisolism. High-dose dexamethasone testing classically demonstrates lack of suppression of the levels of urinary 17-hydroxycorticosteroids in the ectopic Cushing's syndrome. However, in some patients suffering from carcinoid tumors, or in those patients with tumors producing CRF, the steroid dynamics during dexamethasone administration may be indistinguishable from those seen in pituitary Cushing's syndrome, and suppressibility with high-dose dexamethasone may be observed. In such patients, if CT or magnetic resonance imaging (MRI) scans of the pituitary region fail to reveal a pituitary adenoma, petrosal sinus catheterization may be indicated to localize the source of ACTH or CRF production.

The administration of CRF has also recently been shown to be useful in discriminating between the ectopic Cushing's syndrome and pituitary-dependent Cushing's syndrome. Patients with pituitary Cushing's often demonstrate a marked increase in ACTH secretion,

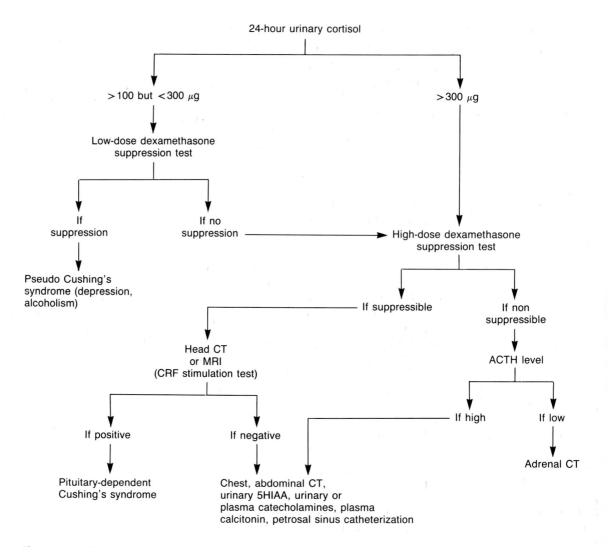

Figure 15-1   Diagnostic approach to the ectopic Cushing's syndrome.

whereas no response is seen in those with ectopic Cushing's syndrome. If dexamethasone and/or CRF tests are negative for the presence of pituitary disease, then anatomic localization of the ectopic source of ACTH or CRF should be pursued. Biochemical tests, as indicated in the flowchart (see Fig. 15–1), should be used to rule out the common tumors associated with the ectopic Cushing's syndrome such as carcinoids, pheochromocytomas, and medullary thyroid carcinomas.

THE SYNDROME OF INAPPROPRIATE ANTIDIURETIC HORMONE (SIADH)

In 1957, Schwartz and colleagues reported two patients with bronchogenic carcinoma who had marked hyponatremia due to persistent urinary sodium loss and an impaired ability to properly reduce urine concentration. It was postulated that these metabolic abnormalities were due to excessive antidiuretic hormone (ADH)

production arising either from tumor impingement on an intrathoracic structure such as the vagus nerve or by invasion, by metastases from the tumor, of a brain area involved in the regulation of ADH secretion. In the early 1960s, Amatruda and co-workers detected, by bioassay, large amounts of antidiuretic activity in a tumor tissue derived from a patient with bronchogenic carcinoma and hyponatremia, thus raising the possibility of ADH synthesis by the tumor. The material extracted from tumors of patients with inappropriate antidiuresis was further characterized and found to be biochemically and immunologically similar to ADH.

Inappropriate ADH secretion is associated predominantly with SCLC, although other tumors, including thymomas, gastrointestinal tumors, genitourinary tumors, and central nervous tissue neoplasms, rarely cause this syndrome. The true frequency of ADH production by tumors is difficult to establish since excess ADH production is not always accompanied by metabolic abnormalities. Indeed, patients with lung tumors who do not have hyponatremia have been shown to have higher plasma levels of ADH than normal subjects. On the other hand, all patients with SIADH do not have high basal levels of ADH. However, in these individuals, the ADH levels are clearly inappropriately high in relation to the hypotonicity of the plasma.

Biologic Aspects

ADH or vasopressin is synthesized in the hypothalamus as a composite precursor, provasopressin, which consists of the hormone vasopressin, its carrier protein neurophysin, and a glycoprotein. Investigation of the biosynthetic pathway for ADH in a transplantable SCLC model revealed that vasopressin is synthesized by post-translational processing from the aforementioned precursor, which is a glycosylated 20,000-dalton protein. The precursor has been detected in the plasma of patients with SCLC, but not in the plasma of patients with inappropriate ADH secretion stemming from overproduction of ADH in the posterior pituitary occurring in the setting of central nervous system disease. This finding suggests that, as for ACTH, ADH may be secreted from tumors as an unprocessed precursor. The detection of this precursor in the circulation strongly suggests the diagnosis of ectopic ADH production by tumor. Studies aimed at characterizing, in tumors, the mRNA encoding ADH and comparing it to its hypothalamic counterpart should provide definitive proof of ADH production by tumors.

Diagnosis

The extent of symptoms of hyponatremia, which include lethargy, confusion, and muscle cramps, depends on the level of serum sodium, its rate of decline, and the age of the patient. The diagnosis of SIADH in a patient with cancer should be entertained whenever hyponatremia is found in concert with serum hypo-osmolarity, hypertonic urine, and elevated urinary sodium (Table 15-5). Other causes of hyponatremia such as hypothyroidism and adrenal insufficiency should be carefully ruled out. Also, the physician should rule out the contribution of drugs that are known to cause SIADH, in particular the antitumor drugs cyclophosphamide and vincristine as well as tranquilizers and antidepressants.

ACROMEGALY

Biologic Aspects

Well-documented instances of acromegaly have occurred in patients with nonpituitary neoplasms and especially with carcinoid and pancreatic islet cell tumors. Acromegaly in these patients is due to the ectopic production by the tumor either of growth hormone itself or of the growth hormone–releasing factor (GRF). GH im-

TABLE 15-5 Diagnostic Signs of SIADH

Hyponatremia (serum sodium <130 mEq/L)
Hypo-osmolarity (<275 mOsm/kg)
Urinary sodium >20 mEq/L
Hypertonic urine
Absence of volume depletion, congestive heart failure, renal failure, cirrhosis, hypothyroidism, hypoadrenalism, and drugs known to cause the syndrome

munoreactivity, even in the absence of symptoms of acromegaly, has been detected in several cancers, including lung, stomach, ovary, and breast carcinomas. Occasionally, however, GH production by nonpituitary tumors can lead to dramatic biologic effects. Recently, Melmed and colleagues reported a patient with acromegaly due to ectopic GH production by a pancreatic tumor. The tumor tissue contained GH-specific mRNA, and the symptoms of acromegaly resolved after resection of the tumor.

The association of excessive GRF production by nonpituitary tumors and clinical signs and symptoms of GH excess were recognized as early as the 1970s. In fact, the structure of GRF was first determined by study of a peptide isolated from pancreatic tumors removed from acromegalic individuals. Cloned cDNA complementary to GRF mRNA became available soon after, and when the human hypothalamic GRF gene was cloned, it was shown to be identical to its pancreatic counterpart.

As mentioned earlier for GH, GRF immunoreactivity has been found in a large variety of tumors that rarely are associated with acromegaly. However, there have been several well-documented cases of acromegaly due to ectopic GRF production by tumors arising primarily from endocrine cells such as SCLCs, carcinoids, pancreatic islet cell tumors, pheochromocytomas, neuroblastomas, and medullary thyroid carcinomas.

Clinical Aspects

The ectopic production of either GH or GRF should be suspected when a patient with cancer develops acromegalic features such as coarsening of the facial features and increased hand or shoe size. The diagnosis of acromegaly can be made by demonstrating elevated levels of GH that are not suppressible by glucose administration. A GH-producing pituitary adenoma should be ruled out by CT or MRI scans of the head. However, in the case of GRF production by the tumor, the pituitary may also be enlarged because of the chronic stimulating effects of GRF.

Since the tumors that have been associated with GRF production are usually endocrine tumors (carcinoids and pancreatic islet cell tumors), the diagnosis of ectopic GRF syndrome must be carefully differentiated from that of multiple endocrine neoplasia (MEN) syndrome Type I and its associated pituitary tumors. MEN-I should be excluded by careful family history and a search for concomitant hyperparathyroidism. Evidence of ectopic GRF production by the endocrine tumor in question should be sought by immunohistochemical analysis of the tumor tissue. Following treatment for the GRF-producing endocrine neoplasm, the patient must be monitored for regression of any pituitary enlargement and of acromegalic features.

TUMOR HYPOGLYCEMIA

Hypoglycemia has been described, as early as the late 1920s, in association with non–islet cell tumors such as hepatomas and fibrosarcomas. Subsequently, it was reported in conjunction with a large variety of tumors, but mostly with other mesenchymal tumors, including leiomyosarcomas, and adrenocortical carcinomas.

Biologic Aspects

Several mechanisms have been proposed to explain the etiology of tumor hypoglycemia. Excessive glucose utilization by tumors and/or failure in patients of mechanisms for reversing hypoglycemia (e.g., deficient glucagon release, inefficient mobilization of glycogen stores) are two of the postulated etiologies of tumor hypoglycemia. However, many patients may have this problem secondary to hormonal output by the neoplastic tissue. Insulin has been detected by bioassays in several tumor types. Definitive proof of true insulin production by extrapancreatic neoplasms is, however, lacking since studies using radioimmunoassays failed to confirm the earlier biologic observations. By contrast, factors with insulin-like biologic activity have been strongly implicated in the pathogenesis of hypoglycemia in tumors. These factors are referred to as nonsuppressible insulin-like activity (NSILA) because they do not cross-react with insulin antibodies in insulin radioimmunoassays. The components of NSILA include insulin-like growth factor I (IGF-I), also known as somatomedin-C, and IGF-II, also known as multiplication-stimulating activity.

The isolation of the preceding factors and the development of specific radioreceptor assays and radioimmunoassays have allowed investigators to study the role of NSILA in tumor hypoglycemia. The results of these studies have been controversial. Some investigators have found high levels of IGF-II in up to 50 percent of patients with extrapancreatic tumors and hypoglycemia, whereas others found no difference in IGF-II levels between these patients and normal subjects. These discrepancies are thought to be due to differences in the assay systems employed. The characterization of the IGF-I and -II genes has made it possible to study the production of these growth factors by tumors at the mRNA level. So far, increased IGF-II expression has been demonstrated only in Wilms' tumors, which are usually not associated with hypoglycemia.

Clinical Aspects

Nonpancreatic tumors associated with hypoglycemia usually present as very large retroperitoneal mass lesions, which are often unresectable. Palliative treatment is then all that can be offered to many patients with tumor-associated hypoglycemia. An adequate caloric intake and constant glucose supplementation are often all that is needed. Glucagon and glucocorticoids that stimulate hepatic glucose production are sometimes of transient benefit.

HUMAN CHORIONIC GONADOTROPIN (hCG) AND ITS SUBUNITS

Sexual precocity in children and gynecomastia in adult males have been known to occur in association with neoplasms, especially hepatoblastomas and large cell lung carcinomas. As early as 1959, the source of the excessive gonadotropic activity was traced to the tumor cells. The development of specific radioimmunoassays for the various human glycoprotein hormones (thyroid-stimulating hormone [TSH], follicle-stimulating hormone, luteinizing hormone, and hCG) has led to the appreciation that hCG is almost exclusively the source of the gonadotropic activity found in nontrophblastic tumors.

With the use of a specific hCG radioimmunoassay, the frequency and types of tumors producing hCG were assessed in a survey of many patients with various types of malignancies. As expected, the incidence of elevated serum hCG levels was very high in trophoblastic tumors (100 percent of choriocarcinomas, 56 percent of testicular embryonal carcinomas, 37.5 percent of seminomas). By contrast, serum levels of hCG were detectable by radioimmunoassay, in only 11 percent of the nontrophoblastic tumors, and these included pancreatic neoplasms, and bronchogenic carcinomas. Interestingly, imbalanced or isolated production of the subunits of hCG, occasionally involving the hCG-specific beta subunit and more often the alpha subunit common to all human glycoprotein hormones, also occurs in patients with various forms of malignancies. In a study of several patients with pancreatic islet cell tumors, Kahn and associates found that up to two-thirds of patients with functioning malignant tumors had elevated serum levels of hCG or one of its subunits, most commonly the alpha subunit. By contrast, none of the patients with benign islet tumors had detectable levels of hCG or one of its subunits in their serum. These data led to the suggestion that hCG and its subunits could be used as specific markers for malignant islet cell tumors.

Patients with carcinoid tumors have also been found to have a significant incidence of increased serum alpha subunit, and elevations are also found in a small percentage of patients with lung cancers and patients with non–islet cell gastrointestinal tract malignancies. However, the alpha subunit has not proved to be a useful marker for cancer screening or for monitoring the course of patients with the vast majority of cancers.

Biologic Aspects

Data about the molecular aspects of hCG production by tumors have been obtained mostly from cell culture systems. Several cell lines derived from human tumors have been shown to produce hCG and/or one of its subunits. The HeLa cell line, derived from a carcinoma of the cervix, is a well-studied example of such tumors. Sodium butyrate induces synthesis of hCG and the alpha subunit in this tumor cell line but represses it in a trophoblastic cell line derived from choriocarcinoma. This would suggest that the regulation of hCG production is different in ectopic versus eutopic sources of this hormone. When the structure of the alpha-subunit gene was compared in normal placenta, hydatidiform moles, and choriocarcinomas, an uncommon DNA polymorphism pattern predominated in choriocarcinoma. These data raise the possibility that a particular DNA rearrangement at the alpha-subunit locus predisposes to malignancy. Also, when hCG-producing HeLa cells are fused with normal fibroblasts, expression of the hCG alpha subunit in the hybrids correlates specifically with the tumorigenicity of these hybrids. These data suggest either that the hCG alpha subunit is involved in cell growth regulation or that a certain DNA rearrangement at the hCG alpha-subunit locus involves closely linked genes that are more directly implicated in the malignant process, similar to the situation seen with the myc oncogene and immunoglobulin loci.

Clinical Aspects

Only rare patients develop signs and symptoms of excessive hCG production by tumors. Tumors associated with precocious puberty in children and gynecomastia in adult males are usually far advanced and respond poorly to treatment. It is important, however, in the evaluation of children with precocious puberty or adult males with gynecomastia to rule out ectopic hCG production, since this may lead to the early recognition and treatment of a potentially fatal tumor.

ERYTHROCYTOSIS

Erythrocytosis has been reported in association with cerebellar hemangiomas, hepatomas, and renal carcinomas and has been attributed to the production of erythropoietin-like substances by these tumors. Several reports of secretion of erythropoietin-like activity by such tumors in culture have appeared in the literature. In these reports, erythropoietin was measured by bioassays. Most radioimmunoassays for erythropoietin, as yet, lack the sensitivity and specificity to confirm the biologic data even though purified erythropoietin has now been available for more than a decade.

The production of erythropoietin-like activity has also been demonstrated by in vitro translation of mRNA extracted from a renal carcinoma. The translation product has the biologic properties of true erythropoietin. Also, an erythropoietin cDNA clone has been isolated from a human kidney carcinoma. The recent cloning of the human genomic erythropoietin gene will allow a more extensive analysis, at the mRNA level, of erythropoietin production by tumors.

The excessive production of erythropoietin-like activity by tumors results in an erythrocytosis that is usually asymptomatic but may require phlebotomy in severe cases. The erythrocytosis usually resolves with successful tumor treatment.

TUMOR-RELATED OSTEOMALACIA

Tumor-related osteomalacia is a rare syndrome believed to be due to the production, by tumors, of factors that cause renal phosphate loss. The tumors associated with this syndrome are usually small mesenchymal tumors located in bone and soft tissue, but instances of prostatic carcinoma and SCLC have also been reported in association with hypophosphatemic osteomalacia.

Biologic Aspects

The exact pathogenic mechanism underlying this tumor-related osteomalacia is still unknown. Renal phosphate loss and decreased levels of 1,25-dihydroxyvitamin D are common features of this syndrome. The mediator of the phosphaturia is still unidentified but is probably secreted by the tumor cells since resection of the tumors results in dramatic cure of the hypophosphatemia and osteomalacia. The decreased levels of 1,25-dihydroxyvitamin D are due to impairment of the renal 1-alpha-hydroxylation of the 25-hydroxyvitamin D metabolite, possibly also by a substance produced by the tumor.

Clinical Aspects

Muscle weakness and bone pain in the presence of profound hypophosphatemia in an adult should lead to the suspicion of tumor-related osteomalacia. The search for a tumor should be diligent since the tumors may be small and difficult to find. Complete tumor resection leads to a dramatic resolution of the hypophosphatemia and osteomalacia. If surgical treatment is not feasible, or if the tumor cannot be localized, treatment with phosphorus and 1,25-dihydroxyvitamin D will produce a marked amelioration of the symptoms.

HYPERTHYROIDISM

Hyperthyroidism can occasionally occur in patients with hydatidiform moles and choriocarcinomas and is believed to be due to the thyrotropic activity associated with the high levels of hCG produced by these tumors. Characteristically, these patients have goiters and increased radioactive iodine uptake due to thyroid stimulation by the TSH-like activity of hCG. Ophthalmopathy and any other stigmata of Graves' disease are absent, and the hyperthyroidism resolves with treatment of the neoplasm. Occasionally, the symptoms of thyrotoxicosis are severe enough to require temporary treatment with antithyroid drugs such as methimazole and propylthiouracil.

Immunoreactive thyrotropin-releasing hormone (TRH) has been identified in human neoplasms. However, the occurrence of thyrotoxicosis with such tumors is unlikely because very slight elevations in serum thyroid hormones can completely inhibit pituitary TSH responses to TRH.

RENIN PRODUCTION AND HYPERTENSION

The rare situation of hypertension secondary to renin production by tumors has been described mostly with renal juxtaglomerular cell tumors but also with pancreatic, ovarian, and pulmonary carcinomas. The renin present in the tumor extracts and plasma of these patients is biochemically similar to that found in normal human kidney. However, a markedly elevated inactive renin (prorenin) to renin ratio is consistently observed in patients with ectopic renin production. This observation suggests that, as in the case of ACTH or ADH, the post-translational processing of large hormone precursors in tumors is inefficient when compared with that in normal tissue.

Ectopic renin production should be suspected when a patient with cancer develops hypertension and hypokalemia. Proof of renin secretion by the tumor should be obtained by examining tissues for renin content. Successful treatment of the underlying tumor can lead to a complete resolution of symptoms. However, since the types of tumors associated with ectopic renin production (pancreatic, ovarian, lung carcinomas) are often not amenable to cure, treatment with the angiotensin-converting enzyme inhibitor, captopril, is indicated for palliation of symptoms.

PROLACTIN

In 1971, Turkington described a patient with undifferentiated bronchogenic carcinoma and another patient with hypernephroma, who had elevated serum levels of prolactin. Prolactin levels declined significantly following irradiation of the lung cancer and surgical excision of the hypernephroma. Also, when maintained in culture, the hypernephroma cells actively secreted prolactin, thus providing evidence for prolactin production by this tumor.

Subsequently, investigators examined the frequency of prolactin production by tumors and reported an incidence of hyperprolactinemia associated with certain tumor types and especially bronchogenic carcinomas. However, when known mechanisms leading to hyperprolactinemia (e.g., several kinds of drugs, chest wall irritation) are excluded, ectopic prolactin production seems to be a rare event. In the largest series reported by Molitch and co-workers (1981), only 2 out of 215 patients with various malignancies had clearly elevated prolactin levels.

In contrast to the patient data, when established cell lines of various tumor types are examined, the frequency of significant prolactin production is 25 percent. Interestingly, in such cultures, prolactin is not detected in the medium, suggesting that the enzymatic machinery of the cells is unable to process the hormone to the mature form for secretion. Similarly, in one study, immunoreactive prolactin was detected in two-thirds of human prostate and breast cancer tissues, yet serum prolactin levels are usually not elevated in patients with these tumors.

In conclusion, although there is clear evidence of prolactin production by tumor cells, serum levels are rarely elevated in patients with cancer, and no cases of galactorrhea in women or gynecomastia and impotence in men have been documented to result from ectopic prolactin secretion.

CALCITONIN

Calcitonin is normally produced by the C cells of the thyroid gland. Levels of this peptide hormone are greatly increased in the serum of patients with MTC. However, calcitonin is not an exclusive marker of MTC and elevated circulating levels are seen in other neoplasms such as lung, breast, pancreas, stomach, and colon cancers. Among the different types of lung cancer, calcitonin production is most often associated with SCLC. However, careful analysis of the various types of lung cancers reveals that calcitonin is produced by 54 percent of SCLC, 50 percent of adenocarcinomas, 55 percent of large cell undifferentiated tumors, and 33 percent of squamous cell carcinomas.

Biologic Aspects

Calcitonin, like other small peptide hormones, is initially synthesized in the form of a large polypeptide precursor. In contrast to the predominantly small molecular-weight forms of calcitonin found in MTC, the immunoreactive calcitonin forms detected in lung tumors are large and presumably represent precursor molecules. The availability of the cloned calcitonin gene has also allowed study at the mRNA level of calcitonin production by tumors. The calcitonin gene comprises six exons or coding domains. By alternative splicing of the primary RNA transcript from this gene, two distinct mRNA molecules are produced. One mRNA encodes calcitonin, and a second mRNA encodes a peptide referred to as calcitonin gene-related peptide (CGRP). The expression of these peptides is tissue-specific. Thus, calcitonin is expressed in the thyroid, and CGRP appears to predominate in the central nervous system. Calcitonin and CGRP mRNA have been detected in several human lung tumor cell lines, including small cell, large cell, adenocarcinomas, and squamous carcinomas. In some of these studies, the ratio of CGRP to calcitonin mRNA seems to be higher than that found in a human MTC cell line. This finding suggests differential processing of the calcitonin gene in these different neoplasms. The size of the predominant calcitonin gene mRNA in non-MTC tumors is identical to that expressed in MTC, although large-molecular-weight mRNA species are occasionally seen. These findings in non-MTC tumors of large forms of calcitonin mRNA, of high CGRP to calcitonin mRNA ratios, as well as of large-molecular-weight calcitonin precursors suggest that the post-transcriptional and post-translational processing of calcitonin may be altered in the non-MTC tumors.

Clinical Aspects

Calcitonin production by non-MTC tumors tends to be asymptomatic. The levels of calcitonin are usually not high enough in the blood to cause flushing, diarrhea, or any of the symptoms that may be associated with the very high calcitonin levels in patients with MTC.

Investigations have been directed at the utility of measuring circulating calcitonin levels to monitor tumor burden and disease activity in patients with SCLC. Although this approach may occasionally be useful in selected patients, in general the calcitonin levels have not tracked well with disease status. This is probably due to the fact, as discussed previously, that neoplasia is a dynamic process and that events in tumor progression may lead to change in the status of endocrine differentiation of tumor cells.

It is interesting to note that, even in MTC, plasma calcitonin is not always a useful tumor marker. Patients with widely disseminated and aggressive MTC do not always have an increase in plasma calcitonin in proportion to their tumor mass. In fact, analysis of tumor tissues by immunohistochemistry from such patients reveals a significant cellular heterogeneity for calcitonin content, as well as a lower tumor tissue calcitonin content than found in tumors from patients with indolent disease. Apparently, in patients with virulent MTC, as well as in patients with ectopic calcitonin production, multiple levels of calcitonin gene expression are altered, including changes in selective RNA splicing during tumor progression.

OTHER NEUROENDOCRINE PEPTIDES

In the past two decades, a great number of small peptides have been discovered in addition to those discussed previously, and these appear to function as neuro-modulators in the brain and/or hormones in the circulation. These hormones are found in a variety of tissues. Thus, the term *ectopic* is particularly inappropriate when referring to the production by tumors of these peptides.

Most of these peptides, such as somatostatin, glucagon, gastrin, and vasoactive intestinal polypeptide, are, like the hormones previously mentioned, derived from large precursor molecules. These precursors can be the source of more than one peptide and thus generate a tremendous diversity of biologic activity. Tissue-specific processing of these precursors or of their corresponding genes appears to be yet another source of complexity in the biosynthesis of these peptides.

Immunoreactivity for peptides such as glucagon, somatostatin, and pancreatic polypeptide has been detected in many tumors and most frequently in carcinoids. Clinical manifestations resulting from the excessive production of these hormones by tumors are rare but can, on occasion, be impressive.

For example, elevated vasoactive intestinal polypeptide levels have been demonstrated in plasma and tumor extracts from patients with the watery diarrhea syndrome and a variety of tumors, including bronchogenic carcinomas and pheochromocytomas. Elevated gastrin levels and the Zollinger-Ellison syndrome have been associated with an ovarian tumor. Also, a high level of pancreatic polypeptide, accompanied by flushing and tachycardia, has been observed in a patient with a gastric tumor. More often, however, these neuropeptides are detected only in tumor tissue, while corresponding plasma levels are not simultaneously increased.

The production of gastrin-releasing peptide (GRP), which is closely related to the amphibian molecule bombesin, has been described in SCLC. GRP production by these tumors has been detected by radioimmunoassays and recently by mRNA analysis. Three distinct mRNAs for GRP are detected in SCLC and are believed to arise from a single primary transcript by an alternative splicing mechanism. Even though the main biologic activity of GRP is gastrin release, none of the patients with ectopic GRP production have been documented to be predisposed to peptic ulcer. However, GRP has generated much interest as a potential autocrine growth factor for SCLC. Antibodies to GRP have been shown to block the growth of this tumor in culture, and this finding opens possible new avenues for treatment approach to patients with SCLC.

CONCLUSION

In this chapter, an attempt has been made to summarize some of the recent biologic and clinical developments in the field of hormone production by neoplasms. Although it is clear that no unifying concept can explain why tumor cells may elaborate high quantities of hormones not produced in great amounts by the corresponding normal cells, recent advances in molecular and cellular biology are beginning to clarify this phenomenon. It seems impossible at present to separate the problem of hormone production by neoplasms from an understanding of the mechanisms underlying the regulatory processes of gene expression, of normal cell differentiation, and of cellular transformation. From the information currently at hand, the following overall conclusions concerning the relationships between tumors and the production of hormones can be made.

Investigators working in this field are now asking questions about the molecular basis of aberrant hormone production by neoplasms. Increasingly sophisticated techniques of peptide and nucleic acid analysis, plus the use of complex cell culture systems, have characterized hormones at the peptide level and led to the delineation of the multiple steps involved in the biosynthesis of hormones both in normal endocrine cells as well as in tumor cells.

The understanding of events in the regulation of hormone gene expression in tumors as well as in normal tissues is now being actively pursued, with emphasis on DNA rearrangements, restriction enzyme site polymorphisms, methylation patterns, as well as the identification of DNA sequences acting as promoters or enhancers and of regulatory events for transcription and translation. Manipulation of cells in culture is also used to examine the process of gene expression by tumors. For example, deletion of specific DNA sequences from a given gene followed by transfer of such a gene into defined cells in culture is likely to provide, in the near future, clues about the specific nucleotide sequences involved in transcriptional control and regulation of proteolytic processing of hormones in different tissues.

More emphasis is being placed on the potential functional role of hormone production by neoplastic cells. Neoplasia is classically thought of as a disorder of cell growth and cell-to-cell communication. Several lines of evidence suggest that the various hormones produced by tumors may be intimately involved in the aberrant growth of cancer cells. For example, insulin acts as a growth factor in some tumors in culture, leading to stimulation of cell proliferation and expression of oncogenes such as c-myc. Also, some of the growth factors produced by tumors are themselves homologous to oncogenes. Thus, platelet-derived growth factor, a potent mitogen for mesenchymal cells, seems to be identical to the product of the oncogene, v-sis. Also, the receptor for EGF is structurally related to the transforming protein encoded by another oncogene, v-erb-B. Some of these growth factors may play a role in the etiology of the well-recognized paraneoplastic syndromes. For example, a role for TGF alpha has been proposed in the development of some cutaneous manifestations associated with cancers such as the multiple skin tags and the acanthosis nigricans that accompany malignant melanomas. Also, a factor produced by endotoxin-stimulated macrophages, cachectin, may play a role in the chronic catabolic state and general cachexia that accompany malignancy. The high frequency with which certain hormones are simultaneously produced in tumors, such as ACTH, GRP, and calcitonin, would suggest that the genes coding for these hormones are linked to one or more genes intimately involved in the establishment and progression of the malignant process such as oncogenes. One can thus imagine a situation in which the expression of combinations of genes could be simultaneously increased in a tumor by activation of a common promoter or enhancer and/or by increased levels of a transcription factor active for a family of hormone genes.

Finally, further dissection of the association between peptide hormone elaboration and tumors could lead to improved therapeutic modalities for cancer. We have stressed in this chapter that the expression of peptide hormone genes may be intimately linked to the neoplastic process itself in several ways. First, such gene expression may mark cellular events in early steps of neoplastic transformation. If so, identification of regulatory mechanisms for expression of peptide hormone genes could elucidate new target points for manipulation of cancer cells. Second, we have outlined relationships between the status of overall cellular differentiation and the degree of endocrine differentiation for cell populations in common neoplasms such as lung cancer. It is now a much sought after goal to use agents that alter the differentiation status of cells to treat different forms of tumors. Endocrine biochemistry could be a potential monitor for the effects of such drugs.

Finally, we have discussed the potential autocrine and paracrine roles that peptide hormones could play in tumors. Altering the levels of such hormones, through changing the differentiation status of the cells and/or directly blocking hormonal effects with antibodies to the hormones themselves or their receptors, could potentially influence neoplastic cell growth. For example, the use of antibodies to GRP has been shown to block the growth the SCLC in culture. It seems likely that the next years of research into the mechanisms underlying "aberrant" hormone production by tumors will include a focus on these possibilities for cancer therapy.

BIBLIOGRAPHY

General

Abe K, Abachi I, Miyakawa, S, et al. Production of calcitonin, adrenocorticotropic hormone and beta-melanocyte-stimulating hormone in tumors derived from amine precursor uptake and decarboxylation cells. Cancer Res 1977; 37:4190.

Abeloff MD, Eggleston JC, Mendelsohn G, et al. Changes in morphologic and biochemical characteristics of small cell carcinoma of the lung—clinicopathologic study. Am J Med, 1979; 66:757.

Abeloff MD, Trump DL, Baylin SB. Ectopic adrenocorticotrophic (ACTH) syndrome and small cell carcinoma of the lung—assessment of clinical implications in patients on combination chemotherapy. Cancer 1981; 48:1082.

Baylin SB, Mendelsohn G. Ectopic (inappropriate) hormone production by tumors: Mechanisms involved and the biological and clinical implications. Endocr Rev 1980; 1:45.

Baylin SB, Mendelsohn G. Medullary thyroid carcinoma: A model for the study of tumor progression and cell heterogeneity. In Owens AH Jr., Coffey DS, Baylin SB, eds. Tumor cell meterogeneity—origins and implications. New York: Academic Press, 1982:9.

Berger CL, Goodwin G, Mendelsohn G, et al. Endocrine-related biochemistry in the spectrum of human lung carcinoma. J Clin Endocrinol Metab 1981; 53:422.

Bodner M, Karin M. A pituitary-specific trans-acting factor can stimulate transcription from the growth hormone promoter in extracts of nonexpressing cells. Cell 1987; 50:267.

Boothby M, Ruddon RW, Anderson C, et al. A single gonadotropin α-subunit gene in normal tissue and tumor-derived cell lines. J Biol Chem 1981; 256:5121.

Borkowski A, Muquardt C. Human chorionic gonadotropin in the plasma of normal, nonpregnant subjects. N Engl J Med 1979; 301:298.

Brereton HD, Mathews MM, Costa J, et al. Mixed anaplastic small-cell and squamous-cell carcinoma of the lung. Ann Intern Med 1978; 88:805.

Brownstein M, Arimura A, Sato H, et al. The regional distribution of somatostatin in the rat brain. Endocrinology 1975; 96:1456.

Chen C-L C, Chang C-C, Krieger DT, et al. Expression and regulation of proopiomelanocortin-like gene in the ovary and placenta: Comparison with the testis. Endocrinology 1986; 118:2382.

DeBold CR, Schworer ME, Conner TB, et al. Ectopic proopiolipomelanocortin: Sequence of cDNA coding for β-melanocyte-stimulating hormone and β-endorphin. Science 1983; 220:721.

de Bustros A, Nelkin BD, Silverman A, et al. The short arm of chromosome 11 is a "hot spot" for hypermethylation in human neoplasia. Proc Nat Acad Sci 1988; 85:5693.

Fisher JA, Tobler PH, Kaufmann M, et al. Calcitonin: Regional distribution of the hormone and its binding sites in the human brain pituitary. Proc Nat Acad Sci USA 1981; 78:7801.

Fusco FD, Rosen SW. Gonadotropin-producing anaplastic large-cell carcinomas of the lung. N Engl J Med, 1966; 275:507.

Gewirtz, G, Yalow RS. Ectopic ACTH production in carcinoma of the lung. J Clin Invest 1974; 53:1022.

Goodwin, G, Baylin SB. Relationships between neuroendocrine differentiation and sensitivity to radiation in culture line OH-1 of human small cell lung carcinoma. Cancer Res 1982; 42:1361.

Gosney JR, Sissons MCJ. Widespread distribution of broncho pulmonary endocrine cells immunoreactive for calcitonin in the lung of the normal adult rat. Thorax 1985; 40:194.

Habener JF, Segre GV. Parathyroid hormone radioimmunoassay. Ann Intern Med 1979; 91:782.

Liddle GW, Nickolson WE, Island DP, et al. Clinical and laboratory studies of ectopic hormonal syndromes. Recent Prog Horm Res 1969; 25:283.

Lippman SM, Mendelsohn G, Trump DL, et al. The prognostic and biological significance of cellular heterogeneity in medullary thyroid carcinoma: A study of calcitonin, L-dopa decarboxylase and histaminase. J Clin Endocrinol Metab 1982; 54:233.

Kilpatrick D, Borland K, Jin DF. Differential expression of opioid peptide genes by testicular germ cells and somatic cells. Proc Nat Acad Sci 1987; 84:5695.

Kolata G. New theory of hormones proposed. Science 1982; 215:1383.

Kyle CV, Evans MC, Odell WD. Growth hormone-like material in normal human tissues. J Clin Endocrinol Metab 1981; 53:1138.

Moore HPH, Walker MD, Lee F, et al. Expressing a human proinsulin cDNA in a mouse ACTH-secreting cell. Intracellular storage, proterolytic processing, and secretion on stimulating. Cell 1983; 35:531.

Pearse AGE. The APUD concept and hormone production. Clin Endocrinol Metab 1980; 9:211.

Pintar JE, Schachter BS, Herman AB, et al. Characterization and localization of proopiomelanocortin messenger RNA in the adult rat testis. Science 1984; 225:632.

Ratcliffe JG, Knight RA, Besser GM, et al. Tumor and plasma ACTH concentrations in patients with and without the ectopic ACTH syndrome. Clin Endocrinol 1972; 1:27.

Rosenzweig JL, Havrankova J, Lesniak MA, et al. Insulin is ubiquitous in extra pancreatic tissues of rats and humans. Proc Nat Acad Sci USA 1980; 77:572.

Said SI, Rosenberg RN. Vasoactive intestinal polypeptide: Abundant immunoreactivity in neural cell lines and normal nervous tissue. Science 1976; 192:907.

Saito E, Iwasa S, Odell WD. Widespread presence of large molecular weight adrenocorticotropin-like substances in normal rat extrapituitary tissues. Endocrinology 1983; 113:1010.

Sporn MB, Todaro GJ. Autocrine secretion and malignant transformation of cells. N Engl J Med 1980; 303:878.

Steenbergh PH, Hoppener JWM, Zandberg J, et al. Expression of the proopiomelanocortin gene in human medullary thyroid carcinoma. J Clin Endocrinol Metab 1984; 58:904.

Stevens RE, Moore GE. Inadequacy of APUD concept in explaining production of peptide hormones by tumours. Lancet 1983; 1:118.

Suda T, Tomori N, Tozawa F, et al. Immunoreactive corticotropin and corticotropin-releasing factor in human hypothalamus, adrenal, lung cancer and pheochromocytoma. J Clin Endocrinol Metab 1984; 58:919.

Wolfsen AR, Odell WD. ProACTH: Use for early detection of lung cancer. Am J Med 1979; 66:765.

Tumor-Related Hypercalcemia

Benson RC Jr., Riggs BL, Pickard BM, et al. Radioimmunoassay of parathyroid hormone in hypercalcemic patients with malignant disease. Am J Med 1974; 56:821.

Breslau NA, McGuire JL, Zerwekh JE, et al. Hypercalcemia associated with increased serum calcitriol levels in three patients with lymphoma. Ann Intern Med 1984; 100:1.

Case records of the Massachusetts General Hospital. N Engl J Med 1941; 225:789.

Eilon G, Mundy GR. Direct resorption of bone by human breast cancer cells in vitro. Nature 1978; 276:726.

Fetchick DA, Bertolini DR, Sarin PS, et al. Production of 1,25-dihydroxyvitamin D_3 by human T cell lymphotropic virus-I-transformed lymphocytes. J Clin Invest 1986; 78:592.

Fisken RA, Health DA, Somers S, et al. Hypercalcemia in hospital patients. Clinical and diagnostic aspects. Lancet 1981; 1:202.

Gowen M, Wood DD, Ihrie EJ, et al. An interleukin-1-like factor stimulates bone resorption in vitro. Nature 1983; 306:378.

Horiuchi N, Caulfield MP, Fisher JE, et al. Similarity of synthetic peptide from human tumor to parathyroid hormone in vivo and in vitro. Science 1987; 238:1566.

Ibbotson KJ, D'Souza SM, Ng Kw, et al. Tumor-derived growth factor increases bone resorption in a tumor associated with humoral hypercalcemia of malignancy. Science 1983; 221:1292.

Kemp BE, Moseley JM, Rodda CP, et al. Parathyroid hormone-related protein of malignancy: Active synthetic fragments. Science 1987; 238:1568.

Mundy GR, Raisz LG, Cooper RA, et al. Evidence for the secretion of an osteoclast-stimulating factor in myeloma N Engl J Med 1974; 291:1041.

Mundy GR, Wilkinson R, Heath DA. Comparative study of available medical therapy for hypercalcemia of malignancy. Am J Med 1983; 74:421.

Salahuddin SZ, Markham PD, Lindner SG, et al. Lymphokine production by cultured human T cells transformed by human T-cell leukemia-lymphoma virus-I. Science 1984; 223:703.

Sato K, Mimura H, Han DC, et al. Production of bone-resorbing activity and colony-stimulating activity in vivo and in vitro by a human squamous cell carcinoma associated with hypercalcemia and leukocytosis. J Clin Invest 1986; 78:145.

Sherwood LM, O'Riordan JLH, Aurbach GD, et al. Production of parathyroid hormone by nonparathyroid tumors. J Clin Endocrinol Metab 1967; 27:140.

Simpson EL, Mundy GR, D'Souza SM, et al. Absence of parathyroid hormone messenger RNA in nonparathyroid tumors associated with hypercalcemia. N Engl J Med 1983; 309:325.

Stewart AF, Horst R, Deftos LJ, et al. Biochemical evaluation of patients with cancer-associated hypercalcemia. Evidence for humoral and nonhumoral groups. N Engl J Med 1980; 303:1377.

Stewart AF, Insogna KL, Goltzman D, et al. Identification of adenylate cyclase-simulating activity and cytochemical glucose-6-phosphate dehydrogenase-simulating activity in extracts of tumors from patients with humoral hypercalcemia of malignancy. Proc Nat Acad Sci USA 1983; 80:1454.

Strewler GJ, Williams RD, Nissenson RA. Human renal carcinoma cells produce hypercalcemia in the nude mouse and a novel protein recognized by parathyroid hormone receptors. J Clin Invest 1983; 71:769.

Valentin-Opran A, Eilon G, Saez S, et al. Estrogens and antiestrogens stimulate release of bone resorbing activity by cultured human breast cancer cells. J Clin Invest 1985; 75:731.

Warrell RP Jr., Bockman RS, Coonley CJ, et al. Gallium nitrate inhibits calcium resorption from bone and is effective treatment for cancer-related hypercalcemia. J Clin Invest 1984; 73:1487.

The Ectopic Cushing's Syndrome

Brown WH. A case of pluriglandular syndrome: "Diabetes of bearded women." Lancet 1928; 2:1022.

Carey RM, Varma SK, Drake CR Jr, et al. Ectopic secretion of corticotropin-releasing factor as a cause of Cushing's syndrome: A clinical, morphological and biochemical study. N Engl J Med 1984; 311:13.

Christy NP. Adrenocorticotrophic activity in the plasma of patients with Cushing's syndrome associated with pulmonary neoplasmas. Lancet, 1961; 1:85.

de Keyzer Y, Bertagna X, Lenne F, et al. Altered proopiomelanocortin gene expression in adrenocorticotropin-producing nonpituitary tumors. J Clin Invest 1985; 76:1892.

Eipper BA, Mains RE. Structure and biosynthesis of pro-adrenocorticotropin/endorphin and related peptides. Endocr Rev 1980; 1:1.

Holub DA, Katz FH. A possible etiological link between Cushing's syndrome and visceral malignancy. Clin Res 1961; 9:194.

Liddle GW, Nicholson WE, Island DP, et al. Clinical and laboratory studies of ectopic humoral syndromes. Recent Prog Horm Res 1969; 25:283.

Nieman LK, Chrousos GP, Kellner C, et al. Successful treatment of Cushing's syndrome with the glucocorticoid antagonist RU486. J Clin Endocrinol Metab 1985; 61:536.

Nieman LK, Chrousos GP, Oldfield EH, et al. The ovine corticotropin-releasing hormone stimulation test and the dexamethasone suppression test in the differential diagnosis of Cushing's syndrome. Ann Intern Med 1986; 105:862.

Pont A, Williams PL, Loose DS, et al. Ketoconazole blocks adrenal steroid synthesis. Ann Intern Med 1982; 97:370.

Tsukada T, Nakai Y, Jingami H, et al. Identification of the mRNA coding for the ACTH-β-lipotropin precursor in a human ectopic ACTH-producing tumor Biochem Biophys Res Commun 1981; 98:535.

Upton GV, Amatruda TT. Evidence for the presence of tumor peptides with corticotropin-releasing factor-like activity in the ectopic ACTH syndrome. N Engl J Med 1971; 285:419.

Vale W, Spiess J, Rivier C, et al. Characterization of a 41-residue ovine hypothalamic peptide that stimulates secretion of corticotropin and β-endorphin. Science 1981; 213:1394.

Syndrome of Inappropriate ADH Secretion

Amatruda TT Jr., Mulrow PJ, Gallagher JC, et al. Carcinoma of the lung with inappropriate antidiuresis. Demonstration of antidiuretic-hormone-like activity in tumor extracts. N Engl J Med 1963; 269:544.

Cherril DA, Stote RM, Birge JR, et al. Demeclocycline treatment in the syndrome of inappropriate antidiuretic hormone secretion. Ann Intern Med 1975; 83:654.

Padfield PL, Morton JJ, Brown JJ, et al. Plasma arginine vasopressin in the syndrome of antidiuretic hormone excess associated with bronchogenic carcinoma. Am J Med 1976; 61:825.

Schwartz WB, Bennett W, Curelop S, et al. A syndrome of renal sodium loss and hyponatremia probably resulting from inappropriate secretion of antidiuretic hormone. Am J Med 1957; 23:529.

Yamaji T, Ishibashi M, Hori T. Propressophysin in human blood: A possible marker of ectopic vasopressin production. J Clin Endocrinol Metab 1984; 59:505.

Yamaji T, Ishibashi M, Katayama S, et al. Neurophysin biosynthesis in vitro in oat cell carcinoma of the lung with ectopic vasopressin production. J Clin Invest 1981; 68:1441.

Acromegaly

Asa SL, Kovacs K, Thorner MO, et al. Immunohistological localization of growth hormone–releasing hormone in human tumors. J Clin Endocrinol Metab 1985; 60:423.

Gubler U, Monahan JJ, Lomedico PT, et al. Cloning and sequence analysis of cDNA for the precursor of human growth hormone–releasing factor, somatocrinin. Proc Nat Acad Sci USA 1983; 80:4311.

Guillemin R, Brazeau P, Bohlen P, et al. Growth hormone–releasing factor from a human pancreatic tumor that causes acromegaly. Science 1982; 218:585.

Mayo KE, Vale W, Rivier J, et al. Expression-cloning and sequencing of a cDNA encoding human growth hormone–releasing factor. Nature 1983; 306:86.

Melmed S, Ezrin C, Kovacs K, et al. Acromegaly due to secretion of growth hormone by an ectopic pancreatic islet-cell tumors. N Engl J Med 1985; 312:9.

Rivier J, Spiess J, Thorner M, et al. Characterization of a growth hormone releasing factor from a human pancreatic islet tumor. Nature 1982; 300:276.

Thorner MO, Perryman RL, Cronin MJ, et al. Somatotroph hyperplasia. Successful treatment of acromegaly by removal of a pancreatic islet tumor secreting a growth hormone–releasing factor J Clin Invest 1982; 70:965.

Calcitonin

Coombes RC, Hillyard C, Greenberg PB, et al. Plasma-immunoreactive-calcitonin in patients with non-thyroid tumors. Lancet 1974; 1:1080.

Edbrooke MR, Parker D, McVey JH, et al. Expression of the human calcitonin/CGRP gene in lung and thyroid carcinoma. EMBO J 1985; 4:715.

Milhaud G, Calmette C, Taboulet J, et al. Hypersecretion of calcitonin in neoplastic conditions. Lancet 1974; 1:462.

Nelkin BD, Rosenfeld KI, de Bustros A, et al. Structure and expression of a gene encoding human calcitonin and calcitonin gene related peptide. Biochem Biophys Res Commun 1984; 123:648.

Rosenfeld MG, Mermod J-J, Amara SG, et al. Production of a novel neuropeptide encoded by the calcitonin gene via tissue-specific RNA processing. Nature 1983; 304:129.

Silva OL, Broder LE, Doppman JL, et al. Calcitonin as a marker for bronchogenic cancer. Cancer 1979; 44:680.

Steenbergh PH, Hoppener JWM, Zandberg J, et al. Calcitonin gene related peptide coding sequence is conserved in the human genome and is expressed in medullary thyroid carcinoma. J Clin Endocrinol Metab 1984; 59:358.

Trump DL, Mendelsohn G, Baylin SB. Discordance between plasma calcitonin and tumor-cell mass in medullary thyroid carcinoma. N Engl J Med 1979; 301:253.

Zajac JD, Martin TJ, Hudson P, et al. Biosynthesis of calcitonin by human lung cancer cells. Endocrinology 1985; 116:749.

Tumor-Related Hypoglycemia

Doege KW. Fibrosarcoma of the mediastinum. Ann Surg 1930; 92:955.

Elliott CA. Hepatogenic hypoglycemia associated with primary liver-cell carcinoma. Trans Assoc Am Physicians 1929; 44:121.

Gorden P, Hendricks CM, Kahn CR, et al. Hypoglycemia associated with non-islet-cell tumor and insulin-like growth factors: A study of the tumor types. N Engl J Med 1981; 305:1452.

Hyodo T, Megyesi K, Kahn CR, et al. Adrenocortical carcinoma and hypoglycemia: Evidence for production of nonsuppressible insulin-like activity by the tumor. J Clin endocrinol Metab 1977; 44:1175.

Megyesi K, Kahn CR, Roth J, et al. Hypoglycemia in association with extrapancreatic tumors: Demonstration of elevated plasms NSILA-S by a new radioreceptor assay. J Clin Endocrinol Metab 1974; 38:931.

Reeve AE, Eccles MR, Wilkins RJ, et al. Expression of insulin-like growth factor II transcripts in Wilms' tumour. Nature 1985; 317:258.

Widmer V, Zapf J, Froesch ER. Is extrapancreatic tumor hypoglycemia associated with elevated levels of insulin-like growth factor II? J Clin Endocrinol Metab 1982; 55:833.

hCG

Braunstein GD, Vaitukaitis JL, Carbone PP, et al. Ectopic production of human chorionic gonadotropin by neoplasms. Ann Intern Med 1973; 78:39.

Chou JY, Robinson JC, Wang S-S. Effects of sodium butyrate on synthesis of human chorionic gonadotropin in trophoblastic and non-trophoblastic tumours. Nature 1977; 268:543.

Dalla-Favera R, Bregni M, Erikson J, et al. Human c-myc oncogene is located on the region of chromosome 8 that is translocated in Burkitt lymphoma cells. Proc Nat Acad Sci USA 1982; 79:7824.

Hoshina M, Boothby MR, Hussa RD, et al. Segregation patterns of polymorphic restriction sites of the gene encoding the α-subunit of human chorionic gonadotropin in trophoblastic disease. Proc Nat Acad Sci USA 1984; 81:2504.

Kahn CR, Rosen SW, Weintraub BD, et al. Ectopic production of chorionic gonadotropin and its subunit by islet-cell tumors: A specific marker for malignancy. N Engl J Med 1977; 297:565.

McArthur JW, Toll GD, Russfield AB, et al. Sexual precocity attributable to ectopic gonadotropin secretion by hepatoblastoma Am J Med 1973; 54:390.

Reeves RL, Tesluk H, Harrison CE. Precocious puberty associated with hepatoma. J Clin Endocrinol Metab 1959; 19:1651.

Stanbridge EJ, Rosen SW, Sussman HH. Expression of the α-subunit of human chorionic gonadotropin is specifically correlated with tumorigenic expresssion in human cell hybrids. Proc Nat Acad Sci USA 1982; 79:6242.

Erythrocytosis

Ascensao JL, Gaylis F, Bronson D, et al. Erythropoietin production by a human testicular germ cell line. Blood 1983; 62:1132.

Hammond D, Winnick S. Paraneoplastic erythrocytosis and ectopic erythropoietins. Ann N Y Acad Sci 1974; 230:219.

Jacobs K, Shoemaker C, Rudersdorf R, et al. Isolation and characterization of genomic and cDNa clones of human erythropoietin. Nature 1985; 313:806.

Miyake T, Kung, C-KH, Goldwasser E. Purification of human erythropoietin. J Biol Chem 1977; 252:5558.

Okabe, T, Urabe A, Kato T, et al. Production of erythropoietin-like activity by human renal and hepatic carcinomas in cell culture. Cancer 1985; 55:1918.

Saito T, Saito K, Trent DJ, et al. Translation of messenger RNA from a renal tumor into a product with the biological properties of erythropoietin. Exp Hematol 1985; 13:23.

Osteomalacia

Drezner MK, Feinglos MN. Osteomalacia due to 1α,25-dihydroxycholecalciferol deficiency. Associated with a giant tumor of bone. J Clin Invest 1977; 60:1046.

Ryan EA, Reiss E. Oncogenous osteomalacia: Review of the world literature of 42 cases and report of two new cases. Am J Med 1984; 77:501.

Salassa RM, Jowsey J, Arnaud CD. Hypophosphatemic osteomalacia associated with "nonendocrine" tumors. N Engl J Med 1970; 283:65.

Hyperthyroidism

Nisula BC, Ketelslegers J-M. Thyroid-stimulating activity and chorionic gonadotropin. J Clin Invest 1974; 54:494.

Wilber JF, Spinella P. Identification of immunoreactive thyrotropin-releasing hormone in human neoplasia. J Clin Endocrinol Metab 1984; 59:432.

Renin and Hypertension

Atlas, SA, Hesson TE, Sealey JE, et al. Characterization of inactive renin ("prorenin") from renin-secreting tumors of non-renal origin. J Clin Invest 1984; 73:437.

Ruddy MC, Atlas SA, Salerno FG. Hypertension associated with a renin-secreting adenocarcinoma of the pancreas. N Engl J Med 1982; 307:993.

Prolactin

Davis S, Proper S, May PB, et al. Elevated prolactin levels in bronchogenic carcinoma. Cancer 1979; 44:676.

Molitch ME, Schwartz S, Mukherji B. Is prolactin secreted ectopically? Am J Med 1981; 70:803.

Purnell DM, Hillman EA, Heatfield BM, et al. Immunoreactive prolactin in epithelial cells of normal and cancerous human breast and prostate detected by the unlabeled antibody peroxidase-antiperoxidase method. Cancer Res 1982; 42:2317.

Rosen SW, Weintraub BD, Aaronson SW. Nonrandom ectopic protein production by malignant cells: Direct evidence in vitro. J Clin Endocrinol Metab 1980; 50:834.

Turkington RW. Ectopic production of prolactin. N Engl J Med 1971; 285:1455.

Neuroendocrine Peptides

Cuttita F, Carney DN, Mulshine J, et al. Bombesin-like peptides can function as autocrine growth factors in human small cell lung cancer. Nature 1985; 316:823.

Long TT III, Barton TK, Draffin R, et al. Conservative management of the Zollinger-Ellison syndrome. Ectopic gastrin production by an ovarian cystadenoma. JAMA 1980; 243:1837.

Moody TW, Pert CB, Gazdar AF, et al. High levels of intracellular bombesin characterize human small-cell lung carcinoma. Science 1981; 214:1246.

Said S, Faloona GR. Elevated plasma and tissue levels of vasoactive intestinal polypeptide in the watery-diarrhea syndrome due to pancreatic, bronchogenic and other tumors. N Engl J Med 1975; 293:155.

Sausville EA, Lebacq-Verheyhen A-M, Spindel ER, et al. Expression of the gastrin-releasing peptide gene in human small cell lung cancer. J Biol Chem 1986; 261:2451.

Solt J, Kadas I, Polak JM, et al. A pancreatic-polypeptide-producing tumor of the stomach. Cancer 1984; 54:1101.

Growth Factors

Beutler B, Greenwald D, Hulmes JD, et al. Identity of tumour necrosis factor and the macrophage-secreted factor cachectin. Nature 1985; 316:552.

Doolittle, RF, Hunkapiller MW, Hood LE, et al. Simian sarcoma virus oncogene, v-sis, is derived from the gene (or genes) encoding a platelet-derived growth factor. Science 1983; 221:275.

Downward J, Yarden Y, Mayes E, et al. Close similarity of epidermal growth factor receptor and v-erb-B oncogene protein sequences. Nature 1984; 307:521.

Ellis DL, Kafka SP, Chow JC, et al. Melanoma, growth factors, acanthosis nigricans, the sign of Leser-Trélat and multiple acrochordons: A possible role for alpha-tranforming growth factor in cutaneous paraneoplastic syndromes. N Engl J Med 1987; 317:1582.

Taub R, Roy A, Dieter R, et al. Insulin as a growth factor in rat hepatoma cells. J Biol Chem 1987; 262:10893.

16 Diseases of Calcium Metabolism

Michael A. Levine, M.D.

The maintenance of constant concentrations of the mineral ions calcium, phosphorus, and magnesium in the extracellular fluid is essential for the functional and structural welfare of many tissues of the body. Of the three principal hormones that regulate mineral homeostasis, the earliest to evolve were calcitonin and vitamin D. Their initial function may have been to conserve phosphorus. With the development of terrestrial forms of life, these hormones were probably adapted to regulate calcium homeostasis. To facilitate more efficient control of calcium metabolism, parathyroid hormone (PTH) evolved later as an adjunctive control. In humans, PTH appears to be the most important hormonal regulator of calcium ion homeostasis.

Although the physiologic importance of PTH to the vital economy of mineral metabolism in general and calcium homeostasis in particular has long been appreciated, the clinical significance of parathyroid dysfunction has emerged more recently. Thus, the advent of automated chemistry procedures for the determination of serum calcium concentrations and the development of radioimmunoassay techniques for the measurement of PTH have changed concepts concerning the frequency and importance of abnormalities of calcium and bone metabolism. For example, primary hyperparathyroidism, once considered to be an uncommon metabolic disorder, is now recognized as an increasingly common clinical problem, with a prevalence of about 0.2 percent in the U.S. population. Secondary hyperparathyroidism, resulting from hypersecretion of PTH in response to a decrease in serum ionized calcium concentrations, complicates chronic renal failure, malabsorption, and various nutritional deficiencies. Finally, disturbed regulation of PTH and vitamin D metabolism may be important etiologic factors in the genesis of some forms of metabolic bone disease and nephrolithiasis.

The diagnostic evaluation of patients with diseases of calcium metabolism requires first a thorough understanding of mineral homeostasis and second an appreciation of the laboratory tests that are used to measure the serum concentrations and the relevant hormones. The purpose of this chapter is to present a logical approach to the laboratory investigation of disorders of calcium metabolism and to outline the application and interpretation of those tests most frequently used in clinical practice.

CALCIUM HOMEOSTASIS

Parathyroid Hormone

The serum calcium concentration is normally maintained within narrow limits despite wide variations in dietary intake, the demands of the skeleton during growth, and losses during pregnancy and lactation. Bone contains 99 percent of total body calcium. Aberrations in the serum calcium concentration and the urinary excretion of calcium thus become important reflections of changes in bone resorption or formation. Net calcium absorption from the gut and its excretion by the kidney are the other organ functions that determine serum and urinary calcium.

The remaining 1 percent of body calcium resides primarily in the extracellular fluid. Approximately 45 percent of total calcium is ionized at normal plasma protein concentrations and is physiologically active. A narrow concentration range of ionized calcium in extracellular fluid is required for normal intracellular transactions. Maintenance of this concentration depends on cellular processes in bone, intestine, and kidney that are responsive to two hormones, PTH and vitamin D. The synthesis and secretion of these hormones are regulated by the concentration of ionized calcium as well as by the reciprocal feedback effects of each hormone on the other.

PTH is synthesized in the four parathyroid glands as a preprohormone (115 amino acids), converted to a prohormone (90 amino acids), and stored as an 84-amino-acid polypeptide. Biologic activity resides in the amino terminal third of the molecule. The sequence 2–25 is the minimum required for biologic activity. Synthetic polypeptides comprising the first 34 amino acids are in general as fully active as the entire 1–84 sequence. Secretion of mature PTH occurs at a rate inversely proportional to the ambient serum ionized calcium concentration. At low levels of serum calcium, secondary to inadequate assimilation of dietary calcium, the parathyroid glands increase secretion of PTH. PTH acts directly on bone and kidney and indirectly, through vitamin D, on the gut. Separately and together these actions raise serum calcium concentrations.

In bone, PTH increases resorption by stimulating the activity of both osteoclasts and osteocytes; this action releases both calcium and phosphorus into the extracellular fluid. PTH has three effects on the kidney: (1) it enhances renal tubular reabsorption of calcium; (2) it increases urinary excretion of phosphate, as well as bicarbonate, potassium, sodium, and amino acids; and (3) it enhances the activity of the 1-α-hydroxylase enzyme and thereby stimulates conversion of 25-hydroxycholecalciferol (25[OH]D) to the more active vitamin D metabolite 1,25-dihydroxycholecalciferol (1,25[OH]$_2$D).

PTH indirectly promotes the absorption of dietary calcium (and to a lesser extent phosphorus) from the gastrointestinal tract through its action on the metabolism of vitamin D.

PTH exerts its effects on its target organs, bone and kidney, by binding to specific membrane receptors, thereby stimulating adenylyl cyclase and phospholipase C. Activation of adenylyl cyclase leads to increased intracellular concentrations of cyclic adenosine 3',5' monophosphate (cyclic AMP). Cyclic AMP activates specific protein kinases that bring about the specific enzymatic reactions that are characteristic of many physiologic effects of PTH in the cell type affected.

Vitamin D

Vitamin D is now considered a prohormone, which must be converted in the body to the active hormone through a series of enzymatic steps. Vitamin D can be synthesized in the skin by conversion of 7-dehydrocholesterol to cholecalciferol (vitamin D$_3$) in response to ultraviolet (sunlight) irradiation. Vitamin D$_3$ and vitamin D$_2$ (ergocalciferol) derived from the diet are then hydroxylated in the 25 position in the liver to form 25-hydroxyvitamin D (25[OH]D). Conversion of vitamin D to 25(OH)D occurs with little or no regulation in adults, and plasma levels of 25(OH)D increase substantially after vitamin D treatment or increased exposure to sunlight. In contrast, in children this reaction is inhibited by elevated plasma levels of 1,25(OH)$_2$D. Degradation of 25(OH)D is enhanced by elevated concentrations of 1,25(OH)$_2$D. In the kidney 25(OH)D is further modified by hydroxylation at either the 24 or 1α position. The 1-α-hydroxylation of 25(OH)D produces 1,25-dihydroxyvitamin D (1,25[OH]$_2$D), the most potent form of vitamin D in stimulating intestinal calcium absorption. The activity of the renal 1-α-hydroxylase is stringently regulated such that production of 1,25(OH)$_2$D is commensurate with the need of the organism. Its activity is enhanced by hypophosphatemia, PTH, and hypocalcemia; its activity is inhibited by hyperphosphatemia, hypercalcemia, and 1,25(OH)$_2$D.

The principal function of vitamin D, which is mediated largely or entirely through 1,25(OH)$_2$D, is to increase intestinal absorption of calcium and phosphorus. In addition, 1,25(OH)$_2$D can increase bone resorption and is required as a permissive agent for PTH to exert its effect in increasing bone resorption and maintaining a normal plasma calcium level. The actions of vitamin D in its target calls require interaction of the hormone with a cytosolic receptor protein in a manner similar to that of other steroid hormones. The activated hormone–receptor complex subsequently regulates expression of specific genes whose protein products ultimately affect the cellular response to vitamin D.

Calcitonin

Calcitonin is a 32-amino-acid polypeptide synthesized and secreted in humans by the parafollicular or C cells of the thyroid gland. The secretion of calcitonin is stimulated by a rise of serum calcium and by gastrin, secretion, and glucagon. Calcitonin acts to decrease osteoclastic bone resorption, which causes a fall in serum calcium concentration. The role of calcitonin in normal physiology in humans is uncertain. In pharmacologic doses it has a hypocalcemic effect and acts on the kidney to increase urinary excretion of sodium, calcium, phosphate, and magnesium.

HYPERCALCEMIA

Automated multichannel procedures in blood chemistry have documented a 1 to 2 percent incidence of hypercalcemia during routine screening. Hypercalcemia may result from a diverse number of pathologic states as well as from inappropriate blood sampling and laboratory errors. Such errors are avoided by the use of calcium-free disposable blood collection materials. The total serum calcium is typically measured, and this value is directly influenced by the level of binding proteins, primarily albumin and globulin. Hemoconcentration secondary to prolonged application of the venipuncture tourniquet, profound dehydration, and prolonged fasting can also result in elevations of serum protein concentrations and thereby cause artifactual hypercalcemia. Direct measurement of the ionized calcium concentration avoids these pitfalls and can confirm the presence of true hypercalcemia. Once a diagnosis of hypercalcemia is achieved, its cause must be established. Although this chapter presents a discussion of the laboratory findings that distinguish between the causes of hypercalcemia, definitive diagnosis in these patients will require a thorough integration of clinical experience, clinical history, physical examination, and knowledgeable interpretation of laboratory data. The differential diagnosis of the hypercalcemic states and the key laboratory findings are presented in Table 16–1. Primary hyperparathyroidism is the most common disorder characterized by hypercalcemia. Recent studies indicate an annual incidence of 25 per 100,000 of the general population, or more than 50,000 new cases per year in the United States. Its biochemical etiology is unknown, but excess secretion of PTH may be produced by a single adenoma, hyperplasia of all glands, or parathyroid carcinoma. The diagnosis is based on hypercalcemia (which may be constant or intermittent), hypophosphatemia, elevated serum concentrations of PTH, and increased urinary excretion of phosphorus, calcium, and cyclic AMP.

Variants of primary hyperparathyroidism include several genetic disorders that are transmitted in an autosomal dominant manner: (1) familial multiple endocrine neoplasia Type I, in which hyperplasia of all parathyroid glands is accompanied by pancreatic tumors (40 to 60 percent) such as gastrinoma or insulinoma and pituitary tumors (25 to 40 percent); (2) familial multiple endocrine neoplasia Type IIa, in which medullary thyroid carcinoma is accompanied by parathyroid hyperplasia (40 to 60 percent) and pheochromocytoma (25 to 50 percent); and (3) familial multiple endocrine neoplasia Type IIb, in which medullary thyroid carcinoma is associated with pheochromocytoma, a marfanoid habitus, and mucosal neuromas; hyperparathyroidism is rare. A final variant of primary hyperparathyroidism is familial hypocalciuric hypercalcemia (also termed benign familial hypercalcemia). This distinct and unique disorder is benign. It is characterized by onset of hypercalcemia by the end of the first decade of life. Serum concentration of PTH and urinary excretion of cyclic AMP are normal or only modestly elevated. In contrast to patients with other forms of primary hyperparathyroidism, patients with familial hypocalciuric hypercalcemia have reduced fractional renal clearance of calcium and magnesium.

Malignancy-associated hypercalcemia is the most common cause of hypercalcemia in hospitalized patients. The etiology of hypercalcemia in patients with underlying malignancies can be divided into two broad groups: osteolytic hypercalcemia and humoral hypercalcemia. Patients with osteolytic hypercalcemia have either widespread skeletal metastases or extensive bone marrow involvement by a primary hematologic malignancy, by increased bone resorption due to direct resorption of bone by invasive malignant cells, or by local production of factors that activate osteoclasts. These patients are characterized biochemically by marked hypercalciuria, parathyroid suppression, reduced urinary cyclic AMP and plasma $1,25(OH)_2D$ concentrations, and normal serum phosphorus concentrations. Patients with most forms of humoral hypercalcemia of malignancy also have a marked degree of bone resorption. In contrast to patients with localized osteolysis, these subjects harbor tumors that elaborate one or more humoral factors that are capable of acting systemically to activate osteoclasts. These patients typically manifest hypophosphatemia and increased urinary cyclic AMP concentrations. These latter findings, in combination with early descriptions of the syndrome

that indicated that plasma concentrations of immunoreactive PTH were not suppressed, suggested that PTH was the humoral mediator. Thus, the terms *ectopic hyperparathyroidism* and *pseudohyperparathyroidism* were frequently used to describe this syndrome. Recent improvements in PTH assays and the isolation of a unique PTH-related peptide from several tumors have now made it clear, however, that PTH is only rarely involved in this syndrome. Patients with humoral hypercalcemia of malignancy are characterized biochemically by hypercalcemia, hypophosphatemia, elevated urine calcium and cyclic AMP excretion, reduced tubular maximum reabsorption capacity for phosphate as a function of the glomerular filtration rate (TmP/GFR), and reduced (or normal) plasma concentrations of PTH and $1,25(OH)_2D$.

A second malignancy-associated hypercalcemic syndrome has been described in several patients with lymphoma, particularly of the diffuse histiocytic type. These patients have been found to have elevated circulating concentrations of $1,25(OH)_2D$ and suppressed concentrations of PTH. The available evidence suggests that the $1,25(OH)_2D$ is produced in an unregulated manner by the malignant lymphoma tissue.

Hypercalcemia and hypercalciuria also occur commonly in patients with sarcoid and other granulomatous disorders. These subjects display increased rates of bone resorption and intestinal absorption of calcium. The pathogenesis of these abnormalities involves the synthesis of $1,25(OH)_2D$ by the granulomatous tissue. Parathyroid secretion is suppressed, and circulating concentrations of $1,25(OH)_2D$ are elevated. The plasma concentration of $25(OH)D$ is characteristically normal, although reduced levels are occasionally seen in patients in whom the rate of conversion of $25(OH)D$ to $1,25(OH)_2D$ is markedly elevated.

Hypercalcemia also is a manifestation of several endocrinopathies (e.g., pheochromocytoma, thyrotoxicosis, and acute adrenal insufficiency) and can result from the injudicious use of medications (e.g., vitamins A and D, absorbable alkali, and lithium).

HYPOCALCEMIA

Hypocalcemia develops when either PTH or vitamin D is deficient or defective, or their target tissues fail to respond. Proof of hypocalcemia may require multiple serum calcium determinations. Because the serum albumin level can influence the concentration of serum calcium, it should be measured concomitantly for accurate interpretation. Alternatively, the plasma concentration of ionized calcium may provide the most meaningful results.

The differential diagnosis of the hypocalcemic states and the key laboratory findings are presented in Table 16-2. Hormonopenic hypoparathyroidism is characterized by normal or undetectable plasma concentrations of PTH. In contrast, patients with pseudohypoparathyroidism

TABLE 16-1 Laboratory Differential Diagnosis of Hypercalcemia

Diagnosis	Plasma Tests					Urine Tests			Comments
	Ca	PO₄	PTH	25(OH)D	1,25(OH)₂D	cAMP	TmP/GFR	Ca	
Primary Hyperparathyroidism	↑	N/↓	↑	N	N/↑	↑	↓	↑	Parathyroid adenoma most common
MEN I									Parathyroid *hyperplasia*; also includes pituitary and pancreatic neoplasms
MEN IIa									Parathyroid *hyperplasia*; also includes medullary thyroid carcinoma and pheochromocytoma
MEN IIb									Parathyroid disease *uncommon*, primarily medullary thyroid carcinoma and pheochromocytoma
FHH	↑	N	N/↑	N	N	N/↑	N/↓	↓↓	Autosomal dominant inheritance; hypercalcemia present within first decade benign
Malignancy									
Solid tumor—humoral	↑	N/↓	↓	N	N	↑	↓	↑↑	Primarily epidermoid tumors; PTH-related protein(s) is mediator
Solid tumor—osteolytic	↑	N/↑	↓	N	N	→	↑	↑↑	
Lymphoma	↑	N/↑	↓	N/↓	↑	→	↑	↑↑	
Granulomatous disease	↑	N/↑	↓	N/↓	↑↑	→	↑	↑↑	Sarcoid most common etiology
Vitamin D intoxication	↑	N/↑	↓	↑↑	N	→	↑	↑↑	
Hyperthyroidism	↑	N	↓	N	N	N	N	↑↑	Plasma concentrations of T₄ and/or T₃ are elevated

MEN, multiple endocrine neoplasia. FHH, familial hypocalciuric hypercalcemia

TABLE 16-2 Laboratory Differential Diagnosis of Hypocalcemia

Diagnosis	Plasma Tests						Urine Tests				Comments
	Ca	PO₄	PTH	25(OH)D	1,25(OH)₂D	cAMP	cAMP After PTH	TmP/GFR	TmP/GFR After PTH	Ca	
Hypoparathyroidism	↓	↑	N/↓	N	↓	↓	↑↑	↑	↓↓	N/↓	Deficiency of PTH
Pseudohypoparathyroidism											
Type I	↓	↑	↑↑	N	↓	↓	→	↑	↑	N/↓	Resistance to PTH; patients may have Albright's hereditary osteodystrophy and resistance to multiple hormones
Type II	↓	N	↑↑	N	↓	↓	↑	↑	↑	N/↓	Renal resistance to cyclic AMP
Vitamin D Deficiency	↓	N/↓	↑↑	↓↓	N/↓	↑	↑	↓	↑	↓	Deficient supply (e.g., nutrition) or absorption (e.g., pancreatic insufficiency) of vitamin D
Vitamin D-dependent rickets											
Type I	↓	N/↓	↑↑	N	↓	↑		↓		↓	Deficient activity of renal 25(OH)D-1α-hydroxylase
Type II	↓	N/↓	↑↑	N	↑↑	↑		↓		↓	Resistance to 1,25(OH)₂D

manifest target organ resistance to PTH and typically have markedly elevated concentrations of circulating PTH. Patients with either form of biochemical hypoparathyroidism have normal or elevated serum levels of phosphorus.

Disorders in which hypocalcemia results from deficient vitamin D supply (nutritional rickets) or activity (vitamin D–dependent rickets Type II) are typically associated with secondary (adaptive) hyperparathyroidism and markedly elevated concentrations of PTH in the circulation. Serum phosphorus levels are typically reduced in response to increased PTH effect at the level of the proximal nephron. Accordingly, urine cyclic AMP excretion is elevated and TmP/GFR is reduced.

TESTS

Calcium

In the plasma, calcium exists within three interconvertible compartments: (1) calcium that is ionized; (2) calcium that is complexed to various anions; and (3) calcium that is bound to plasma proteins. The ionized fraction, which comprises slightly less than one-half the total plasma calcium, is free and physiologically active. A second fraction of calcium, which constitutes 5 to 10 percent of the total plasma calcium, is bound to inorganic anions such as bicarbonate and phosphate and to organic anions such as citrate and lactate. The remaining approximately 50 percent of the total plasma calcium is bound to serum proteins (about four-fifths to albumin and one-fifth to gamma globulins), and as such is nonultrafilterable or nondiffusible (Table 16–3). No physiologic significance has been ascribed to the complexed and protein-bound fractions, and it is generally assumed that only the ionized fraction is physiologically active and under hormone control.

Several factors can affect the reliability and accuracy of a total serum calcium level. Most critical are the technique and timing of venipuncture. Under optimal circumstances, blood samples for serum calcium measurement should be obtained without venous stasis and when the patient is fasting. The tourniquet, if used, should be released when the needle is in the vein, and a pause of 10 seconds should occur before blood is withdrawn. Prolonged application of the tourniquet leads to venosta-

sis, which increases the serum protein concentration, and results in a spuriously elevated total serum calcium level. Similarly, prolonged standing or dehydration can also increase the concentration of plasma proteins and thus of total serum calcium.

The timing of venipuncture is also critical, and only values obtained after an overnight fast should be regarded as reliable. Random, as opposed to fasting, blood specimens introduce the potential of postprandial changes in total serum calcium. These changes may be in either direction and depend on the nature of the meal.

Several other factors can alter the total calcium level without affecting the ionized fraction. Any increase or decrease in serum albumin will alter the protein-bound fraction, and therefore the total serum calcium level, in the same direction. Because globulins bind calcium minimally, only exceptionally large increases in the globulin concentration, or rarely the production of a specific myeloma paraprotein, will raise the total serum calcium level to hypercalcemic levels. The effect of serum protein concentration on total serum calcium concentration is significant. Hence, numerous correction factors, relating measured serum calcium concentration to specific gravity, total protein, and serum albumin concentrations, have been developed. Although no algorithm provides precise values compared with actual measurement of the calcium concentration, it is nevertheless possible to apply a clinically useful formula that is based on the observation that each gram per 100 ml of serum albumin binds approximately 0.8 mg per 100 ml of calcium:

Corrected total serum calcium =
(Measured total serum calcium) −
[Albumin (g per 100 ml)] + 4.0

Routine determination of total serum calcium is performed in most clinical laboratories by colorimetric autoanalyzer techniques. Although these methods are quite dependable, the results obtained are clearly less accurate than those obtained by atomic absorption spectrophotometry. The normal range for total serum calcium must be established for each laboratory, but in general, in the United States, typical normal limits (based on 95 percent confidence limits) are 9.0 to 10.6 mg per deciliter. The mean value for uncorrected total serum calcium is about 0.2 mg per deciliter higher in men than

TABLE 16–3 Physiologic State of Calcium in Plasma

Compartment	Concentration		Percentage of Total
	mg/dl	mmol/L	
Ionized	4.8	2.4	48%
Complexed	0.8	0.4	8%
Protein-bound	4.4	2.2	44%

in women until age 60; thereafter, the values are identical. There does not appear to be significant diurnal variation in the level of total serum calcium.

Ionized Calcium

Because the ionized fraction of the total serum calcium represents the physiologically significant component, it would be highly desirable to measure the ionized calcium for the clinical assessment of patients and dispense with total calcium measurements altogether. Determination of the ionized calcium level can circumvent the problems of interpreting total serum calcium concentrations when there are abnormalities of serum proteins and can confirm the existence of hypercalcemia in patients with so-called normocalcemic primary hyperparathyroidism. Unfortunately, none of the currently available techniques to measure ionized calcium is sufficiently accurate, reliable, or precise to be routinely useful. The equipment most commonly used in clinical hospital laboratories employs flow-through electrodes to measure the calcium ion concentration and the pH of the injected plasma sample. One significant source of error in the determination of ionized calcium is the considerable degree of artifact that can be introduced when blood samples are not collected or handled properly. For some methods, blood samples must be collected anaerobically, maintained on ice, and analyzed within a short time. Accuracy is lessened when blood collection tubes are incompletely filled and when temperature is not rigidly controlled. The pH of the blood sample is also critical. Any increase in blood pH will increase calcium binding to albumin and cause a decrease in the ionized calcium level; conversely, a decrease in blood pH will decrease calcium binding to albumin and cause an increase in the ionized calcium level.

Thus, the concentration of ionized calcium will be significantly influenced by changes in the pH that may occur in vivo or in vitro after the collection of a blood sample.

Parathyroid Hormone

PTH is synthesized in the parathyroid glands as a larger molecular precursor consisting of 115 amino acids, referred to as preproparathyroid hormone. Preproparathyroid hormone is converted to a 90-amino-acid intermediate, proparathyroid hormone, which is then converted by additional proteolytic modification to the mature 84-amino-acid form of the hormone. The major biologically active product secreted from the parathyroid gland represents the 84-amino-acid polypeptide. In addition, considerable evidence suggests that other immunoreactive fragments are released as well. Secretion of intact PTH into the circulation is followed by its rapid uptake into peripheral tissues, primarily liver and kidney, where cleavage of the hormone then generates multiple peptide fragments, some of which reappear in the circulation. Peripheral metabolism and intraglandular proteolytic modification of the hormone result in the production of biologically inactive peptide fragments composed principally of the middle and carboxyl portions of the molecule. Only very low concentrations of the amino terminal fragments, if present in the serum at all, contribute to the circulating pool of immunoreactive PTH. Biologically active PTH 1–84 has a half-life of less than 5 minutes, whereas the middle and carboxyl terminal fragments, which are cleared by the kidneys, have half-lives that are at least 10- to 20-fold longer than the intact hormone. Thus, human serum contains a heterogeneous mixture of PTH molecules, including the intact hormone and much greater concentrations of biologically inactive middle and carboxyl terminal fragments.

Immunoassay of PTH

Measurement of PTH by radioimmunoassay has proved of considerable value in the laboratory diagnosis of disorders of calcium metabolism. Since the introduction of the radioimmunoassay for PTH in 1963 by Berson and Yalow, the test has developed from an esoteric research tool to a practical diagnostic aid with wide-ranging clinical application. The availability of highly sensitive and specific PTH radioimmunoassays is no doubt responsible for the marked change in the diagnostic algorithm applied to patients with hypercalcemia. Whereas in the past a patient with hypercalcemia was likely to undergo an extensive evaluation for the presence of a nonparathyroid disorder, physicians today depend more heavily on the results of radioimmunoassay for PTH to determine whether a patient has primary hyperparathyroidism or another disorder that could cause hypercalcemia.

This new laboratory approach to the diagnosis of hypercalcemia relies on the use of a radioimmunoassay for serum PTH that can consistently distinguish patients with primary hyperparathyroidism from subjects in whom hypercalcemia is due to other causes. The ideal PTH radioimmunoassay for clinical use should provide these desirable features: (1) the ability to detect and measure immunoreactive PTH in greater than 95 percent of normal sera; (2) low or undetectable values in patients with hypoparathyroidism or nonparathyroid hypercalcemia; (3) the ability to measure elevated values in greater than 95 percent of patients with primary hyperparathyroidism; and (4) rapid turnaround time. Unfortunately, few currently available radioimmunoassays for PTH can practically satisfy all of these requirements.

Our current understanding of the complexities of radioimmunoassay has identified several basic difficulties that complicate the measurement and interpretation of PTH radioimmunoassays. Among these problems is a lack of agreement on and/or availability of an accepted PTH reference standard. Thus, although measurement of serum PTH by radioimmunoassay is now performed by many commercial reference laboratories and specialized hospital centers, at present there is no standardized assay technique, nor are assay results expressed as a function of a single reference standard. The standards most frequently employed in commercial assays are synthetic human PTH (1-84) and synthetic fragments. By contrast, many research laboratories continue to express their assay results as a function of purified PTH, PTH extracted from human parathyroid adenomas, or hyperparathyroid serum. To complicate the issue further, some laboratories report their results as mass or volume equivalents to these standards, whereas others express their results in terms of weight (e.g., pg per milliliter) or molarity (e.g., pmol per liter) of their standard. The recent introduction of an international reference standard (WHO 79/500) by the World Health Organization may encourage laboratories to express their assay values in these units or to cross-reference their data in terms of this standard.

A second major difficulty with radioimmunoassay of PTH is due to the complexities involved in the reactions of multivalent antisera with multiple forms of circulating PTH. As noted, human serum contains a complex mixture of PTH molecules, including biologically active intact hormone and biologically inert midmolecule and carboxyl-terminal fragments of the hormone. These latter peptides are derived from peripheral catabolism of intact hormone and, at least in hyperparathyroid patients, secretion from parathyroid tissue itself. Intact PTH 1-84 has a half-life of less than 5 minutes, whereas the inactive middle and carboxyl-terminal fragments, which are cleared by the kidneys, have half-lives that are at least 5 to 15-fold longer than the biologically active native 1-84 peptide. For this reason, the quantity of middle and carboxyl-terminal fragments far exceeds that of intact hormone and constitutes 80 to 90 percent of circulating immunoreactive material. Amino-terminal fragments, if they exist, represent a very small fraction of total serum PTH.

Most of the original PTH radioimmunoassays employed multivalent antisera that were developed by immunization with parathyroid gland extracts. These antisera contained multiple species of antibodies that recognized different regions of the PTH molecule. Subsequent PTH radioimmunoassays have used region-selective antisera that were developed by immunization with synthetic human PTH peptide or fragments. These

assays are thereby directed at specific regions of the PTH molecule and can measure circulating levels of carboxyl-terminal, midmolecule, and amino-terminal hormone. Carboxyl-terminal and midmolecule assays are more sensitive than multivalent assays and, although they detect primarily biologically inactive fragments, are generally adequate for most clinical situations. The midmolecule assays have in general replaced carboxyl-terminal assays because they offer even greater sensitivity (Table 16-4).

The great sensitivity of midmolecule (and carboxyl-terminal) radioimmunoassays derives from the long circulating half-life of the measured fragments. Although this feature improves sensitivity, a desirable feature, the long circulating half-lives of these fragments preclude the use of these assays in dynamic testing. Moreover, because the metabolic clearance of midmolecule and carboxyl-terminal fragments is a function of GFR, a decrease in renal function can reduce clearance of these fragments and lead to their disproportionate accumulation in the circulation. Radioimmunoassays that measure these biologically inactive fragments may provide misleadingly elevated results for PTH concentration in sera from patients with renal insufficiency.

To circumvent the limitations of these assays, in both application and interpretation, several laboratories have developed intact and amino-terminal-specific assays, which measure only the biologically active hormone. The accumulation of these peptides is less influenced by the GFR, and thus these assays provide a more precise assessment of parathyroid function in patients with renal disease as well as in subjects with age-related decreases in glomerular filtration. Furthermore, these assays appear to be useful for dynamic testing, particularly suppression testing, because of the short circulating half-life of the intact hormone. Unfortunately, these antisera are not generally available for nonresearch applications. Accordingly, most PTH radioimmunoassays that are available to clinicians employ antisera that recognize antigenic determinants in the middle portion (i.e., midmolecule-specific) of the PTH sequence.

Midmolecule assays measure both intact PTH and fragments consisting of the middle and carboxyl terminal of the hormone. Under optimal conditions, most of these assays can satisfactorily distinguish patients with primary hyperparathyroidism from normal subjects. Immunoreactive PTH levels are observed to be frankly

TABLE 16-4 Immunoassays for Parathyroid Hormone

Type	PTH Antigen	Specificity	Sensitivity
Radioimmunoassay	Carboxyl-terminal	Intact hormone, carboxyl-terminal fragments	High
	Midmolecule	Intact hormone, carboxyl-terminal fragments	High
	Amino-terminal	Intact hormone	Low
Immunoradiometric assay	Amino-terminal and carboxyl-terminal	Intact hormone	High

elevated in 90 percent or more of patients with primary hyperparathyroidism and generally show a strongly positive correlation with the degree of hypercalcemia. It is not uncommon, however, for commercial reference laboratories to sacrifice these highly desirable assay characteristics in their pursuit of methodology that emphasizes a rapid turnaround time. These modifications not only result in a loss of sensitivity but also produce an increase in assay "noise." These problems may account for the failure of many commercial assays to distinguish adequately between patients with primary hyperparathyroidism and those with other causes of hypercalcemia.

In these assays, normal (or occasionally modestly elevated) rather than suppressed levels of PTH are frequently observed in patients with non-PTH-mediated hypercalcemia. This limitation is most critical when one attempts to use the assay to evaluate patients with suspected malignancy-associated hypercalcemia. Although the humoral hypercalcemic factor (PTH-like peptide) produced by many tumors shares a high degree of homology with the amino-terminal sequence of PTH, there is no immunologic similarity between the two peptides. Moreover, analysis of proteins and mRNA extracted from many tumors indicates that neoplasms associated with hypercalcemia rarely if ever produce "ectopic" PTH. It is therefore likely that elevations of immunoreactive PTH seen in competitive radioimmunoassays are due to nonspecific effects (so called damage or nonspecific binding) from factors present in serum that interfere with binding of the PTH radioligand to its antibody. Indeed, there is a notable lack of correlation between the degree of hypercalcemia and the level of apparent immunoreactive PTH in patients with malignancy-associated hypercalcemia.

To eliminate the false signals from nonspecific effects that appear in competitive radioimmunassays, several groups have developed two-site immunoradiometric assays for intact PTH (Table 16–4). Immunoradiometric assays employ an excess of antibody and offer greater sensitivity and specificity than do competitive radioimmunoassays. One recently introduced immunoradiometric assay for PTH uses two affinity-purified polyclonal antisera—one specific for the amino-terminal (1–34) portion of human PTH and the other for the 39–84 amino acid sequence. The carboxyl-terminal antiserum is immobilized onto polystyrene beads and captures intact hormone and midmolecule and carboxyl-terminal fragments. Hormone bound to the solid phase is detected by an amino-terminal radioiodinated antiserum. Although both intact hormone and midmolecule and carboxyl-terminal fragments are bound to the capture antiserum, the aminoterminal antibody will bind selectively to only intact hormone. Thus, the amount of radioactivity bound to the solid phase will vary as a function of the quantity of intact hormone "sandwiched" between the two antisera. Preliminary results indicate that this assay is highly sensitive and specific for intact hormone and can distinguish patients with primary hyperparathyroidism from patients with hypercalcemia of malignancy.

Bioassay of PTH

PTH can be measured by bioassay (Table 16–5). The in vitro bioassays that are most commonly used to determine PTH in plasma are based on measurement of PTH-dependent activation of adenylyl cyclase in either purified canine renal membranes or intact rat osteosarcoma cells in culture. Unfortunately, neither of these bioassays is sufficiently sensitive to measure biologically active PTH in peripheral plasma without first concentrating the sample. In contrast, a more recently developed cytochemical bioassay is exquisitely sensitive and can detect bioactive PTH at the femtogram level, corresponding to dilutions of plasma that are 100 to 1,000 times greater than those commonly used in immunoassays. The cytochemical bioassay is based on activation of glucose-6-phosphate dehydrogenase activity in distal convoluted tubular cells from guinea pig kidney. The specialized equipment and training required to perform the cytochemical bioassay are significant drawbacks that have limited commercial interest in the technique and have relegated the assay to the research laboratory. A further limitation to the widespread clinical application of this assay (as well as any bioassay) is its failure to distinguish between hypercalcemic patients with hyperparathyroidism and those with humoral hypercalcemia of malignancy.

TABLE 16–5   Bioassays for Parathyroid Hormone

Assay Type	Detector	Sensitivity
Amplified renal membrane adenylyl cyclase	Production of cyclic AMP in response to PTH in patient plasma	10^{-6}–10^{-8} M
Rat osteosarcoma cells (ROS 17/2.8)	Production of cyclic AMP in response to PTH in patient plasma	
Cytochemical bioassay	Glucose-6-phosphate dehydrogenase activity in guinea pig kidney slices is increased by PTH in patient plasma, and causes precipitation of nitroblue tetrazolium (NBT) salts. Particles of NBT are quantified microscopically.	10^{-10}–10^{-14} M

Interpretation of PTH Assay Results

The circulating concentration of intact PTH in normal subjects is less than 50 pg per milliliter. In contrast, the normal range for serum immunoreactive PTH is highly dependent on the immunologic characteristics of the particular immunoassay employed and must be established for each laboratory.

An important step in the interpretation of PTH immunoassay results is to ascertain the renal function of the patient. For reasons outlined previously (e.g., prolongation of circulating half-life of carboxyl-terminal fragments in renal insufficiency), most PTH immunoassays will yield spuriously elevated results in patients with declining renal function. Thus, normal-range values supplied by the reference laboratory must be reviewed with care.

A second note of caution reflects the problem in differential diagnosis of hypercalcemia that occurs frequently in relation to the separation of patients with primary hyperparathyroidism from those with malignancy. Patients with hypercalcemia due to nonparathyroid malignancy should have low immunoreactive PTH values if their hypercalcemia is due to bone metastases or production of humoral factors other than PTH. In many immunoassays (and all bioassays), patients with humoral hypercalcemia of malignancy will have PTH values that are high or high-normal and overlap with values observed in patients with primary hyperparathyroidism. Although some of these cancer patients may have coexistent primary hyperparathyroidism, in most cases the PTH values are artifactually elevated and are not due to ectopic secretion of PTH by the tumor. Because of this overlap and other methodologic modifications that result in noise, many reference laboratories analyze results of plasma PTH and calcium by various statistical means to provide an estimate of probability that the PTH and calcium values for a given patient, when considered in relation to a large data base of normal subjects and patients with proven diagnoses, belong to a specific diagnostic group. In addition, PTH assay results are commonly presented graphically as a function of the serum calcium concentration. Although these nomograms suggest that many hypercalcemic patients with primary hyperparathyroidism will have "normal" values for plasma PTH, it is obvious that the most reliable confirmation of primary hyperparathyroidism derives from a frankly elevated assay value for plasma PTH.

Specimen Collection and Preparation

It is important for the clinician to ascertain what specific guidelines or procedures, if any, need be followed to collect and prepare a blood specimen properly for analysis in a particular PTH immunoassay. In general, the determination of immunoreactive PTH is performed on serum. For the most accurate comparison with normal values, a fasting morning serum sample should be obtained. Moreover, because an elevated dietary calcium intake can reduce circulating levels of biologically active PTH in some patients with primary hyperparathyroidism, it is desirable that blood specimens be obtained from patients who have been on a restricted (about 400 mg per day) calcium diet for 3 to 5 days.

Blood should be collected in a venipuncture tube and allowed to clot quickly at room temperature. The sample should then be placed on ice, centrifuged in a refrigerated centrifuge, and the separated serum stored at $-20\,°C$ until assayed. Improper handling and storage of samples may result in a loss of assayable PTH, particularly when intact hormone is measured.

Cyclic AMP and Tubular Reabsorption of Phosphate

PTH exerts many of its effects on its target organs, bone and kidney, by activating the membrane-bound enzyme adenylyl cyclase and thereby causing an increase in cellular concentrations of cyclic AMP. By increasing the concentration of cyclic AMP in renal tubular cells, PTH decreases the tubular reabsorption of phosphate (TRP) and thereby promotes the urinary excretion of phosphate. Because the quantity of phosphate excreted in the urine is a direct reflection of dietary phosphorus intake, simple determination of the phosphorus excretion rate is rarely useful and provides limited clinical information. Thus, numerous studies have examined the phosphaturic response to endogenous PTH and after exogenous administration of PTH preparations in order to formulate calculated indices that express the renal phosphate clearance as a function of circulating levels of bioactive PTH. The most commonly applied index is the TRP, and it is derived from the following simple formula:

$$TRP = ([\text{Creatinine clearance}]-[\text{Phosphate clearance}]) \div (\text{Creatinine clearance})$$

$$= 1- \frac{[\text{Urine phosphate}]}{(\text{Serum phosphate})} \times \frac{(\text{Serum creatinine})}{(\text{Urine creatinine})}$$

A superior reflection of phosphate clearance is obtained by measurement of the tubular phosphorus threshold (TmP/GFR). This index expresses phosphate reabsorption as function of both serum phosphate concentration and the GFR. The TmP/GFR is derived by use of a reference nomogram that correlates the measured value for serum phosphate and the calculated fractional excretion of phosphate or TRP. When the GFR is above 40 ml per minute, the TmP/GFR provides a reliable estimate of the tubular excretion rate of phosphorus. The normal range of TmP/GFR is 2.5 to 4.2 mg per deciliter and is decreased in hyperparathyroidism. The TmP/GFR is influenced by factors other than PTH, however. Thus, the TmP/GFR is *increased* in states characterized by elevated circulating levels of growth hormone (e.g., growing children and patients with acromegaly) or depressed levels of estrogen (e.g., postmenopausal women). The TmP/GFR is *decreased* in patients who have defects in function of the proximal renal tubule (e.g., Fanconi syndrome).

Because so many dietary and physiologic factors in addition to PTH may influence renal excretion of phosphate, determination of the urinary excretion of cyclic AMP appears to be a superior index of PTH effect on the proximal renal tubule. Normally, the total amount of cyclic AMP excreted in the urine represents cyclic AMP in plasma that is filtered at the glomerulus (50 percent) and that is derived from the kidney (50 percent). Although other agents, notably calcitonin and vasopressin, may activate adenylyl cyclase in the kidney, the proximal tubular effects of PTH account for nearly all of the cyclic AMP produced by the kidney (i.e., nephrogenous cyclic AMP). Thus, the level of nephrogenous cyclic AMP provides a sensitive index of the circulating level of PTH bioactivity. Specifically, more than 90 percent of patients with primary hyperparathyroidism will have elevated levels of nephrogenous cyclic AMP, whereas patients with hypoparathyroidism (or pseudohypoparathyroidism) will have very low values.

Determination of nephrogenous cyclic AMP requires simultaneous measurement of plasma and urinary cyclic AMP and creatinine (Table 16–6). Because measurement of plasma cyclic AMP is technically difficult, in practice the simple determination of total urinary cyclic AMP excretion has been found to be an acceptable (and nearly as accurate) alternative to measurement of nephrogenous cyclic AMP.

Excretion of both the nephrogenous and total urinary cyclic AMP is influenced by the GFR, and results must therefore be expressed as a function of renal clearance (nanomoles of cyclic AMP per deciliter of glomerular filtrate [GF]):

$$\frac{\text{Cyclic AMP } \mu\text{mol}}{L} \times \frac{\text{Serum creatinine (mg/dl)}}{\text{Urine creatinine (mg/dl)}} \times 100$$
$$= \text{nmol/100 ml GF}$$

The normal range for nephrogenous cyclic AMP is 0.34 to 2.70 nmol per 100 ml GF, and for total urinary cyclic AMP it is 1.83 to 4.50 nmol per 100 ml GF.

Urine samples for determination of phosphate clearance or cyclic AMP may be obtained as spot, timed, or 24-hour collections. It is perhaps most convenient to obtain a 2 to 4-hour urine collection in the morning with the patient fasting. Under these conditions the measurement of urinary cyclic AMP can provide a valid index of circulating PTH bioactivity at levels of GFR down to 20 ml per minute.

The reliability of an elevated level of urinary cyclic AMP (or decreased TmP/GFR) as a specific indicator of primary hyperparathyroidism has been challenged recently by the recognition that many nonparathyroid malignancies produce hypercalcemia via elaboration of a humoral factor that activates renal adenylyl cyclase and increases urinary cyclic AMP. In contrast, urinary cyclic AMP determination can be a valuable adjunct in patients with known primary hyperparathyroidism. In this regard, periodic measurement of urinary cyclic AMP values can be used to monitor the course of primary hyperparathyroidism over time. In some highly specialized centers the availability of automated techniques to measure urinary cyclic AMP rapidly (in less than 7 minutes) has permitted the use of intraoperative measurement of urinary cyclic AMP excretion to guide surgery for primary hyperparathyroidism in selected patients. A drop in urinary cyclic AMP excretion to the normal range within 1 to 2.5 hours after parathyroidectomy provides functional confirmation that surgery has been successful.

Another clinical application of urinary cyclic AMP measurement is in the dynamic evaluation of PTH responsiveness. Measurement of urinary cyclic AMP can provide a sensitive method to quantitate the entire spectrum of parathyroid function and has found particular usefulness in assessing the ability of the target organ kidney to respond to PTH in patients in whom the diagnosis of pseudohypoparathyroidism is suspected.

PTH Infusion

The biochemical hallmark of pseudohypoparathyroidism is failure of the target organs bone and kidney to respond to PTH. Accordingly, a diagnosis of pseudohypoparathyroidism should be considered in an individual with biochemical hypoparathyroidism (i.e., hypocalcemia and hyperphosphatemia) who has an elevated plasma concentration of immunoreactive PTH. Because reduced serum concentrations of magnesium have been reported to impair target organ responsiveness to PTH, it is important first to exclude hypomagnesemia in these subjects. Additional evidence of pseudohypoparathyroidism is provided by the presence of a unique constellation of developmental anomalies, termed Albright's hereditary osteodystrophy, that includes obesity, short stature, round facies, subcutaneous ossifications, and brachydactyly. Further testing is indicated only to confirm the diagnosis of pseudohypoparathyroidism or to distinguish between the several variants.

The classic tests for pseudohypoparathyroidism, the Ellsworth-Howard test and later modifications by Chase, Melson, and Aurbach, involved the administration of 200 to 300 USP units of purified bovine PTH or parathyroid extract. Although these preparations are no longer available, the synthetic human PTH (1–34) peptide has recently been approved for human use (Table 16–7). The patient should be fasting, supine except for voiding, and hydrated (250 ml of water hourly from 6:00 AM to noon). Two control urine specimens are collected before 9:00 AM. Synthetic human PTH (1–34) peptide (15 to 25 μg) is administered intravenously from 9:00 to 9:15 AM, and experimental urine specimens are collected from 9:00 to

Table 16–6 Urinary Cyclic AMP Measurement

Method	Radioimmunoassay or protein binding assay for cyclic AMP. Timed spot (2- or 4-hr urinary collections in the morning with the patient in the fasting state) or 24-hr urine collection. Urine collected in a container containing 1 ml of 6 N HCl for each hour of collection. Measurements of serum and urinary creatinine and urinary cyclic AMP made.

$$\frac{\text{Cyclic AMP } \mu\text{mol}}{L} \times \frac{\text{Serum creatinine (mg/dl)}}{\text{Urine creatinine (mg/dl)}} \times 100$$

$$= \text{nmol of cyclic AMP/100 ml GF}$$

Normal	1.83–4.50 nmol/100 ml GF.
Uses	Elevated in 90% of hyperparathyroid patients. Useful in dynamic testing in hyperparathyroidism and in monitoring the course of known hyperparathyroidism.
Problems	Many nonparathyroid malignancies also elevate cyclic AMP.

9:30 AM, 9.30 to 10:00 AM, 10:00 to 11:00 AM, and 11:00 AM to noon. Blood samples should be obtained at 9:00 AM and 11:00 AM for measurement of serum creatinine and phosphorus concentrations. Urine samples are analyzed for cyclic AMP, phosphorus, and creatinine concentrations, and results are expressed as nanomoles of cyclic AMP per 100 ml GF and TmP/GFR. Normal subjects and patients with hormonopenic hypoparathyroidism usually display a 10- to 20-fold increase in urinary cyclic AMP excretion, whereas patients with pseudohypoparathyroidism Type I (Type Ia and Type Ib), regardless of their serum calcium concentration, will show a markedly blunted response. Thus, this test can distinguish patients with so-called normocalcemic pseudohypoparathyroidism (i.e., patients with PTH resistance who are able to maintain normal serum calcium levels without treatment) from subjects with pseudopseudohypoparathyroidism, a genetically related disorder in which patients manifest Albright's hereditary osteodystrophy but do not have hormone resistance.

Patients who have pseudohypoparathyroidism Type II, a much rarer entity, have a normal urinary cyclic AMP

TABLE 16–7 Parathyroid Hormone Infusion Test

Method	Patient in the fasting, supine state. Hydrated with 250 ml of water hourly from 6:00 AM to noon; two control urine samples are collected before 9:00 AM. Synthetic PTH (1-34), 12–25 μg is given IV from 9:00 to 9:15. Urine samples taken from 9:00 to 9:30, 9:30 to 10:00, 10:00 to 10:30, 10:30 to 11:00, and 11:00 to 12:00. Serum samples for creatinine and phosphorus taken at 9:00 and 11:00 AM. Urine cyclic AMP, phosphorus, and creatinine on samples expressed in terms of GFR.
Normal	10 to 20-fold increase in urinary cyclic AMP with a phosphaturic response.
Uses	Diagnosis of pseudohypoparathyroidism Ia and Ib, and pseudohypoparathyroidism type II (see text).
Problems	Requires precise collections and trained personnel.

response to PTH but characteristically fail to show a phosphaturic response.

The plasma calcium response to several hundred units of bovine parathyroid extract given daily for 1 week or more has been used to assess the ability of bone to respond to PTH. Only a few patients with pseudohypoparathyroidism have been tested in this manner, and adequate comparative data from normal subjects are not available. Moreover, recent studies suggest that the calcemic response to PTH may be more a function of plasma concentration of 1,25(OH)$_2$D than of the innate responsiveness of bone to PTH.

Urine Calcium

The determination of fasting urinary calcium clearance rate and measurements of daily calcium excretion require cooperation between physician, patient, and laboratory to ensure reliable results. The physician must explain the method of urine collection, the patient must follow all instructions carefully, and the laboratory must provide accurate measurement. As simple as this guidance may sound, all too frequently uninterpretable results are obtained because of carelessness.

The fasting urinary calcium clearance rate is determined by measuring the concentration of calcium and creatinine in a spot or timed urine sample after an overnight fast (Table 16–8). The corresponding plasma concentrations of calcium and creatine are also measured, and the result is expressed as a function of GFR (calcium clearance divided by creatinine clearance). The normal range for the ratio of calcium clearance to creatinine clearance is approximately 0.02 to 0.15. The fasting urinary excretion rate for calcium is the most clinically useful diagnostic test to discriminate between hypercalcemic patients with familial hypocalciuric hypercalcemia (values typically less than 0.01) and those with typical primary hyperparathyroidism (values typically greater than 0.01). Two or more determinations should be obtained to

TABLE 16-8   Urinary Calcium Clearance

Method	After 12-hr fast and hydration with distilled water, a timed urine collection for calcium and creatinine is made. Serum creatinine and calcium are also determined and the result is expressed as a function of GFR.
Normal	Calcium clearance/creatinine clearance = 0.02 − 0.15.
Uses	Distinguish FHH from primary hyperparathyroidism (see text).
Problems	Values may overlap. Medications such as furosemide and thiazides, as well as intake of sodium and calcium, will affect results.

FHH = familial hypocalciuric hypocalcemia

minimize the variability of this index. Because occasional patients with either disorder will have values that overlap, it is necessary to obtain additional clinical and biochemical data (see previously) to ensure accurate diagnosis.

The fasting calcium excretion rate is influenced by diet and medications—lithium and thiazide diuretics decrease the clearance rate, and the powerful loop diuretics increase the clearance rate. A high calcium and sodium intake can increase the calcium clearance rate. The most reliable results are obtained after several days of a diet that contains moderate quantities of calcium (400 mg per day) and sodium (100 mEq per day).

Determination of the daily urinary excretion of calcium is helpful in differentiating among several forms of hypercalcemia. Its usefulness in the evaluation of patients with nephrolithiasis will not be discussed here. The great variability in dietary intake of calcium and other factors that influence the renal excretion of calcium has complicated attempts to establish a value for the upper limit of normal 24-hour calcium excretion. On a "free diet," which in the United States contains approximately 500 mg of elemental calcium, the upper normal limits are 4 mg or less per kilogram of body weight per day. Indeed, on an undefined diet, most normal men excrete 300 mg or less per day and most normal women excrete 250 mg or less per day. Because the actual dietary intake of calcium may vary considerably on an undefined diet, results that exceed these normal values may occur in individuals who do not have an underlying disorder of mineral metabolism.

Urinary calcium excretion is related to both the filtered load of calcium and the circulating concentration of PTH. Because PTH stimulates reabsorption of calcium from the glomerular filtrate, there is generally less urinary calcium excretion relative to the serum calcium concentration in primary hyperparathyroidism than in other forms of hypercalcemia. Accordingly, in non-PTH-dependent forms of hypercalcemia, such as sarcoidosis, vitamin D intoxication, and malignancy, PTH secretion is inhibited and urinary calcium excretion greatly exceeds normal for any given serum calcium concentration. In contrast, urinary calcium excretion is elevated in only approximately two-thirds of patients with primary hyperparathyroidism.

As noted, because patients with familial hypocalciuric hypercalcemia have a markedly decreased rate of calcium clearance, 24-hour urine calcium excretion is generally low (or normal) in these individuals.

Determination of urine calcium excretion can also provide insight into the pathophysiologic basis for hypocalcemia. Urinary calcium excretion is generally reduced (less than 75 mg per 24 hours in hypocalcemic subjects with secondary hypoparathyroidism, including vitamin D deficiency, vitamin D–dependent rickets Types I and II, and pseudohypoparathyroidism). Owing to the absence of PTH, there is generally more urinary calcium excretion relative to the serum concentration in hypoparathyroidism than in the other aforementioned forms of hypocalcemia.

To obtain more accurate and diagnostic data for calcium excretion, investigators frequently place patients on a defined diet. The two most widely used diets are the low-normal calcium intake (400 mg per day) and the high-normal calcium intake (1,000 mg per day). In general, the 1,000-mg calcium diet is preferred because it provides greater discrimination in defining the presence and degree of hypercalciuria.

For proper evaluation of tests on a 24-hour urine sample it is important that a *complete* and accurate collection be made. The patient should be on a free or defined diet (1,000 mg calcium, 100 mEq sodium). The patient should be instructed to empty his or her bladder upon rising in the morning and to discard this urine. From that point on, the patient is to collect in a clean container all the urine voided during the day and night. The final collection is made when the patient empties his or her bladder the next morning at the same hour. The collected urine should be refrigerated, if possible, and brought to the laboratory as soon as possible after the 24-hour collection is complete. More precise and accurate data for calcium excretion are obtained when several 24-hour urine samples are analyzed.

Vitamin D

The D vitamins are a family of fat-soluble secosteroid hormones that regulate bone resorption and absorption of both calcium and phosphate from the intestine. It is now recognized that vitamin D is biologically inert and that these actions are mediated by the activated metabolite $1,25(OH)_2D_3$. The physiologic roles of other vitamin D metabolites remain to be defined. The production of $1,25(OH)_2D_3$ depends on the availability of precursors and the subsequent hydroxylation of these, first in the liver and then in the kidney.

The daily requirement for vitamin D is generally satisfied by generation of vitamin D_3 (cholecalciferol) in the skin under the influence of the ultraviolet B portion (290- to 315-nm wavelength) of the solar spectrum.

Production of vitamin D in the skin is reduced by skin pigmentation, ultraviolet sun screens, and aging. Thus, adequate sunlight exposure is a critical requirement for endogenous production of vitamin D_3. Vitamin D may also be supplied through ingestion of foods that have been fortified with either vitamin D_3 or vitamin D_2 (ergocalciferol).

In humans, vitamins D_2 and D_3 are similarly metabolized, and for purposes of general discussion, no distinction between these two steroids and their metabolites will be made. Once vitamin D produced in the skin or absorbed from the gastrointestinal tract enters the circulation, it is bound to the serum vitamin D–binding protein (transcalciferin) and transported to the liver. In the liver, vitamin D undergoes hydroxylation to 25(OH)D. Although there is a mild degree of product inhibition of 25-hydroxylase activity, circulating concentrations of 25(OH)D provide a good reflection of the cumulative effects of sunlight exposure and the dietary intake of vitamin D.

The major known physiologic role of 25(OH)D is that of substrate for conversion to $1,25(OH)_2D$, the most potent known natural metabolite of vitamin D. Although 25(OH)D-1-α-hydroxylase activity has been localized principally to the proximal renal tubule, under special circumstances similar enzyme activity can be identified in placenta, bone cells, keratinocytes, and stimulated monocytes. The reaction mediated by renal 25(OH)D-1-α-hydroxylase is the major control point in calciferol metabolism. Enzyme activity is independently increased either by elevated circulating concentrations of PTH or by phosphate depletion. In contrast, renal 25(OH)-1-α-hydroxylase activity is markedly decreased by reduced levels of bioactive PTH or by hyperphosphatemia. Several additional factors have direct or indirect effects on renal 25(OH)-1)α-hydroxylase activity. Enzyme activity is decreased by hypercalcemia and elevated concentrations of $1,25(OH)_2D$, whereas stimulation of enzyme activity has been observed with prolactin, growth hormone, estrogen, insulin, and calcitonin.

Calciferol metabolites may be quantitated by radioligand, spectral, or biologic assays. Highly reliable biochemical and physicochemical assays for most calciferol metabolites are commercially available and can determine the plasma concentration of each of the physiologically important metabolites of vitamin D. Common to all of these assays is the need to separate calciferol metabolites

from each other and from lipids and other substances that interfere in the assay. The most sensitive and specific assays generally require a multistep purification (including organic extraction, column chromatography, and reverse-phase, high-performance liquid chromatography) prior to actual quantitation.

After extensive purification, plasma concentrations of vitamins D_2 and D_3 can be quantitated by either ultraviolet absorption or ligand displacement using rat serum vitamin D–binding protein (Table 16–9). The circulating concentration of the calciferols in normal individuals ranges from 1 to 10 ng per milliliter. Measurement of plasma levels of vitamin D is of little clinical value because the half-life is short (about 2 days), and there can be wide fluctuations in response to exposure to sunlight and vitamin D intake. Because there are few clinical indications for measurement of plasma calciferol concentration, these assays are not generally available commercially. In contrast, there is great clinical interest in measurement of the plasma levels of $25(OH)D_2$ and $25(OH)D_3$, as concentrations of these two metabolites provide a reliable reflection of systemic vitamin D status. Accordingly, highly sensitive and specific assays are available from several commercial reference laboratories. The level of 25(OH)D may be quantitated by competitive displacement ligand assays that employ either rat or human serum vitamin D–binding protein or a cytosolic-binding protein (Table 16–10). These ligand assays do not discriminate between $25(OH)D_2$ and $25(OH)D_3$ when unfractionated plasma samples are used. However, if these metabolites are first separated by high-performance liquid chromatography, the plasma concentrations of each can be quantitated. In the absence of vitamin D supplements, approximately 80 percent of total 25(OH)D is $25(OH)D_3$. The rationale for discriminating between the two metabolites is based on the premise that the concentration of $25(OH)D_2$ is an indication of dietary vitamin D, whereas the concentration of $25(OH)D_3$ is an indication of endogenously synthesized vitamin D due to exposure to sunlight. The use of both vitamins D_2 and D_3 in the fortification of many foods challenges the reliability of this assumption, however, and has reduced enthusiasm for assays that can distinguish between $25(OH)D_2$ and $25(OH)D_3$.

In normal adults, the plasma concentration of 25(OH)D ranges from 10 to 80 ng per milliliter. This wide range no doubt reflects the influence of changes in sun-

TABLE 16-9   Circulating Concentrations of Vitamin D Metabolites

Steroid	Normal Range	Comments
Vitamin D_3 (cholecalciferol)	1–10 ng/ml	Primarily reflects sunlight-dependent synthesis in skin
$25(OH)D_3$ $25(OH)D_2$	10–80 ng/ml	80% of 25(OH)D is $25(OH)D_3$ in subjects who do not ingest vitamin D_2. Elevated levels of $25(OH)D_2$ may indicate excessive consumption of vitamin D_2
$1,25(OH)D_3$	15–60 pg/ml	Most physiologically active vitamin D metabolite

TABLE 16-10   Measurement of 25(OH)D

Method	Competitive displacement ligand assays.
Normal	10–80 ng/ml.
Uses	Diagnosis of hypercalcemia due to vitamin D ingestion; diagnosis of hypocalcemia due to vitamin D deficiency, malabsorption, or severe liver disease.
Problems	Lowered levels in patients with protein deficiency due to loss of vitamin D binding protein.

light exposure and, to a lesser extent, diet. For example, plasma concentrations of 25(OH)D are generally highest at the end of the summer and lowest during midwinter. Plasma levels of calcium and phosphorus do not influence hepatic production of 25(OH)D. In contrast, plasma levels of 25(OH)D are reduced in vitamin D deficiency, intestinal malabsorption syndromes, severe liver disease, and anticonvulsant drug therapy. Moreover, plasma concentrations of 25(OH)D are also decreased (but not below the normal range) in disease states that are associated with enhanced metabolism of 25(OH)D, such as sarcoidosis, primary hyperparathyroidism, tumoral calcinosis, vitamin D–dependent rickets Type II, and obesity. Finally, patients with renal disease who have marked proteinuria (e.g., nephrotic syndrome) or who are undergoing chronic peritoneal dialysis may have decreased plasma concentrations of the vitamin D–binding protein transcalciferin and as a result will have reduced plasma concentrations of 25(OH)D.

Serum concentrations of 25(OH)D are typically elevated in individuals who ingest excessive quantities of vitamin D (or 25[OH]D) and may disclose the etiology of hypercalcemia in surreptitious vitamin D intoxication.

Various methods are used to measure the concentration of 1,25(OH)$_2$D in plasma (Table 16–11). These techniques include radioimmunoassay, bioassay using fetal rat bones, and radioreceptor or protein-binding assays using the cytosolic receptor protein for 1,25(OH)$_2$D isolated from chick intestine. Two recently developed techniques, a protein-binding assay using cytosolic receptor from calf thymus and a cytoreceptor assay using cultured rat osteosarcoma cells, require only minimal purification of plasma samples prior to assay. Over the past several years refinements in 1,25(OH)$_2$D assays have reduced the specimen volume requirements to 2 to 7 ml of serum. This volume is necessary to permit complex extraction procedure as well as purification of 1,25(OH)$_2$D by high-performance liquid chromatography prior to measurement of the steroid by competitive protein-binding assay. Optimally, specimens should be obtained in the morning while fasting. The typical normal range for adults is 15 to 60 pg per milliliter (36 to 144 pmol per liter) but varies considerably from laboratory to laboratory.

The measurement of the plasma concentration of 1,25(OH)$_2$D is of great value in the evaluation of patients with suspected disorders of mineral metabolism, because this metabolite is the active form of the hormone. Serum concentrations of 1,25(OH)$_2$D can be low, normal, or elevated in patients with mild to moderate vitamin D deficiency and will depend on the degree of adaptive (secondary) hyperparathyroidism and the level of 25(OH)D. Serum concentrations of 1,25(OH)$_2$D are reduced in anephric subjects or patients with severe renal failure, in hypoparathyroidism and pseudohypoparathyroidism, in vitamin D–dependent rickets Type I, and in oncogenous osteomalacia. Serum levels of 1,25(OH)$_2$D are normal in subjects with X-linked hypophosphatemic rickets but are inappropriately low relative to the reduced serum phosphorus concentration.

Serum levels of 1,25(OH)$_2$D are elevated (or high-normal) in sarcoidosis and other granulomatous diseases, some lymphomas, primary hyperparathyroidism, idiopathic hypercalciuria, and vitamin D–dependent rickets Type II.

Calcitonin and Provocative Tests

Calcitonin is a 32-amino-acid polypeptide produced by the parafollicular or C cells of the thyroid. Calcitonin is synthesized as part of a larger precursor, preprocalcitonin, which undergoes cotranslational and post-translational processing to yield calcitonin and three other peptides.

The calcitonin molecule of all species examined has an amino-terminal disulfide bridge that links amino acid residues 1 and 7. The reactivity of this disulfide linkage can explain the presence of dimeric and polymeric forms of the hormone in the circulation. Only the monomeric form of calcitonin is biologically active. Comparison of the amino acid sequences of the calcitonin molecule from a variety of species discloses close homologies for only nine of the 32 amino acid residues. Nevertheless, all 32 amino acids are required for bioactivity. This structural diversity most likely accounts for the observation that most radioimmunoassays for calcitonin are species specific.

The precise physiologic role of calcitonin in the regulation of mineral metabolism in humans remains uncertain. Thus, the greatest relevance of calcitonin may be attributed to its clinical usefulness as a pharmacologic agent in the treatment of Paget's disease and its importance as a hormonal marker in the detection of medullary thyroid carcinoma (Table 16–12).

Calcitonin is measured in human plasma by radioimmunoassays that employ synthetic human calcitonin

TABLE 16–11   Measurement of 1,25(OH)$_2$ D

Method	Radioimmunoassay, bioassay, radioreceptor, or protein binding.
Normal	15–60 pg/ml.
Uses	Evaluation of patients with acquired and inherited disorders of 25(OH)D metabolism.
Problems	Changes in levels due to dietary intake of calcium. Large volumes of serum necessary for purification procedures in some of the early assays.

TABLE 16–12 Measurement of Calcitonin

Method	Radioimmunoassay.
Normal	Nonextracted plasma: 20–75 pg/ml Extracted: Men 8.2 ± 5 pg/ml Women 4.8 ± 4 pg/ml
Uses	Diagnosis of medullary thyroid carcinoma.
Problems	Nonspecific increases in normals overlapping patients with medullary carcinoma. Elevated levels with renal failure. 30% of medullary thyroid carcinoma patients have normal levels of basal calcitonin.

as a standard and radioligand and antisera generated against synthetic human calcitonin. Several problems limit the usefulness of conventional calcitonin radioimmunoassays in the diagnosis and management of medullary thyroid carcinoma. For example, nonspecific increases in plasma immunoreactive calcitonin are occasionally found in normal individuals, thus making it difficult to distinguish a seemingly healthy person with a high level of immunoreactive calcitonin from a patient with occult medullary thyroid carcinoma. In healthy subjects, elevated calcitonin values may be due to circulating factors that can interfere in the radioimmunoassay for calcitonin or might reflect the immunochemical influence of dimeric or polymeric forms of calcitonin. This problem can be circumvented by the recent development of a silica-cartridge extraction technique that both isolates and concentrates monomeric calcitonin from plasma prior to radioimmunoassay. This assay is sufficiently sensitive (lower limit of detectability 2 pg per milliliter) to measure basal plasma levels of calcitonin monomer in most normal men (8.2 ± 5 pg per milliliter, $\bar{x}$ ± 2 SD) and women (4.8 ± 4 pg per milliliter). In contrast, calcitonin levels in nonextracted plasma are 20 to 75 pg per milliliter (Table 16–12).

As noted, at all ages basal (and stimulated) levels of calcitonin are higher in men than in women. Moreover, plasma concentrations of calcitonin have been noted to decline with age in both sexes. The basis for these differences, and indeed whether these differences are of any physiologic importance, remains unknown. Because calcitonin is cleared from the circulation via the kidneys, plasma concentrations of immunoreactive calcitonin are elevated in patients with marked renal insufficiency.

The application of calcitonin radioimmunoassay to the early detection of medullary thyroid carcinoma is limited by the observation that more than 30 percent of patients have normal basal concentrations of calcitonin in the plasma. This problem has been largely overcome by the use of provocative tests (Table 16–13). The first provocative test to be introduced was the 4-hour calcium infusion (15 mg per kilogram). This test consistently produces an abnormal rise in calcitonin in patients with medullary thyroid carcinoma, but the test is time-consuming and the marked rise in serum calcium levels produces many side effects. It has been replaced by the development of protocols in which the infusion of calcium occurs over 10 minutes (3 mg per kilogram) or 1 minute (2 mg per kilogram). These procedures produce an increase in serum calcium concentration that is usually less than 1 mg per kilogram, but calcitonin secretion is reliably stimulated (Table 16–14).

Pentagastrin is another widely used provocative agent for calcitonin secretion in patients with medullary thyroid carcinoma (Table 16–15). When administered as a rapid (5-second) intravenous bolus (0.5 μg per kilogram), pentagastrin produces a marked stimulation of calcitonin secretion within a short time (peak plasma calcitonin levels occur within 1 to 5 minutes after injection). Although the rapidity of the pentagastrin test is advantageous, this test does have some drawbacks. For example, patients commonly experience a poorly described but unpleasant sensation of flushing or burning. Also, the use of pentagastrin as a diagnostic test for the suspected diagnosis of medullary thyroid carcinoma is not currently approved by the U.S. Food and Drug Administration.

Two interesting modifications of the pentagastrin stimulation test have been described. The peptide can be administered to patients with suspected medullary thyroid carcinoma while an indwelling catheter is located in the inferior thyroid veins to permit plasma sampling for calcitonin assay. In occasional patients a diagnostic increase in calcitonin concentration has been noted in plasma obtained from the thyroid veins but not the

TABLE 16–13 Provocative Tests for the Diagnosis of Medullary Thyroid Carcinoma

Test	Dose	Comments
Intravenous calcium infusion		
Long—4hr infusion	15 mg/kg	Many side-effects, including hypercalcemia
Short—10-min infusion	3 mg/kg	Easy to perform, reliable
1-min infusion	2 mg/kg	
Pentagastrin infusion		
Bolus—5-sec infusion	0.5 μg/kg	Peak calcitonin levels occur 1–5 min after injection; frequent complaints of "burning" or "flushing"
Combined pentagastrin-calcium infusion		
Pentagastrin—5 sec	0.5 μg/kg	This protocol is experimental and not universally
Calcium—1 min	2 mg/kg	accepted

TABLE 16–14 Short Calcium Infusion Test

Method	Calcium IV at 3 mg/kg over 10 minutes or 2 mg/kg over 1 min. Plasma samples before and 10, 20, and 30 min after the start of the 10-min infusion, and before and 5 and 10 min after the start of the 1-min infusion.
Normal	Calcitonin level < 100 pg/ml
Uses	Diagnosis of medullary carcinoma of the thyroid.
Problems	Small number of false negatives. Combining this test with the pentagastrin test decreases the incidence of false negatives.

peripheral veins. A second modification of the pentagastrin test is the combined pentagastrin (0.5 μg per kilogram per 5 seconds) and calcium (2 mg per kilogram per 1 minute) infusion (Table 16–15).

Differences in opinion have appeared in the literature regarding the relative clinical value of all of the just-described provocative tests in the diagnosis of medullary thyroid carcinoma. All of these infusion procedures have a small incidence of false-negative results, but most tumors (and early cases of C-cell hyperplasia) respond to either pentagastrin or calcium. Therefore, if one procedure fails to provide diagnostic results in a patient suspected of having medullary thyroid carcinoma, an alternative testing protocol should be considered. Overall, the sensitivity and specificity of the calcitonin assay are probably as important as the choice of the specific provocative test protocol.

Plasma samples should be obtained immediately before the intravenous infusion begins and 1.5 and 5 minutes (for pentagastrin infusion) or 5 and 10 minutes (for calcium infusion) later. Peak plasma calcitonin values that are diagnostic of medullary thyroid carcinoma will vary from laboratory to laboratory, but typically they are in excess of 100 pg per milliliter for monomeric calcitonin.

Finally, it is important to recognize that patients at risk for medullary thyroid carcinoma (e.g., members of families in which multiple endocrine neoplasia Type II occurs) should be evaluated periodically for the manifestations of the tumor. In general, screening should begin no later than age 5 and continue until at least age 40 at intervals of approximately 6 to 12 months. Accordingly,

TABLE 16–15 Pentagastrin Test

Method	Rapid IV (5-sec) administration 0.5 μg/kg. Serum samples for calcitonin drawn fasting, 1.5, and 5 min after the start of the pentagastrin infusion.
Normal	Calcitonin level < 100 pg/ml.
Uses	Detection of medullary thyroid carcinoma.
Problems	Flushing or burning sensation following administration. Small false-negative rate. Not approved by US Food and Drug Administration.

it may be most practical to refer such individuals to specialized university centers where the appropriate provocative test protocols and calcitonin assays are available.

PARATHYROID IMAGING

Surgical correction of primary hyperparathyroidism is generally considered the most effective therapy for symptomatic subjects. The success rate for exploratory surgery of the neck is greater than 90 percent when surgery is performed by an experienced operator. In contrast, less favorable results are often achieved when unexperienced surgeons attempt this procedure. Because localizing abnormal parathyroid tissue during surgery can be a problem in 10 percent or more of patients, several diagnostic and localizing methods have been developed to identify the enlarged parathyroid gland prior to surgery (Table 16–16). These approaches include both invasive and noninvasive techniques and are available in many centers.

Noninvasive Imaging Studies

High-resolution ultrasonography with a high-resolution scanner coupled to a 10-MHz transducer provides a sensitive and specific method to identify enlarged parathyroid glands in patients who have had no previous neck surgery. As with all noninvasive techniques, prior neck surgery significantly reduces the overall accuracy. The sensitivity of ultrasonography depends on the size of the enlarged gland as well as its position; glands that weigh less than 200 mg are frequently not identified, particularly if they are localized in the retroesophageal, retrotracheal, or mediastinal areas. Ultrasonography is particularly effective for localizing enlarged parathyroid glands in the neck, especially in the immediate vicinity of the thyroid. However, false-positive results are common in patients who have coexistent thyroid disease or nodules. Ultrasonography offers several advantages over other noninvasive techniques. For example, ultrasonography is readily available in most centers, can be performed with no radiation exposure to the patient, and is relatively inexpensive. Moreover, the ultrasonographic technique can be used to guide fine-needle aspiration biopsy of suspected parathyroid tumors and to facilitate obtainment of material for cytologic analysis and measurement of PTH.

Parathyroid scintigraphy with thallium 201 combined with scanning the thyroid with technetium 99m has emerged as a second noninvasive imaging procedure with great potential usefulness in the localization of parathyroid tumors in the neck. The rationale for the combined thallium-technetium scan derives from the observation that thallium accumulates in both parathyroid and thyroid tissues, whereas uptake of technetium 99m appears more limited to the thyroid gland. After a patient undergoes sequential scanning studies with the two radiochemicals, one can use computer subtraction technology to identify enlarged parathyroid glands and

TABLE 16-16 Parathyroid Imaging Studies

Procedure	Sensitivity(%)		Specificity(%)	
	No Previous Neck Surgery	Previous Neck Surgery	No Previous Neck Surgery	Previous Neck Surgery
Noninvasive Techniques				
High-resolution ultrasonography	69–88	36–82	94–96	86–92
Intraoperative ultrasonography	NA	80	NA	NA
Computed tomography	76	13–65	90	NA
Magnetic resonance imaging	74	NA	88	NA
Invasive Techniques				
Digital subtraction arteriography	80	NA	NA	NA
Selective arteriography	75–90	60–85	NA	NA
Venous sampling	NA	80	NA	NA

NA = No data available.

tumors in and around the thyroid and mediastinum. Early reports of the use of the combined thallium-technetium technique have been encouraging, with an overall sensitivity of 80 to 85 percent and specificity of 90 percent in patients who have not undergone neck surgery previously. The sensitivity of this technique is directly related to the size of the parathyroid adenoma, such that 80 to 85 percent of parathyroid glands that weigh 500 mg or more can be visualized. By contrast, parathyroid glands that weigh less than 500 mg are frequently too small to be identified.

The sensitivity and specificity of the thallium-technetium subtraction technique are reduced in patients who have had previous neck surgery and in individuals with many types of thyroid disease. Misleading results due to disproportionate thallium and technetium uptake are not uncommon in subjects with thyroiditis, thyroid cancer, or thyroid adenomas. Moreover, excessive thallium accumulation may occur in neck or mediastinal lymph nodes that contain metastatic cancer, lymphoma, or sarcoid granulomas.

In general, computed tomography (CT) appears less useful than either high-resolution ultrasonography or thallium- technetium subtraction scanning in the preoperative localization of parathyroid adenomas. In patients who have had no previous neck surgery, high-resolution scanning techniques (e.g., 5-mm overlapping cuts) can identify only 70 to 75 percent of enlarged parathyroid glands. However, because the sensitivity of CT in the identification of parathyroid tumors is not dependent upon anatomic location, this technique is superior to the other noninvasive imaging procedures in the evaluation of the retroesophageal, retrotracheal, and mediastinal areas. CT is particularly well suited in the evaluation of the tracheoesophageal groove in the posterior superior mediastinum. This is one of the most common locations of parathyroid glands missed at initial surgery.

Other noninvasive techniques for localization of abnormal parathyroid tissue include thermography, cer-

vical esophagography, magnetic resonance imaging, and selenomethionine 75 (^{75}Se) scanning. In general, these techniques provide little information that cannot be obtained more readily from ultrasonography or thallium-technetium subtraction scanning.

Invasive Techniques

Invasive techniques for identifying and localizing parathyroid tumors include arteriography (selective and nonselective), venography, venography with selective thyroid venous sampling for PTH, and digital subtraction angiography. Of these techniques, nonselective digital arteriography and highly selective arteriography appear to be the most effective. Selective parathyroid angiography identifies enlarged parathyroid glands in 75 to 90 percent of patients who have had no previous surgery and in 60 to 85 percent of patients who have had unsuccessful initial neck explorations. By comparison, nonselective intra-arterial digital subtraction angiography can demonstrate nearly 90 percent of the enlarged parathyroid glands identified by conventional highly selective arteriographic studies. Although the nonselective intra-arterial digital subtraction technique is less sensitive than is selective parathyroid angiography, it requires no selective catheter position and is therefore safer and easier to perform. Accordingly, it seems most practical to select intra-arterial digital subtraction angiography as the initial vascular localizing procedure. Failure with nonselective angiography signals the need for highly selective arteriography, with catheterization of the interior thyroid, internal mammary, and often the superior thyroid arteries. Visualization of a large parathyroid adenoma by selective arteriography clearly facilitates surgical localization and resection of the tumor. In selected cases, however, arteriographic identification of an abnormal parathyroid can also provide a therapeutic alternative to surgical treatment of hyperparathyroidism. One can attempt to ablate the tumor by forcefully wedging the arteriographic catheter in the feeding artery and slowly infusing 8 to 12 ml of water-soluble contrast dye. This technique produces a dramatic tumor "stain," which, if it persists for at least 12 hours, generally indicates that palliation or cure of hyperparathyroidism has been achieved. This technique is most readily applied to mediastinal parathyroid adenomas, where the blood supply is derived from a single thymic branch of the internal mammary artery. Staining of parathyroid adenomas in the neck is less commonly attempted because wedging a catheter in a branch of the thyrocervical trunk is technically more difficult and involves a greater risk to adjacent structures.

Selective venous sampling and measurement of immunoreactive PTH is often performed in conjunction with selective parathyroid arteriography. This technique requires the greatest experience of all invasive procedures, and is the most poorly performed of all the localizing studies. Great care must be taken to obtain blood samples from the paired superior, middle, and inferior thyroid veins, along with the vertebral, thymic, and internal mammary veins. It is frequently not possible to obtain blood samples from all the pertinent veins, however. This may be due to inexperience of the angiographer or, particularly in patients who have undergone previous neck exploration, surgical ligation of the relevant veins. Under optimal circumstances a unilateral hormone gradient (greater than 1.5×) is demonstrated by venous sampling, and the precise localization of the parathyroid is confirmed by selective arteriography. Failure to obtain a unilateral PTH gradient may indicate that bilateral parathyroid disease is present (e.g., parathyroid hyperplasia) or that collateral venous flow occurs through the inferior thyroid vein plexus.

Recommendations

Parathyroid imaging and localization studies are not to be considered as part of the routine evaluation of the patient with hypercalcemia. Indeed, these studies should not be contemplated until a definitive diagnosis of primary hyperparathyroidism has been established. Because of the expense and risk of invasive angiographic procedures, noninvasive parathyroid localization studies should be considered as the initial imaging procedures. Ultrasonography or CT can be useful both to localize the parathyroid tumor and to guide fine-needle aspiration biopsy of the mass. Absolute histologic confirmation can be obtained through either cytologic examination or PTH assay of the recovered material. Invasive angiographic procedures should be reserved for those patients who have had a previous unsuccessful neck exploration and in whom noninvasive studies have failed to disclose the location of the parathyroid tumor. Few angiographers are highly experienced in the performance of selective arteriography and selective venous sampling. Therefore, it would seem most prudent to refer patients in need of these studies to specialized centers where these techniques are routinely performed.

Although localizing studies have clearly improved the success rate of parathyroid exploration in patients who have previously undergone unsuccessful parathyroid surgery, it is less obvious whether imaging studies are of benefit when performed prior to an initial parathyroid exploration. Inasmuch as a skilled surgeon will be successful in achieving cures in 90 percent of these patients, it would seem practical to reserve preoperative localizing studies for those high-risk patients in whom a more limited surgical approach might be appropriate. In these subjects noninvasive imaging techniques could be used to guide surgical exploration and provide the basis for deciding which side of the neck to explore initially. If successful, the duration of surgery and the risk of surgical complications could be greatly reduced.

BIBLIOGRAPHY

General Reading

Agus SZ, Wasserstein A, Goldfarb S. Disorders of calcium and magnesium homeostasis. Am J Med 1982; 72:473.

Aurbach GD, Marx SJ, Spiegel AM. Parathyroid hormone, calcitonin, and the calciferols. In: Wilson JD, Foster DW, eds. Textbook of endocrinology. Philadelphia: WB Saunders, 1985:1137.

Levine MA. Laboratory investigation of disorders of the parathyroid glands. Clin Endocrinol Metab 1985; 14:257.

Levine MA, Aurbach GD. Pseudohypoparathyroidism. In: DeGroot LJ, Besser GM, Cahill FG Jr, et al, eds. Endocrinology. Vol 2. Philadelphia: WB Saunders, 1989:1065.

Stewart AF, Broadus AE. Mineral metabolism. In: Felig P, Baxter JD, Broadus AE, Frohman LA, eds. Endocrinology and metabolism. New York: McGraw-Hill, 1986:1317.

Measurement of Calcium

Annesley TM, Burritt MF, Kyle RA. Artifactual hypercalcemia in multiple myeloma. Mayo Clin Proc 1982; 57:572.

Berry EM, Gupta MM, Turner ST, Burns RR. Variation in plasma calcium with induced changes in plasma specific gravity, total protein, and albumen. Br Med J 1973; iv:640.

Burman KD, Monchik JM, Earll JM, et al. Ionized and total serum calcium and parathyroid hormone in hyperthyroidism. Ann Intern Med 1976; 84:668.

Jaffe JP, Mosher DF. Calcium binding by a myeloma protein. Am J Med 1979; 67:343.

Keating FR, Jones JD, Elveback CR, Randall RV. The relation of age and sex to distribution of values in healthy adults of serum calcium, inorganic phosphorus, magnesium, alkaline phosphatase, total proteins, albumin, and blood urea. J Lab Clin Med 1969; 73:825.

Ladenson JH, Lewis JW, Boyd JC. Failure of total calcium corrected for protein, albumin, and pH to correctly assess free calcium status. J Clin Endocrinol Metab 1978; 46:986.

Marshall RW. Plasma fractions. In: Nordin BEC, ed. Calcium, phosphate and magnesium metabolism. London: Churchill Livingstone, 1976:162.

McLean FC, Hastings AB. A biological method for the estimation of calcium ion concentration. J Biol Chem 1984; 107:337.

Payne RB, Little AJ, Williams RB, Milner JR. Interpretation of serum calcium in patients with abnormal serum proteins. Br Med J 1973; iv:643.

Measurement of Phosphorus

Bijvoet OLM, Morgan DB, Fourman P. The assessment of phosphate reabsorption. Clin Chim Acta 1969; 26:15.

Nordin BEC, Buluser L. A modified index of phosphate excretion. Postgrad Med J 1968; 44:93.

Nordin BEC, Fraser RR. Assessment of urinary phosphate excretion. Lancet 1960; i:947.

Pak CYC, Townsend J. Chloride-phosphorus in primary hyperparathyroidism. Ann Intern Med 1976; 85:830.

Palmer FJ, Nelson JC, Bacchus H. The chloride-phosphate ratio in hypercalcemia. Ann Intern Med 1974; 80:200.

Walton RJ, Bijvoet OLM. Nomogram for the derivation of renal threshold phosphate concentration. Lancet 1975; ii:309.

Urine Calcium

Law WM, Heath H. Familial benign hypercalcemia (hypocalciuric hypercalcemia). Ann Intern Med 1985; 102:511.

Marx SJ, Attie MF, Levine MA, et al. The hypocalciuric or benign variant of familial hypercalcemia: Clinical and biochemical features in fifteen kindreds. Medicine 1981; 60:397.

Marx SJ, Spiegel AM, Levine MA, et al. Familial hypocalciuric hypercalcemia. N Engl J Med 1982; 307:416.

Miller PD, Dubovsky SL, McDonald KM, et al. Hypocalciuric effect of lithium in man. Min Elect Metab 1978; 1:3.

Measurement of Parathyroid Hormone

Berson SA, Yalow RS. Immunochemical heterogeneity of parathyroid hormone in plasma. J Clin Endocrinol Metab 1968; 28:1037.

Chambers DJ, Dunham J, Zanelli JM, et al. A sensitive bioassay of parathyroid hormone in plasma. Clin Endocrinol 1978; 9:375.

European PTH Study Group. Interlaboratory comparison of radioimmunological parathyroid hormone determination. Eur J Clin Invest 1978; 8:149.

Goltzman D, Henderson B, Loveridge N. Cytochemical bioassay of parathyroid hormone. J Clin Invest 1980; 65:1309.

Klee GG, Preissner CM, Schloegel IW, Kao PC. Bioassay of human parathyrin using a rat osteosarcoma derived cell line. Clin Chem 1985; 31:961.

Lindall AW, Elting J, Ells J, Roos BA. Estimation of biologically active intact parathyroid hormone in normal and hyperparathyroid sera by sequential N-terminal immunoextraction and midregion radioimmunoassay. J Clin Endocrinol 1983; 47:1007.

Mallette LE, Tuma SN, Berger RE, Kirkland JL. Radioimmunoassay for the middle region of human parathyroid hormone using an homologous antiserum with a carboxy-terminal fragment of bovine parathyroid hormone as radioligand. J Clin Endocrinol Metab 1982; 54:1017.

Marx SJ, Sharp ME, Krudy A, et al. Radioimmunoassay for the middle region of human parathyroid hormone: Studies with a radioiodinated synthetic peptide. J Clin Endocrinol Metab 1981; 53:76.

Nissenson RA, Abbott SR, Teitelbaum AP, et al. Endogenous biologically active human parathyroid hormone: Measurement by a guanyl nucleotide-amplified renal adenylate cyclase assay. J Clin Endocrinol Metab 1981; 52:840.

Nussbaum S, Zahradnik R, Lavigne J, et al. Development of a highly sensitive two site immunoradiometric assay for parathyroid hormone and its clinical utility in evaluation of patients with hypercalcemia. Clin Chem 1987; 33:1364.

Raisz LG, Yajnik CH, Bockman RS, Bower BF. Comparison of commercially available parathyroid hormone immunoassays in the differential diagnosis of hypercalcemia due to primary hyperparathyroidism or malignancy. Ann Intern Med 1979; 91:739.

Segre GV. Amino-terminal radioimmunoassays for human parathyroid hormone. In: Clinical disorders of bone and mineral metabolism. Frame B, Potts JT Jr, eds. Amsterdam: Excerpta Medica, 1983:14.

Zanelli IM, Gaines-Ds RE. The first international reference preparation of human parathyroid hormone for immunoassay. J Clin Endocrinol Metab 1983; 57:462.

Measurement of Calcitonin

Austin LA, Heath H. Calcitonin physiology and pathophysiology. N Engl J Med 1981; 304:269.

Body JJ, Heath H. Estimates of circulating monomeric calcitonin: Physiological studies in normal and thyroidectomized man. J Clin Endocrinol Metab 1983; 57:897.

Deftos LJ, Weisman MH, Williams GW, et al. Influence of age and sex on plasma calcitonin in human beings. N Engl J Med 1980; 302:1351.

Gharib H, Kao PC, Heath III HH. Determination of silica-purified plasma calcitonin for the detection and management of medullary thyroid carcinoma: Comparison of two provocative tests. Mayo Clin proc 1987; 62:373.

Goltzman D, Tischler AS. Characterization of the immunochemical forms of calcitonin released by a medullary thyroid carcinoma in tissue culture. J Clin Invest 1978; 61:449.

Parthemore JG, Deftos LJ. Calcitonin secretion in primary hyperparathyroidism. J Clin Endocrinol Metab 1979; 49:223.

Tobler PH, Tschopp FA, Dambacher MA, et al. Identification and characterization of calcitonin forms in plasma and urine of normal subjects and medullary carcinoma patients. J Clin Endocrinol Metab 1983; 57:749.

Urinary Cyclic AMP

Broadus AE. Nephrogenous cyclic AMP as a parathyroid function test. Nephron 1979; 23:136.

Broadus AE. Nephrogenous cyclic AMP. Recent Prog Horm Res 37:667, 1981.

Furlong TJ, Seshadri MS, Wilkinson MR, et al. Clinical experiences with human parathyroid hormone 1–34. Aust NZ J Med 1986; 16:794.

Mallette LE, Kirkland JL, Gagel RF, et al. Synthetic human parathyroid hormone (1–34) for the study of pseudohypoparathyroidism. J Clin Endocrinol Metab 1988; 67:964.

Moses AM, Breslau NA, Coulson R. Renal responses to PTH in hormone-resistant (pseudo) hypoparathyroidism. Am J Med 1976; 61:184.

Rude RK, Sharp CF, Fredericks RS, et al. Urinary and nephrogenous cyclic AMP excretion in the hypercalcemia of malignancy. J Clin Endocrinol Metab 1981; 52:765.

Spiegel AM, Eastman ST, Attie MF, et al. Intraoperative measurements of urinary cyclic AMP to guide surgery for primary hyperparathyroidism. N Engl J Med 1980; 303:1457.

Measurement of Vitamin D

Bouillon R, Auwerx J, Dekeyser L, et al. Serum vitamin D metabolites and their binding protein in patients with liver cirrhosis. J Clin Endocrinol Metab 1984; 59:86.

Clemens TL, Hendy GN, Papapoulos SE, et al. Measurement of 1,25-dihydroxycholecalciferol in man by radioimmunoassay. Clin Endocrinol 1979; 11:225.

Eisman JA, Hamstra AJ, Kream BE, DeLuca HF. 1,25-Dihydroxyvitamin D in biological fluids: A simplified and sensitive assay. Science 1976; 193:1021.

Haddad JG Jr, Walgate J. Radioimmunoassay of the binding protein for vitamin D and its metabolites in human serum. J Clin Invest 1976; 58:1217.

Halloran BP, Portale AA, Castro M, et al. Serum concentration of 1,25-dihydroxyvitamin D in the human: Diurnal variation. J Clin Endocrinol Metab 1985; 61:1104.

Hughes MR, Baylink DJ, Jones PG, Haussler MR. Radioligand receptor assay for 25-hydroxyvitamin D_2/D_3 and 1- alpha 25-dihydroxyvitamin D_2/D_3: Application to hypervitaminosis D. J Clin Invest 1976; 58:61.

Manolagas SC, Culler FL, Howard JE, et al. The cytoreceptor assay for 1,25-dihydroxyvitamin D and its application to clinical studies. J Clin Endocrinol Metab 1983; 56:751.

Reinhardt TA, Horst RL, Orf JW, Hollis BW. A microassay for 1,25-dihydroxyvitamin D not requiring high performance liquid chromatography: Application to clinical studies. J Clin Endocrinol Metab 1984; 58:91.

Stern PH, Hamstra AJ, DeLuca HF, Bell NIH. A bioassay capable of measuring 1 picogram of 1,25-dihydroxyvitamin D₃. J Clin Endocrinol Metab 1978; 46:891.

Parathyroid Localization

Brennan MF, Doppman JL, Krudy AG, et al. Assessment of techniques for preoperative parathyroid gland localization in patients undergoing reoperation for hyperparathyroidism. Surgery 1982; 91:6.

Brennan MF, Marx SJ, Doppman JL, et al. Results of reoperation for persistent and recurrent hyperparathyroidism. Ann Surgery 1981; 194:671.

Doppman JL, Brennan MF, Koehler JO, Marx SJ. Computed tomography for parathyroid localization. J Comput Assist Tomogr 1977; 1:30.

Doppman JL, Krudy AG, Brennan MF, et al. CT appearance of enlarged parathyroid glands in the posterior superior mediastinum. J Comput Assist Tomogr 1982; 6:1099.

Eisenberg H, Pallotta JA. Special localizing techniques for parathyroid disease. In: DeGroot LJ, Cahill GF, Odell WD, et al, eds. Endocrinology. Vol 2. New York: Grune & Stratton, 1979:717.

Gooding GAW, Clark OH, Stark DD, et al. Parathyroid aspiration biopsy under ultrasound guidance in the postoperative hyperparathyroid patient. Radiology 1985; 155:193.

Krudy AG, Doppman JL, Miller DL, et al. Detection of mediastinal parathyroid glands by nonselective digital arteriography. AJR 1984; 142:693.

Mallette LE, Gomez L, Fisher RG: Parathyroid angiography: A review of current knowledge and guidelines for clinical application. Endocrinol Rev 1981; 2:124.

Miller DL, Doppman JL, Krudy AG, et al. Localization of parathyroid adenomas in patients who have undergone surgery. II. Invasive procedures. Radiology 1987; 162:138.

Miller DL, Doppman JL, Shawker TH. Localization of parathyroid adenomas in patients who have undergone surgery. I. Noninvasive imaging. Radiology 1987; 162:133.

Reading CC, Carboneau JW, James EM, et al. High-resolution parathyroid sonography. AJR 1982; 139:539.

Simeone JF, Mueller PR, Ferrucci JT, et al. High-resolution real-time sonography of the parathyroid. Radiology 1981; 141:745.

Stark DD, Clark OH, Moss AA. Magnetic resonance imaging of the thyroid, thymus, and parathyroid glands. Surgery 1984; 96:1083.

Winzelberg GG. Parathyroid imaging. Ann Intern Med 1987; 107:64.

Winzelberg GG, Hydovitz JD, O'Hara KR, et al. Parathyroid adenomas evaluated by T1-201/Tc-99m pertechnetate subtraction scintigraphy and high-resolution ultrasonography. Radiology 1985; 155:231.

Young AE, Gaunt JI, Croft DN, et al. Location of parathyroid adenomas by thallium-²⁰¹ and technetium-⁹⁹m subtraction scanning. Br Med J 1983; 286:1384.

Hypercalcemia of Malignancy

Godsall JW, Burtis WJ, Insogna KL, et al. Nephrogenous cyclic AMP, adenylate cyclase-stimulating activity, and humoral hypercalcemia of malignancy. Rec Prog Horm Res 1986; 42:705.

Lafferty FW. Pseudohyperparathyroidism. Medicine 1966; 45:247.

Powell D, Singer FR, Murray TM, et al. Non-parathyroid humoral hypercalcemia in patients with neoplastic diseases. N Engl J Med 1973; 289:176.

Simpson EL, Mundy GR, D'Souza SM, et al. Absence of parathyroid hormone messenger RNA in nonparathyroid tumors associated with malignancy. N Engl J Med 1983; 309:325.

Stewart AF, Horst R, Deftos LJ, et al. Biochemical evaluation of patients with cancer-associated hypercalcemia. N Engl J Med 1980; 303:1377.

17 Nuclear Medicine

Frederick A. Khafagi, M.B., B.S., F.R.A.C.P.
Brahm Shapiro, M.B., Ch.B., Ph.D.
Milton D. Gross, M.D., F.A.C.P.

The history of the development of clinical nuclear medicine is closely linked with that of endocrinology—specifically, thyroidology. Although the tracer kinetic principle had been described for biologic systems by Gyorgy von Hevesey in 1923, it was the development of artificially produced radioactive isotopes of iodine that gave impetus to the clinical use of radiotracers in humans. The first use of cyclotron-derived iodine 131 (^{131}I) to examine human thyroid physiology was by Hamilton and Soley in 1940. After World War II, ^{131}I became available in relatively large amounts as a nuclear reactor by-product. The first shipment of ^{131}I for medical use was made from Oak Ridge, Tennessee, in August 1946. Werner's studies of the diagnosis and therapy of thyroid disorders using reactor-derived ^{131}I and a handheld Geiger-Müller detector were published shortly thereafter.

The gas-filled Geiger-Müller detector is rather insensitive to penetrating (x-ray and gamma-ray) radiation, which has a low probability of being absorbed and thereby measured; moreover, it provides little directional information as to the source of the radiation. A major step forward was the development of solid crystal detectors of anthracene, naphthalene, calcium tungstate, and later, thallium-activated sodium iodide [NaI(Tl)] coupled to a photomultiplier (PM) tube. Incident x-rays and gamma rays are efficiently absorbed by the crystal, where their energy is converted to a visible light flash (scintillation—hence "scintillation detector"), which, in turn, is converted into an electrical signal by the PM tube. A lead or tungsten shield around the unit with an open channel at the crystal face (i.e., a collimator) limits the field of view of the detector to provide directionality. Detectors of this type were used for laborious, point-by-point counting over the thyroid. In 1950, Cassen mounted such a detector in a device with a stepping motor that permitted automated "step and count" traverses to be made to and fro over the patient and an image of the distribution of administered radioactivity to be built up. Such rectilinear scanners were the workhorses of nuclear medicine until the early to mid-1970s. They are no longer manufactured for imaging purposes, although many remain in use for thyroid scintigraphy. However, the principle on which they were based has been adapted for use in single- and dual-photon absorptiometric measurements of bone mineral (see later). With the development of technetium 99m (^{99m}Tc) and a vast range of ^{99m}Tc-labeled radiopharmaceuticals, and with the ability to grow single NaI(Tl) crystals of up to 50 cm in diameter but only 6.5 mm thick (a thickness better suited to the gamma photon of ^{99m}Tc), the gamma camera has become the main imaging device used in clinical nuclear medicine.

This chapter is devoted to in vivo aspects of nuclear medicine as it applies to endocrinology, with the emphasis on functional imaging. The large field of radioimmunoassay, related ligand assays, and other in vitro techniques is not discussed. We shall not deal with therapeutic nuclear medicine; the interested reader is referred to the outstanding monograph by Harbert. We shall begin by considering the basic physical principles of radioactivity, radiopharmaceuticals, and the generation of an image with the gamma camera.

BASIC PRINCIPLES

Radionuclides, Radiopharmaceuticals, and Radioactive Decay

For our purposes, the most useful atomic model is that of Bohr, which describes the atom as consisting of a dense nucleus containing roughly equal numbers of positively charged protons and uncharged neutrons, surrounded by relatively distant, orbiting, negatively charged electrons that occupy discrete, characteristic "energy shells" (Fig. 17–1). The mass of a neutron (1.6747×10^{-24} g) is approximately equal to that of a proton (1.6724×10^{-24} g); the combined masses of the neutrons and protons account for almost the entire mass of the atom, since the mass of each electron is relatively very small (9.108×10^{-26} g). The positive charge on a proton is exactly equal in magnitude to the negative charge on an electron (1.602×10^{-19} coulomb), and in the non-ionized state, the number of orbital electrons equals the number of nuclear protons. Since the attractive force between the negative electrons and the positive nucleus decreases rapidly with increasing distance from the nucleus, the minimum energy required to remove an electron from any energy shell (the binding energy) is much less for outer than for inner orbital electrons.

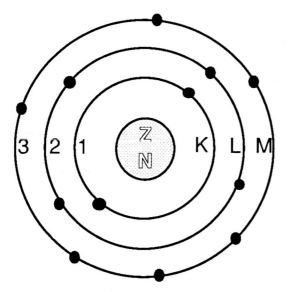

Figure 17-1   The Bohr atomic model. Schematic depiction of an atom with Z protons and N neutrons in the nucleus. The electron shells are designated K, L, M, or numbered (1, 2, 3, . . . , n). Each shell may be occupied by a maximum of $2n^2$ electrons.

The number of protons in a nucleus, designated Z (the atomic number), defines the chemical element, designated $_ZX$. The number of neutrons, N, may vary among different nuclei of the same element; such nuclides, with different N but the same Z, are termed isotopes of the element $_ZX$ ($_ZX^N$, $_ZX^{N-1}$, $_ZX^{N+1}$, and so on). The total number of nuclear particles, i.e., the sum of protons and neutrons, Z+N, is referred to as the mass number, A, of the atom. Thus, different isotopes of the same element have different mass numbers (^AX, ^{A-1}X, ^{A+1}X, and so on). However, since the chemical behavior of an element is determined by its electrons, which are in turn defined by the number of protons in the nucleus, all isotopes of a given element should be chemically identical. This chemical equivalence is fundamental to the use of radionuclides as biologic tracers. Thus, all isotopes of the element iodine have 53 protons ($_{53}I$). (The subscript denoting the atomic number is usually omitted since it is implicit in the chemical symbol for the element.) However, they may have 70, 72, 74, or 78 neutrons to yield ^{123}I, ^{125}I, ^{127}I, or ^{131}I, respectively, all of which behave chemically and biologically as iodine, although they can be separated by nonchemical means. Of the 20 known isotopes of iodine, only ^{127}I is stable; the others are examples of radionuclides and are radioactive isotopes (or radioisotopes) of iodine.

The stable nuclides found in nature generally have even and approximately equal numbers of protons and neutrons, so that a "line of stability" can be constructed relating proton number (Z) to neutron number (N) (Fig. 17-2). An unstable, radioactive nuclide (radionuclide) is any element with an excess of either neutrons or protons in the nucleus that tends toward the line of stability via one or more of several processes collectively termed radioactive decay. The net result of radioactive decay is an alteration of the proportion of neutrons and protons and the emission of energy that may be measurable by an external detector. The important processes in nuclear medicine are β^- emission, electron capture, isomeric transition, and positron emission. Only the first three apply in current, routine practice and are discussed further (Fig. 17-3).

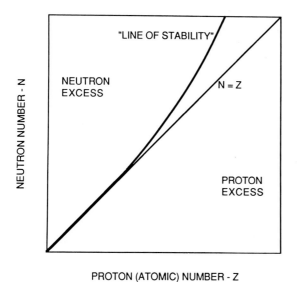

Figure 17-2   Relationship of neutron number (N) to proton (atomic) number (Z) among the stable elements. For low values of Z, N ~ Z; at high Z, N ~ 1.5 Z.

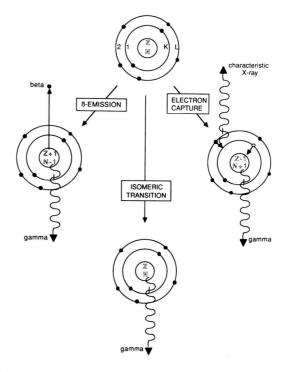

Figure 17-3   Modes of radioactive decay relevant to routine diagnostic nuclear medicine.

β^- Emission

Unstable nuclides with an excess of neutrons may tend toward stability by emitting a high-energy, negatively charged electron from the nucleus, termed a β^- particle, as a result of which N will decrease by 1 and Z will increase by 1. Since Z has changed, the nuclide has been "transmuted" into a new element of atomic number Z+1; note that the mass number has not changed. The β emission may be accompanied by the emission of one or more high-energy photons (gamma rays) from the nucleus, e.g.,

$$^{131}I \rightarrow {}^{131}Xe + \beta^- + \gamma \ (364 \text{ keV}) \qquad (1)$$

Since β^- particles are electrons having a finite, albeit small, mass and unit negative charge, they have a high likelihood of interacting with atoms in their surrounding medium and thus depositing all their energy within a relatively short distance. For example, a β^- particle with an energy of 1 MeV (1.602×10^{-13} J) will have a range in soft tissue of only 4 mm, over which distance it will deposit all its energy chiefly by ionization of atoms in its path. Thus, β^- radiation is undesirable in diagnostic nuclear medicine, since it does not contribute to image formation but adds considerably to the radiation dose to the tissues; this property is exploited in therapy (e.g., ^{131}I for thyroid disease).

Electron Capture

In cases of proton excess, the nucleus may "capture" an inner orbital electron to form a neutron, so that Z will decrease by 1 (and a transmutation will have occurred) although again A will not change. Once again, electron capture may be associated with the emission of one or more gamma photons from the nucleus. In addition, the vacancy left by the captured electron must be filled by an electron from an outer (higher energy) shell; when this occurs, it is accompanied by the emission of a photon equal in energy to the difference between the energy levels of the inner and outer shells (characteristic x-radiation), e.g.,

$$^{123}I \rightarrow {}^{123}Te + \gamma \ (159 \text{ keV}) + X \ (27 \text{ keV}) \quad (2)$$

Isomeric Transition

Any decay process may result in a nucleus with excess energy that may be emitted instantaneously as one or more gamma photons. If the nuclide exists in such an excited state for a measurable period of time ($>10^{-12}$ second), it is said to be metastable. A metastable nucleus also achieves a more stable state by emitting gamma photons, but without any change in Z or N; this process is termed isomeric transition, e.g.,

$$^{99m}Tc \rightarrow {}^{99}Tc + \gamma \ (140 \text{ keV}) \qquad (3)$$

Activity and the Mathematics of Decay

Since the radioactive decay of a radionuclide is a random process (i.e., any one of the radioactive atoms is just as likely as any other to undergo decay), it will occur at a rate that is characteristic for that particular nuclide and proportional to the number of radioactive atoms present. Thus,

$$A = dN/dt = -\lambda N \qquad (4)$$

where A is the activity (rate of decay), N is the number of radioactive atoms of the nuclide, t is time, and λ is the characteristic decay constant (with units of time^{-1}) of the radionuclide. Integrating equation (4) yields

$$N_t = N_0 e^{-\lambda t} \qquad (5)$$

where N_t is the number of radioactive atoms remaining at time t and N_0 is the initial number of radioactive atoms (at time t = 0). Since $A = -\lambda N$,

$$A_t = A_0 e^{-\lambda t} \qquad (6)$$

A radionuclide sample decaying at the rate of one disintegration per second (1 dps or, more correctly, 1 s^{-1}) has an activity of 1 becquerel (Bq)—the SI unit of activity. The older unit of activity, the curie (Ci), was defined as the activity of 1 g of radium 226 (^{226}Ra), which is 3.7×10^{10} s^{-1} or Bq. This unit is still in widespread use in the United States.

The time required for the activity of a sample to decay to half its initial value is referred to as the physical half-life (T_p) of the radionuclide:

$$A_0/2 = A_0 e^{-\lambda T}p$$

$$e^{\lambda T}p = 2$$

$$Tp = \ln2/\lambda = 0.693/\lambda \qquad (7)$$

Hence T_p, like λ (the decay constant), is a characteristic property of the radionuclide.

A radiopharmaceutical is any radioactive compound suitably prepared for in vivo use as a diagnostic or therapeutic agent. It may be simple, such as sodium ^{123}I-iodide, or complex, such as an ^{131}I-labeled monoclonal antibody. Although diagnostic radiopharmaceuticals are given in minute, tracer doses that have no pharmacologic effect, the physicochemical state of the agent will, of course, determine its distribution, localization, disposition, and its biologic half-life (the time required for half the administered chemical quantity of the agent to be eliminated). The biologic half-life, T_b, is another important determinant of the radiation dose from a radiopharmaceutical, since the effective radiobiologic half-life of the agent, T_{eff}, is given by the equation,

$$1/T_{eff} = 1/T_p + 1/T_b \qquad (8)$$

or

$$T_{eff} = T_p \cdot T_b / (T_p + T_b) \qquad (9)$$

Clearly, T_{eff} is largely determined by whichever of the physical or biologic half-lives is the shorter.

Radionuclides for medical use are derived from two sources: nuclear reactors, in which the radionuclides are either fission products of the decay of uranium or the products of neutron bombardment of target nuclides, and accelerators (mainly cyclotrons), in which the radionuclides are the products of the bombardment of target nuclides with high-velocity charged particles (alpha particles [helium nuclei], deuterons [deuterium nuclei], and protons). As a general rule, reactor products are neutron-rich and decay by β^- emission, while accelerator products are proton-rich and decay by electron capture or by positron emission. Accelerator products also tend to be much more expensive than reactor products. Positron-emitting radionuclides have unique physical properties that have led to the development of a new and exciting branch of nuclear medicine, positron-emission tomography (PET); however, they typically have physical half-lives of only minutes, so that their use at present is virtually limited to institutions with an on-site cyclotron. Endocrine applications of PET have, to date, been limited.

The most commonly used radionuclide in current nuclear medicine practice is ^{99m}Tc, introduced in 1963. It decays by isomeric transition (equation 3), and its 140-keV photon has an ideal energy for detection by gamma cameras. Its T_p is 6 hours and it has no beta emissions, so its radiation dosimetry is very favorable. It is generated from a reactor product, molybdenum 99

(^{99}Mo, T_p 67 hours), which is adsorbed to an alumina column (Fig. 17–4); elution of the column with physiologic saline solution yields sodium ^{99m}Tc-pertechnetate (^{99m}TcO$_4^-$) in the eluate. Since the T_p of the "parent" ^{99}Mo is so much longer than the ^{99m}Tc "daughter," ^{99m}Tc accumulates on the column between elutions, approaching a maximum 24 hours after each elution. Thus, a ^{99}Mo generator may be used for several days to produce sufficient quantities of ^{99m}Tc for clinical use at low cost. In its heptavalent form as pertechnetate, ^{99m}Tc(VII) is relatively nonreactive. It may be reduced by one of several cations, usually Sn^{2+}, to a more reactive trivalent, tetravalent, or pentavalent state for incorporation into a variety of pharmaceuticals or for cell labeling.

A list of radionuclides and their associated radiopharmaceuticals relevant to endocrine nuclear medicine appears in Table 17–1.

Instrumentation

The principles of in vivo detection and measurement of penetrating radiation are most simply illustrated by consideration of the scintillation probe, which is still in clinical use for the measurement of thyroid uptake of radioiodine (Fig. 17–5). The probe consists of a circular NaI(Tl) crystal, 5 cm in diameter and 5 to 7.5 cm thick, optically coupled to a single PM tube and shielded with a lead collimator. For a monoenergetic source, the brightness of the scintillations and, therefore, the amplitude of the PM tube output are proportional to the energy of the incident x-rays or gamma rays. The frequency of scintillations is proportional to the intensity of the radiation, which may be defined as the number of photons per unit of area and time, often termed the photon flux (or, more properly, the fluence rate); the radiation intensity, in turn, is proportional to the amount of activity being measured. Unfortunately, not all of the incident photons deposit all of their energy within the probe crys-

Figure 17–4 Schematic diagram of a ^{99}Mo and ^{99m}Tc generator.

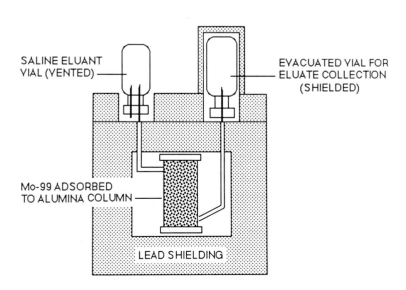

SALINE ELUANT
VIAL (VENTED)

EVACUATED VIAL FOR
ELUATE COLLECTION
(SHIELDED)

Mo-99 ADSORBED
TO ALUMINA COLUMN

LEAD SHIELDING

TABLE 17-1 Radionuclides and Radiopharmaceuticals for Endocrine Scintigraphy

Radionuclide	Source	Mode of Decay	T_p	Principal Photopeak(s)	Radio-pharmaceutical	Clinical Use
^{121}I	C	EC	13.3 hours	159 keV	^{123}I-NaI	Thyroid uptake, thyroid scan
					^{123}I-metaiodo-benzylguanidine	Detection of pheochromo-cytoma and neuroendocrine tumors
^{131}I	R	β^-	8.06 days	364 keV	^{131}I-NaI	Thyroid uptake, treatment of hyperthyroidism; treatment and follow-up of thyroid cancer
					^{131}I-metaiodo-benzylguanidine	Detection and therapy of pheochromocytoma and related tumors
					^{131}I-6β-iodo-methyl-19-nor-cholesterol	Adrenocortical scan
^{75}Se	R	EC	119 days	136 keV 265 keV 280 keV	^{75}Se-6β-seleno-methyl-19-nor-cholesterol	Adrenocortical scan
					Selenomethionine Se75	Obsolete: parathyroid and pancreatic scans
^{99m}Tc	G	IT	6.04 hours	140 keV	^{99m}Tc-NaTcO$_4$	Thyroid scan and uptake; parathyroid scan
^{201}Tl	C	EC	73 hours	68–83 keV	^{201}TlCl	Parathyroid scan

C = cyclotron; G = generator (^{99}Mo); R = reactor by-product; β^- = β^- emission; EC = electron capture; IT = isomeric transition

tal (photoelectric absorption). Some do not interact with the crystal at all. A variable proportion is scattered by interactions with atoms within the crystal (Compton scattering); the scattered photons have lower energies than the incident photons (the decrement depending on the scattering angle) and may or may not be ultimately absorbed by the crystal. In the in vivo situation, photons originating from within the patient may have undergone similar Compton scattering before leaving the body, so that even for a monoenergetic gamma emitter, the radiation reaching the probe has a spectrum of energies up to the original source energy. Analysis of the amplitude of the detector's output likewise reveals a spectrum of voltages, with a maximum amplitude and frequency occurring at the voltage corresponding to the energy of the source, the photopeak (Fig. 17–6). The probe system therefore incorporates a pulse height analyzer, which is set at the center of the photopeak voltage with a "window" of, typically, ±10 percent about the photopeak (20 percent window), so that the majority of events recorded by the instrument are "true" events and the lower-energy, scattered photons are largely ignored.

Although the scintillation probe is used for external counting, it has insufficient spatial resolution (i.e., ability to distinguish between adjacent, discrete sources of radioactivity) to produce an image. The gamma camera is the device used for imaging. It consists of a single, circular (less commonly rectangular) NaI(Tl) crystal coupled to several PM tubes. Typical diameters of circular crystals

in current use are approximately 30 cm (standard or small field of view, SFOV), 40 cm (wide or large field of view, LFOV), and 50 cm (extra-wide field of view); thicknesses range from 6.5 to 9.5 mm. On circular crystals, PM tubes are arranged in concentric hexagonal arrays with a total of 37, 61, or 91 tubes. As well as circuitry for pulse height analysis (the Z pulse) and energy window selection similar to that described previously for the scintillation probe, gamma cameras possess logic circuitry that permits the determination of the spatial (X and Y) coordinates of a scintillation event (Fig. 17–7). Within limits, the thin-

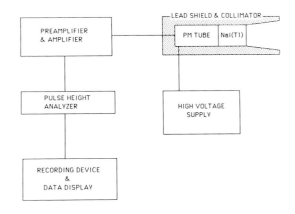

Figure 17–5 Schematic diagram of a typical scintillation probe and associated electronics.

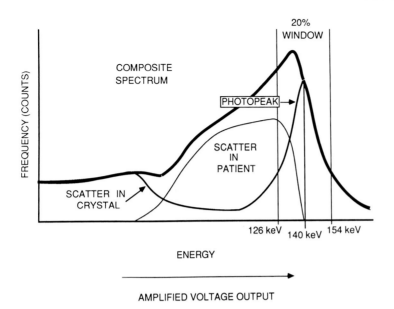

Figure 17–6 Typical, composite pulse-height spectrum for a ^{99m}Tc source at depth in a patient, as detected by a NaI(Tl) probe. The 20 percent window is set at the ^{99m}Tc photopeak energy (140 keV) ± 10 percent.

ner the crystal (i.e., the less the probability of Compton scatter within the crystal) and the greater the number of PM tubes, the better the resolving power of the camera (intrinsic resolution). Thinner crystals also absorb more energetic photons less efficiently, so that crystal thicknesses in current use are a compromise between resolution and detection efficiency, which are optimal for the 140-keV gamma photon of ^{99m}Tc.

Since a radiation source emits energy more or less uniformly in all directions, photons from a gamma emitter strike the crystal face at an infinitely large number of angles of incidence. Since x-rays and gamma rays cannot be optically reflected or refracted, absorptive collimation is used to select rays having a defined trajectory and reject all others, thereby defining the camera's field of view. This is unfortunately an inherently inefficient solution. The only collimators used for endocrine nuclear medicine are multichannel, parallel-hole collimators and the pinhole collimator (Fig. 17–8). A parallel-hole collimator consists of a hexagonal or square array of numerous, parallel, lead-lined channels that may have a round, square, or hexagonal bore. The thickness of the channel walls (septa) is sufficient to absorb photons that would otherwise cross from one channel to the next. Thus, considerably thicker septa are needed to collimate the 364-keV photon of ^{131}I (high-energy collimator) than are necessary for ^{99m}Tc (low-energy collimator). As a result, only photons with trajectories almost perpendicular to the crystal face are allowed to pass. The longer the channels of the collimator, the narrower the permissible deviation from a perpendicular trajectory, and the finer the spatial resolution of the collimator. However, increasing either septal thickness or channel length reduces the fraction of all incident photons that the collimator allows the crystal to "see"—i.e., the geometric efficiency is reduced. The advantages of parallel-hole collimators are that they produce no image distortion (magnification or minifi-

cation) and have constant efficiency regardless of source-collimator distance.

The pinhole collimator, having only one hole, has a very low geometric efficiency that falls rapidly with increasing source-collimator distance. Its major advantage is that it produces image magnification, so that its spatial resolution is potentially high at short source-

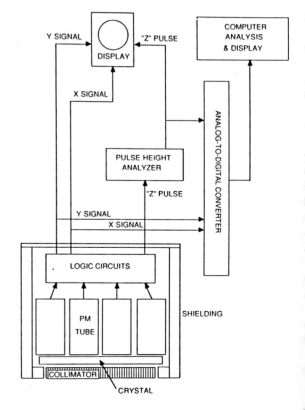

Figure 17–7 Schematic diagram of a gamma camera and associated electronics.

collimator distances. However, the magnification is nonuniform, being maximal at the center of the field, so that a fisheye-lens type of distortion is produced in the image. This can be troublesome when attempting to estimate lesion size or to clarify anatomic relationships (e.g., retrosternal extension of a thyroid).

Most modern gamma cameras are interfaced with dedicated computers that permit the image to be digitized. The operator can select regions of interest within an image by using a joystick or similar device, so that the spatial and temporal distribution of events in the image can be quantified and analyzed. Recent advances in gamma camera gantry design and computer software have permitted the acquisition of data from multiple angles about the patient, with subsequent reconstruction and tomographic display using back-projection algorithms analogous to those used in x-ray computed tomography; this is the basis of emission computed tomography (ECT).

THE THYROID

Radiopharmaceuticals and Rationale

Thyroid physiology as it applies to scintigraphy is outlined in Figure 17–9. Drugs that inhibit various steps in thyroid hormone synthesis and release are also shown. Synthesis of thyroid hormones depends on the thyroid's ability to trap iodide actively and then to oxidize and incorporate it into tyrosyl residues of thyroglobulin (Tg). The last two steps are collectively termed organification. The trapping mechanism is specific neither to the thyroid (it also occurs in the choroid plexus, salivary glands, and gastric mucosa) nor for iodide. Several monoanions (TcO_4^-, ClO_4^-, SCN^-, Br^-) with ionic radii similar to that of I^- can be trapped by the same mechanism, and in pharmacologic doses, they act as competitive inhibitors of iodide trapping. Trapping is also inhibited by exogenous expansion of the iodine pool (see Fig. 17–7).

Although trapping and organification are obviously related, they are distinct processes that may become uncoupled. Congenital or acquired deficiencies of the thyroid peroxidases necessary for iodide oxidation and iodotyrosine coupling are not associated with abnormalities of trapping. Such organification defects are most commonly observed in Hashimoto's thyroiditis and in patients receiving thionamide antithyroid drugs (see Fig. 17–9); the classic congenital defect occurs in Pendred's syndrome (goiter and sensorineural deafness, with autosomal recessive inheritance). Rarely, benign or malignant thyroid neoplasms may have impaired organification but normal or increased trapping. In all these examples, the 20-minute uptake of $^{99m}TcO_4^-$ (a marker of trapping) is normal or increased, whereas the 24-hour uptake of radioiodine (a marker of organification) is low. The clinical significance of this disparity is discussed later.

Since both trapping and organification are dependent on thyroid-stimulating hormone (thyrotropin, TSH), both are reduced by inhibitors of TSH secretion (see Fig.

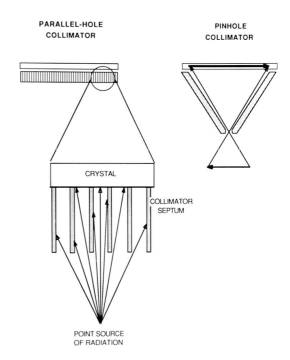

Figure 17–8 Parallel-hole and pinhole collimators. Incident photons with trajectories other than those permitted by the collimator's geometry are absorbed by the lead collimator walls or septa; hence, the term *absorptive collimation*. Note that the pinhole collimator produces a magnified image when the source–pinhole distance is less than the collimator length; at greater distances, the image is minified.

17–9). Conversely, the thyroid-stimulating autoantibodies (TSAb) of Graves' disease enhance both processes by their TSH-mimetic effect on the TSH receptor. The same result occurs very rarely from TSH excess due to a pituitary tumor or from extremely high circulating levels of human chorionic gonadotropin (hCG) associated with trophoblastic malignancies.

The dosimetry of the three major radiopharmaceuticals used for thyroid scintigraphy is summarized in Table 17–2. Because of its β^- emissions and relatively long physical half-life, the dosimetry of ^{131}I is the least favorable, so that it must be given in the smallest practicable dose. If a 5-by-7.5-cm scintillation probe is used, 24-hour thyroid uptake of ^{131}I can be measured after giving as little as 74 kBq (2 μCi) orally. However, in order to obtain a pinhole gamma camera image of the thyroid, at least 1.1 MBq (30 μCi) must be given, because of the low geometric efficiency of the pinhole collimator and the low detection efficiency of the relatively thin gamma camera crystal for 364-keV photons. The absorbed radiation dose to the normal adult thyroid at this level is 24 cGy (rad) (see Table 17–2); it is higher in children in whom, for any given level of iodide uptake, the absorbed dose to the thyroid increases with decreasing age. Even so, the photon flux from such a small administered dose of radioactivity is very low, leading to long imaging times and statistically poor image quality.

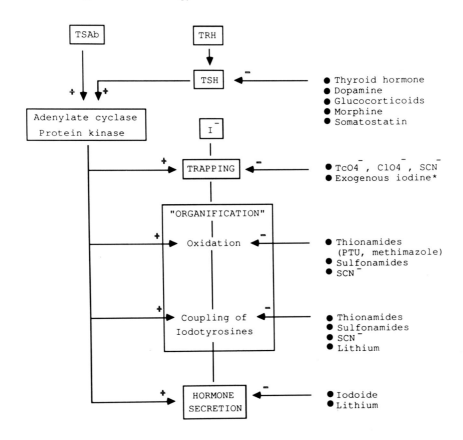

*SOURCES OF EXOGENOUS IODINE:

.Lugol's solution
.Potassium iodide (contained in several "expectorants"
                      and nonprescription cough mixtures)
.Topical iodine preparations
.Kelp (included in many "health food" preparations)
.Seafood, especially shellfish
.Radiographic contrast media
.Iodinated drugs (amiodarone, antiparasitic agents)

Figure 17-9 Simplified diagrammatic representation of thyroid physiology. Drugs that affect thyroid hormone synthesis and their sites of action are shown at right (+: stimulates; − inhibits).

Iodine 123 has no particulate emissions and emits a gamma photon (159 keV) that is efficiently detected by gamma cameras. Therefore, Na^{123}I would seem to be the ideal radiopharmaceutical for in vivo thyroid studies. However, ^{123}I is produced commercially by one of three cyclotron reactions, all of which result in greater or lesser contamination of the product with longer-lived radionuclidic impurities (^{124}I, ^{125}I, ^{126}I, ^{131}I) that add to the absorbed radiation dose. The recommended oral doses of ^{123}I$^-$ are 1.8 MBq (50 μCi) for uptake measurements and 3.7 to 18.5 MBq (100 to 500 μCi) for scintigraphy; taking radionuclidic impurities into account, imaging doses would deliver 2.1 to 10.5 cGy to the normal adult thyroid (see Table 17–2). Since the proportion of radionuclidic impurities per MBq ^{123}I increases as the ^{123}I decays, the useful shelf-life of ^{123}I is limited to the working day for which the dose was calibrated by the manufacturer. Moreover, production facilities for ^{123}I are not widespread and the cost per dose is high. Use of

^{123}I$^-$ is therefore confined to clinics in which thyroid studies can be restricted to certain days of the week.

Advantage is taken of the nonspecificity of the trapping mechanism by using ^{99m}TcO$_4^-$ for thyroid scintigraphy. Sodium ^{99m}Tc-pertechnetate is currently the most widely used radiopharmaceutical for this purpose. It has the advantages of ready availability, simple preparation, low cost, low radiation dose, and virtually ideal physical characteristics for gamma camera scintigraphy. The usual dose is 111 to 185 MBq (3 to 5 mCi) given intravenously, which delivers only 0.39 to 0.65 cGy to the normal adult thyroid (see Table 17–2) yet produces a sufficient photon flux for images of excellent quality. Since it is trapped but not organified, maximal uptake occurs at 20 to 30 minutes after injection (as opposed to 6 to 24 hours for radioiodine); this is very convenient for the patient, since scintigraphy can be performed shortly after tracer administration. A minor disadvantage is that the upper limit of normal pertechnetate uptake is 3.5 t

TABLE 17–2 Thyroid Dosimetry of Radiopharmaceuticals Used for Thyroid Scintigraphy

Radiopharmaceutical	Thyroid Absorbed Dose	
	Adult* cGy/MBq (rad/mCi)‡	Newborn† cGy/MBq (rad/mCi)
[131]I–sodium iodide	21.6 (800.0)	432 (16,000)
[123]I–sodium iodide (100% radionuclidic purity)	0.20 (7.5)	4.3 (160)
[123]I–sodium iodide (with radionuclidic impurities)	0.57 (21.0)	6.3 (233)
[99m]Tc–sodium pertechnetate	0.0035 (0.13)	0.092 (3.4)

* Assuming 24-hour iodine uptake of 13.8% and a 10.6-g thyroid
† Assuming that dose to a newborn is approximately 11 times that to an adult
‡ 1 cGy = 1 rad; 1 cGy/MBq = 37 rad/mCi

4 percent of the administered dose (compared with normal 24-hour iodine uptake of 5 to 25 percent), so that the target-to-background ratio of activity is lower for $^{99m}TcO_4^-$. For this reason, the scintillation probe cannot be used to measure pertechnetate uptake; however, several camera-based algorithms are available for uptake estimation. Much has been made of the occasional discordance between pertechnetate and radioiodine uptake; such clinical situations are in practice relatively uncommon, are usually easily resolved by other means, and rarely have a significant impact on patient management (e.g., increased pertechnetate uptake secondary to organification defect in biochemically hypothyroid patients with Hashimoto's thyroiditis).

Other radiopharmaceuticals have been used for thyroid imaging, mainly in an (unsuccessful) attempt to distinguish scintigraphically between benign and malignant thyroid nodules. Uptake of selenomethionine Se75 is a nonspecific index of protein synthetic activity that might be expected to be higher in malignant nodules. Gallium 67 is taken up by a variety of tumors by poorly understood mechanisms. Neither of these agents has proved sufficiently sensitive or specific for routine clinical use. Gallium 67 also localizes in inflammatory lesions, and ^{67}Ga uptake has been described in patients with active thyroiditis, but this diagnosis is easily made by more conventional means. Uptake of the potassium analogue, $^{201}Tl^+$, is a nonspecific index of perfusion and cellularity; nodules that fail to take up $^{99m}TcO_4^-$ or $^{123}I^-$ but take up $^{201}Tl^+$ are considered to be vascular and cellular and therefore more likely to be malignant. The same information could be obtained more simply and cheaply by incorporating a dynamic flow sequence of images into the $^{99m}TcO_4^-$ scan at the time of injection (i.e., a radionuclide angiogram). The specificity of this finding for malignancy remains low. Whole-body scans with ^{201}Tl (rather than ^{131}I) have also been suggested as a means of following patients with thyroid cancer, with the advantage that withdrawal of thyroid hormone suppressive therapy could be avoided; the sensitivity of this approach compared with that in conventional ^{131}I surveys has been variable in reports published so far.

Technique

Meaningful interpretation of the thyroid scan requires an initial clinical evaluation of the patient and, ideally, the results of recent biochemical thyroid function tests. The history should pay particular attention to symptoms of hyperthyroidism or hypothyroidism, local symptoms (pain, rapid thyroid enlargement, dysphagia, dysphonia), family history of thyroid disease or thyroid cancer, history of craniocervical irradiation, and a dietary and drug history. The recommended period of withdrawal from several agents that interfere with tracer uptake by the thyroid is listed in Table 17–3. In addition to the patient's age and sex, salient features of the physical examination include clinical thyroid status, thyroid size, nodularity, mobility, retrosternal extension, and associated lymphadenopathy.

Scintigraphy is performed with a gamma camera fitted with a 3-mm aperture pinhole collimator. Images are obtained 20 to 30 minutes after the intravenous injection of $^{99m}TcO_4^-$, or 6 to 24 hours after the oral administration of $^{123}I^-$. The patient is positioned supine under the camera with her or his neck extended. The pinhole is centered over the thyroid at such a distance (usually about 4 cm) that the thyroid image occupies at least 75 percent of the camera's field of view. Direct anterior and right and left anterior oblique views are routinely obtained; the anterior view is repeated with radioactive surface markers placed on the suprasternal notch and the tip of the chin, and any clinically palpable nodules are similarly mapped out and marked without changing the patient's position. Because of the anatomic distortion inherent in pinhole imaging, suspected retrosternal extension of a goiter is best evaluated with a parallel-hole collimator or, less satisfactorily, by centering the pinhole over the suprasternal notch.

TABLE 17-3   Recommended Period of Withdrawal of Agents That Interfere With Thyroid Uptake

Agent	Minimum Recommended Delay Before Scan
Amiodarone	1–3 months
Antiparasitic drugs	1 week
Antithyroid drugs (thionamides)	3–5 days
Iodine solutions (e.g., Lugol's, saturated solution of potassium iodide, ''expectorants'')	2 weeks
Kelp	2 weeks
Radiographic Contrast Media	
Angiographic	2–4 weeks
Cholecystographic (oral)	1–4 months
Myelographic: water-soluble;	2–4 weeks
oil-based (obsolete)	6 months–20 years
Urographic	2–4 weeks
Thyroid hormones	
Thyroxine (T_4)	4–6 weeks
Triiodothyronine (T_3)	1–2 weeks

The normal thyroid is butterfly shaped (Fig. 17–10). Each lobe is normally about 5 cm in length, with the right lobe usually slightly longer. The lateral borders of each lobe are smoothly convex; the upper medial borders may be slightly concave owing to the insertions of the strap muscles. Tracer uptake by both lobes is symmetric and uniform; uptake by the isthmus varies widely and may be virtually absent. Uptake by a pyramidal lobe is occasionally seen in normal scans; the pyramidal lobe arises more commonly from the medial aspect of the left lobe. On pertechnetate scans, pyramidal lobe uptake should not be confused with uptake in the esophagus owing to swallowed, labeled saliva; esophageal uptake is also left sided but often extends caudad to the thyroid and can be cleared by having the patient drink water.

Clinical Applications

The major current indications for thyroid scintigraphy to be discussed are listed in Table 17–4. Evaluation of nodular thyroid disease remains the most common rea-

son for requesting a thyroid scan, so this issue is discussed here at some length. The steady improvement in the sensitivity and specificity of assays for thyroid hormones, TSH, Tg, and thyroid autoantibodies (including TSAb) and the increasing use of fine-needle biopsy for cytodiagnosis of palpable thyroid abnormalities are changing the clinical role of thyroid scintigraphy.

The various pharmacologic stimulation and suppression tests of radioiodine uptake using the scintillation probe (TSH stimulation test, triiodothyronine [T_3] suppression test, perchlorate discharge test) are outlined in Chapter 7 and are not discussed further.

Nodular Thyroid Disease

The observation that thyroid carcinoma concentrates radioiodine less well than normal thyroid tissue was first made by Hamilton in 1940. This differential uptake is the basis for using the thyroid scan to differentiate between benign and potentially malignant nodules. Nodules that take up less radioiodine or $^{99m}TcO_4^-$ than

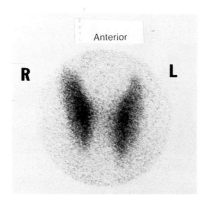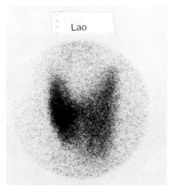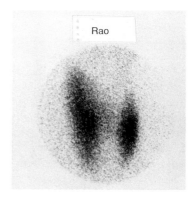

Figure 17-10   Normal $^{99m}TcO_4^-$ pinhole thyroid scan. *Left to right*: anterior, left anterior oblique, and right anterior oblique views.

TABLE 17-4   Indications for Thyroid Scintigraphy

Evaluation of thyroid nodules
Follow-up of differentiated (papillary, follicular) thyroid cancer
Differential diagnosis of hyperthyroidism
Evaluation of anterior neck masses
Evaluation of mediastinal masses and retrosternal goiter
Evaluation of neonatal hypothyroidism (dysembryogenesis
      versus dyshormonogenesis)

surrounding normal thyroid tissue ("cold" nodules—Fig. 17-11) are more likely to be malignant than those that take up more tracer than normal ("hot" nodules); indeed, malignancy in hot nodules is very rare. Indeterminate nodules are palpable nodules that do not distort the shape of the thyroid and are not apparent on scintigraphy; they account for 4 to 6 percent of palpable, solitary nodules and have the same clinical significance, as cold nodules. Malignancy is less common in a multinodular goiter (Fig. 17-12) than in an otherwise normal thyroid with a solitary nodule. A gamma camera fitted with a 3-mm aperture pinhole collimator reliably detects nodules 5 mm in diameter if multiple views are obtained; even smaller nodules can be detected by ECT, and their depth within the gland determined. Thus, a thyroid that appears normal on palpation may prove to harbor one or more nodules on scintigraphy. Although these statements are true as far as they go, their relevance to clinical practice should be evaluated critically.

Nodular thyroid disease is common. Palpable nodules were found in 4.2 percent of the population in the Framingham study, with new nodules appearing at the rate of 0.093 percent per year. However, the annual incidence of thyroid cancer in the United States is 39 per million, so the vast majority of thyroid nodules are benign. Most nodules prove to be cold (or indeterminate) on scans; the frequency of hot nodules in scintigraphic series is no more than 20 percent. The differential diagnosis of cold nodules is extensive (Table 17-5), so that the specificity of this finding for malignancy is low. The reported prevalence of malignancy in surgically excised cold nodules ranges from 1.5 to 38 percent, with a mean of 17 percent.

It is intuitively obvious that applying a sensitive but nonspecific test to detect a disease with a low prevalence is of little diagnostic value. This may be illustrated by the following example (Fig. 17-13). Suppose that the prevalence of malignancy in patients with solitary thyroid nodules presenting to a given clinic is 12 percent. (It is likely that presentation for medical attention biases the population in favor of malignancy.) The pretest probability of disease is therefore 0.12. Suppose, further, that 20 percent of these nodules are hot, that hot nodules are invariably benign, and that 17.5 percent of the cold nodules prove to be malignant at surgery. For the moment, we will ignore the possibility that malignancy could arise in anything other than a solitary, cold nodule. Given all these assumptions, finding a solitary nodule to be cold is 100 percent sensitive but only 23 percent specific for

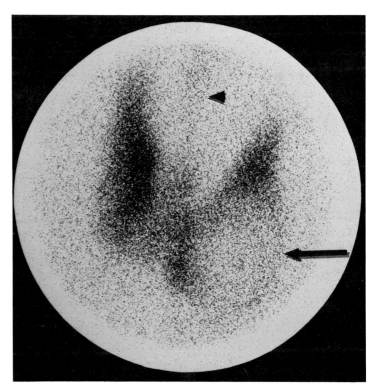

Figure 17-11   Solitary, cold nodule of the left lower pole (*arrow*): $^{99m}TcO_4^-$, anterior pinhole image. Note faint pyramidal lobe uptake (*arrowhead*), a normal variant.

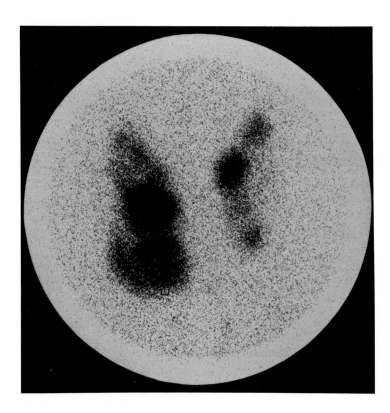

Figure 17-12 Typical, heterogeneous $^{99m}TcO_4{}^-$ uptake by a multinodular goiter.

malignancy, so the post-test probability of malignancy only increases to 0.16 (see Fig. 17–13).

In practice, the gain is even smaller, since not all thyroid cancers manifest as solitary, cold nodules; i.e., the sensitivity of this scintigraphic finding for malignancy is less than 100 percent. Although malignancy is significantly less common in multinodular goiters, the prevalence (3 to 5 percent) is not negligible. Further, the risk of malignancy in a clinically dominant nodule, which is hypofunctioning on the scan, in an otherwise multinodular gland approaches that for a solitary, cold nodule (Fig. 17–14). More than half the clinically solitary nodules that come to surgery prove to be dominant nodules in histologically multinodular glands. Thus, in a patient who presents with a clinically solitary nodule that is cold on scan, the additional ability of scintigraphy to detect clinically impalpable nodules is of doubtful value.

The greater sensitivity of scintigraphy for detecting small nodules has also been invoked by advocates of scintigraphic screening of adults who were exposed to craniocervical irradiation in infancy, childhood, or adolescence and who therefore are at increased risk for thyroid nodules in general and thyroid cancer in particular. However, although radiation-induced thyroid cancer is more frequently multifocal within the thyroid than cancers that arise spontaneously, the natural history is otherwise indistinguishable. Specifically, there is no evidence that radiation-induced thyroid cancer is biologically more aggressive. The prognosis of occult tumors (≤ 1.5 cm) in this subpopulation is no different from the excellent prognosis of similar tumors in the general population, so there appears to be no advantage to detecting subclinical abnormalities. Moreover, the increased likelihood of multifocal malignancy in the irradiated population makes the scintigraphic discovery of unsuspected multinodularity in such a patient with a clinically solitary nodule even less helpful.

The alternative approach to thyroid scintigraphy is to assume that every presenting nodule is potentially malignant and to rule out the possibility by finding it to be hot. The efficiency of this approach is question-

TABLE 17-5   Differential Diagnosis of the Cold Thyroid Nodule

Follicular adenoma—with or without cystic/hemorrhagic degeneration
Hyperplastic nodule
Thyroiditis—subacute, silent, or chronic (rarely acute)
Thyroid carcinoma—papillary, follicular, or anaplastic
Colloid cyst
Previous surgery

Rare causes:
  Hemiagenesis
  Primary thyroid carcinoma
  Medullary thyroid carcinoma
  Branchiogenic cyst
  Parathyroid adenoma, carcinoma, or cyst
  Malignancy metastatic to thyroid
  Tuberculoma
  Amyloidosis
  Postradiation fibrosis
  Marine-Lenhart syndrome

Pre-test Probability of Thyroid Cancer = 0.12

$$Odds = \frac{Probability}{(1 + Probability)}$$

Pre-test Odds of Thyroid Cancer = 0.11

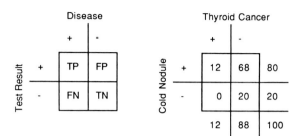

$$Sensitivity = \frac{TP}{TP + FN} = 1.00$$

$$Specificity = \frac{TN}{TN + FP} = 0.23$$

$$\text{Likelihood Ratio of a Positive Result (LR+)} = \frac{Sensitivity}{(1 - Specificity)} = 1.3$$

Post-test Odds of Disease
Given a Positive Result = Pre-test Odds x (LR+) = 0.14

$$Probability = \frac{Odds}{(1 - Odds)}$$

Post-test Probability of Thyroid Cancer = 0.16

---

able in view of the relatively low frequency both of hot nodules and of malignancies in cold nodules. In the example given in Figure 17–13, such a policy would require almost six unnecessary operations to find each malignant nodule. The definition of a hot nodule in this context needs to be quite clear. It will be recalled that occasional thyroid neoplasms retain the ability to trap pertechnetate but lose the ability to organify iodine. Therefore, they appear to be functioning with $^{99m}TcO_4{}^-$ but nonfunctioning with $^{123}I^-$. Such discordant imaging has been reported in only 2 to 3 percent of apparently functioning nodules; it is not specific for malignancy but has the same significance as any cold (or indeterminate) nodule. The issue does not arise if, in the absence of routine ^{123}I scintigraphy, the term *hot nodule* is limited to those nodules that show evidence of autonomy, namely, suppression of tracer uptake by the remainder of the thyroid.

A detailed discussion of fine-needle biopsy (FNB) of the thyroid is beyond the scope of this chapter. However, FNB is rapidly replacing scintigraphy as the first diagnostic procedure for evaluating palpable thyroid abnormalities. It is relatively simple to perform and well tolerated by the patient, with no known mortality and virtually no morbidity. Some technical skill is required to obtain consistently adequate specimens, but the main determinant of the diagnostic utility of the test is the interpretative expertise of the cytopathologist. Given an adequate specimen, the specificity of frankly malignant or suspicious cytologic findings for thyroid cancer is high. Follicular neoplasia presents a problem, since follicular adenomas cannot reliably be distinguished cytologically from follicular carcinomas. An inadequate specimen is indeterminate; i.e., it does not alter the pretest, clinical probability of disease. The ultimate role of FNB remains somewhat controversial since many subjects with benign or normal cytologic findings do not come to surgery. Thus, the true false-negative rate (and hence the sensitivity) of FNB is uncertain. Nevertheless, institutions that have adopted FNB as the primary modality generally report a halving of their thyroidectomy rates, but no decrease in the number of thyroid cancers found. One suggested approach to the diagnosis of nodular thyroid disease is outlined in Figure 17–15.

The schema in Figure 17–15 makes no reference to other imaging modalities, particularly ultrasonography. High-resolution thyroid ultrasound using a 7.5-MHz or 10-MHz transducer provides excellent anatomic detail of the thyroid, but the clinical utility of detecting very small nodules has already been questioned. True cysts of the thyroid, which are virtually never malignant yet are cold on scintigrams, can be distinguished by ultrasound with a fair degree of confidence, but they represent only a small minority of cold nodules and are, in any case, managed by aspiration. Ultrasonography cannot otherwise contribute to the differentiation between benign and malignant nodules. Although ultrasound can be used to guide FNB, it remains to be shown that this improves the diagnostic yield of FNB. Ultrasonography is the most precise, objective method of measuring serial nodule size during attempted thyroid hormone suppression, but the diagnostic and therapeutic usefulness of suppression is in doubt. X-ray computed tomography (CT) and magnetic resonance imaging (MRI) of the thyroid likewise provide high-resolution anatomic information but do not resolve the issue of whether a nodule is malignant. They cannot be recommended for routine use.

Follow-Up of Patients with Thyroid Cancer

After the surgical eradication of macroscopically evident papillary or follicular thyroid cancer, with or without postoperative ^{131}I ablation of remnant tissue, ^{131}I whole-body radionuclide surveys have long been the most important means of following patients with this disease. Success with this technique requires total or near-total thyroidectomy in the first instance, and a sufficiently long abstinence from suppressive thyroid hormone therapy to stimulate endogenous TSH secretion and thereby max-

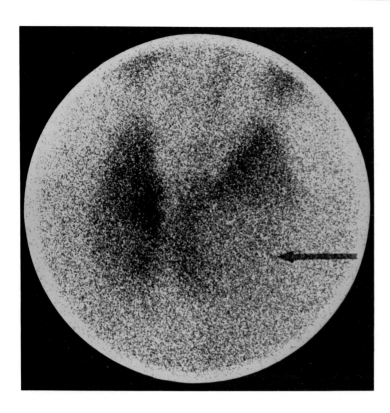

Figure 17-14   Poorly defined, dominant, cold nodule of the left lower pole in a multinodular goiter (*arrow*). Mixed papillary and follicular carcinoma.

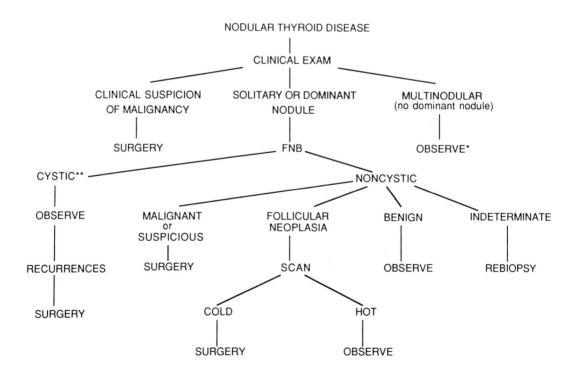

*"Observation" may include attempted suppression with thyroid hormone.
**Disappears completely after aspiration. Aspiration of fluid with only partial reduction in nodule size implies a noncystic nodule.

Figure 17-15   One cost-effective approach to the management of nodular thyroid disease.

imize ^{131}I uptake by residual or metastatic thyroid tissue. Clearly, drugs that interfere with radioiodine uptake (see Fig. 17–9) must be avoided; restriction of dietary iodine intake may help to enhance uptake by reducing iodine pool size.

Withdrawal of thyroxine (T_4) for 5 to 6 weeks before the scan reliably elevates serum TSH levels to more than 30 IU per liter (more than 50 IU per liter in most cases), even in elderly patients or in patients who have received long-term T_4. As a result, clinically, patients will become moderately to severely hypothyroid; this not only is uncomfortable for the patient but also poses some risks, particularly in patients who are receiving drugs that are cleared predominantly by the liver. The discomfort of hypothyroid symptoms can be alleviated in some patients by substituting the shorter-lived T_3 for the withdrawn T_4 and stopping the T_3 no later than 2 weeks before scanning. However, the duration of abstinence from thyroid hormone may be the most important single factor for successful post-thyroidectomy scintigraphy, although this remains an empirical observation. The additional administration of bovine TSH has not been shown to produce any useful increment in ^{131}I uptake over that attributable to endogenous TSH, but it has frequently caused allergic reactions.

Imaging is best performed 48 to 72 hours after tracer administration, when background levels of activity have fallen, so ^{131}I$^-$ is used. The sensitivity of the survey for metastases clearly increases with higher doses of tracer, but since these patients are likely to require repeated scans, the likely cumulative radiation dose must be taken into consideration. Accordingly, an oral dose of 74 to 185 MBq (2 to 5 mCi) of ^{131}I is now used in most centers. On the whole-body scan, physiologic uptake is seen in the nasopharynx, salivary glands, stomach, bowel, and bladder. Uptake outside these sites should be evaluated further (Fig. 17–16). Pinhole camera views of activity in the neck, together with appropriate surface markers, help resolve the number and distribution of cervical lesions; other foci are better evaluated radiographically. Faint, diffuse hepatic uptake of ^{131}I is seen only when sufficiently functioning normal or malignant thyroid tissue is present to synthesize ^{131}I-labeled thyroid hormones and iodoproteins (which are metabolized in the liver).

The first whole-body survey is usually performed 6 weeks after definitive surgery. If an ablative dose of ^{131}I is given, a post-therapy study is done 72 to 96 hours later to document any foci that may not have been apparent with the tracer dose. Successive scans are performed at progressively increasing intervals (assuming each study is negative for recurrent or metastatic disease)—e.g., annually for the first 3 years, then after a further 3-year interval, and at 5-year intervals thereafter. Life-long follow-up is generally recommended. However, patients who have no evidence of extracervical disease at diagnosis or on their first whole-body survey have a very low likelihood of late recurrence after a 10-year disease-free interval.

In recent years, the serum level of Tg has proved to be a useful marker of the presence of residual or recurrent thyroid tissue. Monitoring of Tg has the major advantage that it can be done in patients while they are taking T_4. It is of greatest value in the patient who has had a true total thyroidectomy or postoperative ablation of thyroid remnants with ^{131}I. In these cases, Tg should be undetectable while the patient is taking T_4. Measurable or rising Tg levels mandate a careful examination of the neck for clinical evidence of local disease recurrence and FNB of any suspicious masses, a chest radiograph, and withdrawal of T_4 in preparation for a whole-body scan with ^{131}I. In patients who are known to have thyroid remnants but in whom a decision has been made against remnant ablation, interpretation of TG levels is more problematic; nevertheless, a significant deviation from the usual T_4-suppressed Tg level established

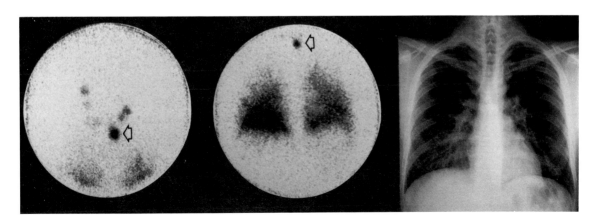

Figure 17–16   Metastatic papillary thyroid carcinoma. Anterior camera views of the head and neck (*left*) and the chest (*center*) obtained after the oral administration of 74 MBq (2 mCi) ^{131}I, 6 weeks following near-total thyroidectomy. There is residual activity in the thyroid remnant (*arrow*), in multiple, bilateral cervical lymph nodes, and diffusely throughout both lungs. The chest radiograph (*right*) underestimates the extent of pulmonary metastases. The patient was treated successfully with a total of 22.2 GBq (600 mCi) of ^{131}I.

for an individual patient should trigger a similar search for metastatic disease. Given a sufficiently reliable Tg assay, this approach has proved at least as sensitive as serial whole-body scans for detecting recurrences of thyroid cancer. Indeed, rising Tg levels have frequently preceded the development of scintigraphically demonstrable disease by several months, and occasional patients have been reported with biopsy-proven, scintigraphically "nonfunctioning" metastases and elevated Tg. Significant titers of antithyroglobulin antibodies invalidate the Tg radioimmunoassay; such patients must be identified early and followed up with serial scans.

Medullary Thyroid Carcinoma

Medullary thyroid carcinoma (MTC) is considered separately since it arises from tissue that is embryologically and functionally distinct from thyroid follicular epithelium. The parafollicular cells (C cells) are neuroectodermal derivatives that produce calcitonin and a number of proven and putative neurotransmitters; they do not trap or organify iodide. Thus, discrete primary medullary tumors (the usual sporadic type) appear as cold lesions on thyroid scans—classically as bilateral, nonfunctioning nodules. In this circumstance, a cytologic diagnosis of MTC may be made by FNB. However, MTC may involve the thyroid diffusely, particularly in the familial, autosomal dominant type (which may be associated with Type 2 multiple endocrine neoplasia [MEN-2] syndromes), in which case its presence may not be appreciated on routine scintigraphy.

The pentagastrin-stimulated serum level of calcitonin is an extremely sensitive marker of residual or recurrent MTC. Several radiopharmaceuticals have been used to try to localize tumor deposits scintigraphically in patients with positive pentagastrin tests. Skeletal and hepatic metastases may be located in the usual way with ^{99m}Tc–methylene diphosphonate (MDP) and ^{99m}Tc–sulfur colloid, respectively. In addition, primary or metastatic MTC may occasionally contain sufficient calcitonin-derived amyloid to take up ^{99m}Tc-MDP actively. In common with other cellular thyroid tumors, both the primary tumor and metastases may be detectable with ^{201}Tl. Presumably because of their neuroectodermal origins, a significant proportion of MTCs and their metastases have been shown to take up ^{123}I- or ^{131}I-metaiodobenzylguanidine (MIBG), more commonly in familial than in sporadic cases. However, the most promising radiopharmaceutical to date has been pentavalent ^{99m}Tc–dimercaptosuccinic acid (99mTc[V]DMSA), which has been reported to have 95 percent overall sensitivity for lesion detection; the mechanism by which this agent localizes in MTC is unknown.

Hyperthyroidism

The diagnosis of hyperthyroidism is a clinical and biochemical one. Thyroid scintigraphy is useful for distinguishing among the various causes of hyperthyroidism (Figs. 17–17 to 17–21). One advantage of ^{99m}TcO$_4$$^-$ scintigraphy over ^{123}I scans is that an image can be obtained, if necessary, while the patient is taking antithyroid drugs since trapping is not blocked.

Some estimate of thyroid uptake is necessary for hyperthyroid patients who are to receive a therapeutic dose of ^{131}I, in order to ensure that an adequate dose of radiation can be delivered to the gland and to exclude patients with hyperthyroidism due to clinically unsuspected subacute or "silent" thyroiditis—or factitious—in whom uptake will be markedly reduced. An impression of uptake can be gained from a visual estimate of the thyroid-to-background and thyroid-to-salivary ratios of activity on the ^{99m}TcO$_4$$^-$ image. Pertechnetate uptake can be quantified by using computer-assisted definition of thyroid and background regions and by comparing the background-corrected thyroid counts with the counts

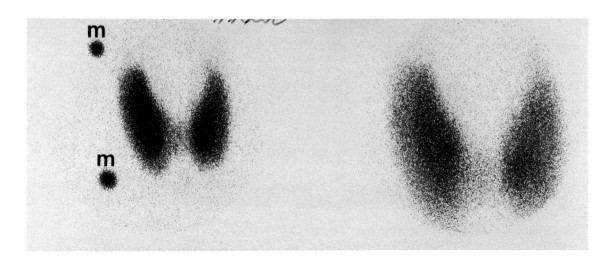

Figure 17–17   Graves' disease: diffuse, toxic goiter. Twenty-four-hour ^{131}I uptake is 66 percent (m: surface markers 6 cm apart).

from a known standard dose in a neck phantom, in much the same way as described in Chapter 7 for radioactive iodine uptake measurement using a scintillation probe.

The advantages of measuring $^{99m}TcO_4^-$ uptake are that it can be done 20 to 30 minutes after administration of the tracer, and an image is obtained at the same time. However, $^{99m}TcO_4^-$ uptake cannot be used directly in the various formulas for calculating the therapeutic dose of ^{131}I to be given, since they are all based on the 24-hour radioiodine uptake. This is not a problem if it is the clinic's policy to administer empirical or relatively fixed doses of ^{131}I.

Miscellaneous Applications

The follicular elements of the thyroid are derived from the embryonic endoderm of the floor of the primitive pharynx. The primordial thyroid migrates caudally together with the developing heart but maintains its connection with its pharyngeal origin by means of the thyroglossal duct, which extends to the foramen cecum of the tongue. Thus, in addition to the usual site in the lower anterior neck, foci of thyroid tissue may be found anywhere between the base of the tongue and the middle mediastinum (rarely as far caudad as the diaphragm). Thyroid scintigraphy is therefore helpful in the differential diagnosis of anterior and anterolateral neck masses in children and mediastinal masses in adults. Iodine 123 is theoretically superior for the investigation of mediastinal masses, since the high mediastinal blood-pool activity 20 to 30 minutes after injection of $^{99m}TcO_4^-$ may ob-

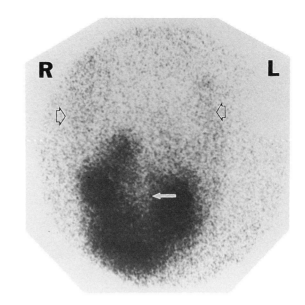

Figure 17-18 Autonomous (hot) nodule. Decreased $^{99m}TcO_4^-$ uptake at the center (*white arrow*) corresponds with an area of cystic degeneration. Uptake by the remainder of the gland is suppressed (*open arrows*). Twenty-four-hour ^{131}I uptake is 35 percent.

scure uptake by substernal thyroid tissue. However, in practice, retrosternal extension of a thyroid is almost never present if the size and contour of the cervical portion of the gland are normal (Fig. 17-22).

Figure 17-19 Left lobe nodule in a hyperthyroid patient. Twenty-four-hour ^{131}I uptake is 70 percent. The $^{99m}TcO_4^-$ scan shows a diffuse, toxic goiter with a solitary, cold nodule in the left lobe (*open arrow*) that proved to be a papillary carcinoma. Note the prominent pyramidal lobe uptake (*closed arrows*).

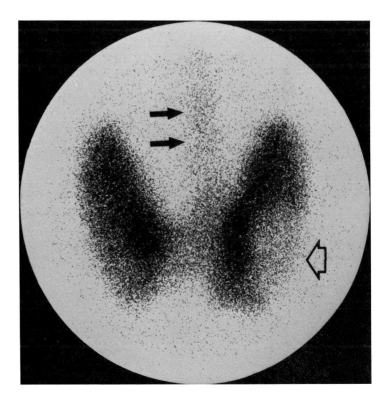

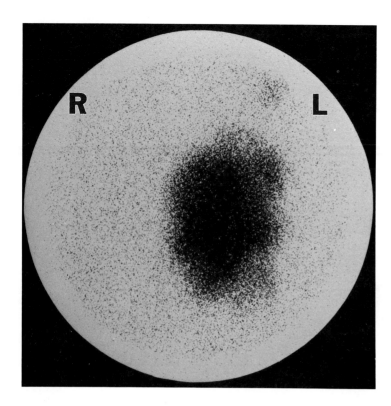

Figure 17-20 Toxic, multinodular left thyroid remnant (previous right hemithyroidectomy). Twenty-four-hour ^{131}I uptake is 43 percent.

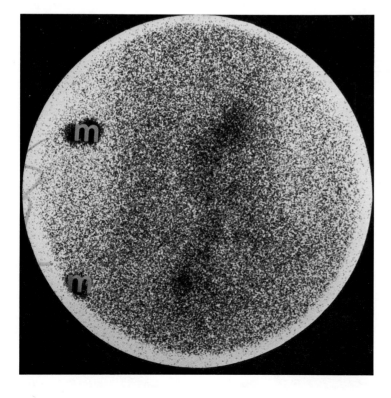

Figure 17-21 Painless thyroiditis. Hyperthyroid patient with a nontender, multinodular gland. Minimal, irregular [99m]TcO₄⁻ uptake (m: surface markers). Twenty-four-hour ^{131}I uptake is 1.2 percent. The patient was not taking thyroid hormone.

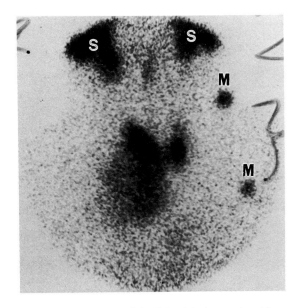

Figure 17-22 Large, cold nodule of the right lower pole, with retrosternal extension (S = salivary glands; M = surface markers).

As an adjunct to the general use of neonatal mass-screening for hypothyroidism, scintigraphy is a simple method of distinguishing between abnormalities of embryogenesis (thyroid ectopia, hemiagenesis, or agenesis) and hormonogenic defects (in which the thyroid is entopic but dysfunctional). Although both types of disorder require thyroid hormone replacement, the former group is sporadic and the latter is inherited, with different implications for genetic counseling. Technetium 99m pertechnetate is the agent of choice; scintigraphy must be performed before replacement therapy has begun.

THE PARATHYROIDS

Radiopharmaceuticals and Rationale

Hyperparathyroidism is recognized more frequently in asymptomatic patients as a result of the widespread use of "screening panels" of automated biochemical tests on blood. Primary hyperparathyroidism is usually caused by a single parathyroid adenoma; about 15 percent of cases are due to diffuse parathyroid hyperplasia and 2 percent to parathyroid carcinoma. Treatment is surgical.

The somewhat complex embryogenesis of the parathyroids from the third and fourth branchial clefts accounts for the potentially wide range of distribution of these glands. In particular, the inferior parathyroids (which originate from the third branchial cleft) may be found anywhere from the angle of the mandible to the pericardium. With such anatomic variability, a reliable, noninvasive method of preoperatively locating abnormal parathyroids should be attractive. This sentiment should be tempered by the fact that a highly experienced parathyroid surgeon will operate successfully in 95 percent of patients on the first attempt without the benefit of any preoperative localizing procedure.

No radiopharmaceutical that is specific for parathyroid tissue has been found. There were several reports in the mid 1960s of success with selenomethionine Se75, but subsequent experience has shown it to be both insensitive and nonspecific. Attempted stimulation of parathyroid hormone synthesis by pretreatment of patients with the calcium-chelating agent ethylenediaminetetraacetic acid (EDTA) produced only a modest improvement in sensitivity. Toluidine blue and methylene blue have long been used by surgeons as aids for intraoperative localization of the parathyroids. The mechanism of uptake is uncertain, but ^{131}I-labeled toluidine blue has been reported as a specific agent for parathyroid scintigraphy, particularly for small adenomas and hyperplastic glands. Experience with this radiopharmaceutical is very limited, but uptake by lymph nodes and thyroid nodules has been documented.

Uptake of ^{201}Tl by parathyroid tumors was first reported from Japan in the late 1970s. It is presumed to reflect vascularity and cellularity nonspecifically, as already suggested for thyroid nodules. Cesium 131 is another potassium analogue that is distributed similarly to ^{201}Tl, but it has less favorable physical characteristics for gamma camera imaging. Thallium 201 is, of course, also taken up by the normal (vascular, cellular) thyroid. Interest in parathyroid scintigraphy has been rekindled by the development of computer-assisted subtraction of a ^{99m}TcO$_4{}^-$ image of the thyroid from a ^{201}Tl image of the neck (^{201}Tl/^{99m}Tc subtraction scintigraphy). Since the first description of this technique, there have been numerous enthusiastic reports hailing its sensitivity and specificity. However, re-examination of many of these series shows a selection bias against operating on patients with negative scans, so that sensitivity is overestimated. It must be emphasized that, if parathyroid scintigraphy is to be used at all, it should be as a localizing procedure and not as a diagnostic test. The diagnosis of hyperparathyroidism must be made on biochemical grounds (not always a straightforward matter) and the decision to operate should then be made independently of the scan.

A realistic estimate of the sensitivity of ^{201}Tl/^{99m}Tc subtraction scanning for parathyroid adenomas is 70 to 85 percent—far short of that of a skilled surgeon. Adenoma size seems to be the major determinant of detectability, so that tumors weighing less than 250 mg are almost never demonstrated. For the same reason, sensitivity for detecting hyperplastic glands is substantially less than for adenomas—about 50 to 60 percent. Normal parathyroids are not visualized. Specificity is much higher, on the order of 90 to 95 percent, in the absence of associated thyroid disease. This reservation is important, and careful palpation of the patient's neck is essential before scintigraphy is planned. Patients with palpably abnormal thyroids, particularly multinodular glands, should be excluded, since most cold thyroid nodules are cellular and take up ^{201}Tl to produce a false-positive (or uninterpretable) subtraction scan. Other reported causes of false-positive scans have been lymph nodes involved with sarcoidosis, Hodgkin's disease, and various metastatic malignancies.

The preceding data should discourage the routine preoperative use of parathyroid scintigraphy. In selected patients, such as those who are likely to tolerate anesthesia poorly, a positive preoperative study may be very useful for directing the neck exploration and reducing operating time. The most challenging problem for the parathyroid surgeon remains the patient with persistent or recurrent hyperparathyroidism after one or more previous neck explorations. It is generally agreed that preoperative localization is worthwhile in this situation. Although selective venous sampling remains the standard procedure, it is technically demanding, is not without risk to the patient, and has a sensitivity, at best, of 75 to 80 percent. Scintigraphy alone has a sensitivity of only 30 to 50 percent in such patients, but the sensitivity of a combination of noninvasive tests—namely, scintigraphy, high-resolution ultrasonography, and x-ray CT scanning—

approaches that of venous sampling. This adjunctive role is probably the most useful one for parathyroidscintigraphy in its present form (Fig. 17–23).

Technique

The methods of acquiring and analyzing ^{201}Tl/^{99m}Tc scans have not been standardized. There are two main divisions based on the order in which the radiopharmaceuticals are administered (Table 17–6). Each approach has its advantages, disadvantages, and passionate advocates, but neither is demonstrably superior to the other. A prerequisite of both methods is immobilization of the patient's head and neck throughout the procedure. Patient cooperation and comfort and a quiet environment are therefore paramount. Patient movement results in misregistration of the ^{201}Tl and the ^{99m}Tc data, producing artifacts on the subtracted image. It is helpful to have one or more ^{99m}Tc surface markers, so positioned on the patient as to be on the edge of the camera's field of view, to serve as a check for patient movement. Computer programs are available that track the position of such markers and realign each image frame if movement has

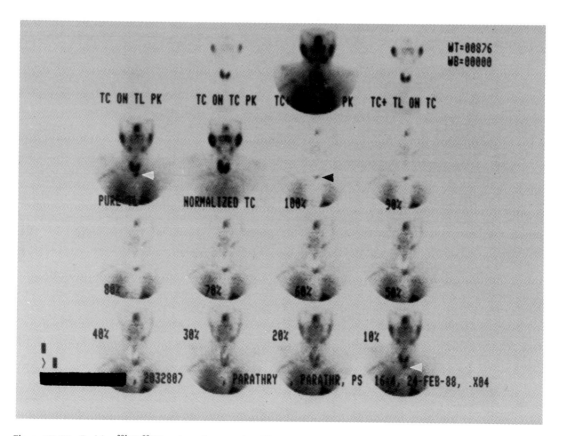

Figure 17-23   Positive ^{201}Tl/^{99m}Tc subtraction parathyroid scan in a patient with recurrent hypercalcemia 12 years after parathyroid adenomectomy. Left superior mediastinal parathyroid adenoma was confirmed at reoperation. The adenoma is clearly visible below the left lower pole of the thyroid gland on the pure Tl image (*second row left, arrowhead*). Progressively less subtraction of the normalized Tc image from the pure Tl image, from 100 percent subtraction to 10 percent subtraction, confirms this as the only focus of disparity between the Tl and Tc images (*arrowheads*).

TABLE 17–6   Techniques of ^{201}Tl ^{99m}Tc Subtraction Parathyroid Scintigraphy

"Thallium First"	"Technetium First"
1. 20% window on ^{201}Tl photopeak. 2. Position patient under camera. 3. Inject 74 MBq (2 mCi) ^{201}Tl IV. 4. Acquire ^{201}Tl image. 5. 20% window on ^{99m}Tc photopeak. 6. Inject 111 MBq (3 mCi) ^{99m}TcO$_4^-$ IV. 7. Acquire ^{99m}Tc image 15–20 minutes after injection.	1. Inject 37 MBq (1 mCi) ^{99m}TcO$_4^-$ IV. 2. 20% window on ^{99m}Tc photopeak. 3. Position patient 15–20 minutes after injection. 4. Acquire ^{99m}Tc image. 5. 20% window on ^{201}Tl photopeak. 6. Acquire image of ^{99m}Tc downscatter into ^{201}Tl window. 7. Inject 74 MBq (2 mCi) ^{201}Tl IV. 8. Acquire ^{201}Tl image.
Analysis 1. Define thyroid region from ^{99m}Tc image. 2. Determine counts in thyroid region for each radionuclide. 3. Normalize* ^{201}Tl image to ^{99m}Tc image. 4. Subtract ^{99m}Tc image from normalized ^{201}Tl image.	1. Define thyroid region from ^{99m}Tc image. 2. Determine counts in thyroid region for each radionuclide and downscatter counts. 3. Subtract downscatter image from ^{201}Tl image. 4. Normalize ^{99m}Tc image to downscatter-subtracted ^{201}Tl image 5. Subtract normalized ^{99m}Tc image from downscatter-subtracted ^{201}Tl image.

* Multiply the counts in each pixel in the lower-count image by the ratio of the counts in the thyroid region for each radionuclide.

occurred, but they are not in general use. The patient is positioned as for thyroid scintigraphy. The camera is fitted with a parallel-hole rather than a pinhole collimator to improve counting efficiency and to avoid spatial distortion, and the images are electronically magnified ("zoomed") if an LFOV camera is used. The image field should extend from the jaw to the xiphoid; it is essential that mediastinal foci of abnormal ^{201}Tl uptake be identified.

The advantages of the "thallium first" approach are that the ^{201}Tl image is free of scatter from ^{99m}Tc (see later) and that the later administration of a higher dose of ^{99m}TcO$_4^-$ permits better definition of the thyroid. The major disadvantage is that the period of immobilization required is somewhat longer, particularly if ^{99m}Tc data acquisition is delayed for the usual 20 to 30 minutes required for peak thyroid pertechnetate uptake to occur.

With the "technetium first" approach, sufficient time can be allowed to elapse for maximum pertechnetate uptake before the patient is positioned for imaging. The main disadvantage is a technical one, which can be appreciated by reference to Figure 17–6. The principal photopeak used for ^{201}Tl imaging (69- to 83-keV characteristic x-rays) falls in the Compton scatter region of the ^{99m}Tc spectrum. Hence the need for correction of the ^{201}Tl image for the contribution from so-called ^{99m}Tc downscatter. A relatively low dose of ^{99m}TcO$_4^-$ is therefore used to reduce downscatter as much as possible.

Published variations in technique have included use of a pinhole collimator or a converging collimator, substitution of ^{123}I$^-$ for ^{99m}TcO$_4^-$ (in which case the ^{201}Tl must be given second and a correction made for ^{123}I downscatter), image subtraction without normalization, graduated subtraction of ^{99m}Tc from ^{201}Tl, and a sophisticated, color-coded subtraction routine.

THE ADRENAL CORTEX

Radiopharmaceuticals and Rationale

From the functional standpoint, the adrenal cortex behaves as two more or less distinct organs—the subcapsular zona glomerulosa and the deeper zona fasciculata and zona reticularis. A simplified outline of adrenocortical physiology, and of drugs that modify it, is presented in Figure 17–24. The early steps in steroid hormone biosynthesis are common to all three zones of the cortex. The major hormone precursor is circulating low-density lipoprotein (LDL) cholesterol, which is internalized into cortical cells by way of specific cell-surface LDL receptors. Expansion of the intracellular cholesterol pool and, indirectly, of the extracellular pool of LDL cholesterol results in feedback reduction ("down-regulation") in the number of LDL receptors.

The zona glomerulosa is primarily under the control of the renin-angiotensin system. Angiotensin II and III (and K$^+$) stimulate the later steps in aldosterone synthesis; angiotensin II also exerts a trophic effect on the zona glomerulosa in the long term. The zonae fasciculata and reticularis are under the control of adrenocorticotropic hormone (corticotropin, ACTH), which not only is trophic to these zones and directly stimulates hormone biosynthesis but also increases the number of membrane LDL receptors.

Cholesterol labeled with ^{131}I (^{131}I-19-iodocholesterol) was the first successful radiopharmaceutical for adrenocortical scintigraphy. It has been supplanted by the cholesterol analogues, ^{131}I-6β-iodomethyl-19-norcholesterol (NP-59) and ^{75}Se-6β-selenomethyl-19-norcholesterol (SMC) (Fig. 17–25), which provide better adrenal-to-background ratios of activity. As might be anticipated

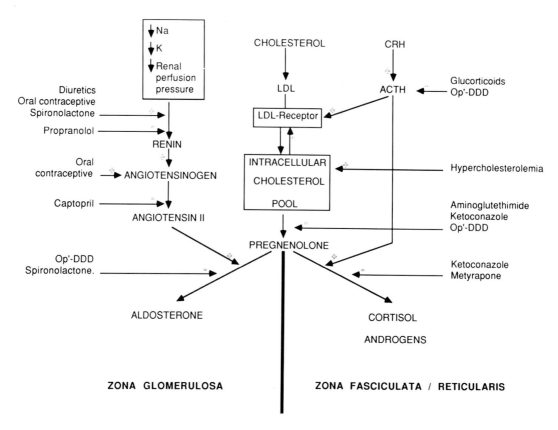

Figure 17–24 Simplified scheme of adrenocortical physiology. The effects of drugs and hypercholesterolemia, and their sites of action, are summarized (+: stimulates; −: inhibits).

from their structural similarity, both analogues behave virtually identically in vivo. SMC has some practical advantages over NP-59. The photopeaks of ^{75}Se (see Table 17–1) are more efficiently detected by gamma cameras; SMC undergoes less radiolysis, which, combined with the long physical half-life of ^{75}Se, means that the shelf-life of SMC is 6 weeks at room temperature (compared with 2 weeks frozen for NP-59); and thyroid blockade is not required when SMC is used. Although ^{75}Se is a pure gamma emitter, its very long physical half-life means that the dosimetry for SMC is similar to that of NP-59 (Table

17–7). NP-59 is the only agent currently available for clinical use in the United States and the agent for which the greatest body of clinical experience exists.

After intravenous injection, approximately 20 percent of the dose of NP-59 is carried in the LDL fraction of plasma. LDL-bound NP-59 is taken up by the adrenal cortical cell, but unlike native cholesterol, it does not undergo any further significant metabolism. NP-59 that is not taken up by the adrenals is largely excreted unchanged by the liver, and there is an active enterohepatic circulation; a small fraction is excreted as ^{131}I-labeled bile acid analogues.

Uptake by the zona fasciculata normally accounts for 80 to 90 percent of total adrenocortical NP-59 uptake. The administration of exogenous ACTH increases uptake of NP-59. Conversely, suppression of endogenous ACTH production by dexamethasone reduces NP-59 uptake by 50 percent, and sodium loading with resultant inhibition of the renin-angiotensin system reduces NP-59 uptake by a further 10 percent. The profound reduction of NP-59 uptake by normal, ACTH-dependent adrenocortical tissue after the administration of pharmacologic doses of dexamethasone has been exploited to enhance the ability of NP-59 scintigraphy to distinguish between adenomas and bilateral hyperplasia in cases of primary hyperaldosteronism and adrenal hyperandrogenism (dexamethasone-suppression adrenocortical scintigraphy).

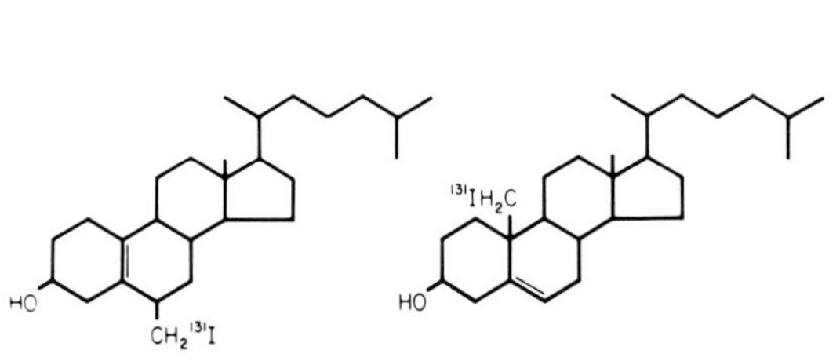

Figure 17–25 Structural formulas of NP-59 and ^{131}I-19-iodocholesterol. ^{75}Se-6β-selenomethyl-19-norcholesterol is structurally identical to NP-59 but for the substitution of ^{75}Se for ^{131}I.

TABLE 17-7   Dosimetry of Adrenocortical Scintigraphic Agents

	^{131}I-6β-iodomethyl-19-norcholesterol (NP-59)		^{75}Se-6β-selenomethyl-19-norcholesterol	
	cGy/MBq	(rad/mCi)	cGy/MBq	(rad/mCi)
Whole body	0.032	(1.2)	0.038	(1.4)
Adrenals	0.70	(26.0)	0.16	(6.1)
Ovaries	0.22	(8.0)	0.05	(1.9)
Testes	0.062	(2.3)		
Liver	0.065	(2.4)	0.095	(3.5)
Adult dose	37 MBq	(1.0 mCi)	9.25 MBq	(250 μCi)

The effects of hypercholesterolemia and of several drugs on NP-59 uptake can be predicted from the physiologic outline given in Figure 17-24.

Technique

The procedural details of adrenocortical scintigraphy are outlined in Table 17-8. Drugs known to interfere with NP-59 uptake must be identified and withdrawn 3 to 4 weeks before injection of the tracer. The clinical and biochemical diagnosis must be reviewed; if dexamethasone-suppression scintigraphy is indicated, dexamethasone must be started 1 week before injection. Since NP-59 contains trace amounts of free ^{131}I, thyroid blockade with stable iodine must be started 1 to 2 days before injection and for 2 weeks thereafter; potassium perchlorate (200 mg every 8 hours) or T_3 (20 μg every 8 hours) may be substituted in patients who are allergic to iodine. The dose of NP-59 is 37 MBq (1.0 mCi) per 1.7 m² of body surface area; the tracer is dissolved in an alcoholic vehicle containing Tween 80, so it should be injected intravenously slowly. Potentially confusing colonic retention of excreted NP-59 can be reduced by the routine prescription of bisacodyl to start 2 to 3 days before the first scan; this laxative does not interfere significantly with the enterohepatic circulation of NP-59.

Quantitation of adrenal NP-59 uptake is, in principle, similar to the measurement of $^{99m}TcO_4^-$ uptake by the thyroid, described previously, with the important additional requirement of correction for photon attenuation because of adrenal depth. The injection syringe must be counted both before and after injection to calculate the precise dose administered. The sensitivity and efficiency for the specific gamma camera–collimator system to be used must be established for known activities of ^{131}I at different depths in a tissue-equivalent phantom. Adrenal depth may be determined from the lateral view obtained with an external marker on the skin of the back (in which case the length represented by each pixel must be known for the computer system); depth may be more simply and accurately calculated from a recent x-ray CT scan through the patient's adrenals. Adrenal and background regions are defined, and the net counts for each adrenal (corrected for background, depth, and radioactive decay since the time of injection) are determined, translated into activity, and expressed as a percentage of the administered dose. The entire procedure is semiautomated.

Normal adrenal cortical uptake of NP-59 is approximately symmetric, with normal mean uptake per adrenal of 0.16 percent of the injected dose (range, 0.07 to 0.26 percent). On posterior scintiscans, uptake by the normal right adrenal appears to be greater than that by the left, owing both to the more posterior position of the right gland (less attenuation of photons by interposed soft tissue) and to a higher background activity contributed by the liver; however, when appropriate attenuation and

TABLE 17-8   Procedure for NP-59 Scintigraphy

No Dexamethasone Suppression	Dexamethasone Suppression
• SSKI 1 drop t.i.d. to start 1–2 days before injection and continue for 14 days	• Dexamethasone 1 mg q.i.d. to start 7 days before injection and continue through study
• Inject 37 MBq (1.0mCi) NP-59 IV	• SSKI 1 drop t.i.d. to start 1–2 days before injection and continue for 14 days
• Posterior, anterior, lateral and marker images from days 5–7 postinjection	• Inject 37 MBq (1.0 mCi) NP-59 IV
	• Posterior, anterior, lateral and marker images from days 3–5 postinjection; specific pelvic views if indicated

SSKI = saturated solution of potassium iodide

background corrections are made, the normal right-to-left uptake ratio ranges from 0.9 to 1.2. In patients with syndromes of adrenal cortical hyperfunction, total (right + left) adrenal uptake of NP-59 correlates with integrated biochemical indices of disease activity; i.e., in Cushing's syndrome, primary hyperaldosteronism, and adrenal hyperandrogenism, NP-59 uptake correlates with 24-hour urinary excretion of free cortisol, aldosterone, and 17-ketosteroids, respectively. However, the scintigraphic *patterns* of uptake, taken together with the biochemical findings in plasma and urine and the anatomic findings from x-ray CT or MRI of the adrenals, permit the differential diagnosis of these disorders on functional grounds.

Clinical Applications

The patterns of NP-59 uptake seen in adrenal cortical disorders are summarized in Table 17-9. It is immediately apparent that the repertoire of possible scintigraphic findings is narrow, re-emphasizing the fundamental importance of rigorously defining the biochemical abnormality.

Cushing's Syndrome

Operationally, Cushing's syndrome may be ACTH-dependent, resulting from overproduction of ACTH by the pituitary (owing to a pituitary adenoma or ectopic production of corticotropin-releasing hormone [CRH]) or ectopically by an extrapituitary, benign, or malignant tumor; or it may be ACTH-independent, resulting from autonomous adrenal overproduction of cortisol. ACTH-dependent Cushing's syndrome is characterized biochemically by inappropriately high circulating levels of ACTH,

whereas in ACTH-independent variants, ACTH production is suppressed by the high cortisol levels. The distinction is important, since the optimal current treatment of ACTH-independent disease is surgical attack on the involved adrenal(s), which is no longer the treatment of choice for ACTH-dependent disease. Pituitary Cushing's syndrome (Cushing's disease) accounts for approximately two-thirds of all cases; ectopic ACTH secretion accounts for 15 percent of cases. Adrenal cortical adenomas account for a further 10 percent, and adrenal carcinomas and autonomous cortical nodular hyperplasia (CNH) each for about 5 percent.

The pathophysiology of Cushing's syndrome predicts the scintigraphic patterns of its variants (Fig. 17-26). ACTH-dependent adrenal hyperplasia is characterized by bilaterally, symmetrically increased NP-59 uptake; as might be expected, total measured uptake tends to be higher in patients with the ectopic ACTH syndrome than in those with Cushing's disease. Unilateral uptake is seen on the side of an adrenocortical adenoma, with suppression of contralateral uptake as a result of feedback inhibition of pituitary ACTH secretion. Although a similar pattern might be anticipated for adrenocortical carcinomas, it is seen only rarely since these (usually large) tumors synthesize cortisol inefficiently and take up insufficient NP-59 per gram of tissue to produce an image; however, since the tumor as a whole produces excess cortisol, ACTH secretion and contralateral NP-59 uptake are again suppressed. Thus, the characteristic scintigraphic pattern of adrenocortical carcinomas is "bilateral nonvisualization." Like ACTH-dependent adrenal hyperplasia, autonomous CNH is also characterized by bilaterally increased NP-59 uptake; however, the disease is typically, though not invariably, asymmetric. Ultimately, the distinction hinges on the ACTH level.

TABLE 17-9 Summary of Scintigraphic Findings in Adrenocortical Disorders

Disorder	Pathology	Scintigraphy
Cushing's syndrome		
ACTH-dependent	Hyperplasia	Bilaterally increased uptake (symmetric)
ACTH-independent	Adenoma	Ipsilaterally increased uptake, contralateral suppression
	Hyperplasia	Bilaterally increased uptake (may be asymmetric)
	Carcinoma	Bilateral nonvisualization
Primary hyperaldosteronism	Adenoma	Ipsilateral early visualization*
	Hyperplasia	Bilateral early visualization*
Hyperandrogenism	Adenoma	Ipsilateral early visualization*
	Hyperplasia (Ovarian)	Bilateral early visualization* (Ovarian visualization)*
"Incidental" nodule	Nonfunctioning	Ipsilaterally decreased uptake (discordant NP-59 and CT)
	Functioning	Ipsilaterally increased uptake (concordant NP-59 and CT)

* Dexamethasone-suppression scans

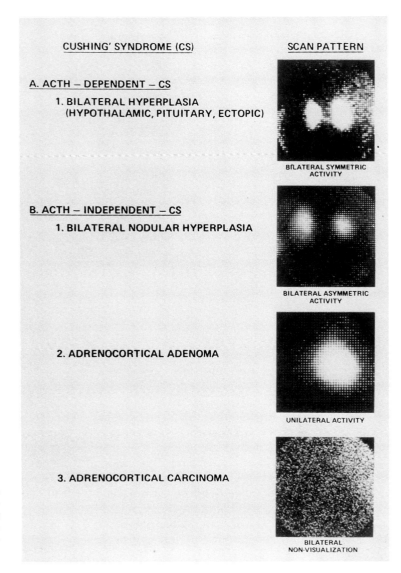

Figure 17-26 Spectrum of scintigraphic findings with NP-59 in Cushing's syndrome. (From Gross MD, Beierwaltes WH, Thompson NW, et al. Scintigraphic approach to the localization of adrenal lesions causing hypertension. Urol Radiol 1982; 3:241; with permission.)

In practice, the major clinical role of NP-59 scintigraphy in Cushing's syndrome is to characterize the functional abnormality in ACTH-independent disease. X-ray CT of the adrenals consistently identifies tumors larger than 2 cm in diameter and, in cases of adrenal carcinoma, may demonstrate anatomic evidence of the malignant nature of the tumor. However, CT is relatively insensitive for lesions smaller than 1 cm, which poses a major difficulty when one is trying to discriminate between a small, unilateral adenoma and a dominant nodule in adrenals bilaterally but asymmetrically affected by CNH. The management is different; the distinction is readily made by scintigraphy. MRI of the adrenals has proved no more sensitive than CT for this purpose.

Primary Hyperaldosteronism

Once again, the distinction between an adrenocortical adenoma (aldosteronoma) and bilateral zona glomerulosa hyperplasia as the cause of primary hyperaldosteronism (PHA) is critical to the patient, since the treatment is surgical in the former case and medical (spironolactone) in the latter. Reliance on an anatomic diagnosis through x-ray CT or MRI is fraught with the same pitfalls just described for CNH, since aldosteronomas are usually small (less than 2 cm) and zona glomerulosa hyperplasia is frequently nodular.

As already mentioned, dexamethasone suppression is used to increase the proportion of NP-59 taken up by the relatively ACTH-independent zona glomerulosa. When the regimen in Table 17-8 is used, the adrenals are not normally visualized earlier than 5 days after NP-59 injection. Visualization of both adrenals before the fifth day suggests bilateral zona glomerulosa hyperplasia (Fig. 17-27); it is vital that the biochemical diagnosis of PHA be certain for this interpretation to hold true, since the same appearance is seen in some patients with low-renin essential hypertension or secondary hyperaldosteronism. Unilateral early visualization or marked asymmetry of NP-59 uptake indicates an aldosteronoma (see Fig.

PRIMARY ALDOSTERONISM   SCAN PATTERN

1. ADRENAL ADENOMA

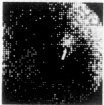

EARLY UNILATERAL
ACTIVITY (DAY 3)

2. BILATERAL ADRENAL HYPERPLASIA

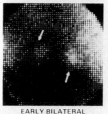

EARLY BILATERAL
ACTIVITY (DAY 3)

Figure 17–27 Primary hyperaldosteronism. Findings on dexamethasone-suppression NP-59 scintigraphy. (From Gross MD, Beierwaltes WH, Thompson NW, et al. Scintigraphic approach to the localization of adrenal lesions causing hypertension. Urol Radiol 1982; 3:241; with permission.)

17–27). Spironolactone, diuretics, and the combination oral contraceptive pill can enhance contralateral zona glomerulosa uptake in patients with unilateral adenomas to such a degree that a false scintigraphic diagnosis of hyperplasia may be made. Hence it is necessary to discontinue these drugs several weeks before scintigraphy.

NP-59 scintigraphy is at least as sensitive and specific as CT for the differential diagnosis of PHA. The final arbiter may still be adrenal vein sampling, but this is a difficult, invasive technique associated with adrenal hemorrhage and infarction in 5 percent of cases and therefore should be avoided if possible. If both scintigraphy and CT (or MRI) demonstrate a unilateral adenoma, adrenalectomy can proceed without recourse to adrenal vein sampling. Adrenal vein sampling should be reserved for cases in which the NP-59 scan is equivocal, or when scintigraphy and CT disagree as to the side of unilateral disease.

Hyperandrogenism

The majority of cases of hyperandrogenism encountered in clinical practice are due to relatively subtle abnormalities of sex steroid metabolism or end-organ sensitivity that are best diagnosed biochemically and managed pharmacologically. In practice, localization studies are necessary only in women with clinically or biochemically impressive hyperandrogenism.

The most common identifiable disorder in hirsute, oligomenorrheic, and amenorrheic women is the polycystic ovary (Stein-Leventhal) syndrome. Adrenal NP-59 uptake tends to be increased bilaterally in these patients, the mean total uptake being similar to that measured in patients with Cushing's disease. This is a scintigraphic reflection of the secondarily abnormal adrenal androgen metabolism that has often been documented in this disorder.

Dexamethasone-suppression scintigraphy in patients with biochemical evidence of adrenal hyperandrogenism produces results analogous to those in patients with PHA, namely, bilateral visualization before day 5 following injection in patients with bilateral adrenal hyperplasia (classical congenital adrenal hyperplasia [CAH] and its late-onset variants) and unilateral early visualization in patients with adenomas. Attention is again drawn to the fact that estrogens and oral contraceptive pills are frequently used to manage women with hirsutism and menstrual disturbances and, unless they are withdrawn, may lead to a false scintigraphic diagnosis of adrenocortical hyperplasia. Ovarian uptake of NP-59 following dexamethasone suppression of adrenal cortical uptake has also been documented in patients with ovarian hyperandrogenism.

Hyperandrogenism that is sufficiently severe to cause frank virilization is much more likely to be due to an underlying tumor, usually ovarian. The anatomy of the adnexa can be displayed by ultrasound, CT, or, optimally, MRI. Dexamethasone-suppression NP-59 scintigraphy of both the adrenals and the pelvis may be useful for establishing the functional significance of demonstrable pelvic abnormalities, particularly in cases in which the biochemical findings favor an adrenal source of hyperandrogenism (e.g., high circulating levels of dehydroepiandrosterone sulfate). Vigorous bowel cleansing may be necessary in this circumstance to ensure that an apparent pelvic focus of NP-59 uptake does not represent retained colonic activity. Selective adrenal and ovarian vein sampling studies should then be reserved for patients with equivocal findings on these noninvasive localizing tests.

The Incidentally Discovered Adrenal Nodule

The widespread availability and steadily improving resolution of abdominal x-ray CT have resulted in the discovery of asymptomatic abnormalities of adrenal morphology in approximately 1 percent of all examinations.

The frequency approaches 10 percent in patients with known primary extra-adrenal malignancies, since the adrenal is a frequent site of metastasis, particularly from carcinomas of the lung, breast, stomach, and kidney. The likelihood that an adrenal nodule represents a primary or metastatic malignancy is low in patients without a known malignancy; even in patients with known malignancies, fewer than half such nodules prove to be malignant. Unless there is clear evidence of spread beyond the adrenal on the CT scan to indicate malignant behavior, the morphologic findings are nonspecific. Although adrenal masses greater than 5 cm in diameter are more likely to be malignant, size alone is a poor discriminator. Nor has MRI permitted consistent separation of benign from malignant nodules on the basis of tissue characteristics (relative water and lipid content).

The overwhelming majority of these abnormalities are endocrinologically "silent" inasmuch as they are not associated with any clinical or biochemical evidence of adrenal hyperfunction. Nevertheless, the first step in the evaluation of such an incidentally discovered nodule is the exclusion of cortical or medullary hyperfunction by appropriate screening tests. If these tests prove negative, then the functional significance of the nodule is best evaluated scintigraphically, without dexamethasone suppression. In our experience, increased NP-59 uptake in the morphologically abnormal adrenal (concordant NP-59 and CT scans; Fig. 17–28) invariably signifies that the nodule consists of benign, functioning, adenomatous, or hyperplastic adrenocortical tissue. Adrenal vein sampling in such cases has shown that these lesions produce increased quantities not only of cortisol but also of aldosterone and androgens in comparison with the morphologically normal, contralateral gland, despite the normal peripheral venous levels of these hormones. In contrast, markedly reduced or absent NP-59 uptake on the side

of the mass (discordant NP-59 and CT; Fig. 17–29) denotes a nonfunctioning, space-occupying lesion that has proved to be a primary or secondary malignancy in the majority of our cases; thus, discordance between the functional and anatomic studies warrants further evaluation of the lesion, usually by CT-guided needle biopsy.

The analogy between adrenocortical and thyroid scintigraphy for the functional evaluation of nodules is obvious: functioning adrenal nodules are seldom, if ever, malignant, whereas nonfunctioning nodules are more likely to be malignant. There are important differences. First, cold adrenal nodules in our experience are more likely to be malignant than cold thyroid nodules; second, needle biopsy of the adrenal is not a simple procedure and is associated with a significant morbidity and a low, but recognizable, mortality. Since the natural history of functioning nodules is unknown insofar as we are unable to predict which, if any, will ultimately become frankly autonomous, periodic re-evaluation of such patients is advised. Finally, the finding of normal, symmetric NP-59 uptake despite a unilateral adrenal abnormality is indeterminate since small lesions (<1.5 cm in diameter) may not produce an appreciable change in NP-59 uptake, but it should at least prompt a re-evaluation of the morphologic studies to confirm that the mass is, indeed, intra-adrenal and not juxta-adrenal, particularly if it is larger than 2 cm.

THE ADRENAL MEDULLA AND NEUROENDOCRINE TUMORS

Radiopharmaceuticals and Rationale

The major mechanism for uptake of biogenic amines (including the catecholamines) into adrenal medullary cells, presynaptic sympathetic neurons, and presumably,

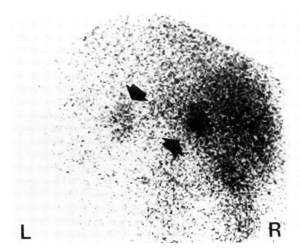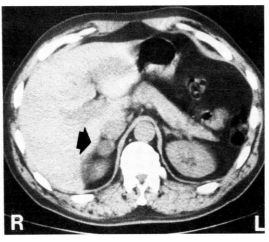

Figure 17–28 Incidental adrenal nodule with concordant NP-59 (*left*) and CT (*right*) scans. The 2-cm right adrenal nodule (*right panel, arrow*) demonstrates higher uptake of NP-59 (*left panel, arrow*) than the morphologically normal left adrenal gland. No biochemical evidence of adrenocortical dysfunction is found. (From Gross MD, Wilton GP, Shapiro B, et al. Functional and scintigraphic evaluation of the silent adrenal mass. J Nucl Med 1987; 28:1401; with permission.)

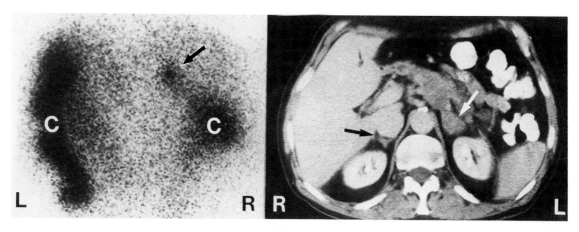

Figure 17–29 Discordant pattern of adrenocortical imaging. The incidental left adrenal nodule (*right panel, white arrow*) failed to take up NP-59. Biopsy showed metastatic adenocarcinoma. The right adrenal was morphologically and scintigraphically normal (*black arrows*). (C = NP-59 in colon.) (From Khafagi FA, Shapiro B, Gross MD. The adrenal gland. In: Maisey MN, Britton KE, Gilday DL, eds. Clinical nuclear medicine. 2nd ed. London: Chapman & Hall, 1988; with permission.)

ontogenically related tissues of neural crest origin is a relatively stereospecific, energy-requiring, saturable pathway termed *uptake-1*. This process is classically inhibited by cocaine and the tricyclic antidepressants (Fig. 17–30). Once inside the cell, the amines are taken up by a second stereospecific active transport process into membrane-bounded vesicles, where they are stored in association with chromogranins and adenosine triphosphate (ATP). This second mechanism is specifically blocked by reserpine and tetrabenazine (see Fig. 17–30). Unstored catecholamines are rapidly degraded by cytoplasmic monoamine oxidase (MAO). Catecholamines that "escape" into the circulation are nonspecifically taken up by extraneuronal tissues (*uptake-2*) where they are catabolized predominantly by catechol-*O*-methyl transferase (COMT).

A protracted search for a suitable adrenomedullary scintigraphic agent at the University of Michigan culminated in the development and successful clinical use of radioiodinated MIBG for the scintigraphic detection of pheochromocytomas. MIBG is an aralkylguanidine that structurally resembles norepinephrine sufficiently to be recognized by uptake-1 and to be taken up into neurosecretory storage vesicles (Fig. 17–31). Because it has a halogenated benzyl ring (like bretylium) and a guanidino side-chain (like guanethidine), MIBG is resistant to metabolism by COMT and MAO, respectively. Thus, after the intravenous injection of ^{131}I-MIBG, up to 80 percent of the administered radioactivity is recovered in the urine within 4 days as unaltered MIBG; ^{131}I-metaiodohippuric acid and free ^{131}I-iodide account for most of the remainder.

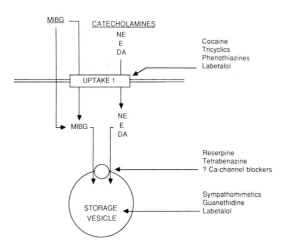

Figure 17–30 Schematic representation of catecholamine and MIBG uptake and storage in adrenergic cells. Note that MIBG enters the cell both by uptake-1 and by passive diffusion. Interfering drugs and their sites of action are shown at right.

Figure 17–31 Structural formula of MIBG, compared with those of norepinephrine and guanethidine.

Pharmacologic blockers of uptake-1 and of storage vesicle uptake have been shown to inhibit MIBG uptake both in vitro and in vivo (Fig. 17–32). Drugs that deplete storage vesicle contents, such as guanethidine and sympathomimetic agents, have the same net effect; the latter group includes pseudoephedrine and phenylpropanolamine, which are frequently present in a wide variety of nonprescription cough medicines, decongestants, and anorectic agents. There is in vitro evidence that pretreatment with calcium-channel-blocking drugs, particularly verapamil, also reduces MIBG uptake. All these agents should be discontinued at least 2 weeks before MIBG injection. Alpha- and beta-adrenergic-blocking drugs have not been shown to affect MIBG uptake significantly, which is of some clinical importance since they need not be discontinued prior to scintigraphy in patients with suspected pheochromocytomas. An important exception is labetalol, a combined alpha- and beta-blocker introduced relatively recently into the United States. Although labetalol appears theoretically attractive for the management of pheochromocytoma, it both blocks uptake-1 and depletes catecholamine storage vesicle contents; it should accordingly be discontinued at least 1 week before MIBG scintigraphy and conventional alpha- and beta-blocking drugs should be substituted.

MIBG may be labeled with ^{131}I or ^{123}I; the dosimetry for both agents is given in Table 17–10. Since ^{123}I-MIBG is given in a dose up to 20-fold larger than ^{131}I-MIBG and since the 159-keV photon is more efficiently detected, spatial resolution and lesion detection are improved and ECT is possible; the disadvantages of ^{123}I-MIBG are its high cost, limited availability, and brief shelf-life.

Technique

Procedures for ^{131}I- and ^{123}I-MIBG scintigraphy are outlined in Table 17–11. As with NP-59, thyroid blockade is required but need continue for only 6 days after MIBG injection.

MIBG is normally taken up by the liver, spleen, salivary glands, and myocardium—in the last three organs, by virtue of their rich sympathetic innervation (Fig. 17–33). Myocardial uptake is inversely related to circulating levels of norepinephrine. The normal adrenal medullae are seen uncommonly with ^{131}I-MIBG, but they are regularly visualized with ^{123}I-MIBG. Intraluminal colonic activity is occasionally present and may be confusing; it may be cleared with bisacodyl or an enema. Since the principal route of MIBG excretion is urinary, activity in the bladder may obscure vesical or pelvic tumors. In ad-

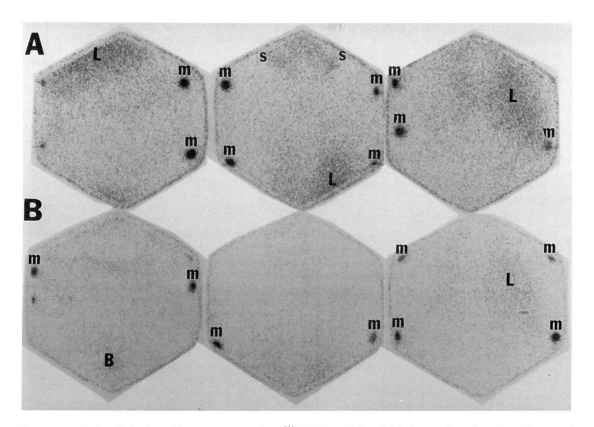

Figure 17–32   Effect of tricyclic antidepressants on uptake of ^{131}I-MIBG. *A (left to right)*, Camera views of anterior abdomen and pelvis, posterior neck and chest, and posterior mid-abdomen 24 hours after ^{131}I-MIBG injection. *B,* Corresponding views at 48 hours. Uptake is markedly reduced in all tissues. Compare with Figure 17–33. (L = liver; m = surface markers; s = salivary glands; B = bladder.)

TABLE 17-10   Dosimetry of MIBG

	131I-MIBG		123I-MIBG	
	cGy/MBq	(rad/mCi)	cGy/MBq	(rad/mCi)
Whole body	0.006	(0.22)	0.0005	(0.02)
Adrenals	0.95	(35.0)	0.075	(2.76)
Ovaries	0.027	(1.0)	0.0019	(0.07)
Liver	0.011	(0.4)	0.0014	(0.05)
Adult dose	18.5 MBq	(0.5 mCi)	74–370 MBq	(2–10 mCi)

dition to radioactive surface markers for orientation, other radiopharmaceuticals can be used as internal markers to clarify the anatomic relationship of sites of abnormal MIBG uptake to the urinary tract (^{99m}Tc-diethylenetri-aminepentaacetic acid [DTPA]), the skeleton (^{99m}Tc-MDP), the liver (^{99m}Tc–sulfur colloid), or the heart (^{201}Tl or ^{99m}Tc-labeled red blood cells).

Clinical Applications

Pheochromocytoma

Since the first reported scintigraphic portrayal of pheochromocytomas with ^{131}I-MIBG in 1981, extensive worldwide experience has shown MIBG to be a safe, sensitive (87 percent), and, in the appropriate clinical setting, highly specific (97 percent) radiopharmaceutical for locating both adrenal (Fig. 17–34) and extra-adrenal (Fig. 17–35) tumor deposits and metastases of malignant pheochromocytomas (Fig. 17–36). Whereas abdominal x-ray CT can detect virtually all adrenal pheochromocytomas larger than 2 cm in diameter, MIBG scintigraphy is clearly superior for smaller tumors, for extra-adrenal tumors or metastases, and in patients who have undergone previous surgery (Fig. 17–37), and it can detect preneoplastic adrenal medullary hyperplasia in the MEN-2 syndromes. The principle we have emphasized repeatedly in the discussions of parathyroid and adrenocortical scintigraphy applies equally to adrenomedullary scintigraphy—namely, MIBG should

not be used as a diagnostic test for possible pheochromocytoma; rather, the diagnosis should be established as confidently as possible on biochemical grounds before scintigraphy is requested. The sequence of localizing procedures depends to some extent on local availability, so that abdominal CT is frequently performed first. However, in patients with a reasonably certain biochemical diagnosis of pheochromocytoma, MIBG scintigraphy is indicated even if a CT scan has demonstrated an intra-abdominal tumor, both to confirm the functional nature of the anatomic abnormality and to rule out the possibility of multifocal or metastatic disease—each of which may be expected to occur in 10 percent or more of cases.

Neuroblastoma and Other Neuroendocrine Tumors

Several tumors of neural crest origin, other than pheochromocytomas, possess the property of amine precursor uptake and decarboxylation (APUD tumors); tissues from these tumors fluoresce when exposed to hot formaldehyde vapor, they take up silver stains, and ultrastructurally they can be shown to contain typical, dense-core, neurosecretory granules. A number of such tumors, most consistently neuroblastomas, and their metastases have been detected scintigraphically with MIBG (Table 17–12).

Neuroblastomas are highly malignant childhood tumors for which prognosis and correct treatment are critically dependent on adequate staging. MIBG scintigra-

TABLE 17-11   Procedures for MIBG Scintigraphy

	131I-MIBG	123I-MIBG
Thyroid blockade	2 days before to 6 days after injection	2 days before to 4 days after injection
Image acquisition	24, 48, 72 hours after injection	2–3, 24, (48) hours after injection
Camera	Wide field of view, interfaced with a computer	
Collimator	High energy	Medium energy
Minimum views	Posterior abdomen; overlapping anterior views from pubis to skull	
	Surface markers on iliac crests, lateral costal margins, axillae	
	Internal markers as necessary (see text)	
Time/counts (per view)	20 minutes/100,000 counts	20 minutes/1,000,000 counts ± emission computed tomography

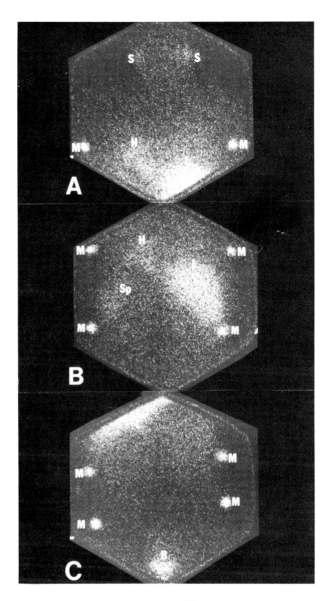

Figure 17-33 Normal distribution of ^{131}I-MIBG 48 hours after injection. Overlapping camera views of *A* (posterior head and chest), *B* (posterior mid-abdomen), and *C* (anterior abdomen and pelvis) are shown. Note tracer accumulation in salivary glands (S), heart (H), liver (L), spleen (Sp), and bladder (B). (M = surface markers.) (From Nakajo M, Shapiro B, Copp J, et al. The normal and abnormal distribution of the adrenomedullary imaging agent *m*[I-131]iodobenzylguanidine (131-I-MIBG) in man. Evaluation by scintigraphy. J Nucl Med 1983; 24:672; with permission.)

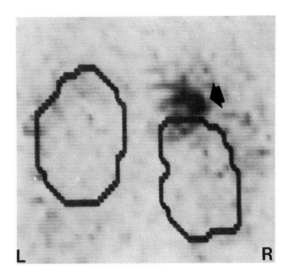

Figure 17-34 Recurrent right adrenal pheochromocytoma (*arrow*): posterior ^{131}I-MIBG scan. The renal outlines were drawn from a simultaneously acquired ^{99m}Tc-DTPA scan. (From Gross MD, Shapiro B, Thral JH. Adrenal scintigraphy. In: Gottschalk A, et al, eds. Golden's diagnostic radiology: diagnostic nuclear medicine. 2nd ed. Baltimore: Williams & Wilkins, 1988; with permission.)

EVALUATION OF BONE MINERAL

Radiokinetic studies of calcium turnover using radioisotopes of calcium and strontium (Sr) are among the oldest studies in nuclear medicine and a classic embodiment of the tracer principle. The mathematical modeling for such analyses, which are combined with metabolic calcium balance studies, is complex. Imaging is not involved, and data are generated for the total body calcium pool, both skeletal and extraskeletal, with no regional differentiation possible. Studies with ^{85}Sr require measurements of tracer retention to be made over several months with a whole-body counter, an instrument that is not generally available in most clinical nuclear medicine departments. A somewhat simpler alternative is to measure the whole-body retention of the conventional bone scanning agent, ^{99m}Tc-MDP, which provides an index of bone turnover rate or, more precisely, of total skeletal osteoblastic activity. Unfortunately, since MDP is excreted by glomerular filtration, retention is markedly affected by variations in hydration and renal function; although a correction for renal status can be made by incorporating a simultaneous measurement of glomerular filtration rate such as (chromium 51)-EDTA clearance, it renders the test too complex for other than research purposes.

The suggestion that fractures are more common among elderly individuals because their bones are thinner was made by Sir Astley Cooper in 1824. Destructive testing of isolated cadaveric bones has shown that the ability of bone to resist fracture at any given level of mechanical stress correlates best with its mineral (predominantly calcium) content. This mechanical fact, coupled with

phy appears to be approximately 90 percent sensitive and almost 100 percent specific for neuroblastoma. Skeletal uptake of MIBG is a more sensitive marker of bone and bone-marrow involvement than conventional ^{99m}Tc-MDP bone scans (Fig. 17-38). The high specificity of MIBG uptake for neuroblastoma is occasionally useful to separate this tumor from other small, round cell malignancies of childhood.

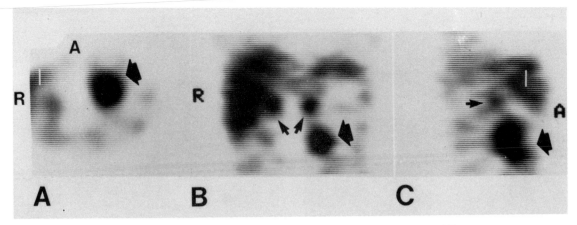

Figure 17-35 Extra-adrenal pheochromocytoma of left renal hilum (*large arrow*) demonstrated by ^{123}I-MIBG and emission computed tomography (ECT). *A*, Transverse; *B*, coronal; and *C*, sagittal reconstructions. The normal adrenal medullae are clearly seen (*small arrows*). (A = anterior; R = right; l = liver.) (From Khafagi FA, Shapiro B, Gross MD. The adrenal gland. In: Maisey MN, Britton KE, Gilday DL, eds. Clinical nuclear medicine. 2nd ed. London: Chapman & Hall, 1988; with permission.)

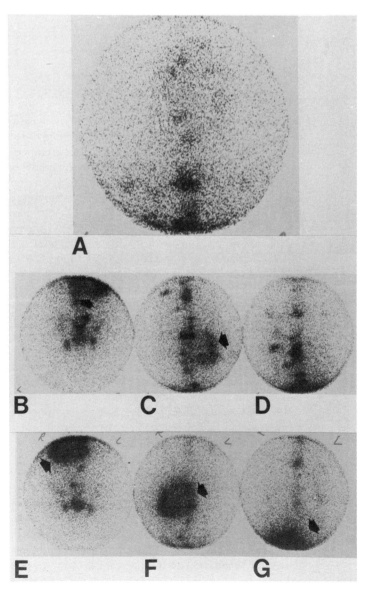

Figure 17-36 Malignant pheochromocytoma. Widespread skeletal metastases demonstrated with ^{131}I-MIBG. *A*, Anterior head and neck; *B*, posterior pelvis; *C*, posterior abdomen; *D*, posterior chest; *E*, anterior pelvis; *F*, anterior abdomen; *G*, anterior chest. Arrows (*C, E, F, G*) indicate the right adrenal primary; note the cool, necrotic center. (From Shapiro B, Sisson JC, Lloyd R, et al. Malignant phaeochromocytoma: clinical, biochemical and scintigraphic characterisation. Clin Endocrinol (Oxf) 1984; 20:189; with permission.)

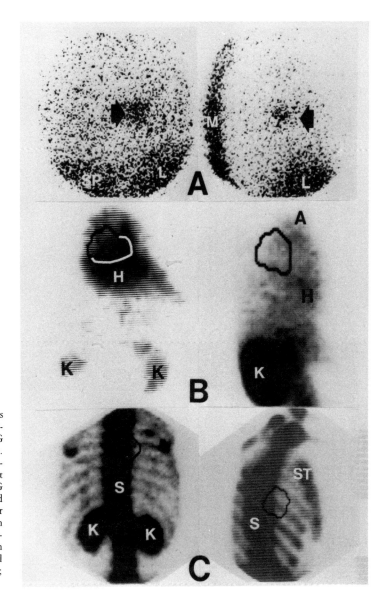

Figure 17-37 Left atrial pheochromocytoma. Previous thoracic CT scan and exploratory thoracotomy had been normal. *A,* Posterior (*left*) and right lateral (*right*) ^{131}I-MIBG scans of the chest, with an area of abnormal uptake (*arrow*). (M = marker on spine; L = liver; SP = spleen.) *B,* ^{99m}Tc-labeled red cell blood pool images (anterior [*left*] and right lateral [*right*] views), with region of abnormal ^{131}I-MIBG uptake superimposed. (A = aortic arch; H = cardiac blood pool; K = kidney.) *C,* ^{99m}Tc-MDP bone scan (posterior [*left*] and right posterior oblique [*right*] views) with region of abnormal ^{131}I-MIBG uptake superimposed. (K = kidney; S = spine; ST = sternum.) (From Shapiro B, Sisson JC, Kalff V, et al. The location of middle mediastinal pheochromocytomas. J Thorac Cardiovasc Surg 1984; 87:814; with permission.)

the rising awareness of the enormous socioeconomic burden imposed by the high prevalence of fractures in an increasingly aging population and the accumulating evidence that estrogen replacement is an effective means of preventing postmenopausal osteoporosis, has prompted the development of several noninvasive means of measuring bone mineral content.

TABLE 17-12   Neuroendocrine Tumors Reported to Take Up MIBG

Pheochromocytoma
Neuroblastoma
Nonfunctioning paraganglioma
Carcinoid tumor
Medullary thyroid carcinoma
Atypical schwannoma
Merkel cell tumor of skin
Pancreatic islet cell tumor

Earlier techniques, such as radiogrammetry and photodensitometry, attempted to correlate the cortical thickness of tubular bones on radiographs (usually of the hand), obtained under carefully standardized conditions, against the risk of sustaining a fracture of the wrist, spine, or femoral neck. Statistically significant correlations were obtained for large population groups, and a mass of useful epidemiologic data relating cortical thickness to demographic, dietary, medical, and other characteristics was generated. However, these methods are too insensitive for the clinical evaluation of individual patients.

Three techniques are currently employed for bone mineral measurement: single-photon absorptiometry (SPA), dual-photon absorptiometry (DPA), and quantitative x-ray computed tomography (QCT). Their accuracy, reproducibility (precision), and radiation dosimetry are compared in Table 17-13. SPA and DPA are discussed here in some further detail. These procedures use external, sealed sources of radioactivity and, unlike the other

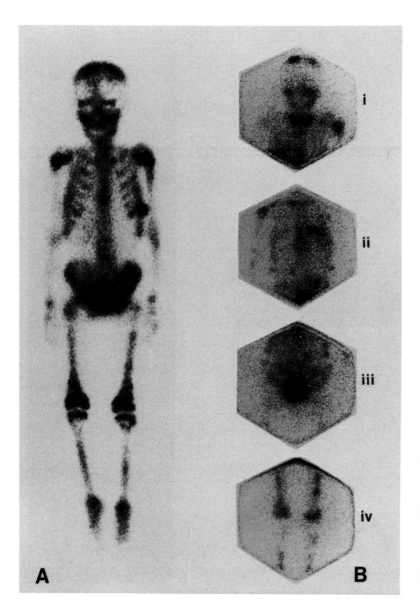

Figure 17–38 Metastatic neuroblastoma. *A*, ^{99m}Tc-MDP bone scan showing multiple skeletal metastases. *B*, ^{131}I-MIBG scan showing more extensive skeletal and bone marrow involvement than suggested by the bone scan (anterior views of: i, head and neck; ii, chest and abdomen; iii, pelvis and proximal femora; iv, lower extremities). (From Geatti O, Shapiro B, Sisson JC, et al. ^{131}I-metaiodobenzylguanidine (^{131}I-MIBG) scintigraphy for the localization of neuroblastoma: preliminary experience in 10 cases. J Nucl Med 1985; 26:736; with permission.)

TABLE 17–13   Comparison of Single-Photon Absorptiometry (SPA), Dual-Photon Absorptiometry (DPA), X-ray Absorptiometry (XRA), and Quantitative Computed Tomography (QCT) for Bone Mineral Measurement

Technique	Accuracy*	Reproducibility†	Radiation Dose mGy	(mrad)
Lumbar spine series	—	—	6.0	(600)
SPA (radius)	0.93–0.96	1.4–2.0%	0.05	(5)
(calcaneus)		0.8–0.9%	0.05	(5)
DPA	0.94–0.98	1.4–4.0%	0.15	(15)
XRA	—	0.4–1.0%	<0.03	(<3)
QCT	0.81–0.96	1–3%	0.9–20	(90–2000)

* Correlation (r) with mineral content of ashed bone
† % Coefficient of variation

nuclear medicine procedures described so far, do not involve radiotracer administration. A radiologic counterpart of DPA, dual-energy x-ray absorptiometry (XRA), has recently become commercially available.

Single-Photon Absorptiometry

An ^{125}I or americium 241 source is collimated to provide a narrow beam of monoenergetic photons ("single" photon; 27 keV for ^{125}I, 60 keV for ^{241}Am) of known initial intensity (Fig. 17–39). In passing through the bone to be measured, the beam is attenuated. The attenuated, transmitted beam is detected by an opposed NaI(Tl) scintillation detector; both source and detector traverse the limb synchronously in a rectilinear fashion, and an attenuation map of the bone and surrounding soft tissues is stored in a microcomputer. Newer systems incorporate automated repositioning algorithms based on the radioulnar distance at the measurement point in order to improve long-term reproducibility. Since the degree of attenuation of the beam is proportional to both the width and the mineral content of the bone (the attenuation coefficient of which is known for the photon energy used), bone mineral content can be calculated, corrected for bone width, and expressed in units of grams per square centimeter.

SPA has been applied to the radius and the calcaneum. Progressively distal radial sites contain progressively greater proportions of trabecular (cancellous) bone, and the calcaneum is made up predominantly of trabecular bone. In large groups of subjects, appendicular measurements of bone mineral content made at trabecular sites such as the calcaneum and the ultradistal 3 to 5 percent of the radius correlate better with vertebral bone miner-

al density than bone mineral content at predominantly cortical sites such as the mid-radius. However, the correlation coefficients are sufficiently low (0.6 to 0.8) and the confidence intervals sufficiently broad that, in individual cases, appendicular SPA measurements do not reliably predict bone mineral density in the spine or the femoral neck. Since SPA assumes that the soft tissue surrounding the bone to be measured has a regular geometry and uniform, water-equivalent composition, it cannot be used to measure spinal or femoral-neck bone mineral directly. Its major advantages are high reproducibility and relatively low cost.

Dual-Photon Absorptiometry

Like SPA systems, a DPA system consists of a modified rectilinear scanner opposed to a collimated radiation source and interfaced with a minicomputer. However, in this case, the radiation beam consists of two different energies. The usual source in commercial DPA systems is 37 GBq (1 Ci) of gadolinium 153, which has photopeaks at 44 keV and 100 keV ("dual" photons). Each photon is simultaneously attenuated to a different degree by the bone and soft-tissue combination through which the beam passes. The attenuation of the photons can therefore be described mathematically by two separate equations (one for each energy), which are then solved simultaneously for the bone term. Thus, no assumptions need be made about soft-tissue geometry or composition (water, fat, gas content), so that DPA can directly measure bone mineral in the spine and the femoral neck, sites of complex and nonuniform soft-tissue geometry and composition. The T_p of ^{153}Gd is 242 days, and the useful working life of the source is 13 to 15 months.

Figure 17–39 Schematic diagram of a single-photon absorptiometer. The dual-photon device is mechanically similar but differs in principle (see text). (From Riggs BL, Jowsey J, Kelly PS, Wahner HW. Special procedures for assessing metabolic bone disease. Med Clin North Am 1970; 54:1061; with permission.)

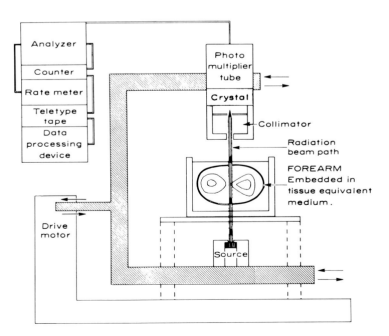

XRA systems exploit the same theoretic principle as DPA and are mechanically similar, except that the photon source is an x-ray tube capable of delivering a highly collimated beam at two well-defined effective energies—43 and 110 keV in one system and 40 and 70 keV in the other. The major advantage of XRA over DPA is that a much higher photon flux is achievable, permitting faster scan speeds, statistically better transmission data, higher image resolution, and consequently more reproducible region of interest selection, at a lower radiation dose to the patient. In addition, the XRA devices are readily adaptable for measuring bone mineral content at appendicular sites. Finally, the need for costly replacement of spent radionuclide sources is eliminated. Although clinical experience with these new instruments is limited at present, correlation with DPA measurements has been excellent.

Scans of the lumbar spine (L1–L4) are obtained with the patient supine with hips slightly flexed to flatten the lumbar lordosis and increase the intervertebral separation. Scans of the hip are obtained on the same instrument with the patient's femur held in slight internal rotation. The computer defines the lateral margins of the vertebral bodies (excluding the transverse processes), the greater trochanter, the femoral neck, and Ward's triangle; the computer-defined regions can be manually modified or overridden if necessary. Output is expressed as "areal bone mineral density" in units of grams per square centimeter, which represents an integral of both trabecular and cortical bone in the beam path. It is essential that the computer-generated pictograms of the spine and hip (Fig. 17–40) be inspected for abnormalities such as scoliosis, vertebral compression fracture, large osteophytes, evidence of Paget's disease, or overlying vascular or other soft-tissue calcification that will affect mineral density. If such an abnormality is suspected, a plain radiograph should be obtained, and if this is confirmatory, an attempt should be made to redefine the regions for measurement of bone mineral density. A "hard copy" of the patient's previous studies should be available to ensure consistent region definition.

Whereas DPA, XRA, and QCT can all be used to measure vertebral bone mineral, current QCT technology does not lend itself readily to measurement at the femoral neck. Since QCT isolates samples of purely trabecular bone at the centers of L1–L4, this technique is capable in principle of detecting changes in axial bone mineral earlier than DPA, but the slightly greater sensitivity of QCT over DPA is offset by its lower accuracy and reproducibility (see Table 17–13). In practice, there is little to choose between these two methods for the spine, although the substantially higher radiation dose delivered by QCT must be considered when serial measurements are contemplated.

Clinical Applications

In any consideration of the clinical application of bone mineral measurement to individual patients, a clear distinction must be made between *screening* of asymptomatic individuals who may be at risk for osteoporosis and *monitoring* of patients with established metabolic bone diseases (including osteoporosis) to document disease progression and the effects of therapy. The first type of application is highly controversial and is discussed here at some length.

Trabecular bone, which predominates in the axial skeleton, has a much larger metabolically active surface area than cortical bone, which predominates in the appendicular skeleton. Age-related loss of bone mass is first evident in the spine from the ages of 30 to 35 years in both men and women, and it progresses at a faster rate in the spine than in the distal radius or the proximal femur. It was therefore hoped that screening of asymptomatic individuals would permit the early identification of those at risk of developing osteoporotic fractures so that appropriate treatment could be started to retard or arrest bone loss and, ultimately, prevent fractures. To be

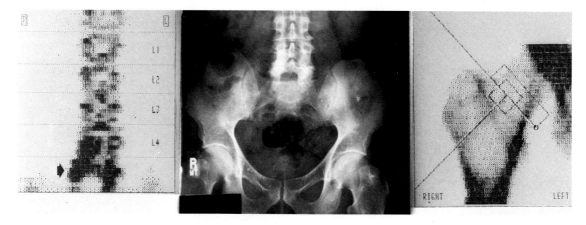

Figure 17–40 Typical DPA output from the lumbar spine (*left*) and the hip (*right*). The area of increased bone mineral density in the pictogram of the lumbar spine (*left panel, arrow*) is due to facet-joint osteoarthritis, as shown on the radiograph (*center panel*).

successful, such a program must fulfill several requirements.

First, adequate normal ranges that take account of race, sex, age (or, in women, menopausal age) and local conditions must be established. Although data have been published for normal U.S., Scandinavian, and Australian populations, they are not internationally or interracially transferable. Indeed, in the absence of industry-wide standards for instrument and software quality control, normal ranges established on one brand of instrument are not transferable to other brands.

Second, the precision of measurement must be such that clinically relevant changes can be detected with confidence. Women have less bone mass on average than men at all ages; after the attainment of peak bone mass, age-related bone loss proceeds at about 1 percent per year in both sexes, with a relatively abrupt acceleration in women to about 3 percent per year during the 10 to 15 years following menopause, after which the rates for men and women resume their roughly parallel courses. Monitoring by DPA with a reproducibility of 2 percent would require a change in bone mineral density of at least 5.6 percent between two consecutive measurements in order to be detectable with 95 percent confidence. Clearly, even during the rapid postmenopausal phase of bone loss, the significance of smaller differences found over intervals of less than 1 to 2 years would be difficult to interpret.

Third, a threshold value of bone mineral density, below which fracture risk rises significantly, needs to be defined. Retrospective analyses of regional mineral values in patients who have already sustained fractures of the spine or femoral neck indicate that the 90th centile of bone mineral density (by DPA) for both the spine and the femoral neck in these groups is 1.0 g per square centimeter; the equivalent value for the spine by QCT is 110 mg per cubic centimeter. Although these values are widely cited as fracture thresholds, their derivation, from individuals who have already declared themselves to have significant disease by virtue of having actually sustained a fracture, is fundamentally flawed. Studies aimed at establishing fracture thresholds prospectively are under way, but their results are unlikely to be available for several years. Even if the retrospectively derived fracture thresholds were to be accepted for the time being, it must be re-emphasized that, in the individual case, whether the threshold has been reached at one site cannot be predicted reliably from a measurement made at another site. For example, patients with femoral neck fractures have significantly lower femoral neck BMD values than age- and sex-matched controls, but their vertebral BMD is not significantly different from that of controls.

Finally, screening for any disease is pointless unless effective therapy is available. In the case of postmenopausal osteoporosis, it is now abundantly clear that estrogen administered from the time of menopause reduces or abolishes the accelerated phase of bone loss and reduces the incidence of vertebral compression fractures (although such fractures are associated with relatively low morbidity). Calcium supplements are of no proven benefit in the absence of estrogen replacement. Postmenopausal estrogen therapy probably has additional beneficial effects, including reduction of mortality from cardiovascular causes. The development of reliable transcutaneous estrogen delivery systems, which short-circuit the first-pass hepatic metabolism inherent in oral therapy, is likely to reduce the incidence of troublesome estrogen side effects. Nevertheless, except for patients who have had total hysterectomies, estrogen must be given cyclically with progestogens to minimize the risk of endometrial cancer; not only might many women be reluctant to prolong the inconvenience of menses, but also the addition of progestogens may attenuate the cardiovascular benefit of estrogen. The optimal duration of estrogen replacement has not been established. Although accelerated bone loss will occur upon estrogen withdrawal, it is not certain that the beneficial effects of estrogen on bone mass will be sustained if therapy is continued indefinitely. Neither estrogen nor any other therapy is of clearly proven value once the phase of accelerated postmenopausal bone loss is complete, although the use of calcitonin has recently been approved for this indication. Whether estrogen after natural (as opposed to surgical) menopause has a significant impact on the incidence of femoral neck fractures remains to be proved; although these devastating fractures account for most of the morbidity and mortality associated with osteoporosis, bone density is only one of many complex factors in their pathogenesis.

It should be clear from the foregoing discussion that current technology for measuring bone mineral content falls short of the requirements of an effective mass screening test for osteoporosis, particularly when considered against the cost of the procedures (typically, $150 to $300 for DPA and QCT) and the lingering uncertainties about the ultimate effectiveness of therapy. Indeed, in a recent position paper, the American College of Physicians argued forcefully against any screening application of these tests. We favor a less conservative approach. If a perimenopausal woman is prepared to undertake estrogen replacement therapy, she should be encouraged to do so. If she is unsure, measurement of vertebral mineral by DPA or QCT will place our advice and her decision on a more rational, objective footing. A clearly normal value, for example, would allow her to defer treatment for 2 or more years. Such a patient should be re-evaluated periodically, but no more frequently than every 2 years. Although we are mindful of the imperfect state of our present knowledge, a strong recommendation for therapy should be made when vertebral BMD values approach or fall below 1.0 g per square centimeter (by DPA) or 110 mg per cubic centimeter (by QCT). Once therapy has been instituted in such a case, the patient's response should be monitored either by DPA or more cheaply ($50 to $150 per examination) and with somewhat greater precision by appendicular SPA, since all skeletal sites appear to respond equally to estrogen replacement. XRA may eventually prove to be superior to either DPA or SPA in flexibility, reproducibility, radiation dose, and cost, but further clinical experience with the technique is necessary.

Monitoring of patients with established metabolic bone disease is a much less controversial topic. The ability to evaluate objectively the efficacy of any therapeutic intervention is both reasonable and desirable, particularly if the treatment is experimental, inconvenient (e.g., calcitonin injections), or potentially toxic (e.g., fluoride, 1,25[OH]$_2$-vitamin D). In such a setting, the patient acts as his or her own control, and normal population data are not essential to management. The magnitude of changes in bone mineral values is likely to be greater than "normal" age-related changes and therefore well within the detection capabilities of current techniques.

MISCELLANEOUS APPLICATIONS

The use of conventionally labeled radiopharmaceuticals for the detection of pituitary and pancreatic tumors is of historical interest only, since the superior anatomic resolution of x-ray CT and MRI clearly makes them the current imaging modalities of choice for these applications. CT and MRI have also superseded the use of ^{67}Ga citrate or (indium 111)–bleomycin for the staging of seminomas.

Immunoscintigraphy of malignant ovarian, prostatic, testicular, and thyroid tumors has been investigated using a variety of relatively tumor-specific monoclonal antibodies (MAb) and their Fab or F(ab)$_2$' fragments labeled with ^{131}I, ^{111}In, or ^{99m}Tc. Problems with the specificity and immunogenicity of MAb preparations, nonspecific hepatic and reticuloendothelial uptake of MAb, and persistent circulating MAb activity in the blood pool are slowly being resolved. Despite occasional reports of the detection by MAb of tumor deposits missed by other means, immunoscintigraphy has some way to go before it can be considered routine or clinically superior to more conventional staging methods.

The search continues for adrenocortical tracers that can be labeled with ^{123}I or ^{99m}Tc in order to improve dosimetry and imaging characteristics. Such agents would need to achieve adequate target-to-background ratios of activity within 12 to 24 hours of injection. Radioiodinated 11β-hydroxylase inhibitors and pregnenolone esters have been promising in animal studies but have not been used clinically.

To manage patients with endocrine disorders, particularly diabetic patients, the endocrinologist must often call upon the full diagnostic armamentarium of general internal medicine. Diagnostic applications of nuclear medicine other than endocrine imaging that are frequently applicable to endocrinology are summarized in Table 17–14.

Just as endocrinology has reached beyond the classical ductless glands to claim every organ system—most recently the heart—as its own, so clinical nuclear medicine has extended far beyond the evaluation of thyroid disease to have a significant impact on the practice of every medical and surgical subspecialty. However, the functional study of the thyroid using radioiodine remains the clinical paradigm to which all subsequent nuclear medicine techniques have aspired. In a sense, the wheel has come full circle with the ability to label trace quantities

TABLE 17–14 Nonendocrine Applications of Nuclear Medicine Relevant to Endocrinology

System	Radiopharmaceutical	Application
Cardiovascular	^{99m}Tc-labeled red blood cells	Radionuclide ventriculography: evaluation of cardiac function and regional wall motion at rest and with exercise
	^{201}TlCl	Evaluation of myocardial perfusion and viability at rest and with exercise
	^{133}Xe; ^{201}TlCl	Evaluation of skin perfusion: prediction of ulcer and amputation site healing
Cerebrovascular	^{123}I-iodoamphetamine; ^{99m}Tc-HMPAO	Evaluation of cerebral perfusion
Genitourinary	^{99m}Tc-DTPA; ^{131}I or ^{123}I Hippuran	Evaluation of native and transplant renal perfusion, differential function, and outflow tract patency
	^{99m}TcO$_4$$^-$	Differential diagnosis of the "acute scrotum": e.g., testicular torsion vs. epididymo-orchitis
Gastrointestinal	^{99m}Tc-labeled meal	Evaluation of esophageal motility, gastro-esophageal reflux, and gastric emptying
Skeletal	^{99m}Tc-MDP	Diagnosis of osteomyelitis complicating peripheral ulcers or cellulitis
Infectious disease	^{111}In-labeled leukocytes; ^{67}Ga citrate	Localization of infection

HMPAO = Hexamethylpropyleneamine oxime

of endogenous compounds and therapeutic drugs with the short-lived, positron-emitting radioisotopes of carbon, nitrogen, and oxygen (^{11}C, ^{13}N, ^{15}O)—the biologic building blocks—for true in vivo autoradiography using PET.

BIBLIOGRAPHY

Introduction and Basic Principles

Beierwaltes WH. The history of the use of radioactive iodine. Semin Nucl Med 1979; 9:151.

Blahd WH. History of external counting procedures. Semin Nucl Med 1979; 9:159.

Erikson JJ, Rollo FD, eds. Digital nuclear medicine. Philadelphia: JB Lippincott, 1983.

Gelfand MJ, Thomas SR, eds. Effective use of computers in nuclear medicine: practical clinical applications in the imaging laboratory. New York: McGraw-Hill, 1978.

Gross MD, Shapiro B, Thrall JH, et al. The scintigraphic imaging of endocrine organs. Endocr Rev 1984; 5:221.

Harbert JC. Nuclear medicine therapy. New York: Thieme, 1987.

McAfee JG, Subramanian G. Radioactive agents for imaging. In: Freeman LM, ed. Freeman and Johnson's clinical radionuclide imaging. 3rd ed, Vol 1. Orlando, FL: Grune & Stratton, 1984:55.

Patton JA, Rollo FD. Basic physics of radionuclide imaging. In: Freeman LM, ed. Freeman and Johnson's clinical radionuclide imaging. 3rd ed, Vol 1. Orlando, FL: Grune & Stratton, 1984:13.

The Thyroid

Radiopharmaceuticals and Technique

Keyes JW, Thrall JH, Carey JE. Technical considerations in in vivo thyroid studies. Semin Nucl Med 1978; 8:43.

Lee WP, Siegel JA, Harpen MD, et al. In vivo evaluation of intrathyroidal iodide metabolism. J Clin Endocrinol Metab 1982; 55:1131.

Pinsky S, Ryo UY. Thyroid imaging: a current status report. In: Freeman LM, Weissmann HS, eds. Nuclear medicine annual 1981. New York: Raven Press, 1981:157.

Ryo UY, Vaidya PV, Schneider AB, et al. Thyroid imaging agents: a comparison of ^{123}I and ^{99m}Tc pertechnetate. Radiology 1983; 148:819.

Tonami N, Bunko H, Michigishi T, et al. Clinical application of ^{201}Tl scintigraphy in patients with cold thyroid nodules. Clin Nucl Med 1978; 3:217.

Clinical Applications

Nodular Thyroid Disease

Ashcraft MW, Van Herle AJ. Management of thyroid nodules. I. History and physical examination, blood tests, x-ray tests, and ultrasonography. Head Neck Surg 1981; 3:216.

Ashcraft MW, Van Herle AJ. Management of thyroid nodules. II. Scanning techniques, thyroid suppressive therapy, and fine needle aspiration. Head Neck Surg 1981; 3:297.

Gharib H, James EM, Charboneau JW, et al. Suppressive therapy with levothyroxine for solitary thyroid nodules. A double-blind controlled clinical study. N Engl J Med 1987; 317:70.

Hamberger B, Gharib H, Melton LS, et al. Fine-needle aspiration biopsy of thyroid nodules: impact on thyroid practice and cost of care. Am J Med 1982; 73:381.

Miller JM, Kini SR, Hamburger JI. Needle biopsy of the thyroid. New York: Praeger, 1983.

Molitch ME, Beck JR, Dreisman M, et al. The cold thyroid nodule: an analysis of diagnostic and therapeutic options. Endocr Rev 1984; 5:185.

Nagai GR, Pitts WE, Basso L, et al. Scintigraphic hot nodules and thyroid carcinoma. Clin Nucl Med 1987; 12:123.

Ramaciotti CE, Pretorius HT, Chu EW, et al. Diagnostic accuracy and use of aspiration biopsy in the management of thyroid nodules. Arch Intern Med 1984; 144:1169.

Reeve TS, Delbridge L, Sloane D, Crummer P. The impact of fine-needle aspiration biopsy on surgery for single thyroid nodules. Med J Aust 1986; 145:308.

Rojeski MT, Gharib H. Nodular thyroid disease. Evaluation and management. N Engl J Med 1985; 313:428.

Samaan NA, Schultz PN, Ordonez NG, et al. A comparison of thyroid carcinoma in those who have and have not had head and neck irradiation in childhood. J Clin Endocrinol Metab 1987; 64:219.

Vander JB, Gaston EA, Dawber TR. The significance of nontoxic thyroid nodules: final report of a 15 year study of the incidence of thyroid malignancy. Ann Intern Med 1968; 69:537.

Van Herle AJ. UCLA conference: the thyroid nodule. Ann Intern Med 1982; 96:221.

Vorne M, Jarvi K. ^{99m}Tc-pertechnetate in the detection of thyroid carcinoma in a ten year period. Eur J Nucl Med 1987; 13:362.

Follow-Up of Thyroid Cancer

Ashcraft MW, Van Herle AJ. The comparative value of serum thyroglobulin measurements and iodine 131 total body scans in the follow-up study of patients with treated differentiated thyroid cancer. Am J Med 1981; 71:806.

Beierwaltes WH, Rabbani R, Dmuchowski C, et al. An analysis of "ablation of thyroid remnants" with I-131 in 511 patients from 1947–1984: experience at the University of Michigan. J Nucl Med 1984; 25:1287.

Black EG, Sheppard MC, Hoffenberg R. Serial serum thyroglobulin measurements in the management of differentiated thyroid carcinoma. Clin Endocrinol (Oxf) 1987; 27:115.

Freitas JE, Gross MD, Ripley S, Shapiro B. Radionuclide diagnosis and therapy of thyroid cancer: current status report. Semin Nucl Med 1985; 15:106.

Galligan JP, Winship J, Van Doorn T, Mortimer RH. A comparison of serum thyroglobulin measurements and whole body ^{131}I scanning in the management of treated differentiated thyroid carcinoma. Aust N Z J Med 1982; 12:248.

Hurley JR, Becker DV. The use of radioiodine in the management of thyroid cancer. In: Freeman LM, Weissmann HS, eds. Nuclear medicine annual 1983. New York: Raven Press, 1983:329.

Medullary Thyroid Carcinoma

Clarke SEM, Lazarus CR, Edwards S, et al. Scintigraphy and treatment of medullary carcinoma of the thyroid with iodine-131 metaiodobenzylguanidine. J Nucl Med 1987; 28:1820.

Clarke SEM, Lazarus CR, Wraight P, et al. Pentavalent [^{99m}Tc]DMSA, [^{131}I]MIBG, and [^{99m}Tc]MDP—an evaluation of three imaging techniques in patients with medullary carcinoma of the thyroid. J Nucl Med 1988; 29:33.

Hyperthyroidism and Miscellaneous Applications

Fogelman I, Cooke SG, Maisey MN. The role of thyroid scanning in hyperthyroidism. Eur J Nucl Med 1986; 11:397.

Lecklitner ML. Neonatal and pediatric thyroid imaging. In: Sandler MP, Patton JA, Partain CL, eds. Thyroid and parathyroid imaging. Norwalk, CT: Appleton-Century-Crofts, 1986:149.

Ripley SD, Freitas JE, Nagle CE. Is thyroid scintigraphy necessary before I-131 therapy for hyperthyroidism? Concise communication. J Nucl Med 1984; 25:664.

Sostre S, Parikh S. A visual index of thyroid function. Clin Nucl Med 1979; 4:59.

The Parathyroids

Clark OH, Okerlund MD, Moss AA, et al. Localization studies in patients with persistent or recurrent hyperparathyroidism. Surgery 1985; 98:1083.

Ferlin G, Borsato N, Camerani M, et al. New perspectives in localizing enlarged parathyroids by technetium-thallium subtraction scan. J Nucl Med 1983; 24:438.

Fine EJ. Parathyroid imaging: its current status and future role. Semin Nucl Med 1987; 27:350.

Miller DL, Doppman JL, Shawker TH, et al. Localization of parathyroid adenomas in patients who have undergone surgery. I. Noninvasive imaging techniques. Radiology 1987; 162:133.

Miller DL, Doppman JL, Krudy AG, et al. Localization of parathyroid adenomas in patients who have undergone surgery. II. Invasive procedures. Radiology 1987; 162:138.

Okerlund MD, Sheldon K, Corpuz S, et al. A new method with high sensitivity and specificity for localization of abnormal parathyroid glands. Ann Surg 1984; 200:381.

Winzelberg GG. Parathyroid imaging. Ann Intern Med 1987; 107:64.

Young AE, Gaunt JI, Croft DN, et al. Localisation of parathyroid adenomas by thallium-201 and technetium-99m subtraction scanning. Br Med J 1983; 286:1384.

Zwas ST, Czerniak A, Boruchowsky S, et al. Preoperative parathyroid localization by superimposed iodine-131 toluidine blue and technetium-99m pertechnetate imaging. J Nucl Med 1987; 28:298.

The Adrenal Cortex

Radiopharmaceuticals and Technique

Beierwaltes WH, Wieland DM, Yu T, et al. Adrenal imaging agents: rationale, synthesis, formulation and metabolism. Semin Nucl Med 1978; 8:5.

Gross MD, Freitas JE, Swanson DP, et al. The normal dexamethasone-suppression adrenal scan. J Nucl Med 1979;20:1131.

Gross MD, Valk TW, Swanson DP, et al. The role of pharmacologic manipulation in adrenal cortical scintigraphy. Semin Nucl Med 1981; 9:128.

Hawkins LA, Britton KE, Shapiro B. [75]Se selenomethyl cholesterol; a new agent for quantitative functional scintigraphy of the adrenals: physical aspects. Br J Radiol 1980; 53:883.

Koral KF, Sarkar SD. An operator-independent method for background subtraction in adrenal uptake measurements. Concise communication. J Nucl Med 1977; 18:925.

Lynn MD, Gross MD, Shapiro B, Bassett D. The influence of hypercholesterolaemia on the adrenal uptake and metabolism of [131]I-6 beta-iodomethyl-19-norcholesterol (NP-59). Nucl Med Commun 1986; 7:631.

Shapiro B, Nakajo M, Gross MD, et al. Value of bowel preparation in adrenocortical scintigraphy with NP-59. J Nucl Med 1983; 24:732.

Clinical Applications

Copeland PM. The incidentally discovered adrenal mass. Ann Intern Med 1983; 98:940.

Fig LM, Gross MD, Shapiro B, et al. Adrenal localization in ACTH-independent Cushing's syndrome. Ann Intern Med 1988; 109:547.

Fischer M, Vetter W, Winterberg B, et al. Adrenal scintigraphy in primary aldosteronism. Spironolactone as a cause of incorrect classification between adenoma and hyperplasia. Eur J Nucl Med 1982; 7:222.

Glazer HS, Weyman PJ, Sagel SS, et al. Nonfunctioning adrenal masses: incidental discovery on computed tomography. AJR 1983; 139:81.

Gross MD, Shapiro B, Bouffard JA, et al. Distinguishing benign from malignant euadrenal masses. Ann Intern Med 1988; 109:613.

Gross MD, Shapiro B, Freitas JE, et al. The relationship of I-131 6 beta-iodomethyl-19-norcholestrol (NP-59) adrenal cortical uptake to indices of androgen secretion in women with hyperandrogenism. Clin Nucl Med 1984; 9:264.

Gross MD, Shapiro B, Grekin R, et al. Scintigraphic localization of adrenal lesions in primary aldosteronism. Am J Med 1984; 77:839.

Gross MD, Shapiro B, Grekin RJ, et al. The relationship of adrenal gland iodomethylnorcholesterol uptake to zona glomerulosa function in primary aldosteronism. J Clin Endocrinol Metab 1983; 57:477.

Gross MD, Valk TW, Freitas JE, et al. The relationship of adrenal iodomethylnorcholesterol uptake to indices of adrenal cortical function in Cushing's syndrome. J Clin Endocrinol Metab 1981; 52:1062.

Gross MD, Wilton GP, Shapiro B, et al. Functional and scintigraphic evaluation of the silent adrenal mass. J Nucl Med 1987; 28:1401.

Gross MD, Wortsman J, Shapiro B, et al. Scintigraphic evidence of adrenal cortical dysfunction in the polycystic ovary syndrome. J Clin Endocrinol Metab 1986; 62:197.

Shapiro B, Britton KE, Hawkins LA, Edwards CRW. Clinical experience with ^{75}Se selenomethylcholesterol adrenal imaging. Clin Endocrinol (Oxf) 1981; 15:19.

Taylor L, Ayers JW, Gross MD, et al. Diagnostic considerations in virilization: iodomethyl-norcholesterol scanning in the localization of androgen secreting tumors. Fertil Steril 1986; 49:1005.

The Adrenal Medulla and Neuroendocrine Tumors

Radiopharmaceuticals and Technique

Khafagi FA, Shapiro B, Mallette S, Sisson JC. Reduction of (I-131)-metaiodobenzylguanidine uptake by labetalol. J Nucl Med (in press).

Lynn MD, Shapiro B, Sisson JC, et al. Pheochromocytomas and the normal adrenal medulla: improved visualization with I-123 MIBG scintigraphy. Radiology 1985; 155:789.

Mangner TJ, Tobes MC, Wieland DM, et al. Metabolism of iodine-131 metaiodobenzylguanidine in patients with metastatic pheochromocytoma. J Nucl Med 1986; 27:37.

Nakajo M, Shapiro B, Copp J, et al. The normal and abnormal distribution of the adrenomedullary imaging agent m[I-131]iodobenzylguanidine (131-I-MIBG) in man. Evaluation by scintigraphy. J Nucl Med 1983; 24:672.

Sisson JC, Frager MS, Valk TW, et al. Scintigraphic localization of pheochromocytoma. N Engl J Med 1981; 305:12.

Tobes MC, Jaques S, Wieland DM, Sisson JC. Effect of uptake-one inhibitors on the uptake of norepinephrine and metaiodobenzylguanidine. J Nucl Med 1985; 26:897.

Clinical Applications

Pheochromocytoma

Ackery DM, Tippett PA, Condon BR, et al. New approach to the localization of phaeochromocytoma: imaging with iodine-131-meta-iodobenzyl guanidine. Br Med J 1984; 288:1587.

Chatal JF, Charbonnel B. Comparison of iodobenzylguanidine imaging with computed tomography in locating pheochromocytoma. J Clin Endocrinol Metab 1985; 61:769.

McEwan AJ, Shapiro B, Sisson JC, et al. Radioiodobenzylguanidine for the scintigraphic location and therapy of adrenergic tumors. Semin Nucl Med 1985; 15:132.

Shapiro B, Copp JE, Sisson JC, et al. Iodine-131 metaiodobenzylguanidine for the locating of suspected pheochromocytoma: experience in 400 cases. J Nucl Med 1985; 26:576.

Shapiro B, Sisson JC, Lloyd R, et al. Malignant phaeochromocytoma: clinical, biochemical and scintigraphic characterization. Clin Endocrinol (Oxf) 1984; 20:189.

Swensen SJ, Brown ML, Sheps SG, et al. Use of I-131 MIBG scintigraphy in the evaluation of suspected pheochromocytoma. Mayo Clin Proc 1985; 60:299.

Valk TW, Frager MS, Gross MD, et al. Spectrum of pheochromocytoma in multiple endocrine neoplasia. A scintigraphic portrayal using 131I-metaiodobenzylguanidine. Ann Intern Med 1981; 94:762.

Neuroblastoma and Other Neuroendocrine Tumors

Geatti O, Shapiro B, Sisson JC, et al. ^{131}I-metaiodobenzylguanidine (^{131}I-MIBG) scintigraphy for the localization of neuroblastoma: preliminary experience in 10 cases. J Nucl Med 1985; 26:736.

Hoefnagel CA, Voute PA, De Kraker J, Marcuse HR. Radionuclide diagnosis and therapy of neural crest tumors using iodine-131-metaiodobenzylguanidine. J Nucl Med 1987; 28:308.

Kimmig B, Brandeis WE, Eisenhut M. Scintigraphy of neuroblastoma with ^{131}I-MIBG. J Nucl Med 1984; 25:773.

Munkner T. ^{131}I-metaiodobenzylguanidine scintigraphy of neuroblastoma. Semin Nucl Med 1985; 15:154.

Shulkin BL, Shen SW, Sisson JC, et al. Iodine-131 MIBG scintigraphy of the extremities in metastatic pheochromocytoma and neuroblastoma. J Nucl Med 1987; 28:315.

Von Moll L, McEwan AJ, Shapiro B, et al. Iodine-131 MIBG scintigraphy of neuroendocrine tumors other than pheochromocytoma and neuroblastoma. J Nucl Med 1987; 28:979.

Evaluation of Bone Mineral

Cummings SR, Black D. Should perimenopausal women be screened for osteoporosis? Ann Intern Med 1986; 104:817.

Fogelman I, Bessent RG. Age-related alterations in skeletal metabolism—24 hour whole-body retention of diphosphonate in 250 normal subjects. Concise communication. J Nucl Med 1982; 23:296.

Genant HK, ed. Osteoporosis update 1987. San Francisco: Radiology Research and Education Foundation, 1987.

Goodwin PN. Methodologies for the measurement of bone density and their precision and accuracy. Semin Nucl Med 1987; 27:293.

Gross MD, Shapiro B. New aspects of osteoporosis: bone mineral content (BMC) measurement in osteoporosis associated with drugs, arthritis and related conditions. Nucl Compact 1987; 18:17.

Health and Public Policy Committee, American College of Physicians. Position paper: bone mineral densitometry. Ann Intern Med 1987; 107:932.

Melton LJ, Wahner HW, Richelson LS, et al. Osteoporosis and the risk of hip fracture. Am J Epidemiol 1986; 124:254.

Riggs BL, Melton LJ. Involutional osteoporosis. N Engl J Med 1986; 314:1676.

Riggs BL, Wahner HW. Bone densitometry and clinical decision-making in osteoporosis. Ann Intern Med 1988; 108:293.

Sartoris DJ, Resnick D. Digital radiography may spark renewal of bone densitometry. Diagn Imaging 1988; 16:145.

Seldin DW, Esser PD, Alderson PO. Comparison of bone density measurements from different skeletal sites. J Nucl Med 1988; 29:168.

Shapiro B, Gross MD, Fig LM. Bone mineral content measurement in metabolic bone disease. Nucl Compact 1987; 18:11.

Slemenda CW, Johnston CC. Bone mass measurement: which site to measure? Am J Med 1988; 84:643.

Wahner HW. Single- and dual-photon absorptiometry in osteoporosis and osteomalacia. Semin Nucl Med 1987; 27:305.

Wahner HE, Dunn WL, Mazess RB, et al. Dual-photon Gd-153 absorptiometry of bone. Radiology 1985; 156:203.

Wahner HW, Dunn WL, Riggs BL. Assessment of bone mineral. Parts 1 and 2. J Nucl Med 1984; 25:1134; 1241.

18 Pituitary Imaging

Samuel M. Wolpert, M.B., B.Ch.

The advent of computed tomography (CT) in the 1970s, resulting in the diagnosis of suprasellar growth of pituitary adenomas without the need for pneumoencephalography, can be said to have ushered in the modern era of the radiologic management of these tumors (Gyldensted and Karle, 1977; Hatam et al, 1979; Naidich et al, 1976; Wolpert, 1980). Intrasellar tumors, however, were seldom detected by the first- or second-generation scanners, and pluridirectional tomography was still necessary.

Improvement in CT scan technology led to enhanced spatial resolution with demonstration of both the pituitary gland and microadenomas within the gland (Syvertsen et al, 1979). Furthermore, small sellar floor erosions and sella enlargement could be seen on the CT scans, and the significance of these sella changes, i.e., whether they were contiguous with the microadenomas or not, could now be determined. Pluridirectional tomography was largely abandoned.

Although high-detail CT scanning has proved an excellent radiologic test for the detection of macroadenomas, unfortunately experience has taught us that it is not the hoped-for panacea for the detection of microadenomas. Many of the CT features of microadenomas initially considered to be diagnostic have also been found with other pituitary lesions such as developmental and necrotic cysts as well as necrotic tumors. The next major imaging advance in the diagnosis of pituitary adenomas occurred in the 1980s with the development of magnetic resonance imaging (MRI). The high detail available with this new technology and the avoidance of x-rays have led to rapid acceptance of the new modality. However, experience with MRI indicates that it probably has many of the same drawbacks as CT. The last word in the radiologic diagnosis of pituitary microadenomas has clearly not been written, and further research on this diagnostic dilemma is still necessary.

HIGH-DETAIL DIRECT CORONAL COMPUTED TOMOGRAPHY

To appreciate fully the relationships between the sphenoid sinus, sella turcica, pituitary gland, and suprasellar cistern by CT, sagittal and coronal views are necessary. Sagittal views can be obtained by reformatting either multiple axial images or multiple coronal images. Unfortunately, some sacrifice of soft-tissue detail and of spatial resolution occurs with reformatted images. Coronal images are best obtained by scanning the patient supine or prone with the neck extended. The supine position appears easier for most patients to tolerate, and if this position is used with a scanner with a gantry that can tilt to approximately 20 degrees, scans almost perpendicular to the canthomeatal line can be obtained (Fig. 18–1). With maximal gantry tilt and a flexible neck, artifacts from teeth fillings are seldom a problem. A scan obtained midway between the outer canthus of the eye

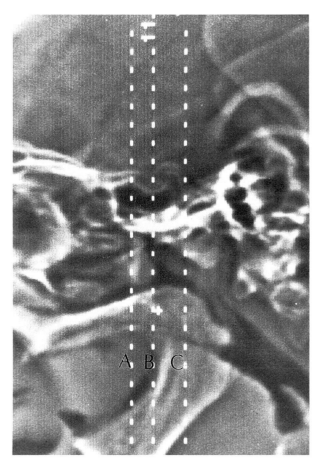

Figure 18–1 Lateral scanogram of the skull demonstrates scan planes at approximately right angles to the Reid base line. Plane A is through the anterior clinoid process; plane B is through the sella turcica; plane C is slightly posterior to the dorsum sellae. (From Wolpert SM: The radiology of pituitary adenomas. Semin Roentgenol 1984; 29:53; with permission.)

and the external auditory canal usually passes through the sella turcica.

Scans are done from the level of the anterior clinoid processes at 2-mm intervals posteriorly until the apex of the basilar artery is seen (the hypothalamus lies above the basilar artery and should be examined in all patients with suspected pathology of the pituitary gland). If the patient cannot maintain neck hyperextension, axial scans with reformatted images are performed. Scans are started during and concluded after the intravenous administration of a drip infusion of 300 ml of Reno-M-30. Nonenhanced scans are not routinely obtained but may be necessary later if there is difficulty in determining whether a high-density lesion contains calcium or is hypervascular.

DIRECT CORONAL SCANNING OF THE PITUITARY GLAND AND ADJACENT STRUCTURES

Vascular Structures

After the intravenous administration of an iodinated contrast agent, the internal carotid arteries, proximal anterior cerebral arteries, basilar artery, pituitary gland, infundibulum, and cavernous sinuses are seen (Fig. 18–2). Some authors advise a bolus injection with immediate imaging of the gland (dynamic scanning) to maximize visualization of the pituitary gland, which is enhanced in parallel with the level of iodine in the serum (Taylor, 1982).

Gland Density

The pituitary gland usually is enhanced as densely as the cavernous sinuses, and distinction between the two structures is difficult. Usually, the gland is moderately homogenous in density, but artifacts on the images due to noise can easily be mistaken for cystic change. Comparison of the gland density with that of the adjacent brain should aid in this distinction, since the brain and gland appearances are usually equally noisy. Image noise is inversely proportional to scan thickness, and since high-detail imaging necessitates thin sections, noise often is a problem in determining pituitary gland density. Some researchers have suggested that it may be possible to distinguish the anterior from the posterior lobe by differences in densities, the posterior lobe being lower in density.

Originally, the hallmark of a pituitary microadenoma (a tumor 10 mm or smaller in diameter) was thought to be a low-density cystic area within the gland (Syvertsen et al, 1979). Unfortunately, many types of nonneoplastic cysts such as neuroepithelial cysts (colloid cysts), Rathke cleft cysts, and arachnoid cysts may be present within the gland (Baskin and Wilson, 1984; Chambers et al, 1982; Shuangshoti, et al, 1970; Spaziante et al, 1981) and mimic tumors (Baskin and Wilson, 1984)(Fig. 18–3). The incidence of cysts, microinfarcts, and small metastases in the pituitary gland in autopsy series varies between 8.7 and 33 percent (McGrath, 1971; Muhr et al, 1981; Ring and Waddington, 1966).

It is apparent, therefore, that there are many potential causes of low-density areas within the pituitary gland.

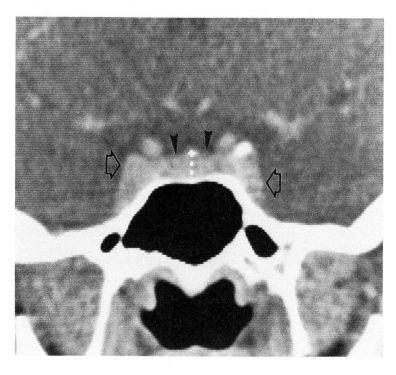

Figure 18–2 Normal midsellar scan. The pituitary gland (*arrowheads*) is opacified. The height of the pituitary gland (note cursor measurement) is 6 mm. The cavernous sinus (*open arrows*) and vascular structures such as the carotid arteries, middle cerebral arteries, and proximal anterior cerebral arteries are also identified. (From Wolpert SM: The radiology of pituitary adenomas. Endocrinol Metab Clin North Am 1987; Vol 16, No 3; with permission.)

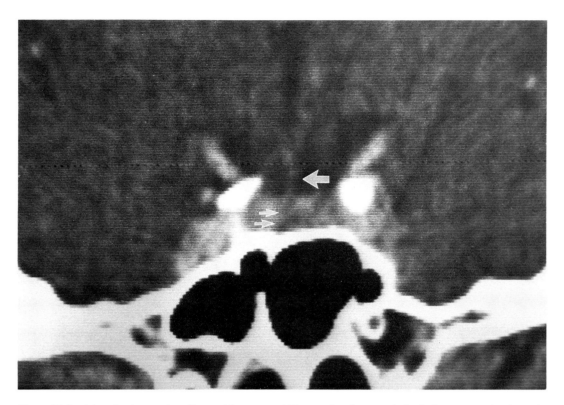

Figure 18-3   A low-density area (*small arrows*) is present within an otherwise normal gland. A cyst measuring 3 mm in diameter was found at surgery. The infundibulum (*large arrow*) is also identified. Septa are present in the sphenoid sinus. (From Wolpert SM: The radiology of pituitary adenomas. Endocrinol Metab Clin North Am 1987; Vol 16, No 3; with permission.)

In a series of CT scans in 107 females from the New England Medical Center, aged 18 to 65, who were referred for suspected intracranial lesions other than pituitary tumors, low-density areas measuring 3 mm or more in diameter were seen in seven patients (Wolpert, 1984). Possibly some of these lesions represent silent microadenomas. In a series of 50 pituitary studies in patients scanned for orbital symptoms and with no endocrinologic complaints, there were ten low-density areas 3 mm in diameter or larger seen in the pituitary glands (Chambers et al, 1982). A low-density area may also be due to an empty sella (Rozario, et al 1977), which, however, should be diagnosable if the infundibulum extends to the floor of the sella (Haughton, 1980) (Fig. 18-4).

High-density areas may also occur within the sella turcica in the normal patient. Tortuous cavernous carotid arteries extending into the sella turcica and transsellar communicating channels between the carotid arteries exist (Rhotan, 1977) and can conceivably cause areas of enhancement higher than that of the adjacent normal pituitary gland. Rhotan and colleagues found the lateral aspect of the pituitary gland to be indented by the carotid arteries in 14 of 50 cadaver specimens (1977). Bonneville and co-workers performed dynamic scans in 100 patients and found a central high-density pituitary blush in 39 patients (1983). They attributed this blush to the hypophyseal-portal venous plexus.

The same pituitary gland may have different densities on separate examinations, and sequential comparisons may therefore be difficult to make. The size of the intravascular and interstitial spaces within the pituitary gland, the degree of diffusibility of contrast material from the vessels into the interstitial spaces (the gland does not have a blood-brain barrier and therefore opacifies in parallel with the blood-iodine level), the glomerular filtration rate, and the rate of shift of the contrast material from the interstitial spaces back to the intravascular spaces can all influence the concentration of iodine and thus the degree of enhancement of the gland at any one time (Gardeur et al, 1981; Hirano et al, 1972).

Gland Height

Because the border between the pituitary gland and the cavernous sinus cannot be defined, whereas the border between the gland and the chiasmatic cistern is easily seen, an increase in gland size can best be determined by assessing the height of the gland. Ideally, the height of the gland should be measured at right angles to the diaphragma sellae, but with CT this probably necessitates an unobtainable degree of neck hyperextension. The height of the gland as measured by coronal CT, therefore, is at best an approximation of the size of the gland. The height as measured by CT was reported as not ex-

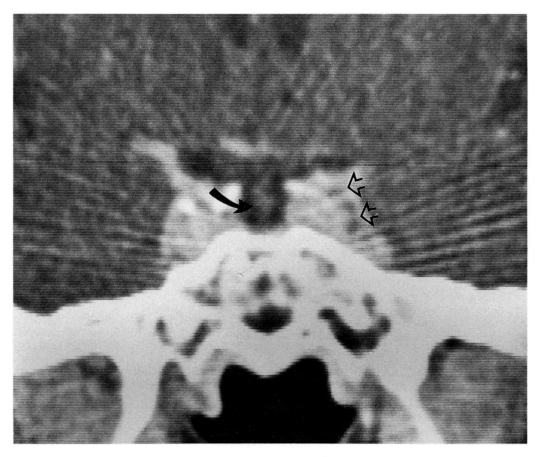

Figure 18-4 Empty sella on a midsellar scan. The infundibulum extends inferiorly to the floor of the sella (*curved arrow*). There are three lucencies within the left cavernous sinus (*open arrows*). The upper lucency is the combined third and fourth cranial nerves; the middle and lower lucencies are the first and second divisions of the fifth cranial nerve. The terminal internal carotid arteries and the proximal anterior cerebral arteries are also demonstrated. Note that the right lateral margin of the cavernous sinus bulges slightly, a normal variation. (From Wolpert SM: The radiology of pituitary adenomas. Semin Roentgenol 1984; 29:53; with permission.)

ceeding 7 mm in females and 6 mm in males in 20 normal patients in one series (Syvertsen et al, 1979). A mean height of 5.3 mm ± 1.7 mm was found in 50 normal patients in another series (Chambers et al, 1982), and a mean height of 4.4 mm ± 1.1 mm in 28 normal men were found in a third series (Brown et al, 1983).

In the series of 107 asymptomatic females from the New England Medical Center, two patients had gland heights of 9 mm (Fig. 18-5) and eight patients had gland heights of 8 mm, as measured by direct coronal CT (Wolpert, 1984) (measured from the center of the floor of the sella as determined with a bone window of 2,000 H units to the top of the gland viewed with a window of 256 H units). Both patients with 9-mm gland heights (aged 21 and 65) had normal serum prolactin levels. Possibly asymptomatic tumors are present in the two patients. The gland heights also varied with age, being larger in the younger patients and decreasing with age. Gland heights in excess of 9 mm are probably always abnormal (Cusick et al, 1980; Peyster et al, 1986; Swartz et al, 1983). Peyster and associates also found that the height of the pituitary

gland as measured by CT depended on the age of the patient, being usually greater in adolescents aged 8 to 21 years than in a comparison group of adults aged 24 to 91 years (1983). The gland height has been shown to decrease post partum, indicating that an enlarged gland may be seen during the latter months of pregnancy (Hinshaw et al, 1984).

Superior Surface of the Gland

The weight of the normal pituitary gland can vary between 450 and 900 mg in females and between 350 and 800 mg in males (Rasmussen, 1968). During pregnancy and with multiparity, the weight increases progressively. The superior surface of the normal gland can bulge and have a round convexity (Muhr et al, 1981), although usually it is flat or concave (Brown et al, 1983; Chambers et al, 1982). The diaphragma sellae cannot be distinguished from the top of the gland and also may bulge superiorly normally. The superior surface bulged in 19 of the 107 asymptomatic female patients investigated at

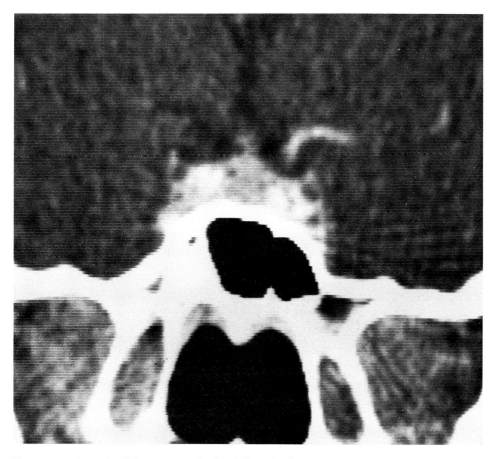

Figure 18-5 Convexity of the upper margin of a pituitary gland in an asymptomatic 21-year-old woman with a cervical cord ependymoma. There were no symptoms or signs of pituitary disease, and the prolactin and serum growth hormone levels were normal.

the New England Medical Center (Wolpert, 1984). Bulging occurred more frequently in the larger glands than in the smaller glands. The superior surface may be tented if the carotid siphons are relatively close together (Renn and Rhoton, 1975; Rhotan et al, 1977). Often, a small bulge is present at the point where the infundibulum inserts on the pituitary gland.

Infundibulum

The infundibulum should be seen extending between the gland and the infundibular recess of the third ventricle in almost all normal patients (see Figs. 18-3 and 18-5). It is usually seen on the more posterior scans, lying immediately anterior to the dorsum sellae in patients with a postfixed chiasm. If the chiasm is prefixed, the infundibulum is more anteriorly located. Since the anterior margin of the dorsum sellae may be slightly concave anteriorly, a single coronal scan may show the two posterior clinoid processes and lateral struts of the dorsum sellae with the infundibulum superiorly and the posterior lobe of the pituitary gland inferiorly. The infundibulum is generally in the midline but may be slightly off midline in some normal cases (Syvertsen et al, 1979),

particularly if the patient is rotated. On an axial view, the cross-sectional diameter of the infundibulum should not exceed that of the basilar artery (Peyster et al, 1984). In children, the infundibulum enlarges with age (Seidel et al, 1985), and as with adults, the diameter should not exceed that of the basilar artery. If the infundibulum is enlarged, numerous pathologic conditions, including histiocytosis X, pituitary adenoma, hypothalamic tumors, Rathke cleft cysts, metastases, sarcoidosis, hyperthyroidism, and infection, should all be considered.

Cavernous Sinus

Following contrast administration, the cavernous sinuses enhance simultaneously with the intravascular blood-pool iodine content (Kline et al, 1981). The cranial nerves are usually seen as filling defects in the lateral wall of the cavernous sinus (see Figs. 18-4 and 18-5). Superolaterally, the third and fourth cranial nerves are seen as a single lucency lying between the two folds of dura that form the lateral walls of the cavernous sinus. Slightly inferiorly in the same dural plane, the first and second divisions of the fifth nerve may be seen. The third division does not lie within the cavernous sinus but extends forward from Meckel's cave below the sinus. The cave is identified as an oval, low-density area owing to its cerebrospinal fluid content posterior and lateral to the dorsum sellae. The sixth nerve is rarely seen within the cavernous sinus. The lateral wall of the cavernous sinus is usually straight, and according to Kline and associates (1981), if it bulges laterally, a pituitary adenoma or cavernous sinus lesion is present. I have, however, seen convex lateral cavernous sinus walls in normal patients and in those with empty sellae (see Figs. 18–4 and 18–5).

Suprasellar Structures

The chiasmatic cistern is seen as a low-density area immediately above the sella turcica. The optic chiasm is often seen on direct coronal scans but is better defined on axial scans using thicker sections (4 or 5 mm). The anteroinferior portion of the third ventricle is seen above the optic chiasm. Laterally, the internal carotid arteries are defined with the A1 segments of the anterior cerebral arteries extending anteromedially.

More posteriorly, the interpeduncular cistern lies behind and above the dorsum sellae and extends superiorly to the hypothalamus. The apex of the basilar artery, the proximal posterior cerebral arteries, and occasionally the superior cerebellar arteries can also be seen.

Sellar Floor and Subsellar Structures

With direct coronal CT scanning, details of both the pituitary gland and the bony floor of the sella turcica are seen simultaneously, and a more accurate correlative analysis of normal variations and pathologic changes is possible than with polytomography (Taylor, 1982). Pituitary adenomas may lie in parts of the pituitary gland other than where cortical thinning or a depressed sellar floor is present (Burrow et al, 1981; Muhr et al, 1981; Turski et al, 1981). Inferiorly, the sphenoid sinus, its septa, and the degree of sinus pneumatization are defined. The anatomy of the septa is important if transsphenoidal adenomectomy is planned (see Fig. 18–3).

AXIAL COMPUTED TOMOGRAPHIC SCANNING

If the patient cannot tolerate the hyperextended neck position or if artifacts from teeth fillings degrade the images, axial scanning can be done. Axial scans are also preferred to direct coronal scans if a suprasellar mass is clinically suspected. Unfortunately, axial scans at the level of the sella turcica are not free from linear artifacts, which by crisscrossing the sella may mask intrasellar lesions or mimic an empty sella (Earnest et al, 1981). Because of the noisy images obtained by thin-section axial scanning, thicker scans (4 or 5 mm) are desirable to demonstrate the suprasellar structures, although if sagittal or coronal reformatted images are needed, thinner scan sections are preferable. Scans parallel to the base of the skull (20 degrees craniad to the canthomeatal line) have fewer artifacts than scans parallel to the canthomeatal line. All axial scans should include the sphenoid sinus. The chiasmatic and interpeduncular cisterns, optic chiasm, floor of the third ventricle, and circle of Willis are all easily defined in this projection.

MAGNETIC RESONANCE IMAGING

In the years since the early reports of MRI of the sella appeared (Hawkes et al, 1983; Oot et al, 1984), the quality of the images has improved remarkably. Soft-tissue contrast, absence of bone artifact, and multiplanar imaging are recognized important advantages of the new modality over CT (Kucharczyk et al, 1986). However, only recently, with the development of higher-strength magnets has good spatial resolution permitting high-detail analysis of the pituitary gland with adequate signal-to-noise ratios been achieved. To compete with CT, 3-mm-thick sections with a maximum of 1-mm-square pixels are necessary for detailed intrasellar evaluation, although thicker scans obtained with lower-strength magnets are certainly useful for suprasellar work.

Our routine technique is initially to obtain T_1-weighted, 3-mm-thick sagittal and coronal images using a 1 tesla Magnatom scanner. This technique highlights the anatomic detail of the gland and surrounding structures. Subsequently, a second series of scans is obtained in the coronal plane using T_2-weighted techniques that accent pathologic changes in the pituitary gland. On T_1-weighted images the sella turcica is seen to contain tissue of two intensities. The major component almost fills the sella and has a signal intensity isointense with cerebral white matter (Fig. 18–6). Posteriorly, a curvilinear sliver of tissue at a much higher intensity is usually seen (Colombo et al, 1987). The nature of this sliver of tissue is controversial. Some consider it to represent fat either within the dorsum sellae or posterior to the pituitary gland within the confines of the sella (Haughton and Prost, 1986). Current opinion, however, is that the high-intensity tissue is possibly due to fat within the pituicytes of the neurohypophysis (Colombo et al, 1987; Fujisawa et al, 1987). The intensity of the gland on the T_2-weighted series is identical to that of cerebral white matter.

The size, morphology, and appearance of the pituitary gland on MR scans corresponds to those seen with CT (Wiener et al, 1985). In addition, parasellar structures such as the optic chiasm are accurately depicted (see Fig. 18–6). Vascular structures such as the carotid arteries in the cavernous sinus and in the suprasellar cisterns are recognized by characteristically low signals. The cavernous sinus has an intensity identical to that of the pituitary gland. On occasion, the dural division between the sella turcica and the cavernous sinus can be defined. Cranial nerves III, V^1, and V^2 may also be seen (Daniels et al, 1985).

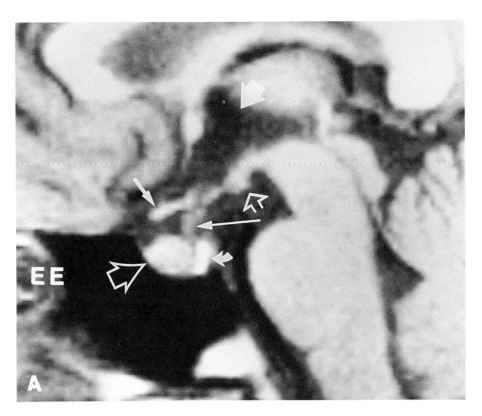

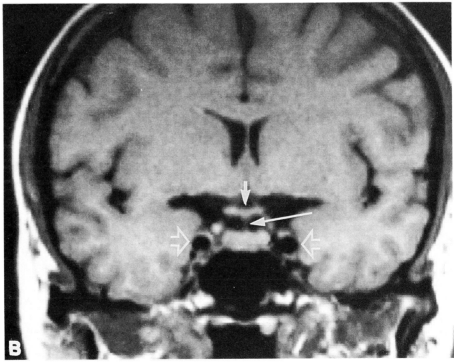

Figure 18–6 *A*, Sagittal T₁-weighted (TR = 600 msec, TE = 17 msec) MR demonstrates the anterior lobe of the pituitary gland (*large open arrow*), the high-intensity posterior lobe (*curved arrow*), and the infundibulum (*long straight arrow*). Note also the third ventricle (*large upper arrow*) and mamillary bodies (*small open arrow*). *B*, Coronal T₁-weighted (TR = 600 msec, TE = 17 msec) MR scan demonstrates the optic chiasm (*short arrow*) and the infundibulum (*long arrow*) extending inferiorly into the pituitary gland. Note also the cavernous carotid arteries bilaterally (*open arrows*) within the cavernous sinuses.

The diagnostic potential for MRI in the evaluation of the pituitary gland has improved with the development of the contrast agent gadolinium-diethylenetriaminepentaacetic acid (Gd-DTPA). The new agent has a role similar to that of the iodinated contrast agent used in conjunction with CT. After intravenous injection, the agent, which is paramagnetic, causes marked shortening of both the T₁ and T₂ relaxation times of the pituitary gland and infundibulum. Since the pituitary gland and the infundibulum both lie outside the blood-brain barrier, after injection of Gd-DTPA the normal gland and infundibulum become hyperintense owing to the marked

T_1 effect (Fig. 18–7). Although the T_2 effect also causes a decrease in the signal intensity of the gland, the T_1 effect predominates, and with relatively low doses of Gd-DTPA, T_2 shortening is not apparent. With increasing doses of Gd-DTPA, the T_2 effect becomes more significant. Gd-DTPA also enhances the venous sinuses, which are well seen on the T_1-weighted scans. There is no alteration of the signal intensity of the parasellar arteries, which remain visible as structures of low-signal intensity. The enhancement occurs promptly, is maximal within one-half hour after injection of the gadolinium, and then slowly fades (Kilgore et al, 1986).

PATHOLOGY OF PITUITARY ADENOMAS

Robert found that 80 percent of pituitary tumors are hormone producing (1979). The common secretory tumors are prolactinomas, growth hormone–secreting (GH-secreting) tumors, and adrenocorticotropic-hormone–secreting (ACTH-secreting) tumors. Prolactinomas are considered to be the most common pituitary disease in clinical practice (Frantz, 1978). As yet, it is not clear whether the work-up of patients with suspected microadenomas should commence with high-detail iodinated-contrast-enhanced CT or with high-detail Gd-DTPA-enhanced MRI, particularly since false-positive and false-negative studies have been reported with both techniques.

Patients with nonsecreting tumors or with tumors producing insufficient hormone to elevate serum hormone levels may not seek medical attention until the tumors have enlarged sufficiently to cause visual field abnormalities or hypopituitarism. Since these tumors have probably enlarged the sella turcica and have grown into the suprasellar and parasellar regions and because of the excellent soft-tissue detail obtained with MRI, the radiologic work-up should commence with MR scanning. The ability of contrast-enhanced CT to diagnose these tumors is, however, almost certainly equivalent to that of MRI.

MICROADENOMAS

Hardy divided pituitary tumors into microadenomas and macroadenomas (1973). Today, the radiologic diagnosis of macroadenomas is not difficult, and the radiologist, when faced with a CT or MR scan showing

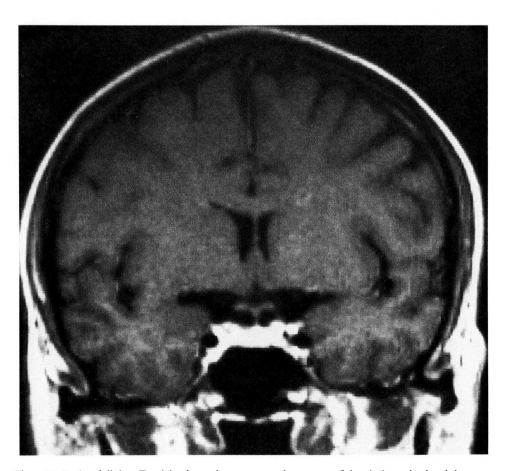

Figure 18–7   A gadolinium T_1-weighted scan demonstrates enhancement of the pituitary gland and the cavernous sinuses (same case as Fig. 18–6B). Note that the pituitary gland cannot be distinguished from the cavernous sinus.

a suprasellar mass, in most cases must differentiate between an adenoma, an aneurysm, and a meningioma. With microadenomas, however, the radiologist's role is considerably more difficult. Microadenomas may exist silently in the general population, with an incidence varying between 2.7 and 27 percent (Bonafe et al, 1981; Burrow et al, 1981; Hemminghytt et al, 1983; Kovacs et al, 1980; Sakoda et al, 1981) and 40 to 50 percent of the tumors being prolactinomas. Unfortunately, the fact that microadenomas are so prevalent can affect the radiologist's index of suspicion when viewing the scans, particularly in a patient with galactorrhea and amenorrhea and a moderately elevated serum prolactin level. Since a small tumor is probably present in such a case, there is a tendency to overread the scan. Overenthusiastic acceptance of polytomography without an assessment of normal variations led to its demise. This error must not be repeated with CT and MR scanning.

Enhancement Patterns

Direct coronal high-detail CT scanning of the sella turcica can demonstrate tumors 3 or 4 mm in diameter (Cusik et al, 1980; Taylor, 1982). Most microadenomas appear as low-density or even cystic lesions (Bonafe et al, 1981; Cusik et al, 1980; Hemminghytt et al, 1983; Taylor, 1982) (Fig. 18–8). As mentioned, because the pituitary gland enhances in parallel with the blood-iodine level, scanning should commence as the intravenous contrast agent is being administered in order to "highlight"

the prolactinoma. Carrying out this dynamic technique, Bonneville and colleagues found displacement or absence of the central high-density pituitary blush in four of 15 macroadenomas and in 17 of 26 microadenomas (Bonneville et al, 1983). Unfortunately, as already mentioned, pituitary blushes were seen only in the minority of their normal patients (39 of 100), and since there was no indication of whether the tumors were surgically verified, the value of dynamic scanning in patients with suspected prolactinomas has not as yet been established.

Often, the infundibulum is displaced by the tumor (see Fig. 18–8), but this is not a completely reliable sign, since the infundibulum may normally be off midline. It is important to image the CT scans with both soft-tissue and bone techniques. Thinning and depression of the sellar floor are strong confirmatory indices for a pituitary adenoma if the bony changes are contiguous with the soft-tissue tumor (Fig. 18–9).

Not all microadenomas are of a low density. Gardeur and co-workers (1981) described focal hypodensity in 12 and focal hyperdensity in 15 of 63 microprolactinomas. Unfortunately, surgical proof was not available in all these patients. Sakoda and associates, using an early-generation scanner, found that 20 of 25 surgically proven prolactinomas were enhanced and that small zones of decreased attenuation found in four of these patients represented cystic degeneration or necrosis within the tumor (1981). The variability in tumor density has not been adequately explained as yet, but it may be due to how soon the pituitary glands are imaged after contrast

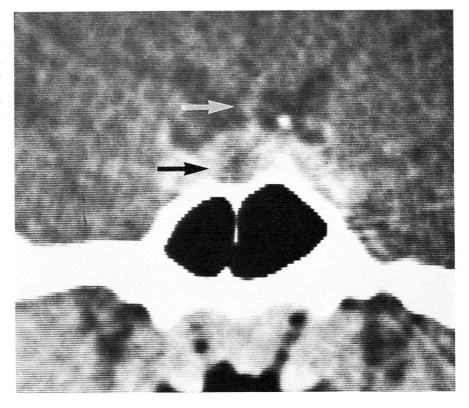

Figure 18–8 Prolactinoma with a hypodense center (*black arrow*). The superior margin of the pituitary gland is convex upward, and the infundibulum (*white arrow*) is displaced away from the tumor at its insertion into the gland. (From Wolpert SM: The radiology of pituitary adenomas. Semin Roentgenol 1984; 29:53; with permission.)

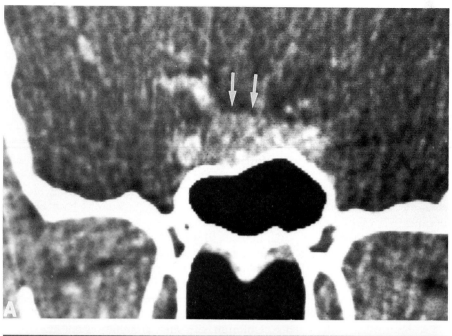

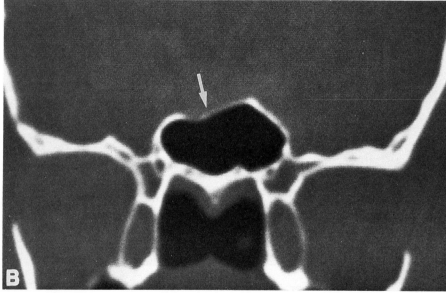

Figure 18-9 Pituitary adenoma. *A*, The low-density tumor (*arrows*) is eccentrically situated in the gland. *B*, With bone technique imaging, thinning and erosion of the floor of the sella (*arrow*) are seen at the tumor site. (From Wolpert SM: The radiology of pituitary adenomas. Semin Roentgenol 1984; 29:53; with permission.)

administration, since with time, contrast can leak into a tumor, increasing its density. There is a strong correlation between the serum prolactin level and the presence of a tumor (Fluckiger et al, 1982). There is also a correlation between the prolactin level and the size of the tumor, although cavernous sinus invasion rather than the size of the tumor may best correlate with the height of the serum prolactin (Fluckiger et al, 1982; Shucart, 1980).

The sensitivity and specificity of the CT scan in the diagnosis of pituitary adenomas have recently been addressed. Davis and co-workers examined the gland heights, presence of focal lesions, sellar floor erosions, infundibula displacements, and configuration of the superior surfaces of the glands in 51 patients with suspected

microadenomas, all surgically proved (1984). The only statistically significant CT criterion for a microadenoma was the presence of a focal hypodense area, at least 2 mm in size. All the hypodense lesions were asymmetrically situated in the gland. Davis and co-workers also concluded that patients with several abnormalities—i.e., focal hypodensities, increase in height of the sellar contents, infundibulum displacement, bulging of the glands, and sellar erosions—were most likely to have an adenoma. They also concluded that the radiologist cannot by CT alone exclude the presence of a clinically significant functioning microadenoma. Similar skepticism was expressed by Teasdale and associates, who considered that high-detail CT is sufficiently unreliable as to preclude its routine use in patients with hyperprolactinemia or Cushing's syndrome (1986). These authors found that a normal CT scan does not exclude a microadenoma, nor does a focal abnormality demonstrated by high-resolution CT establish unequivocally the presence or the site of a microadenoma.

As yet, there are no large series devoted to the value of MRI in the diagnosis of microadenomas. Microprolactinomas usually appear as low-intensity focal lesions on T_1-weighted scans (Fig. 18–10A and B) and as high-intensity lesions on T_2-weighted scans (Pojunas et al, 1986). In one series, ten of 11 microadenomas, all 3 mm or larger in size, were correctly diagnosed on T_1-weighted images (Kucharczyk et al, 1986). In another series, all eight microadenomas found at surgery were correctly identified by MRI preoperatively (Kulkarni et al, 1988). As with CT, the most common morphologic change is asymmetric, upward convexity of the glands on the side of the tumors (see Fig. 18–10A). Displacement of the infundibulum is a useful ancillary sign. In studies in which CT and MRI were compared, MRI was found to be not as sensitive as CT for identifying discrete focal lesions with the minimally enlarged or normal-sized pituitary gland (Davis et al, 1987; Pojunas et al, 1986).

After the administration of Gd-DTPA, pituitary microadenomas may appear on T_1-weighted scans as low-intensity lesions within a high-intensity enhancing gland. Some tumors may appear as isointense lesions and be obscured after the administration of the contrast agent. Other tumors may be hyperintense. This variability, similar to that found after the injection of contrast media for CT, is probably due to the difference in the enhancement patterns of the normal pituitary gland and adenomas. The normal gland enhances promptly, and adenomas enhance slowly. Thus, there may be a window during which time adenomas will be obscured by the presence of Gd-DTPA (Dwyer et al, 1987). More research into the use of paramagnetic-enhanced MRI for the diagnosis of pituitary microadenomas is necessary before its value and efficiency as compared with CT can be determined.

MACROADENOMAS

Despite some skepticism about the value of CT and MRI for the diagnosis of microadenomas, there is no doubt about the value of CT and MRI in the evaluation of macroadenomas. With macroadenomas, the sella turcica is enlarged, part or all of the suprasellar cistern is obliterated, and the tumor or its capsule enhances on CT following intravenous iodinated contrast administration (Houser, 1982; Taylor, 1982). Because of the excellent visualization of the basal cisterns on the axial CT scan, direct coronal scanning is usually not necessary, although the combination of axial and coronal views can provide a comprehensive three-dimensional demonstration of the tumor size. With suprasellar growth, compression or obliteration of the third ventricle causes obstructive

hydrocephalus. The tumor can also grow laterally into the cavernous sinuses, posteriorly into the pontine or cerebellopontine-angle cisterns, or, after breaking through the sellar floor, inferiorly into the sphenoid sinus. Cavernous sinus extension can be recognized by sinus expansion and encasement of the carotid artery (Ahmadi et al, 1985). Intracavernous cranial nerve compression, obliteration or displacement as well as invasion of the lateral walls of the cavernous sinus, and bone destruction may also indicate sinus invasion.

Most macroadenomas appear as low-intensity lesions on T_1-weighted MR scans and as high- or mixed-intensity lesions on T_2-weighted scans (Fig. 18–11) (Karnaze et al, 1986). In addition, the superior margin of the gland may bulge symmetrically or asymmetrically and the infundibulum is usually displaced away from the tumor. Usually, the posterior pituitary high-intensity signal is not seen, presumably because of compression by the expanding neoplasm. The excellent soft-tissue detectability of MRI easily defines the relationship of the tumor to the optic chiasm (see Fig. 18–11). On occasion, macroadenomas may be of high intensity on both T_1- and T_2-weighted scans. There is no definitive correlation between the appearances of these tumors and their pathology, although the signal intensities may indicate that the tumors are cystic and have a proteinaceous content or contain clinically silent hemorrhages. Whereas suprasellar extension of macroadenomas is easily seen on MR scans (Fig. 18–11), cavernous sinus involvement is often difficult to diagnose (Kucharczyk et al, 1986). After Gd-DTPA administration, cavernous sinus extension can be diagnosed if a low-intensity tumor is seen extending into a high-intensity cavernous sinus. However, usually macroadenomas enhance, and then with cavernous sinus extension, the tumor may be masked by the high-intensity signal of the sinus.

The term *invasive prolactinoma* has been used for the tumors with extensive capsular penetration as well as dural, sinus, and osseous invasion. These tumors should not be grouped clinicopathologically with those macroadenomas demonstrating expansile and compressive but not destructive growth (Scheithauer, 1982). Such local invasion, although a reflection of aggressive potential, is considered insufficient evidence by some to designate the tumor as malignant (Russell and Rubinstein, 1971). The diffuse bone destruction from invasive prolactinomas can involve the sella, the sphenoid bone, and adjacent petrous temporal bones. These destructive changes and the tumor extension into the adjacent soft tissues are well seen on the CT scan (Virapongse et al, 1984). With MR, however, although extension into the sphenoid sinus can easily be seen, the lack of signal from cortical bone makes discontinuity of the sella walls difficult to diagnose. Differentiating an invasive adenoma from a chordoma, chondroma, chondrosarcoma, craniopharyngioma, metastasis, or nasopharyngeal carcinoma may be impossible with CT or MRI.

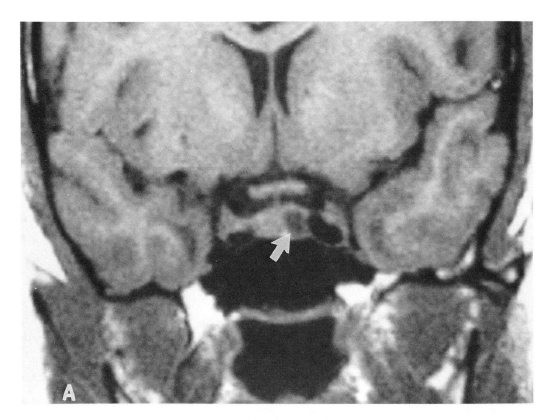

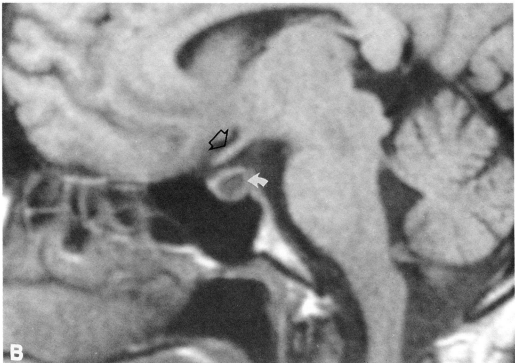

Figure 18-10   Pituitary microadenomas on MR scan. *A*, Coronal T_1-weighted image demonstrates a low-intensity tumor in the lateral margin of the gland (*arrow*) with eccentric enlargement of the pituitary gland. *B*, A sagittal T_1-weighted scan taken through the adenoma (*white arrow*) demonstrates its proximity to the optic nerve (*open arrow*). (From Wolpert SM: The radiology of pituitary adenomas. Endocrinol Metab Clin North Am 1987; Vol 16, No 3; with permission.)

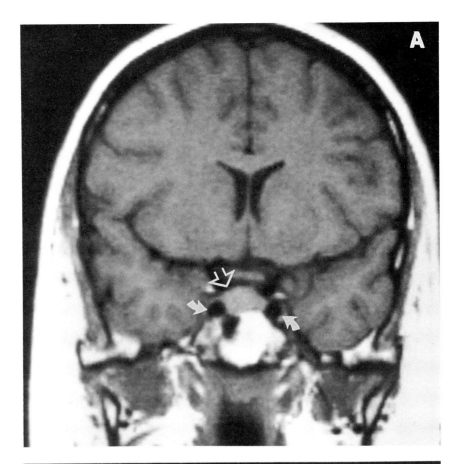

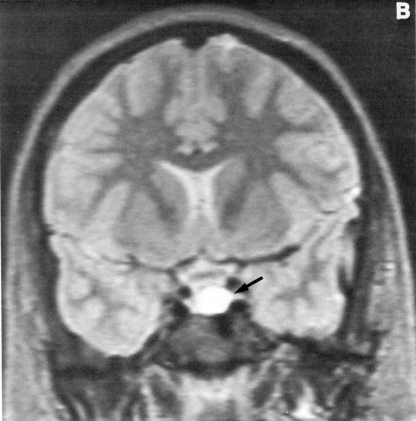

Figure 18-11 Pituitary microadenoma on MR scan. *A*, On the T₁-weighted image, note the enlarged pituitary gland (*open arrow*) extending superiorly into the suprasellar cistern. Note also the flow void due to the carotid artery within the cavernous sinus (*curved arrow*). *B*, On the T₂-weighted image, the tumor (*arrow*) has a prolonged T₂, as evidenced by its high intensity. (From Wolpert SM: The radiology of pituitary adenomas. Endocrinol Metab Clin North Am 1987; Vol 16, No 3; with permission.)

PITUITARY CALCIFICATIONS

Microscopic calcifications were seen in 51 of a surgical series of 755 pituitary adenomas (6.75 percent) and by x-ray film (plain films and tomography) in 13 of these adenomas (1.72 percent) (Rillet et al, 1981). The majority of the tumors were prolactinomas. Pituitary calcifications are nonspecific, since they can also be physiologic (called pituitary stones) (Ozanoff, 1971) or can be seen in the newborn only to disappear during the first postnatal months (Plaut and Galenson, 1944). The key differential diagnosis is with craniopharyngiomas, which by CT cannot be distinguished from calcified adenomas. Calcification cannot be seen on MR scans unless it is massive.

ADENOMAS AND PITUITARY APOPLEXY

Pituitary apoplexy is characterized by a sudden onset of neurologic symptoms and signs such as headache, diplopia, or visual defects occurring in a patient with a preexisting secretory or nonsecretory pituitary adenoma (David et al, 1975; Ebersold et al, 1983). On occasion, the apoplexy may be the first indication of an adenoma. The clinical presentation is due either to infarction of the tumor with swelling, secondary hemorrhage, and necrosis or to acute bleeding into the tumor. Hemorrhage into pituitary adenomas is not infrequent; the incidence has been reported as varying between 0.6 and 9 percent (Cardoso and Peterson, 1984), and there is an even higher percentage of asymptomatic hemorrhages (diagnosed by CT scans). Pituitary hemorrhages and infarcts are as frequent in prolactinomas as in nonsecretory adenomas. On CT, the demonstration of a suprasellar mass containing a high-density area or, more frequently, a mottled mixed-density area (Ebersold et al, 1983; Post and Kasdon, 1980) suggests the diagnosis. On occasion, CT may show a fluid-blood density level in the suprasellar mass (Fujimoto et al, 1981).

Hemorrhages, at least when they are 48 hours old or more, are easily diagnosed by MRI (Fig. 18–12). Typically, high-intensity areas due to methemoglobin are seen on both the T_1- and T_2-weighted scans (Gomori et al, 1985). Chronic pituitary hemorrhage does not exhibit the

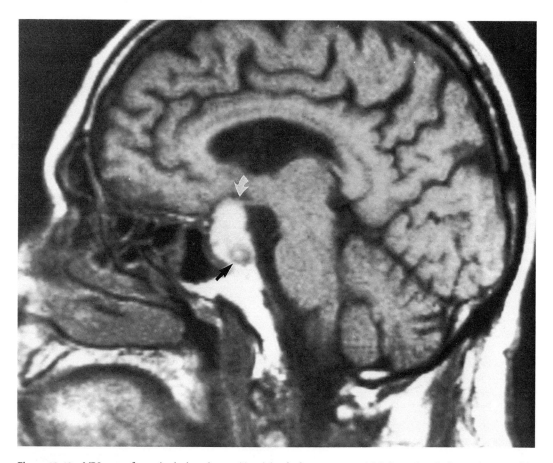

Figure 18–12   MRI scan of a sagittal plane image, T_1-weighted, demonstrates a high-intensity pituitary adenoma with some areas of low intensity at its base (*black arrow*). Note the approximation of the tumor to the optic nerve (*white arrow*). In view of the history of sudden acute blindness and the classic appearance of a hemorrhage into a pituitary adenoma, the diagnosis of pituitary apoplexy was made and confirmed at surgery. (From Wolpert SM: The radiology of pituitary adenomas. Endocrinol Metab Clin North Am 1987; Vol 16, No 3; with permission.)

low-intensity appearance suggestive of hemosiderin (as seen with intracerebral hemorrhages) on T_2-weighted images, presumably because of more efficient macrophage removal of the blood products in the extracerebral pituitary gland.

MEDICALLY TREATED PROLACTINOMAS

The ergot derivative bromocriptine has been used effectively for the treatment of hyperprolactinemia for a number of years, with clinical and hormonal improvements as well as radiographic evidence of prolactinoma regression (Baskin and Wilson, 1984; Bonneville et al, 1982; Chernow et al, 1982; Horowitz et al, 1983; Scotti et al, 1982) (Fig. 18–13). Favorable responses have been seen with both microadenomas and macroadenomas. The responses can be very rapid, with clinical improvement and decrease in tumor sizes being seen within 2 to 3 days after the initiation of treatment. On CT, hypodense areas often develop within the tumors. When the treatment is stopped, there may be a rapid regrowth of the tumors (Bonneville et al, 1982; Thorner et al, 1980), the treatment being suppressive, not curative. Bromocriptine may be more effective in the treatment of larger and faster-growing macroadenomas than in the treatment of the smaller and generally slower growing microadenomas. This difference in drug efficacy may be due to different biologic characteristics of the two types of tumors, with increased mitotic rates occurring in the larger tumors (Fluckiger et al, 1982). The drug is also more effective in secretory than in nonsecretory tumors (Chakera et al, 1985).

At the New England Medical Center, 20 patients (ten female and ten male) with suspected prolactinomas were treated with the ergot derivative (Wolpert, 1986). Fifteen of the patients had macroadenomas, and five had microadenomas. Noteworthy in this series was a decrease in the heights of the tumors of at least 2 mm in 14 of the 15 macroadenomas but in none of the microadenomas, although substantial serum prolactin decreases occurred in all the patients. In nine of the 15 macroadenomas, low-density areas appeared within the tumors (Fig. 18–13); in none of the microadenomas did such a pattern occur. Two of the patients came to surgery—one after 15 months of treatment and the other after 12 months of treatment. Neither had fibrotic changes, which are cited as occurring in some tumors after chronic ergot therapy.

Areas of decreased density within pituitary adenomas treated with ergot derivatives have also been described by others (Bonneville et al, 1982; Scotti et al 1982) and are possibly due to the cellular degeneration that occurs after this type of treatment (Baskin and Wilson, 1984). An increase in the tumor size with the development of eye signs indicative of a compressive neuropathy has been reported in two of a series of 30 patients with macroprolactinomas treated with bromocriptine (Bonneville et al, 1982). In both patients, the CT scans showed areas of high density, possibly due to hemorrhages. Increase in tumor size was not seen in any of the patients in the series from the New England Medical Center. Pergolide, a new long-acting ergot derivative, may be as effective as or more effective than bromocriptine in causing tumor shrinkage (Horowitz et al, 1983).

Initial reports on the MR appearance of pituitary adenomas after treatment with bromocriptine describe the development of high-intensity signals within the tumor on T_1-weighted scans and low-intensity signals on T_2-weighted scans (Pojunas et al, 1986). The cause for these appearances is unclear although hemorrhage is the probable cause.

ADENOMAS AND THE EMPTY SELLA

Adenomas can coexist with the primary empty sella syndrome (Domingue et al, 1978; Molitch et al, 1977). If nodular areas of increased density partly surrounded by cerebrospinal fluid density are seen within the sella, the diagnosis of an empty sella coexisting with a tumor is suggested (Smaltino et al, 1980). The empty sella may also be associated with hyperprolactinemia without an associated tumor (Gharib et al, 1983).

Empty sella is easily diagnosed on MR scans by the demonstration of cerebrospinal fluid signal intensities on all sequences extending into the sella turcica.

ACTH-PRODUCING TUMORS

There is little information in the literature about the CT enhancement patterns of microadenomas other than prolactinomas. Hyperdense and hypodense GH-secreting and ACTH-secreting adenomas were reported in one study (Gardeur et al, 1981). In another study, such tumors were usually but not invariably hypodense (Hemminghytt et al, 1983). Both the sensitivity and diagnostic accuracy of CT in the detection of ACTH-producing pituitary tumors are low. In three series reviewed, abnormal CT scans (all high resolution) were found in less than 50 percent of patients with surgically confirmed ACTH-producing tumors (Chandler et al, 1987; Marcovitz et al, 1987; Saris et al, 1987). However, early reports indicate that MRI may be very useful in the diagnosis of this tumor type. Tumors were seen in eight of 12 patients after precontrast MRI and in ten of 12 patients after postcontrast Gd-DTPA scans (Dwyer et al, 1987). Sampling of serum from the inferior sinus can localize the source of elevated ACTH (Doppman et al, 1985).

GROWTH-HORMONE-PRODUCING TUMORS

Patients with GH-secreting tumors present clinically with acromegaly usually when the disease is well advanced and sella enlargement and erosion are already present. The excessive growth of the skeletal tissue is manifested

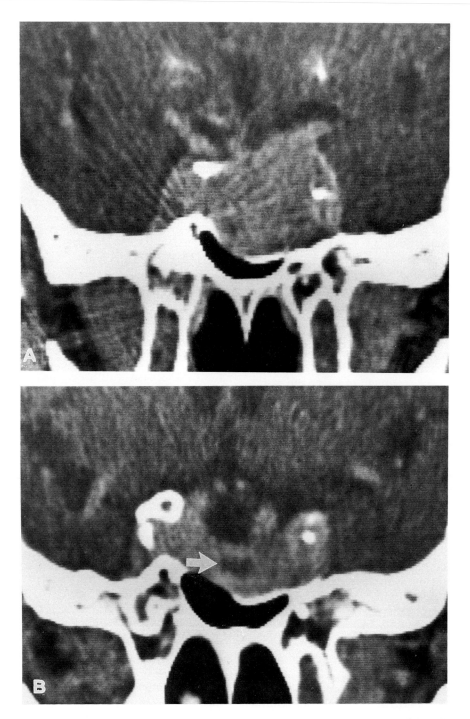

Figure 18–13 Prolactinoma treated with bromocriptine. *A*, Before treatment. Erosion of the sellar floor and extension of the tumor superiorly into the suprasellar cistern are shown. The serum prolactin level was 3,580 ng per milliliter. The tumor decreased in size 6 weeks after bromocriptine therapy was started. *B*, After 1 year of therapy. The tumor has markedly decreased in size. Focal low-density areas have developed within the tumor (*arrow*). The serum prolactin level was normal. (From Wolpert SM: The radiology of pituitary adenomas. Semin Roentgenol 1984; 29:53; with permission.)

by thickening of the skull vault, increased bone density, and enlargement of all the paranasal sinuses and of the mastoid air cells. When sellar enlargement and prognathism accompany the skull vault changes, the diagnosis is easily established. The role of CT or MRI in patients with acromegaly is to confirm the presence of the sellar tumor and to demonstrate parasellar extension, if any.

GONADOTROPIN-PRODUCING TUMOR ON CT

Prominent suprasellar extension of enhancing tumors was described in five patients with the rare gonadotropin-producing tumor in one series (Miura et al, 1985).

PREDICTIVE FACTORS IN THE MANAGEMENT OF PATIENTS WITH PITUITARY ADENOMAS

Biologic cures have been found to be higher with enclosed GH-secreting tumors than with invasive tumors (Garcia-Urea et al, 1978; Giovanelli et al, 1976; Hardy, 1973). The absence of suprasellar extension rather than the effect of the tumor on the sellar walls may be the best prognostic factor (Sang et al, 1977). The unreliability of CT to predict surgically verified sphenoid sinus invasion in patients with acromegaly has been reported (Balagura et al, 1981). Similar doubts about the relationship between the appearance of the sella and the prognosis following surgical treatment of patients with Cushing's syndrome have also been reported. The original optimism that surgical removal of functioning pituitary tumors may be curative has not been confirmed (Ciric et al, 1983; Rodman et al, 1984). In a series of 95 surgically treated pituitary tumors, persistence or evolution of pituitary stalk enlargement or parasellar extension on the preoperative CT scan indicated surgical failure (Kaplan et al, 1985). Conversely, resolution of pituitary stalk enlargement was a sign of successful surgery.

ANGIOGRAPHY OF ADENOMAS

Angiography is not used for the diagnosis of adenomas but is necessary for asymmetrically positioned suprasellar masses as seen by CT or MRI and for masses having uniformly dense enhancement by CT, suggesting the diagnosis of meningioma or aneurysm.

DIFFERENTIAL DIAGNOSIS OF PITUITARY ADENOMAS—RADIOLOGIC FEATURES

Many sellar lesions, neoplastic and nonneoplastic, may mimic pituitary adenomas clinically, endocrinologically, and radiologically. A modestly elevated prolactin level with an enlarged sella does not always indicate that the patient has a prolactinoma. The hyperprolactinemia may be due to interference with the hypothalamic-prolactin-inhibiting mechanism, which in turn may be due to any one of a number of lesions in the suprasellar area.

Aneurysms

The importance of distinguishing an aneurysm in the suprasellar parasellar area from an adenoma is exemplified by descriptions of rupture of aneurysms during surgery for anticipated adenomas (Scotti et al, 1982). Bone destruction together with abnormal calcification, usually curvilinear, should alert the radiologist to the possibility of an aneurysm. The bone destruction is eccentric, and there may be widening of the superior orbital fissure. CT may show a far larger lesion than is apparent on angiography (Fig. 18–14), since there may be a considerable amount of blood clot, unseen on the angiogram, within the aneurysm (Pinto et al, 1982). Dynamic CT with visualization of the different parts of the aneurysm (lumen and clot) during the rapid injection of contrast material can help demonstrate the true vascular anatomy (Pinto et al, 1982). MRI can demonstrate the decreased signal of flowing blood (Bradley et al, 1984; Karnaze et al, 1986; Olsen et al, 1987) and thereby demonstrate the aneurysm. Thrombus in the aneurysm may be recognized by high-intensity signals on T_1 and T_2 sequences, indicating the presence of methemoglobin (Fig. 18–15). Angiography is diagnostic, and the aneurysm may originate from the cavernous carotid artery or the circle of Willis. The demonstration of a parasellar aneurysm does not exclude the presence of a pituitary adenoma since the two conditions can coexist (Jakubowski and Kendall, 1978).

Tuberculum Sellae Meningiomas

The region of the sella, particularly at the dural attachments, is a common site for meningiomas. The tumors can arise from the tuberculum sellae, diaphragma sellae, cerebellopontine-angle cistern, cavernous sinus, or medial sphenoidal ridge and spread as parasellar masses (Fig. 18–16). Hyperostosis of the adjacent bone, which may be seen on the CT scans, was seen on skull x-ray films in 50 percent of the patients reported by DiChiro and Lindgren (1952). The sella may be enlarged. Calcium may be seen in the lesion on the nonenhanced scan. On CT, after contrast administration, the lesion enhances in a mottled or homogeneous manner (Naidich et al, 1976). The diagnosis of meningiomas by MRI may be difficult, since these tumors are often isointense with gray matter on both T_1- and T_2-weighted sequences (Lee and Deck, 1985). However, the space-occupying features of the lesion are usually well seen (Fig. 18–17), and the diagnosis is seldom a problem (Yeakley et al, 1988). Gd-DTPA is an excellent contrast agent for the MR diagnosis of meningiomas, causing marked shortening of the T_1 relaxation

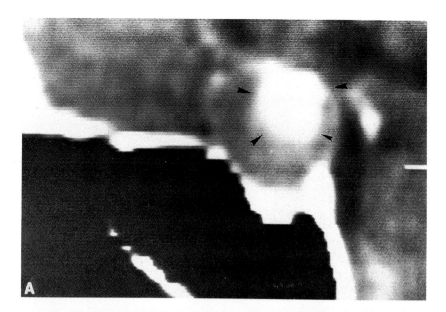

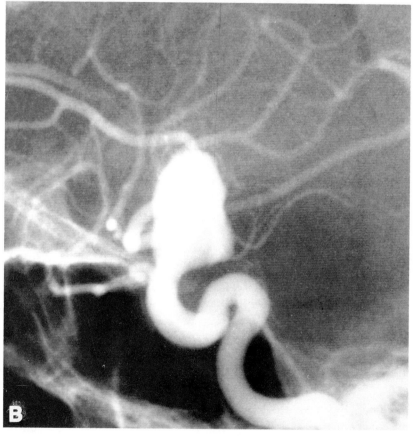

Figure 18-14   *A*, Sagittal reconstruction after a series of contiguous scans demonstrates a suprasellar lesion with central enhancement (*arrowheads*). *B*, Right carotid angiogram, lateral projection, demonstrates an aneurysm corresponding in size to the enhancing lesion seen on the CT scan. The part of the lesion seen on *A* that does not enhance represents blood clot within the aneurysm. (From Wolpert SM: The radiology of pituitary adenomas. Semin Roentgenol 1984; 29:53; with permission.)

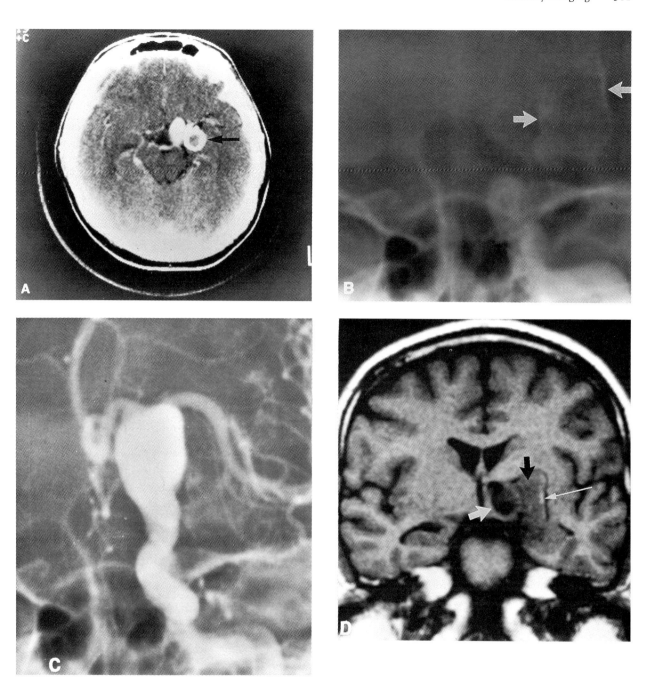

Figure 18–15   *A*, Contrast-enhanced CT scan at the suprasellar level. Note the contrast-enhancing lesion immediately medial to a dense, calcified ring (*arrow*) representing calcification of part of the aneurysm. *B*, Anteroposterior view of the first film of a left carotid arteriogram. Calcification can be seen within the walls of the aneurysm (*arrows*). *C*, Left carotid arteriogram demonstrates a giant aneurysm of the terminal internal carotid artery. *D*, MR scan, coronal T₁-weighted image, demonstrates flow void within the aneurysm (*short white arrow*) immediately medial to the thrombosed portion of the aneurysm (*black arrow*), which is of a slightly higher intensity than the surrounding white matter. Note also the high-intensity tissue (*long arrow*) due to methemoglobin immediately medial to the low-intensity calcification of the aneurysm. (From Wolpert SM: The radiology of pituitary adenomas. Endocrinol Metab Clin North Am 1987; Vol 16, No 3; with permission.)

time with hyperintensity of the tumors. Angiography with selective internal carotid studies and subtraction may in about one-third of cases show either a characteristic blush or feeding arteries derived usually from the meningohypophyseal trunk, which is a branch of the precavernous carotid artery (Post and Kasdon, 1980).

Craniopharyngiomas

Craniopharyngiomas account for about 5 to 10 percent of brain tumors in children. They arise from embryonic squamous cell nests which are the residua of upward migration of stomodeal epithelium to the up-

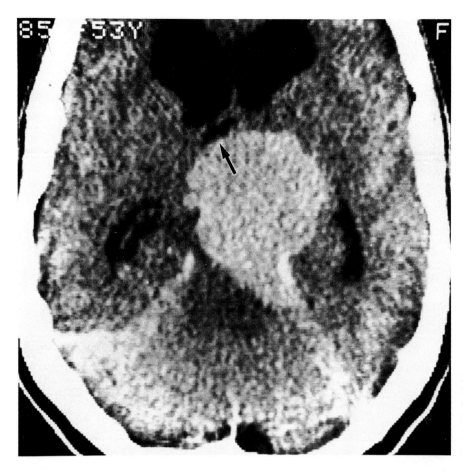

Figure 18-16 Axial contrast-enhanced CT scan demonstrates a large suprasellar contrast-enhancing lesion extending into the middle and posterior cranial fossae. Note the indentation on the third ventricle (*arrow*). Hydrocephalus is also present.

per part of the anterior lobe of the pituitary gland (Post and Kasdon, 1980). The tumors generally originate above the sella but often extend down into the sella, causing enlargement. They usually present as calcific suprasellar tumors with or without sellar erosion (Fig. 18–18). The majority occur in the younger age groups, but a second peak incidence in middle-aged patients is also seen. Calcification is seen more frequently in the younger patients (70 to 90 percent) than in the older patients (40 to 60 percent).

Diagnostically, CT scanning is very useful, since the scan can detect minute amounts of calcium. The calcification, which can be flocculent or curvilinear, if seen in conjunction with a low-density cystic midline tumor in a child, is almost pathognomonic of a craniopharyngioma. Enhancement is rare, according to one series, but was seen in six of eight children in another (Fitz et al, 1978). Once the CT scan shows these abnormalities, seldom are any other radiologic studies necessary. Craniopharyngiomas have variable signal characteristics of MRI. Some report that they are usually hyperintense or isointense on MR T_1-weighted images and hyperintense on T_2-weighted images (Lee and Deck, 1985; Pusey et al, 1987)(Fig. 18–19). Others (Karnaze et al, 1986) have reported that the tumors are usually hypointense on T_1-weighted images. The calcification cannot be seen by

MRI unless it is massive in amount. Often, the tumors extend posteriorly into the interpeduncular and prepontine cisterns.

Hypothalamic Gliomas

Hypothalamic and optic nerve gliomas should be considered conjunctively, since both pathologically and radiologically they can be almost identical in appearance. The hypothalamic glioma often presents clinically in children with the diencephalic syndrome, since the tumor arises in the anterior hypothalamus in the floor of the third ventricle. When the suprasellar cistern is examined by axial or direct CT coronal scanning, the lesion appears as a mass indenting the cistern from above and the third ventricle from below. The lesion may enhance slightly.

Optic nerve gliomas are situated immediately anterior to the hypothalamus and present clinically with visual loss (Post and Kasdon, 1980). Visual loss may not be appreciated in very young children, and the tumors may not become evident until they have grown posteriorly to involve the hypothalamus. There is a well-known association between optic nerve gliomas and neurofibromatosis. Skull x-ray films may show enlargement of the optic foramen, which can be easily diagnosed by thin-

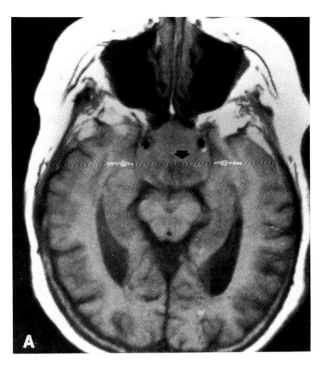

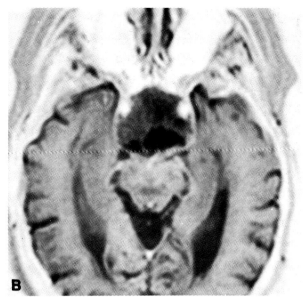

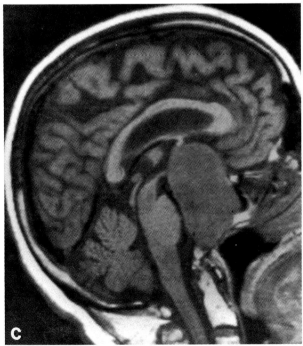

Figure 18–17 *A,* Axial T₁-weighted MR scan demonstrates a tumor *(white arrows)* in the suprasellar area enveloping the carotid arteries. Note the low-intensity area within the tumor *(black arrow). B,* T₂-weighted scan at the same level demonstrates the tumor with a high-intensity area posteriorly. *C,* Sagittal scan demonstrates a large tumor centered on the sella growing into the third venticle and also inferiorly through the sphenoid sinus. At surgery, a meningioma was found. Different intensities on tissues within the meningioma were due to cystic changes in the tumor. (From Wolpert SM: The radiology of pituitary adenomas. Endocrinol Metab Clin North Am 1987; Vol 16, No 3; with permission.)

section, high-detail CT scanning of the optic canals. Usually, the sella is normal, but there may be undercutting of the anterior clinoid process with deepening of the chiasmatic groove. The tumor is usually isodense on the nonenhanced scan and shows moderate enhancement. When a chiasmatic or optic nerve glioma is clinically suspected but is not seen on the standard axial CT scans, MRI is usually diagnostic (Fig. 18–20). On MRI, optic nerve and hypothalamic gliomas usually mirror the pat-

tern of gliomas elsewhere in the brain, i.e., hypointensity on T₁-weighted images and hyperintensity on T₂-weighted images (Karnaze et al, 1986; Lee and Deck, 1985). Extension of the tumor posteriorly along the optic tracts is easily defined by MRI. In patients with neurofibromatosis, an incidental finding has been the demonstration of focal high-signal lesions in the brain stem, centrum semiovale, thalamus, corpus callosum, or globus pallidus on T₂-weighted images (Brown et al, 1987) (Fig.

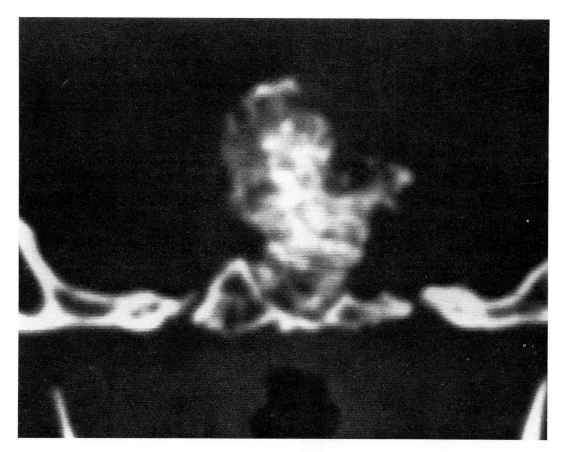

Figure 18-18   Direct coronal CT scan demonstrates a large high-density lesion extending superiorly out of the sella turcica. (From Wolpert SM: The radiology of pituitary adenomas. Endocrinol Metab Clin North Am 1987; Vol 16, No 3; with permission.)

18–21). It is unclear whether these lesions represent hamartomas, areas of gliosis, or preclinical gliomas.

Metastases

Metastases to the pituitary gland may originate from carcinomas of the breast, bronchus, kidney, and colon (Frantz, 1978). In one series, clinically silent pituitary metastases were seen in 3.6 percent of 500 patients dying from cancer (Max et al, 1981). Radiographically, the sella is destroyed, and the lesion on CT appears as an enhancing mass lesion. The differentiation from other causes of sellar enlargement may be impossible. The diagnosis is usually considered when the patient presents with a pituitary tumor and a known primary tumor. Metastases in one small series were seen as slightly hypointense or isointense lesions on T_1-weighted MR images and hyperintense on T_2-weighted images (Karnaze, 1986). Metastases to the infundibulum can be diagnosed by stalk enlargement (Peyster and Hover, 1984). Metastases may also seed into the suprasellar subarachnoid space and be visible on MR scanning. This can occur in patients with medulloblastomas, germinomas, or ependymomas.

Rathke Cleft Cysts

The majority of sellar and parasellar epithelial cysts are remnants or derivatives of Rathke clefts. The cyst can enlarge and compress the pituitary gland, stalk, optic chiasm, or hypothalamus (Kucharczyk et al, 1987). By CT these cysts are usually hypodense on nonenhanced scans and hyperdense after contrast administration (Kucharczyk et al, 1987). The MR pattern is variable. The cysts can have the same signal characteristics as cerebrospinal fluid or be isointense to slightly hyperintense on T_1-weighted images and have decreased intensity on T_2-weighted images.

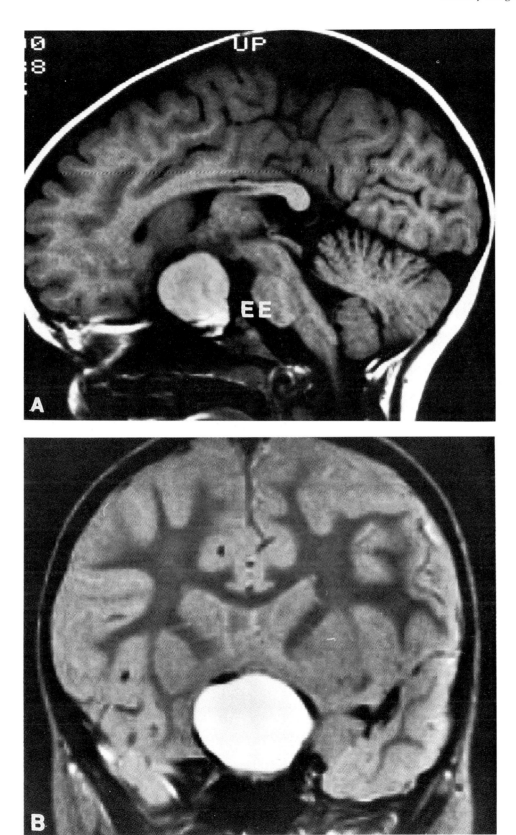

Figure 18–19 *A*, Sagittal T₁-weighted MR scan demonstrates a large high-intensity tumor extending out of the sella turcica into the suprasellar cistern. *B*, Coronal T₂-weighted MR scan (TR = 3,000 msec, TE = 45 msec) also demonstrates a high-intensity tumor extending superiorly out of the sella turcica into the suprasellar cistern.

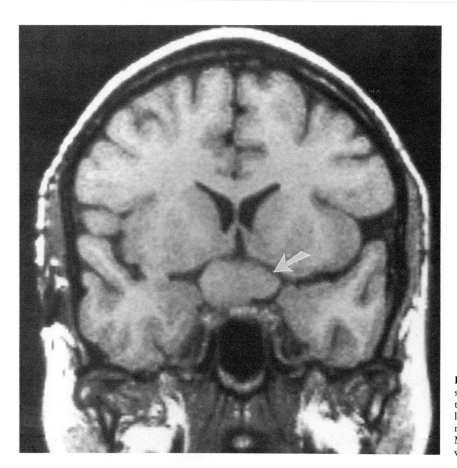

Figure 18–20 Coronal T₁-weighted MR scan demonstrates a tumor isointense with the gray matter of the brain in the suprasellar cistern (*arrow*). (From Wolpert SM: The radiology of pituitary adenomas. Endocrinol Metab Clin North Am 1987; Vol 16, No 3; with permission.)

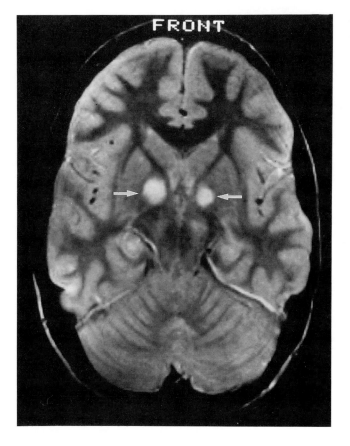

Figure 18–21 Note the bilateral high-intensity lesions within the posterior limbs of the internal capsule and globi pallidus (*arrows*).

Other

A number of other lesions in the sellar and suprasellar regions also must be considered in the differential diagnosis of pituitary adenomas. These include arachnoid cysts, chordomas, germinomas, dermoids, epidermoids, hamartomas, sarcoid granulomas, eosinophilic granulomas, and sphenoid sinus mucoceles (Post and Kasdon, 1980).

BIBLIOGRAPHY

Ahmadi J, North CM, Segall HD, et al. Cavernous sinus invasion by pituitary adenomas. AJNR 1985; 6:893.

Balagura S, Derone P, Guiot G. Acromegaly: Analysis of 132 cases treated surgically. Neurosurgery 1981; 8:413.

Baskin DS, Wilson CB. Transsphenoidal treatment of nonneoplastic intrasellar cysts. J Neurosurg 1984; 60:8.

Bonafe A, Sobel D, Manelfe C. Relative value of computed tomography and hypocycloidal tomography in the diagnosis of pituitary microadenoma. A radio-surgical correlative study. Neuroradiology 1981; 22:133.

Bonneville J-F, Moussa-Bacha K, Portha C. Dynamic computed tomography of the pituitary gland: The "Tuft sign." Radiology 1983; 149:145.

Bonneville J-F, Poulignot D, Cattin F, et al. Computed tomography demonstration of the effects of bromocriptine on pituitary microadenoma size. Radiology 1982; 143:451.

Bradley WG, Waluch V, Lai K-S, et al. The appearance of rapidly flowing blood on magnetic resonance imaging. AJR 1984; 143:1167.

Brown SB, Irwin KM, Enzman DR. CT characteristics of the normal pituitary gland. Neuroradiology 1983; 24:259.

Brown EW, Riccardi VM, Mawad M, et al. MR imaging of optic pathways in patients with neurofibromatosis. AJNR 1987; 8:1031.

Burrow GN, Wortzman G, Rewcastle NB, et al. Microadenomas of the pituitary and abnormal sellar tomograms in an unselected autopsy series. N Engl J Med 1981; 304:156.

Cardoso ER, Peterson EW. Pituitary apoplexy: A review. Neurosurgery 1984; 14:363.

Chakera TMJ, Khangure MS, Pullen P. Assessment by computed tomography of the response of pituitary macroadenomas to bromocriptine. Clin Radiol 1985; 36:223.

Chambers EF, Turski PA, LaMasters D, et al. Regions of low density in the contrast-enhanced pituitary gland: Normal and pathologic processes. Radiology 1982; 144:109.

Chandler WF, Schteingart PE, Lloyd RV, et al. Surgical treatment of Cushing's disease. J Neurosurg 1987; 66:204.

Chernow B, Buck DR, Early CB, et al. Rapid shrinkage of a prolactin-secreting pituitary tumor with bromocriptine: CT documentation. AJNR 1982; 3:443.

Ciric I, Mikhael M, Stafford T, et al. Transsphenoidal microsurgery of pituitary macroadenomas with long-term follow-up results. J Neurosurg 1983; 59:395.

Colombo N, Berry I, Kucharczyk J, et al. Posterior pituitary gland: Appearance on MR images in normal and pathologic states. Radiology 1987; 165:481.

Cusick JF, Haughton VM, Hagen TC. Radiological assessment of intrasellar prolactin-secreting tumors. Neurosurgery 1980; 6:376.

Daniels DL, Pech P, Mark L, et al. Magnetic resonance imaging of the cavernous sinus. AJNR 1985; 6:187.

David NJ, Gargano FP, Glaser JS. Pituitary apoplexy in clinical perspective. Neurophthalmology 1975; 8:140.

Davis PC, Hoffman JC Jr, Spencer T, et al. MR imaging of pituitary adenoma: CT, clinical, and surgical correlation. AJNR 1987; 8:107.

Davis PC, Hoffman JC, Tindall GT, et al. Prolactin secreting pituitary microadenomas: Inaccuracy of high-resolution CT imaging. AJNR 1984; 5:721.

DiChiro G, Lindgren E. Bone changes in cases of suprasellar meningiomas. Acta Radiol 1952; 38:133.

Domingue JN, Wing SD, Wilson CB. Coexisting pituitary adenomas and partially empty sellas. J Neurosurg 1978; 48:23.

Doppman JL, Krudy AG, Girton ME, et al. Basilar venous plexus of the posterior fossa: A potential source of error in petrosal sinus sampling. Radiology 1985; 155:375.

Dwyer AJ, Frank JA, Doppman JL, et al. Pituitary adenomas in patients with Cushing's disease: Initial experience with Gd-DTPA-enhanced MR imaging. Radiology 1987; 163:421.

Earnest FIV, McCullough EC, Frank DA. Fact or artifact: An analysis of artifact in high-resolution computed tomographic scanning of the sella. Radiology 1981; 140:109.

Ebersold MJ, Law ER, Scheithauer BW, et al. Pituitary apoplexy treated by transsphenoidal surgery. A clinicopathological and immunocytochemical study. J Neurosurg 1983; 58:315.

Fitz CR, Wortzman G, Harwood-Nash DC, et al. Computed tomography in craniopharyngiomas. Radiology 1978; 127:687.

Fluckiger E, de Pozo E, von-Werder K. Prolactin. In: Gross F, Grumbach MM, Labhart A, eds. Monographs in endocrinology. Berlin: Springer Verlag, 1982:191.

Frantz AG. Prolactin. N Engl J Med 1978; 298:201.

Fujimoto M, Yoshino E, Vegushi T, et al. Fluid blood density level demonstrated by computerized tomography in pituitary apoplexy. Report of two cases. J Neurosurg 1981; 55:143.

Fujisawa I, Asato R, Nishimura K, et al. Anterior and posterior lobes of the pituitary gland: Assessment by 1.5T MR imaging. J Comput Assist Tomogr 1987; 11:214.

Garcia-Urea J, del Pozo JM, Bravo G. Functional treatment of acromegaly by transsphenoidal microsurgery. J Neurosurg 1978; 49:36.

Gardeur D, Naidich TP, Metzger J. CT analysis of intrasellar pituitary adenomas with emphasis on patterns of contrast enhancement. Neuroradiology 1981; 20:241.

Gharib H, Frey HM, Laws ER, et al. Coexistent primary empty sella syndrome and hyperprolactinemia. Arch Intern Med 1983; 143:1383.

Giovanelli MA, Motti EDF, Paracchi A, et al. Treatment of acromegaly by transsphenoidal microsurgery. J Neurosurg 1976; 44:677.

Gomori JM, Grossman RI, Goldberg HI, et al. Intracranial hematomas: Imaging by high-field MR. Radiology 1985; 157:87.

Gyldensted C, Karle A. Computed tomography of intra- and juxtasellar lesions. Neuroradiology 1977; 14:5.

Hardy J. Transsphenoidal surgery of hypersecreting pituitary tumors. In: Kohler PO, Ross GT, eds. Diagnosis and treatment of pituitary tumors. Amsterdam: Elsevier, 1973:179.

Hatam A, Bergstrom M, Greitz T. Diagnosis of sellar and parasellar lesions by computed tomography. Neuroradiology 1979; 18:249.

Haughton VM, Prost R. Pituitary fossa: Chemical shift effect in MR imaging. Radiology 1986; 158:461.

Haughton VM, Rosenbaum AE, Williams AL, et al. Recognizing the empty sella by CT: The infundibulum sign. AJNR 1980; 1:527.

Hawkes RC, Holland GN, Moore WS, et al. The applications of NMR imaging to the evaluation of pituitary and juxtasellar tumors. AJNR 1983; 4:221.

Hemminghytt S, Kalkhoff RK, Daniels DL, et al. Computed tomographic study of hormone secreting microadenomas. Radiology 1983; 146:65.

Hinshaw DBJ, Hasso AN, Thompson JR, et al. High resolution computed tomography of the postpartum pituitary gland. Neuroradiology 1984; 26:299.

Hirano A, Tomiyasu U, Zimmerman HM. The fine structure of blood vessels in chromophobe adenoma. Acta Neuropathol (Berl) 1972; 22:200.

Horowitz BL, Hamilton DJ, Sommers CJ, et al. Effects of bromocriptine and pergolide on pituitary tumor size and serum prolactin. AJNR 1983; 4:415.

Houser OW, Baker HL, Reese DF, et al. Radiographic evaluation of the sella turcica and the pituitary gland. In: Laws ER, Randall RV, Kern EB, et al, eds. Management of pituitary adenomas and related lesions with emphasis on transsphenoidal microsurgery. New York: Appleton-Century-Crofts, 1982:81.

Jakubowski J, Kendall B. Coincidental aneurysms with tumors of pituitary origin. J Neurol Neurosurg Psychiatry 1978; 41:972.

Kaplan HC, Baker HL, Houser OW, et al. CT of the Sella turcica after transsphenoidal resection of pituitary adenomas. AJNR 1985; 6:723.

Karnaze MG, Sartor K, Winthrop JD, et al. Suprasellar lesions: Evaluation with MR imaging. Radiology 1986; 161:77.

Kilgore DP, Breger RK, Daniels DL, et al. Cranial tissues: Normal MR appearance after intravenous injection of Gd-DTPA. Radiology 1986; 160:757.

Kline LB, Acker JD, Post MJD, et al. The cavernous sinus: A computed tomographic study. AJNR 1981; 2:299.

Kovacs K, Ryan N, Horvath E, et al. Pituitary adenomas in old age. J Gerontol 1980; 35:16.

Kucharczyk W, Davis DO, Kelly WM, et al. Pituitary adenomas: High-resolution MR imaging at 1.5 T. Radiology 1986; 161:761.

Kucharczyk W, Peck WW, Kelly WM, et al. Rathke cleft cysts: CT, MR imaging, and pathologic features. Radiology 1987; 165:491.

Kulkarni MV, Lee KF, McArdle CB, et al. 1.5-T MR imaging of pituitary microadenomas: Technical considerations and CT correlation. AJNR 1988; 9:5.

Lee BCP, Deck MDF. Sellar and juxtasellar lesion detection with MR. Radiology 1985; 157:143.

Marcovitz S, Wee R, Chan J, et al. The diagnostic accuracy of preoperative CT scanning in the evaluation of pituitary ACTH-secreting adenomas. AJNR 1987; 8:641.

Max MB, Deck MDG, Rottenberg DA. Pituitary metastasis: Incidence in cancer patients and clinical differentiation from pituitary adenoma. Neurology 1981; 31:998.

McGrath P. Cysts of sellar and pharyngeal hypophyses. Pathology 1971; 3:123.

Miura M, Matsukado Y, Kodama T, et al. Clinical and histopathological characteristics of gonadotropinal-producing pituitary adenomas. J Neurosurg 1985; 62:376.

Molitch ME, Hieshima GB, Marcovitz S, et al. Coexisting primary empty sella syndrome and acromegaly. Clin Endocrinol (Oxf) 1977; 7:261–263.

Muhr C, Bergstrom K, Grimelius L, et al. A parallel study of the roentgen anatomy of the sella turcica and the histopathology of the pituitary gland in 205 autopsy specimens. Neuroradiolog 1981; 21:55.

Naidich TP, Pinto RS, Kushner MJ, et al. Evaluation of sellar and paraseller masses by computed tomography. Radiology 1976; 120:91.

Olsen WL, Brant-Zawadzki M, Hodes J, et al. Giant intracranial aneurysms: MR imaging. Radiology 1987; 163:431.

Oot R, New PFJ, Buonanno FS, et al. MR imaging of pituitary adenomas using a prototype resistive magnet: Preliminary assessment. AJNR 1984; 5:131.

Ozanoff MB. Intracranial calcification. In: Newton TH, Potts DG, eds. Radiology of the skull and brain. Vol 1. St. Louis: CV Mosby, 1971:823.

Peyster RG, Adler LP, Vixcarello RR, et al. CT of the normal pituitary gland. Neuroradiology 1986; 28:161.

Peyster RG, Hoover ED. CT of the abnormal stalk. AJNR 1984; 5:49.

Peyster RG, Hoover ED, Adler LP. CT of the normal pituitary stalk. AJNR 1984; 5:45.

Peyster RG, Hoover ED, Viscarello RR, et al. CT appearance of the adolescent and preadolescent pituitary gland. AJNR 1983; 4:411.

Pinto RS, Cohen WA, Kricheff II, et al. Giant intracranial aneurysms: Rapid sequential computed tomography. AJNR 1982; 3:495.

Plaut A, Galenson E. Concretions in the anterior pituitary lobe of the human embryo and the newborn. Am J Pathol 1944; 20:223.

Pojunas KW, Daniels DL, Williams AL, et al. MR imaging of prolactin-secreting microadenomas. AJNR 1986; 7:209.

Post KD, Kasdon DL. Sellar and paraseller lesions mimicking adenomas. In: Post KD, Jackson IMD, Reichlin S, eds. The pituitary adenoma. New York: Plenum, 1980:159.

Pusey E, Kortman KE, Flannigan BD, et al. MR of craniopharyngiomas: Tumor delineation and characterization. AJNR 1987; 8:439.

Rasmussen AT. Cited by Bergland RM, Ray BS, and Torack RM. Anatomical variations in the pituitary gland and adjacent structures in 225 human autopsy cases. J Neurosurg 1968; 28:93.

Renn WH, Rhoton AL. Microsurgical anatomy of the sellar region. J Neurosurg 1975; 43:288.

Rhotan AL, Harris FS, Renn WH. Microsurgical anatomy of the sellar region and cavernous sinus. Clin Neurosurg 1977; 24:54.

Rillet B, Mohr G, Robert R, et al. Calcification in pituitary adenomas. Surg Neurol 1981; 15:249.

Ring BA, Waddington M. Primary arachnoid cysts of the sella turcica. AJR 1966; 98:611.

Robert F. Electron microscopy of human pituitary tumors. In: Tindall GT, Collins WF, eds. Clinical management of pituitary disorders. New York: Raven Press, 1979:113.

Rodman EF, Molitch ME, Post KD, et al. Long-term follow-up of transsphenoidal selective adenomectomy for prolactinoma. JAMA 1984; 252:921.

Rozario R, Hammerschlag SB, Post KD, et al. Diagnosis of empty sella with CT scan. Neuroradiology 1977; 13:85.

Russell DS, Rubinstein LJ. Adenohypophysis. In: Russell DS, Rubinstein LJ, eds. Pathology of tumours of the nervous system. 2nd ed. Edinburgh: Edward Arnold, 1971:184.

Sakoda K, Mukada K, Yonezawa M, et al. CT scan of pituitary adenomas. Neuroradiology 1981; 20:249.

Sang H, Wilson CB, Tyrrel JB. Transsphenoidal microhypophysectomy in acromegaly. J Neurosurg 1977; 47:840.

Saris SC, Patronas NJ, Doppman JL, et al. Cushing syndrome: Pituitary CT scanning. Radiology 1987; 162:775.

Scheithauer BW. Surgical pathology of the pituitary and sellar region. In: Laws ER, Randall RV, Kern EB, et al, eds. Management of pituitary adenomas and related lesions with emphasis on transsphenoidal microsurgery. New York: Appleton-Century-Crofts, 1982:129.

Scotti G, Scialfa G, Pieralli S, et al. Macroprolactinomas: CT evaluation of tumor size after medical treatment. Neuroradiology 1982; 23:123.

Seidel FG, Towbin R, Kaufman RA. Normal pituitary stalk size in children: CT study. AJNR 1985; 6:733.

Schuangshoti S, Netsky MG, Nashold B. Epithelial cysts related to the sella turcica. Arch Pathol Lab Med 1970; 90:444.

Shucart WA. Implications of very high serum prolactin levels associated with pituitary tumors. J Neurosurg 1980; 52:226.

Smaltino F, Bernini FP, Muras I. Computed tomography for diagnosis of empty sella associated with enhancing pituitary microadenomas. J Comput Assist Tomogr 1980; 4:592.

Spaziante R, de Divitiis E, Stella L, et al. Benign Intrasellar cysts. Surg Neurol 1981; 15:274.

Swartz JD, Russell KB, Basile BA, et al. High resolution computed tomographic appearances of intrasellar contents in women of childbearing age. Radiology 1983; 147:115.

Syvertsen A, Haughton VM, Williams AL, et al. The computed tomographic appearance of the normal pituitary gland and pituitary microadeonomas. Radiology 1979; 133:385.

Taylor S. High resolution computed tomography of the sella. Radiol Clin North Am 1982; 20:207.

Teasdale E, Teasdale G, Mohsen F, et al. High-resolution computed tomography in pituitary microadenoma: Is seeing believing? Clin Radiol 1986; 37:227.

Thorner MO, Perryman RL, Rogol AD, et al. Rapid changes of prolactinoma volume after withdrawal and reinstitution of bromocriptine. J Clin Endocrinol Metab 1980; 53:480.

Turski PA, Newton TH, Horten BH. Sellar contour: Anatomic-polytomographic correlation. AJNR 1981; 2:331.

Virapongse C, Bhimani S, Sarwar M. Prolactin-secreting pituitary adenomas: CT appearance of diffuse invasion. Radiology 1984; 152:447.

Wiener SN, Rzeszotarski MS, Droege RT, et al. Measurement of pituitary gland height with MR imaging. AJNR 1985; 6:717.

Wolpert SM. The radiology of pituitary adenomas—an update. In: Post KD, Jackson IMD, Reichlin S, eds. The pituitary adenoma. New York: Plenum, 1980:287.

Wolpert SM. The radiology of prolactinomas. In: Olefsky JM, Robbins RJ, eds. Prolactinomas. New York: Churchill Livingston, 1986:131.

Wolpert SM. Size, shape, and appearance of the normal female pituitary gland. AJNR 1984; 5:263.

Yeakley JW, Kulkarni MV, McArdle CB, et al. High-resolution MR imaging of juxtasellar meningiomas with CT and angiographic correlation. AJNR 1988; 9:279.

Index